Relative Values for Physicians

Relative Value Studies, Inc.

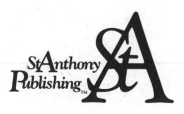

St. Anthony Publishing™

Disclaimer

Relative Values for Physicians is designed to provide accurate and authoritative information in regard to the subject covered. Every reasonable effort has been made to ensure the accuracy of the information within these pages. However, the ultimate responsibility for accuracy lies with the user.

St. Anthony Publishing, Inc., its employees, agents and staff make no representation, guarantee or warranty, expressed or implied, that this compilation is error-free or that the use of this publication will prevent differences of opinion or disputes with Medicare or third-party payers, and will bear no responsibility for the results or consequences of its use.

Contents

Introduction

User Guide

Its long history and careful development make Relative Values for Physicians (RVP) the most accurate and comprehensive relative value system. Use of RVP spans North America and several European countries. In this relative value system, values are provided for physician services contained in the American Medical Association's Current Procedural Terminology (CPT) system, as well as Medicare's HCPCS Level II codes. Additional codes, as recommended by physicians, have been included in this system and assigned relative values in order to address special reimbursement issues.

RVP provides a user-friendly coded listing of physician services with unit values. The accompanying instruction guidelines and modifiers explain the application of these procedure descriptors and unit values in medical practice. All sections of the book may be used by any or all physicians. Appropriate surgery descriptors are not confined to use by surgeons, nor is the medicine section confined to use by internists or primary care physicians.

Definitions of Terms in Relative Values for Physicians

RVP Column Descriptions

(1) UPD	(2) TYPE	(3) CPT	(4) DESCRIPTION	(5) UNITS	(6) FUD	(7) ANES
94.1	M	27126	Arthroplasty, cup (CCR 27999)	30.0	120	6

1) UPD — This column indicates the date the procedure was updated for RVP. The numbers preceding the decimal indicate the year in which the update was made. The number following the decimal indicates whether the change occurred in the first or second official update of that year. The update stamp is removed after three years.

2) TYPE — Indicates code type or AMA change:

M — Indicates a code which is not found in CPT published by the AMA. The code has either been deleted from CPT or is a newly developed code by Relative Value Studies, Inc./St. Anthony Publishing, Inc. CPT copyright remains with the American Medical Association.

▲ — The triangle indicates a CPT code identifier reflecting a change in the CPT code description in the year listed for AMA copyright appearing at the bottom of the page.

● — This circle indicates a CPT code identifier reflecting that the code was added to CPT in the year listed for the AMA copyright at the bottom of the page.

+ — Indicates an add-on code. Add-on codes describe additional intra-service work associated with the primary procedure. They are performed by the same physician on the same date of service as the primary service/procedure, and must never be reported as a stand-alone code.

⊘ — Indicates the procedure is modifier -51 exempt. Codes identified as exempt from modifier -51 are not subject to multiple procedure rules. No reimbursement reduction or modifier -51 is applied.

If the column is blank, no special consideration for the code is required.

3) CPT — Indicates the numerical code for the procedure. An asterisk (*) to the right indicates a surgical procedure only. See Surgery Value Guidelines at the beginning of the surgery section of this manual.

4) DESCRIPTION — Provides a description of the procedure.

5) TOTAL UNITS	The numerical relative value assigned to the procedure. Special notations for this column include:
BR	By Report. For some procedures, RVSI has been unable to obtain sufficient data to establish a value.
RNE	Relativity Not Established. Procedures denoted RNE in the unit value column indicate a procedure that is new or uncommon.
(I) xx.x	Interim Value. Interim relative values (designated by a box and the letter "I") are preliminary and may change when additional data have been gathered from practitioners.
(I-97) xx.x	Date stamped value. Some procedures flagged as an interim value (e.g., codes 63050 and 63051) will have a date stamp, i.e., I-97, which means:

1) The procedure is new and considered to be technically difficult.

2) Physicians may require special training to perform the procedure.

3) The value of the procedure will automatically decline at the end of the year of the date stamp.

6) FUD	Follow-up days. Number of days for postoperative care when any subsequent care should be considered part of the original procedure. (See Surgery Value Guidelines.)
7) ANES	Anesthesia Unit Value. Base value for general anesthesia, if required, for the procedure. (See Anesthesia Value Guidelines.)
PROF	In the Radiology and Pathology/Laboratory sections of this manual, these figures identify relative values for the professional component of the service.
TECH	In the Radiology and Pathology/Laboratory sections of this manual, these figures identify the technical component of the service.

Historical Background

The use of relative values in determining physician's compensation began during the early 1950s in California. The first study was published in 1956. Relative values were derived from survey results of large samples of physicians. The study incorporated a three-digit code with medical nomenclature. Later, four- and five-digit code systems were used to provide for the expansion of procedures through technological advances. The California Standard Nomenclature became the norm for medical practice.

During the 1970s, several courts questioned the legality of relative value systems (see next section). At issue was the close involvement of medical associations in setting relative values that were closely linked to minimum or maximum prices in a geographic area. Only large insurers continued to produce such studies for internal use.

In order to make this type of data more widely available, Relative Value Studies, Inc. began to research and compile existing information and collect new data for publication of the Relative Value System. The results were completed in 1983 and published in 1984.

In 1986, the federal government authorized the development of a relative value study for use with the Medicare program. The first phase of implementing the Medicare's Resource Based Relative Value System began Jan. 1, 1992. The implementation of the Medicare relative value system has completed its initial phase to mixed reviews. The impact of this study has reached beyond Medicare. It is important to note that differences between the Medicare system and the Relative Values and Relative Values for Physicians are significant in some areas and not so great in others.

The most significant difference is that in Relative Values for Physicians the relative values for one section of the CPT coding system are not set in relation to another section. For example, relative values for surgical codes are not set in relation to office visits. Accordingly, RVP consists of five independent relative value scales.

Financial pressure on the Medicare system has, in the opinion of many, resulted in inequitable payments to providers. Relative Values for Physicians, however, remains free from federal budgetary interference. Relative Values for Physicians' statistical integrity has long been recognized by insurers who have made this the most widely used relative value study for commercial insurance claims.

Relative Value Studies — Legal and Fair

Relative value studies are legal, acceptable, and necessary systems for determining rational fees. It is also important to recognize that the use of a relative value study is proper. Only the professional agreement to set minimum or maximum fees in a geographic area is disapproved by the Courts.

A history of antitrust law in this area begins with Goldfarb vs. Virginia State Bar, 421 US 773 (1975). There, a minimum fee schedule developed, disseminated, and recommended by a peer group of attorneys was struck down as anticompetitive. This principle, that professional associations must not control fees, has been reiterated several times, in National Society of Professional Engineers vs. United States, 435 US 679 (1978) and in Arizona vs. Maricopa County Medical Society, 457 US 332 (1982).

In United States vs. American Society of Anesthesiologists, 473 F. Supp. 147 (1979), a relative value study promulgated and disseminated by a professional association was upheld as lawful. The Court stated that the study was intended to serve as a methodology for arriving at fees and as an aid in computing bills. Even in Goldfarb (supra), the Court suggested that a purely advisory fee schedule may be proper.

A long-standing antitrust principle is that while prices may not be fixed, competitors may exchange price information; see Rosebrough Monument Co. vs. Memorial Park Cemetery Association, 666 F2d 1130 (1981). The information itself is quite appropriate and given certain First Amendment constitutional protection. Again, only the conspired attempt to fix fees in a geographic area is impermissible and a violation of the Sherman Act-Section I.

The Federal Trade Commission (FTC), an administrative enforcement body created in 1914 by the federal government, has not prohibited the use of a relative value study by independent physicians as an informational tool. In its 1976 consent decree with the California Medical Association (CMA), the FTC used its authority to stop publication of the CRVS because it did appear that the CMA might be found guilty of price fixing as a professional association.

Insurance payers and nonphysician groups are also permitted to use a relative value study. Any insuring entity performing within the "business of insurance" is insulated from antitrust. The "business of insurance" umbrella means an analysis and sharing of risk.

In fact, a relative value is only one component in the creation of a fee. As long as no conspiracy exists among practitioners to fix conversion factors in a particular geographic area, a relative value scale can be used. "Relative Values for Physicians" is an invaluable tool for all health care systems.

The Research Behind Relative Value Units

The research and data collection required to produce this relative value scale began in 1980. A research group of medical and legal professionals incorporated as Relative Value Studies, Inc. (RVSI) in 1982 and, in 1984, published the first edition of Relative Values for Physicians.

The early research included compiling existing relative value scales from state medical societies, insurance groups and academic journals. The state medical societies, following the lead of California, had developed relative value scales by various methods. Further development of these relative values was halted, however, when the Federal Trade Commission (FTC) took action against the California Medical Association. The RVSI research group gathered the available studies and statistically normalized each scale for a reliable comparison. Procedures for which there was 75 percent consensus among the relative value scales were accepted as valid representations of value. Procedures with consensus exceeding 85 percent were used as anchor codes for further review.

Since that time, the value setting methodology has been refined and currently evaluates the relative value based on five criteria:

1.   Time

2.   Skill

3.   Severity of illness

4.   Risk to patient

5.   Risk to physician (medico-legal)

In a random sample of physicians across the country, physicians are asked to use the above five criteria in evaluating those medical procedures they frequently perform and/or feel qualified to evaluate.

Because individual criteria are not weighted, our methodology results in a more accurate accounting of actual relative values. Weighted criteria could distort the findings from the surveys. For example, if an individual element were limited to a fixed proportion of the total relative value (e.g., if time were limited to only 10 percent of the final value) lengthy procedures would be undervalued. Our surveys and independent sources show that practicing physicians are consistent in their assessment of relative value without weighting for individual criteria.

Evaluations of procedures are collected annually from thousands of individual practitioners from all specialties across the country. The results of these surveys are presented to the editorial board of RVSI who set interim relative values after considering the variance, standard deviation, and mean of survey responses.

Selected values are then reviewed by a cross-specialty group for adjustment. Their recommendations are presented to the editorial board for a final decision.

RVP with CPT

In addition to the current year CPT codes, RVP includes some codes and modifiers not found in CPT to help users address reimbursement issues CPT may not cover. These codes are clearly marked by a bold M in the column preceding the code.

RVP will continue to expand the coding system to further simplify the reimbursement process. RVP will maintain such codes under separate numerical designation. Payers and physicians may use either the separate code or the CPT code indicated, including the description and value listed in RVP. Many new or uncommon procedures may require an operative report, dependent upon the individual case, physician, and payer. (Note: Payers and providers may or may not contractually require specific use of nomenclature. Please communicate your questions to the individual payer or physician as appropriate.)

The editors of RVP will gladly accept suggestions for additional coding to clarify procedural definitions where no CPT exists. Each suggestion will be carefully considered and surveyed. All responses are confidential and should be addressed to Relative Value Studies, Inc. (see address under Customer Comments in this Introduction).

How to Use This Relative Value Scale

This book is organized into seven sections. These are:

1.   Anesthesia

2.   Surgery/Anesthesia

3.   Radiology

4.   Pathology

5.   Medicine

6.   Evaluation and Management

7.   HCPCS Level II

Each section begins with a guideline to define particular values or processes as applicable. Section 7, "HCPCS Level II," provides a complete listing of non-CPT codes that are developed and maintained by the Health Care Financing Administration (HCFA). Each section of the book has been developed on a different scale. Therefore, one section of the book cannot yet be fully compared to another without adjusting the values.

The value guidelines in each section reprint similar information from section to section as is appropriate. Modifiers are provided in a comprehensive list at the end of this User Guide. Modifiers of particular importance to a specific section are referenced in that section's guidelines.

Determining Fees

The formula for setting a fee is:

Relative Value Unit (UNITS) x Conversion Factor (CF) = Fee

The relative values listed under UNITS for each procedure are determined by physician input as described in Research Behind Relative Value Units, in this Introduction. The Conversion Factor (CF) should be determined by taking into consideration current fees (if available); prevailing area rates; and overhead costs, including malpractice insurance, rent, salaries, and the cost of living.

Conversion Factor Development

A conversion factor is required to use the Relative Values to develop a fee schedule. Individual practices should have a customized conversion factor that reflects practice type, its clinical reputation, and local market pricing. Discounts and participation in lower paying plans are at the discretion of the practice; therefore, it is a sound and legal business practice to maintain more than one fee schedule.

The easiest method to determine a conversion factor is to use your current charges. A medical practice that has no established fee schedule could use Medicare's fee schedule, or fee schedules from managed care groups, or other payers as a starting point.

Note: Fee schedules for Medicare and managed care groups are usually discounted from customary charges.

To develop the individual monetary CF, the following basic process is recommended:

1.   List 20 to 30 basic procedures (those that constitute a high volume of practice) for each of the seven sections of the book. In compiling your list of codes do not use any that show BR or RNE instead of a Relative Value.

2.   List the relative value opposite the procedure.

3.   List the fee next to the relative value.

4.   Add the column of relative values.

5.   Add the column of fees.

6.   Divide the total fees by the total relative values. The result is known as a "gross conversion factor."

7.   A "gross conversion factor" should be developed for each of the seven sections: Anesthesia, Surgery, Radiology, Pathology, Medicine, Evaluation and Management, and the HCPCS Level II.

8.   Multiply the "gross conversion factor" by any relative value within the appropriate section and an appropriate dollar amount will result.

If you have been using some relative value study other than Relative Values for Physicians, it is important to note that you cannot apply the conversion factor you have been using with that other study to the values in Relative Values for Physicians.

When developing a conversion factor, go back through your fee schedule (20-30 basic procedures) and divide your fee by the relative value unit for each procedure. If the procedure specific conversion factor is significantly different—either higher or lower—from the average conversion factor (refer to steps above), you may wish to remove these procedures from your list of basic procedures and recalculate the conversion factor. This additional step will yield a conversion factor that is more reflective of your practice.

The following pages illustrate the calculation of conversion factors. These examples are not meant to be representative of any specialty and in no way reflect a suggested pricing for procedures.

Anesthesia
Example Gross Conversion Factor Worksheet

	Procedure Description	Code	RVU	Your Base Fee ($)
1	Corneal Transplant	00144	6.0	245.00
2	Thyroid Biopsy	00322	3.0	105.00
3	Breast Reconstruction	00402	5.0	175.00
4	Bronchoscopy	00520	6.0	175.00
5	Open Heart	00560	15.0	525.00
6	Laminectomy, Sitting	00604	13.0	455.00
7	Pancreatectomy	00794	8.0	280.00
8	Endoscopy	00810	6.0	210.00
9	Hernia, lower side	00830	4.0	140.00
10	TURP	00914	5.0	175.00
11	Hysterectomy	00944	6.0	210.00
12	Total Hip	01214	10.0	350.00
13	Knee, Arthroscopy	01382	3.0	105.00
14	Bone, Lower Leg	01480	3.0	105.00
15	Closed Humerus	01730	3.0	105.00
16				
17				
18				
19				
20				
21				
22				
23				
24				
25				
	SUM TOTAL		96.0	3360.00

Divide the Total Fee by the Total Relative Value Units

$$\frac{\$3360.00 \text{ (Total Fee)}}{96 \text{ (Total RVU)}} = \$35.00 \quad \text{Gross Conversion Factor}$$

Surgery
Example Gross Conversion Factor Worksheet

	Procedure Description	Code	RVU	Your Base Fee ($)
1	Lesion	11604	3.0	310.00
2	Graft Trunk	15734	19.0	1700.00
3	Breast reconstruction	19361	35.0	2400.00
4	Arthroplasty TMJ	21242	28.0	2500.00
5	Fracture	25560	2.9	250.00
6	Total Hip	27130	32.5	3600.00
7	Arthroscopy, Knee	29876	16.0	1750.00
8	Ethmoidectomy	31254	6.8	1000.00
9	Triple Bypass	33512	48.0	5200.00
10	Appendectomy	44950	10.0	950.00
11	Cholecystectomy	47600	14.2	1500.00
12	Hernia	49500	8.0	740.00
13	TURP	52601	20.0	1900.00
14	Total OB	59400	20.0	2100.00
15	Burr Hole	61140	22.0	2340.00
16	Foreign Body Eye	65205	0.7	65.00
17	Myringotomy	69420	1.0	89.00
18				
19				
20				
21				
22				
23				
24				
25				
	SUM TOTAL		287.10	28394.00

Divide the Total Fee by the Total Relative Value Units

$$\frac{\$28394.00 \text{ (Total Fee)}}{287.10 \text{ (Total RVU)}} = \$98.90 \text{ Gross Conversion Factor}$$

Radiology
Example Gross Conversion Factor Worksheet

	Procedure Description	Code	RVU	Your Base Fee ($)
1	Nose Prof Comp	70160-26	1.0	20.00
2	Cat Scan, Neck Tech Comp	70490-27	16.3	295.00
3	MRI Limited, Brain	L 70551	40.0	880.00
4	Chest	71010	2.4	72.00
5	CAT Scan Spine Prof Comp	72128-26	6.8	150.00
6	Hand	73120	2.2	42.00
7	Aortography	75605	14.4	235.00
8	Child G I	76010	2.5	55.00
9	Mammography	76090	4.5	95.00
10	Echography, uterus	76805	11.5	150.00
11	Bone Marrow Prof Comp	78102-26	3.3	60.00
12	Liver imaging (SPECT)	78205	21.1	465.00
13	Cardiac shunt detection	78428	11.0	210.00
14	Bladder, Residual	78730	6.3	95.00
15				
16				
17				
18				
19				
20				
21				
22				
23				
24				
25				
	SUM TOTAL		143.3	2824.00

Divide the Total Fee by the Total Relative Value Units

$$\frac{\$2824.00 \text{ (Total Fee)}}{143.3 \text{ (Total RVU)}} = \$19.71 \quad \text{Gross Conversion Factor}$$

Pathology
Example Gross Conversion Factor Worksheet

	Procedure Description	Code	RVU	Your Base Fee ($)
1	Chemistry 7 tests	80007	1.2	14.00
2	Urinalysis	81000	.7	9.00
3	Alcohol, Blood	82055	3.0	34.00
4	Cholesterol Total P C	82465-26	.2	3.00
5	Iron Binding	83550	1.9	20.00
6	CBC	85022	1.4	16.00
7	Bone Marrow Prof Comp	85102-26	2.9	31.00
8	Clot Reaction Prof Comp	85170-26	.3	4.00
9	HBSAg Tech Comp	86287-27	1.9	20.00
10	Blood Culture	87040	1.7	17.00
11	Chlamydia	87110	3.0	33.00
12	Tissue Exam	87220	1.1	10.00
13	Cytopathology	88160	3.6	32.00
14	Sperm Antibodies	89325	1.8	20.00
15	Water Load	89365	2.3	25.00
16				
17				
18				
19				
20				
21				
22				
23				
24				
25				
	SUM TOTAL		27.0	288.00

Divide the Total Fee by the Total Relative Value Units

$$\frac{\$288.00 \ (\text{Total Fee})}{27.0 \ (\text{Total RVU})} \quad = \quad \$10.67 \quad \text{Gross Conversion Factor}$$

Copyright © 1999 St. Anthony Publishing

Medicine
Example Gross Conversion Factor Worksheet

	Procedure Description	Code	RVU	Your Base Fee ($)
1	Esophageal Motility	91010	26.0	158.00
2	Ophthalmological Exam	92002	11.0	72.00
3	Screening Test	92551	3.5	24.00
4	CPR	92950	37.0	234.00
5	Spirometry	94010	10.5	60.00
6	EEG Sleep Only	95822	19.0	110.00
7	Chemotherapy	96400	3.7	20.00
8	Physical Med–Traction	97012	4.5	23.00
9	Add On for After Hours	99050	4.0	27.00
10	Established Patient	99212	6.0	40.00
11	Consult, Office	99244	28.0	172.00
12	Critical Care	99291	42.0	250.00
13	Telephone Brief	99371	2.0	15.00
14				
15				
16				
17				
18				
19				
20				
21				
22				
23				
24				
25				
	SUM TOTAL		197.20	1205.00

Divide the Total Fee by the Total Relative Value Units

$$\frac{\$1205.00 \text{ (Total Fee)}}{197.20 \text{ (Total RVU)}} = \$6.11 \quad \text{Gross Conversion Facot}$$

Gross Conversion Factor Worksheet For:_____

	Procedure Description	Code	RVU	Your Base Fee ($)
1				
2				
3				
4				
5				
6				
7				
8				
9				
10				
11				
12				
13				
14				
15				
16				
17				
18				
19				
20				
21				
22				
23				
24				
25				
SUM TOTAL				

Divide the Total Fee by the Total Relative Value Units

$$\frac{\text{(Total Fee)}}{\text{(Total RVU)}} \quad = \quad \$ \quad \text{Gross Conversion Facot}$$

NOTE: Keep this form as a master copy for producing other worksheets

Conversion Factors by Payer

The following worksheet is provided to assist in comparing the conversion factors of individual payers.

		1997	1998	1999
1)	Workers' Compensation			
	Medicine	_____	_____	_____
	Anesthesia	_____	_____	_____
	Surgery	_____	_____	_____
	Pathology	_____	_____	_____
	Radiology	_____	_____	_____
2)	Blue Cross/Blue Shield			
	Medicine	_____	_____	_____
	Anesthesia	_____	_____	_____
	Surgery	_____	_____	_____
	Pathology	_____	_____	_____
	Radiology	_____	_____	_____
3)	Medicare			
	Medicine	_____	_____	_____
	Anesthesia	_____	_____	_____
	Surgery	_____	_____	_____
	Pathology	_____	_____	_____
	Radiology	_____	_____	_____
4)	Medicaid			
	Medicine	_____	_____	_____
	Anesthesia	_____	_____	_____
	Surgery	_____	_____	_____
	Pathology	_____	_____	_____
	Radiology	_____	_____	_____
5)	Insuror #1			
	(Name) _____			
	Medicine	_____	_____	_____
	Anesthesia	_____	_____	_____
	Surgery	_____	_____	_____
	Pathology	_____	_____	_____
	Radiology	_____	_____	_____

	1997	1998	1999
6) Insuror #2			
(Name) _____			
Medicine	_____	_____	_____
Anesthesia	_____	_____	_____
Surgery	_____	_____	_____
Pathology	_____	_____	_____
Radiology	_____	_____	_____
7) Insuror #3			
(Name) _____			
Medicine	_____	_____	_____
Anesthesia	_____	_____	_____
Surgery	_____	_____	_____
Pathology	_____	_____	_____
Radiology	_____	_____	_____

Productivity Measurement

Productivity is measured for a variety of reasons, some of which include general office efficiency, distribution of the workload between partners and incentive payments under capitation contracts. Relative values can provide a reasonable measurement of work performed for each of these applications.

Productivity within the office can be measured by work performed rather than fees generated. By tracking actual work performed, resources can be properly allocated within the practice. A relative value system can help you determine which procedures are responsible for most of your practice cost or profit.

One of the most confusing aspects of work measurement in the medical office concerns time. While a physician's office is remunerated for procedures performed, few procedures include extra monies for time spent to accomplish them. Quality service does take time to render. How does one account for that time? Some practices compensate by measuring productivity on a system that is purely time based. This system, however, encourages practitioners to take as much time as possible to complete a procedure. Time becomes more important than the procedure performed. With all of this confusion, how does one include time in the productivity measurement equation?

Any practice attempting to measure productivity must consider time in relation to the actual performance of a procedure. This will help reduce the effect any variable may have on the outcome. An experience-based relative value system allows one to do this rather easily.

The relative values for each procedure in RVP are determined by physician input as described on page 4 of the Introduction, in Research Behind Relative Value Units. Time is one component in the relative value development process. Because time is considered to be one of the five criteria inherent to the provision of physician services, the relative value can be used as a productivity factor.

Some things to consider when using relative values to measure productivity:

1.   How does one address services for which no unit value is assigned?

2.   How is the time between services (not related to actual set up or performance of the procedure) to be handled?

The time for any service for which there is no unit value should be taken out of the calculation completely or a unit value must be assigned (see BR and RNE value explanation in Using Relative Values section) if the measurement is to be accurate.

All practices have "down" time, and it is recommended that this time be acknowledged in the productivity monitoring. A comparison between relative value production with "down" time and without "down" time can prove very educational.

Remember—in order to get the most accurate measurements for your practice, it is important to remain consistent. Keep the time variables in mind, and adhere to the following outline.

Outline for Productivity Measurement

The following basic process is recommended for measuring office productivity:

1. Determine the frequency of each procedure performed for one month.

2. When multiplying the number of times a given service was provided that month by the relative value for each code, each section's relative values must also be adjusted by a comparative factor to create a single scale of relative value units. Remember that all relative value units in RVP are not equivalent. For example, 10 relative value units for surgical services are not the same as 10 relative value units for radiology services.

A practice-specific comparative factor can be developed by dividing the lowest conversion factor used in the practice by the other conversion factors used. For example, Dr. Smith has the following existing conversion factors:

Specific	Conversion Factor	Divide by the Lowest Conversion Factor	Practice Comparative Factor
Surgery	72.00	72.00/6.00	12
Anesthesia	36.00	36.00/6.00	6
Pathology	12.00	12.00/6.00	2
Radiology	24.00	24.00/6.00	4
Medicine	6.00	6.00/6.00	1

Alternatively, the following general comparative factors may be used:

	Medicare Equivalent Factor	Average Conversion Factor
Surgery	10.23	15.78
Anesthesia	4.46	5.67
Pathology	1.67	2.29
Radiology	2.44	3.24
Medicine	1.00	1.00

3. Once the single scale relative values have been calculated, multiply the frequency of each procedure performed by the corresponding adjusted relative value.

4. Add the monthly adjusted relative values and divide the total by the number of days (or hours) your practice was in operation that month.

Fictitious example for measuring productivity:

Code	Unit Value	x	Commercial Comparative Factor	x	Frequency March	=	Total Work Value for March
00120	5.0		5.67		7		198.45
01460	3.0		5.67		5		85.05
21325	5.0		15.78		2		157.80
25560	2.9		15.78		3		137.29
59410	12.5		15.78		1		197.25
75665	5.0		3.24		15		243.00
76090	1.4		3.24		12		54.43
80500	3.1		2.29		6		42.59
94060	6.0		1.00		10		60.00
90788	2.5		1.00		3		7.50
							1183.36

March: 1183.36 divided by 23 working days of practice = 51.45

Code	Unit Value	x	Commercial Comparative Factor	x	Frequency April	=	Total Work Value for April
00120	5.0		5.67		5		141.75
01460	3.0		5.67		3		51.03
21325	5.0		15.78		1		78.90
25560	2.9		15.78		6		274.57
59410	12.5		15.78		3		591.75
75665	5.0		3.24		20		324.00
76090	1.4		3.24		8		36.29
80500	3.1		2.29		12		85.19
94060	6.0		1.00		15		90.00
90788	2.5		1.00		9		22.50

April: 1695.89 divided by 20 working days of practice = 84.80   1695.98

Productivity measurement can be compared year to year, month to month, day to day, or even hour to hour. This process can also analyze the productivity of individuals by simply using the Total Work Value for each individual instead of the Total Work Value for the practice.

Applications for productivity analysis include the following:

- Allocating bonuses;

- Setting incentive-based payment programs;

- Creating internal productivity goals for optimum efficiency;

- Anticipating patient volume and time required for treatments

Cost and Profitability Analysis

Because many expenditures in a practice are fixed, relative values can be used to examine cost of practice. Regardless of the practice case mix, relative values can be used to generate a per procedure cost analysis.

Cost analysis can be performed by using a case mix calculation similar to productivity measurement. Although the case mix can be derived from daily, monthly, or yearly periods, cost allocation is better addressed over a longer period of time. As in productivity measurement, each section's relative values must be adjusted by a comparative factor to create a single scale of relative value units. Special consideration should also be given to services for which no unit value is assigned. However, unlike productivity measurement, cost analysis should consider long breaks and vacation days in its calculations, as many of these aspects incur cost to the practice. Once a single scale relative value total is obtained for the practice case mix (see Productivity Measurement), this sum should be divided by the total cost outlay for that time period. Total service cost should include all expenditures that are not separately billable (i.e., rent, salaries, individual office supplies, and utilities). This will give you an average cost per unit value for your practice.

The formula for determining Average Cost per Unit Value is:

$$\frac{\text{Total Cost Outlay}}{\text{Total Relative Value Units (using single scale)}} = \text{Average Cost per Unit Value}$$

An average cost for any given procedure can be derived by multiplying the average cost per unit by any one procedure's relative value.

The formula for deriving an Average Cost for a procedure is:

Average Cost per Unit Value x Procedure Unit Value = Average Cost per Procedure

When used in connection with service time, the cost per procedure can be adapted to determine procedure profitability. To determine the profitability of a service, simply subtract the average cost for the service from the reimbursed amount.

The formula is:

Reimbursement-Average Total Service Cost = Profitability

Other uses for the average cost per unit include determining a conversion factor to develop fees and evaluating payment proposals. In either case, a percentage increase above cost, depending upon the components included in your gross cost calculation, is used to develop or explain the conversion factor desired by the practice. For example, if one wanted to set their fees to include the cost of providing care, plus 20 percent, the conversion factor that reflects cost would be increased by 20 percent.

The percentage variation for cost is dependent upon gross cost inclusion by either including or excluding "salaries" for providers. Obviously, the exclusion of provider salaries would necessitate a greater cost percentage increase than a calculation including provider "salaries."

When similar provider "salaries" are used in the calculation of gross cost, average cost per unit can be used for comparison between practices as well. Comparison of this type may prove educational but should not dictate a specific practice's charges. In other words, each practice should be considerate of cost, but cost should also be determined by considering other target market needs.

Internal average cost comparison can be derived to determine profitability within capitated programs. In order to measure this, the average cost per unit for the entire practice should be calculated first. Then the case mix relative value total for all services provided to those treated under a capitation agreement should be calculated. The next step is to multiply the cost per unit by the relative value total and compare the result to the gross revenue under the program. The difference between the two amounts is the relative profit or loss under the system. This calculation should include the provider salary for accurate comparison.

Capitation

The payment for health care via capitation is becoming more common. It is estimated that over half of all health care insurance will function under a capitated system by the year 2005. Given the potential savings a capitated system can provide, many believe that this projection is low. In this section, RVSI will provide some insight to concerns received from providers and payers about functioning profitably in a capitated system.

Capitation transfers much of the financial risk from the payer to the provider. In a capitated system, the payment remains constant regardless of the services provided to the patient. Therefore the obvious way to increase income is to control costs. One must consider, however, that a patient who is not provided a service may return at a later date in a more advanced disease state and therefore cost the provider more. The provider now faces an increased risk—financially, legally, and professionally.

Providers and payers want to know what role CPT and ICD-9 coding will play in a capitated system. Because data analysis is very critical, CPT and ICD-9 coding will play a major role in both the set-up and maintenance of this system. Resource allocation and treatment guidelines need careful monitoring. Not only do the CPT and ICD-9 systems already collect and compare current data, but they also provide a method for tracking resource allocation and can also be used to provide reasonable treatment guidelines.

There are some concerns, however, that these systems are inadequate. The most notable criticism is that CPT and ICD-9 are too slow in adopting changes. Additionally, many feel that pressure from the Medicare system to maintain budget neutrality will slow the system even further.

Providers and payers would also like to know whether or not a relative value system can be used in a capitated system. The answer is yes.

RVUs and the Capitation Contract

Careful evaluation of a capitated contract is imperative. The provider must look at the type of service he/she is responsible for providing. Looking at the CPT codes listed in the contract can help in determining what those services will be. If codes are included for services that a provider is not prepared to perform, it is important to remove them from the contract. This is more commonly known as a carveout.

Patient mix is another area that must be scrutinized when considering capitation. An older, sicker population can dramatically affect utilization. A significant increase in the amount of services may be required for the more acutely ill patient.

In order to determine whether the office can even afford to sign a particular capitation contract, the per member/per month (PMPM) fee must be examined very carefully. Given an increased number of patients requiring additional costs, it is necessary to assess the cost of doing business vs. the reimbursement received. By using a relative value system, you can compare the capitation rate to your fee-for-service rate. (Remember: variables such as changes in incentives to providers, demographics, and relative environmental factors are unknown and should be taken into account when addressing per member/per month fees.)

EXAMPLE   (use data for at least a six month period—preferably for a year—for a more reliable assessment of each capitated plan)

Step 1:   Determine the total number of RVUs for all services predicted for all capitated patients for one year. This information should be available from the payer.

For comparison of relative values between sections, the relative value must be adjusted. A discussion of relative value adjustments is contained in this section. For example:

Cysto is 2.0 RVUs, thus 80 cystos =	2 x 80	= 160
Office visit is 2.0 RVUs, thus 40 OV =	2 x 40	= 80
Total RVUs =	160 + 80	= 240

Step 2:   Multiply the number of capitated patients signed to cover by the annual dollar amount for each patient. For example:

20 patients at $.50 per patient/per month x 12 months = $120.00

Step 3:   Divide the dollar amount from Step 2 by the total RVUs from Step 1, and the result is the dollar amount per RVU. For example:

$120.00 divided by 240 = $.50 per RVU

Step 4:   To compare your capitation contract with your current fee-for-service contract, compare the dollars per RVU in Step 3 to your current conversion factor per RVU. You can also compare this to your current fee schedule by multiplying your conversion factor obtained in Step 3 by the appropriate RVU for any procedure. (Refer to the Conversion Factor Development section on page 9 of this introduction to determine your conversion factor.)

An alternative method for evaluating a capitated payment proposal uses the premium paid by an individual as the starting point for estimating the number of RVUs that a patient panel will consume. Note that each physician's share of the premium and relative values varies and that the estimate of RVUs that results from this technique gives a total RVU of primary care and specialist services.

In this example, we assume that an HMO's monthly single premium rate is $156.25.

Step 1:   Subtract 20 percent from the premium for HMO administration. What remains is the unadjusted medical cost.

$156.25 x 0.2 = $125

Step 2:   Subtract from the medical cost the "Adult-to-Member Cost Ratio." Because the actual amount of the medical costs depends upon the ratio of adults to children in the plan, and the cost for each, an adult-to-member cost ratio is used to find that portion of the premium that represents the mix of adult and child medical costs.

Here's how we can estimate the Adult-to-Member Ratio when the actual number of adults and children is not known.

a)   Assume that an HMO has 300 members

b)   Assume that 1/3 or 100 are children, and 200 are adults

c)   Assume that monthly medical costs are $125 for adults and $50 for children

d)   So the HMO's total medical costs are

$125 x 200 + $50 x 100 = $30,000

e)   So medical costs per member are $30,000 divided by 300 or $100

f)   Therefore the adult to member cost ratio is $125 divided by $100 or 1.25

The HMO monthly PMPM for medical costs is $125 divided by 1.25 = $100. If we did not account for this factor, the amount we use for medical costs would be too large; i.e. $125

Step 3:   To find the portion of medical costs that are physician services, assume that 36 percent is for physician services. This figure is from the American Association of Health Plans.

$100 multiplied by 36 percent = $36

Step 4:   Divide the physician service cost by an average conversion factor. For example, using $7 as a conversion factor (an average conversion factor for evaluation and management services) yields the following:

$36/$7 = 5.14 relative value units per month, or 60.2 relative value units per year.

More important is the total number of relative value units for the proposed patient panel. For example, if the patient panel were 2,000, then the number of RVUs per year would be

60.2 RVUs x 12 months x 2,000 persons = 1,444,800 RVUs per year

This calculation provides an estimate of the number of relative value units for all physician services, which will then be shared by both primary care and specialists.

Product and Sales Information

If you have questions or would like information about conversion factor reports for your state or local area, contact St. Anthony Publishing, Inc., toll free (800) 632-0123 or write to:

Relative Values for Physicians
St. Anthony Publishing, Inc.
11410 Isaac Newton Square
Reston, VA 20190

Customer Comments

For questions and comments concerning this study and the use of relative value units, please write to:

Relative Value Studies, Inc.
1675 Larimer, Suite 410
Denver, Colorado 80202

or call (303) 534-0506. Your suggestions will be given serious consideration by the Editors.

Example:

Procedure number (90050) should receive a value of _____ or should be re-evaluated for the following reasons:

_____

_____

_____

_____

_____

_____

Comprehensive Listing of Modifier Codes

Listed values may be modified under certain circumstances. When applicable, the modifying circumstance should be identified by the addition of the appropriate "modifier code number" (including the hyphen) after the usual procedure number. The modifier may also be listed using the modifier code along with 099 in front of the modifier (i.e., 09922 for -22). No dash is needed in this case. The fee should be listed as a single modified total for the procedure. Any modifier may be used in conjunction with any procedure, if appropriate.

Carriers will vary on the use and acceptance of modifiers. Some carriers will accept all modifiers listed here. Others may accept only CPT compatible codes or some CPT compatible codes. You may wish to determine which carriers will accept modifiers and which do not. Most carriers will accept "-22" with a report. This modifier may be used in place of unaccepted modifiers.

Modifier codes listing additional value show customary increases when available. Carriers may vary in actual reimbursement values.

When multiple modifiers are used, see modifier code -99.

-10   **Endoscopic Surgery:** When the surgical procedure is performed through any type of endoscope for which there is no endoscopic code, attach this modifier to the open surgery procedure code. (This modifier is not CPT compatible.) Attachment of this modifier should warrant no reduction or increase in value for the interim. Values established for laparoscopic procedures will be given a separate listing in the Body of RVP. Please check the code range for both the correct open procedure and codes 56300-56399 for possible CPT compatible codes.

-21   **Prolonged Evaluation and Management Services:** When the face-to-face or floor/unit service(s) provided is prolonged or otherwise greater than that usually required for the highest level of evaluation and management service within a given category, it may be identified by adding modifier '-21' to the evaluation and management code number or by use of the separate five digit modifier code 09921. A report may also be appropriate.

-22   **Unusual Procedural Services:** When the service(s) provided is greater than that usually required for the listed procedure, it may be identified by adding modifier '-22' to the usual procedure number or by use of the separate five digit modifier code 09922. A report may also be appropriate.

-23   **Unusual Anesthesia:** Occasionally, a procedure, which usually requires either no anesthesia or local anesthesia, because of unusual circumstances must be done under general anesthesia. This circumstance may be reported by adding the modifier '-23' to the procedure code of the basic service or by use of the separate five digit modifier code 09923.

-24   **Unrelated Evaluation and Management Service by the Same Physician During a Postoperative Period:** The physician may need to indicate that an evaluation and management service was performed during a postoperative period for a reason(s) unrelated to the original procedure. This circumstance may be reported by adding the modifier '-24' to the appropriate level of E/M service, or the separate five digit modifier 09924 may be used.

-25   **Significant, Separately Identifiable Evaluation and Management Service by the Same Physician on the Same Day of the Procedure or Other Service:** The physician may need to indicate that on the day a procedure or service identified by a CPT code was performed, the patient's condition required a significant, separately identifiable E/M service above and beyond the other service provided or beyond the usual preoperative and postoperative care associated with the procedure that was performed. The E/M service may be prompted by the symptom or condition for which the procedure and/or service was provided. As such, different diagnoses are not required for reporting of the E/M services on the same date. This circumstance may be reported by adding the modifier '-25' to the appropriate level of E/M service, or the separate five digit modifier 09925 may be used. Note: This modifier is not used to report an E/M service that resulted in a decision to perform surgery. See modifier '-57.'

NOTE: This modifier is not used to report an E/M service that resulted in a decision to perform surgery. See modifier '-57.' Service must be substantiated by report and listed value should be allowed 100%.

-26   **Professional Component:** Certain procedures are a combination of a physician component and a technical component. When the physician component is reported separately, the service may be identified by adding the modifier '-26' to the usual procedure number or the service may be reported by use of the five digit modifier code 09926.

-27   **Technical Component:** Under certain circumstances, a charge may be made for the technical component alone. (This modifier is not CPT compatible.)

-28   **Debridement and/or Decontamination** are considered of additional value when appreciable amounts of devitalized or contaminated tissue are removed. Report required. (This modifier is not CPT compatible.)

-29   **Services Provided by Other Than Physician:** When a service is performed by a licensed physician assistant or personnel other than the physician under direct supervision of a physician. (This modifier is not CPT compatible.)

-30   **Anesthesia Services:** Add this modifier for normal, uncomplicated anesthesia. Medicare and some other carriers may require reporting of specific anesthesia code section. Otherwise, use the value indicated in the anesthesia column. (This modifier is not CPT compatible.)

-32   **Mandated Services:** Services related to mandated consultation and/or related services (eg, PRO, 3rd party payor) may be identified by adding the modifier '-32' to the basic procedure or the service may be reported by use of the five digit modifier 09932.

-47   **Anesthesia by Surgeon:** Regional or general anesthesia provided by the surgeon may be reported by adding the modifier '-47' to the basic service or by use of the separate five digit modifier code 09947. (This does not include local anesthesia.) Note: Modifier '-47' or 09947 would not be used as a modifier for the anesthesia procedures 00100-01999.

NOTE: Modifier '-47' or 09947 would not be used as a modifier for the anesthesia procedures 00100–0199.

-48   **Reduced Anesthesia Value for Supervision:** When the anesthesiologist is supervising the services of the nurse anesthetist and is involved in medical direction of the patient, including pre- and post-operative evaluation and care, but is not personally administering the anesthesia. (This modifier is not CPT compatible.)

-49   **Significant, Separately Identifiable Evaluation and Management Service by the Same Physician during a pre-operative period and prior to the Day of a Procedure:** The physician may need to indicate that during a pre-operative period and prior to the day of a procedure or service identified by a CPT code was performed, the patient's condition required a significant, separately identifiable E/M service above and beyond the usual preoperative care associated with the procedure that was performed. This circumstance may be reported by adding the modifier '-49' to the appropriate level of E/M service. The use of the modifier requires substantiation by report and 100% of the listed value should be allowed. (This modifier is not CPT compatible.)

-50   **Bilateral Procedure:** Unless otherwise identified in the listings, bilateral procedures that are performed at the same operative session should be identified by adding the modifier '-50' to the appropriate five digit code or by use of the separate five digit modifier code 09950.

-51   **Multiple Procedures:** When multiple procedures, other than Evaluation and Management Services, are performed at the same session by the same provider, the primary procedure or service may be reported as listed. The additional procedure(s) or service(s) may be identified by appending the modifier '-51' to the additional procedure or service code(s) or by the use of the separate five digit modifier 09951. Note: This modifier should not be appended to designated "add-on" codes (see Appendix E).

            NOTE: This modifier should not be appended to designated "add-on" codes (e.g., 22612, 22614). See Surgery Value Guidelines for Rules.

-52   **Reduced Services:** Under certain circumstances a service or procedure is partially reduced or eliminated at the physician's discretion. Under these circumstances the service provided can be identified by its usual procedure number and the addition of the modifier '-52', signifying that the service is reduced. This provides a means of reporting reduced services without disturbing the identification of the basic service. Modifier code 09952 may be used as an alternative to modifier '-52.' Note: For hospital outpatient reporting of a previously scheduled procedure/service that is partially reduced or cancelled as a result of extenuating circumstances or those that threaten the well-being of the patient prior to or after administration of anesthesia, see modifiers '-73' and '-74' (see modifiers approved for ASC hospital outpatient use).

-53   **Discontinued Procedure:** Under certain circumstances, the physician may elect to terminate a surgical or diagnostic procedure. Due to extenuating circumstances or those that threaten the well being of the patient, it may be necessary to indicate that a surgical or diagnostic procedure was started but discontinued. This circumstance may be reported by adding the modifier '-53' to the code reported by the physician for the discontinued procedure or by use of the separate five digit modifier code 09953. Note: This modifier is not used to report the elective cancellation of a procedure prior to the patient's anesthesia induction and/or surgical preparation in the operating suite. For outpatient hospital/ambulatory surgery center (ASC) reporting of a previously scheduled procedure/service that is partially reduced or cancelled as a result of extenuating circumstances or those that threaten the well being of the patient prior to or after administration of anesthesia, see modifiers '-73' and '-74' (see modifiers approved for ASC hospital outpatient use).

            NOTE: This modifier is not used to report the elective cancellation of a procedure prior to the patient's anesthesia induction and/or surgical preparation in the operating suite. Value for a discontinued procedure should be based on actual work performed. A report may be required for value approval.

-54   **Surgical Care Only:** When one physician performs a surgical procedure and another provides preoperative and/or postoperative management, surgical services may be identified by adding the modifier '-54' to the usual procedure number or by use of the separate five digit modifier code 09954.

-55   **Postoperative Management Only:** When one physician performs the postoperative management and another physician has performed the surgical procedure, the postoperative component may be identified by adding the modifier '-55' to the usual procedure number or by use of the separate five digit modifier code 09955.

-56   **Preoperative Management Only:** When one physician performs the preoperative care and evaluation and another physician performs the surgical procedure, the preoperative component may be identified by adding the modifier '-56' to the usual procedure number or by use of the separate five digit modifier code 09956.

-57   **Decision for Surgery:** An evaluation and management service that resulted in the initial decision to perform the surgery may be identified by adding the modifier '-57' to the appropriate level of E/M service, or the separate five digit modifier 09957 may be used.

-58   **Staged or Related Procedure or Service by the Same Physician During the Postoperative Period:** The physician may need to indicate that the performance of a procedure or service during the postoperative period was: a) planned prospectively at the time of the original procedure (staged); b) more extensive than the original procedure; or c) for therapy following a diagnostic surgical procedure. This circumstance may be reported by adding the modifier '-58' to the staged or related procedure, or the separate five digit modifier 09958 may be used. Note: This modifier is not used to report the treatment of a problem that requires a return to the operating room. See modifier '-78.'

NOTE: This modifier is not used to report the treatment of a problem that requires a return to the operating room. See modifier '-78.'

-59   **Distinct Procedural Service:** Under certain circumstances, the physician may need to indicate that a procedure or service was distinct or independent from other services performed on the same day. Modifier '-59' is used to identify procedures/services that are not normally reported together, but are appropriate under the circumstances. This may represent a different session or patient encounter, different procedure or surgery, different site or organ system, separate incision/excision, separate lesion, or separate injury (or area of injury in extensive injuries) not ordinarily encountered or performed on the same day by the same physician. However, when another already established modifier is appropriate it should be used rather than modifier '-59.' Only if no more descriptive modifier is available, and the use of modifier '-59' best explains the circumstances, should modifier '-59' be used. Modifier code 09959 may be used as an alternative to modifier '-59.'

-60   **Add-on Procedure:** Procedures for which the editor's note indicates the service is an add-on procedure and therefore is already reduced by multiple procedure rules should be identified by adding modifier (-60) to the code. Bill at 100% of the previously reduced value.

NOTE: This modifier is not CPT compatible.

-62   **Two Surgeons:** When two surgeons work together as primary surgeons performing distinct part(s) of a single reportable procedure, each surgeon should report his/her distinct operative work by adding the modifier '-62' to the single definitive procedure code. Each surgeon should report the co-surgery once using the same procedure code. If additional procedure(s) (including add-on procedure(s)) are performed during the same surgical session, separate code(s) may be reported without the modifier '-62' added. Modifier code 09962 may be used as an alternative to modifier '-62'. Note: If a co-surgeon acts as an assistant in the performance of additional procedure(s) during the same surgical session, those services may be reported using separate procedure code(s) with the modifier '-80' or modifier '-81' added, as appropriate.

-66   **Surgical Team:** Under some circumstances, highly complex procedures (requiring the concomitant services of several physicians, often of different specialties, plus other highly skilled, specially trained personnel, various types of complex equipment) are carried out under the "surgical team" concept. Such circumstances may be identified by each participating physician with the addition of the modifier '-66' to the basic procedure number used for reporting services. Modifier code 09966 may be used as an alternative to modifier '-66.'

-68   **Related Procedure Performed During The Post-Operative Period In The Office Or Outpatient Setting (Non Operating Room):** The physician may need to report another procedure that was performed during the post-operative period of the initial procedure. When this subsequent procedure is related to the first, it may be reported by adding -68 to the related procedure. In these circumstances 70% of the listed value is warranted. Note: This modifier is not CPT compatible.

-73   **Discontinued Out-Patient Hospital/Ambulatory Surgery Center (ASC) Procedure Prior to the Administration of Anesthesia:** Due to extenuating circumstances or those that threaten the well being of the patient, the physician may cancel a surgical or diagnostic procedure subsequent to the patient"s surgical preparation (including sedation when provided, and being taken to the room where the procedure is to be performed), but prior to the administration of anesthesia (local, regional block(s) or general). Under these circumstances, the intended service that is prepared for but cancelled can be reported by its usual procedure number and the addition of the modifier "-73" or by use of the separate five digit modifier code 09973. Note: The elective cancellation of a service prior to the administration of anesthesia and/or surgical preparation of the patient should not be reported. For physician reporting of a discontinued procedure, see modifier "-53."

-74   **Discontinued Out-Patient Hospital/Ambulatory Surgery Center (ASC) Procedure After Administration of Anesthesia:** Due to extenuating circumstances or those that threaten the well being of the patient, the physician may terminate a surgical or diagnostic procedure after the administration of anesthesia (local, regional block(s), general) or after the procedure was started (incision made, intubation started, scope inserted, etc).

Under these circumstances, the procedure started but terminated can be reported by its usual procedure number and the addition of the modifier "-74" or by use of the separate five digit modifier code 09974. Note: The elective cancellation of a service prior to the administration of anesthesia and/or surgical preparation of the patient should not be reported. For physician reporting of a discontinued procedure, see modifier "-53."

-75   **Concomitant Care:** Services rendered by more than one physician. When the patient's condition requires the services of more than one physician, each physician may identify his or her services by adding this modifier to the basic service he or she performed. (This modifier is not CPT compatible.)

-76   **Repeat Procedure by Same Physician:** The physician may need to indicate that a procedure or service was repeated subsequent to the original procedure or service. This circumstance may be reported by adding the modifier "-76" to the repeated procedure or service or the separate five digit modifier code 09976 may be used.

-77   **Repeat Procedure by Another Physician:** The physician may need to indicate that a basic procedure or service performed by another physician had to be repeated. This situation may be reported by adding modifier '-77' to the repeated procedure/service or the separate five digit modifier code 09977 may be used.

-78   **Return to the Operating Room for a Related Procedure During the Postoperative Period:** The physician may need to indicate that another procedure was performed during the postoperative period of the initial procedure. When this subsequent procedure is related to the first, and requires the use of the operating room, it may be reported by adding the modifier '-78' to the related procedure, or by using the separate five digit modifier 09978. (For repeat procedures on the same day, see '-76'.)

-79   **Unrelated Procedure or Service by the Same Physician During the Postoperative Period:** The physician may need to indicate that the performance of a procedure or service during the postoperative period was unrelated to the original procedure. This circumstance may be reported by using the modifier '-79' or by using the separate five digit modifier 09979. (For repeat procedures on the same day, see '-76'.)

-80   **Assistant Surgeon:** Surgical assistant services may be identified by adding the modifier '-80' to the usual procedure number(s) or by use of the separate five digit modifier code 09980.

-81   **Minimum Assistant Surgeon:** Minimum surgical assistant services are identified by adding the modifier '-81' to the usual procedure number or by use of the separate five digit modifier code 09981.

-82   **Assistant Surgeon (when qualified resident surgeon not available):** The unavailability of a qualified resident surgeon is a prerequisite for use of modifier '-82' appended to the usual procedure code number(s) or by use of the separate five digit modifier code 09982.

-90   **Reference (Outside) Laboratory:** When laboratory procedures are performed by a party other than the treating or reporting physician, the procedure may be identified by adding the modifier '-90' to the usual procedure number or by use of the separate five digit modifier code 09990.

-99   **Multiple Modifiers:** Under certain circumstances two or more modifiers may be necessary to completely delineate a service. In such situations modifier '-99' should be added to the basic procedure, and other applicable modifiers may be listed as part of the description of the service. Modifier code 09999 may be used as an alternative to modifier '-99.'

Anesthesia

Guidelines

I.   **General:** Values for anesthesia services are listed for each procedure in the surgical section under ANES and by CPT code in the anesthesia section. These values are to be used only when the anesthesia is legally administered by or under the responsible supervision of a licensed physician. These values include usual pre- and postoperative visits, the administration of the anesthetic, and administration of fluids and/or blood incident to the anesthesia or surgery. Anesthesia services may be billed under the appropriate anesthesia code or by using the surgical code with modifier -30 ANES value in the surgical section. Use the methodology most acceptable to the payer/anesthesiologist. Discussion of values as derived from the base unit and time increment are discussed under Calculations of Total Anesthesia Values.

II. **Unlisted Service or Procedure:** When an unlisted service or procedure is provided, the value should be substantiated "by report" (BR).

III. **Procedures Listed Without Specified Unit Values**

     By Report "BR" Items: "BR" in the value column indicates that the value of this service is to be determined "by report," because the service is too unusual or variable to be assigned a unit value. A detailed clinical record is generally not necessary.

IV. **Materials Supplied By Physician:** Identify as 99070 or the appropriate HCPCS Level II code. The list of appropriately billable supplies for each CPT code is variable by contract. RVUs are not based on supply costs. However, traditional fees or conversion factors may be constructed to account for supplies required for a given code.

V.   **Stand-by Anesthesia:** When an anesthesiologist is requested by the attending physician to be present in the operating room to monitor vital signs and manage the patient from an anesthesia standpoint, even though the actual surgery is being done under local anesthesia, calculation will be the same as if the general anesthesia had been administered (time + base value).

     Stand-by anesthesia is generally accepted without justifying documentation for the following:

     A.   Deliveries;

     B.   Subdural hematomas;

     C.   Femoral or brachial arterial embolectomies;

     D.   Patients with physical status 4 or 5 — the physician must document the patient's condition (e.g., severe systemic disease, moribund patient);

     E.   Insertion of a cardiac pacemaker;

     F.   Cataract extraction and/or lens implant;

     G.   Stand-by anesthesia for other than the above generally requires documentation.

VI. **More Than One Anesthesiologist:** When it is necessary to have a second anesthesiologist, the necessity should be substantiated by report "BR." It is recommended that the second anesthesiologist receive 5.0 base units plus time units (calculation of total ANES value).

+ Add-on Code   ⊘ Modifier -51 Exempt   ▲ Revised code   ● New code   **M** RVSI code or deleted from CPT   **(I)** Interim Value

CPT codes and descriptions only copyright © 1998 American Medical Association   Copyright © 1999 St. Anthony Publishing

VII. All anesthesia services are reported by use of the surgical code with the addition of modifier -30 or the anesthesia five-digit procedure code (00100-01999) plus the addition of a physical status modifier. These modifying units may be added to the basic values. The use of other modifiers may be used if appropriate. A comprehensive listing of modifiers is provided in the introduction.

Physical status modifiers are represented by the letter P followed by a single digit defined below:

		Unit Values
1.	Healthy patient	0
2.	Patient with mild systemic disease	0
3.	Patient with severe systemic disease	1
4.	Patient with severe systemic disease that is a constant threat to life	2
5.	A moribund patient who is not expected to survive without the operation	3
6.	A declared brain-dead patient whose organs are being removed for donor purposes	0

The above six levels are consistent with the American Society of Anesthesiologists (ASA) ranking of patient physical status.

Examples: 00100-P1 or 11510-30-P1

VIII. **Qualifying Circumstances:** Some circumstances warrant additional value due to unusual events. The following list of CPT-4 codes and the corresponding anesthesia unit values may be listed if appropriate. More than one code may be necessary. The value listed is added to the existing anesthesia base.

CPT-4		Unit Values
99100	Anesthesia for patient of extreme age, under one year or over seventy	1
99116	Anesthesia complicated by utilization of total body hypothermia	5
99135	Anesthesia complicated by utilization of controlled hypotension	5
99140	Anesthesia complicated by emergency conditions (specify) (An emergency is defined as existing when delay in treatment of a patient would lead to a significant increase in the threat to life or body part.)	2

IX. For the following codes the base Anesthesia unit is used for valuation of the procedure. (No time unit is allowed)

01995	36600	62280	64412	64440	64530
01996	36620	62281	64413	64441	64600
20550	36625	62282	64415	64442	64605
31500	36660	62288	64417	64443	64610
36400	62273	62289	64418	64445	64620
36420	62274	64400	64420	64450	64622
36425	62275	64402	64421	64505	64623
36488	62276	64405	64425	64508	64630
36489	62277	64408	64430	64510	64640
36490	62278	64410	64435	64520	64680
36491	62279				

Calculations of Total Anesthesia Values

The **total anesthesia value** is calculated by **adding the separately listed basic value** and **time value**.

A **basic** value is listed for most procedures. This includes the value of all anesthesia services except the value of the actual time spent administering the anesthesia or in unusual detention with the patient. When multiple surgical procedures are performed during the same period of anesthesia, only the greater basic anesthesia value of the various surgical procedures will be used as the base.

The **time** value is computed by allowing 1.0 unit for each 15 minutes of anesthesia time for the **first four hours** and, **thereafter** (obstetrical anesthesia excluded), by allowing 1.0 unit for each **10 minutes** of anesthesia time. For obstetrical anesthesia, 15 minute time increments are applicable for the entire duration of the service. In each instance, 5 minutes or greater is considered a significant portion of a time unit.

Anesthesia time begins when the anesthesiologist physically starts to prepare the patient for the induction of anesthesia in the operating room (or its equivalent) and ends when the anesthesiologist is no longer in constant attendance (when the patient may be safely placed under post-operative supervision).

The following examples illustrate the calculation of TOTAL ANESTHESIA VALUES:

1. PROCEDURE NUMBER + ANESTHESIA MODIFIER OR ANESTHESIA CODE

    Basic Value
    + Time Value
    Total Anesthesia Value
    (sum of basic value and time value)

2. For an incisional breast biopsy performed in 48 minutes (3 time units):

    19101   Basic Value 3
                         + Time Value 3
            Total Anesthesia Value 6

    Note: Modifiers and additional or reduced values should be used when appropriate.

Anesthesia Section

UPD	Code	Description	Units
		Head	
	00100	Anesthesia for procedures on integumentary system of head and/or salivary glands, including biopsy; not otherwise specified	5.0
	00102	plastic repair of cleft lip	6.0
	00103	blepharoplasty	(I) 5.0
	00104	Anesthesia for electroconvulsive therapy	4.0
	00120	Anesthesia for procedures on external, middle, and inner ear including biopsy; not otherwise specified	5.0
	00124	otoscopy	4.0
	00126	tympanotomy	4.0
	00140	Anesthesia for procedures on eye; not otherwise specified	5.0
97.1	00142	lens surgery	6.0
	00144	corneal transplant	6.0
	00145	vitrectomy	6.0
97.1	00147	iridectomy	6.0
	00148	ophthalmoscopy	4.0
	00160	Anesthesia for procedures on nose and accessory sinuses; not otherwise specified	5.0
	00162	radical surgery	7.0
	00164	biopsy, soft tissue	4.0
	00170	Anesthesia for intraoral procedures, including biopsy; not otherwise specified	5.0
	00172	repair of cleft palate	6.0
	00174	excision of retropharyngeal tumor	6.0
	00176	radical surgery	7.0
	00190	Anesthesia for procedures on facial bones; not otherwise specified	5.0
	00192	radical surgery (including prognathism)	7.0
	00210	Anesthesia for intracranial procedures; not otherwise specified	11.0
	00212	subdural taps	5.0
	00214	burr holes	9.0
	00215	elevation of depressed skull fracture, extradural (simple or compound)	(I) 9.0
	00216	vascular procedures	15.0
	00218	procedures in sitting position	13.0

UPD	Code	Description	Units
	00220	spinal fluid shunting procedures	10.0
	00222	electrocoagulation of intracranial nerve	6.0

Neck

UPD	Code	Description	Units
	00300	Anesthesia for all procedures on integumentary system of neck, including subcutaneous tissue	5.0
	00320	Anesthesia for all procedures on esophagus, thyroid, larynx, trachea and lymphatic system of neck; not otherwise specified	6.0
	00322	needle biopsy of thyroid	3.0
	00350	Anesthesia for procedures on major vessels of neck; not otherwise specified	10.0
	00352	simple ligation	5.0

Thorax (Chest Wall and Shoulder Girdle)

UPD	Code	Description	Units
	00400	Anesthesia for procedures on anterior integumentary system of chest, including subcutaneous tissue; not otherwise specified	3.0
	00402	reconstructive procedures on breast (eg, reduction or augmentation mammoplasty, muscle flaps)	5.0
	00404	radical or modified radical procedures on breast	5.0
	00406	radical or modified radical procedures on breast with internal mammary node dissection	13.0
	00410	electrical conversion of arrhythmias	4.0
	00420	Anesthesia for procedures on posterior integumentary system of chest, including subcutaneous tissue	5.0
	00450	Anesthesia for procedures on clavicle and scapula; not otherwise specified	5.0
	00452	radical surgery	6.0
	00454	biopsy of clavicle	3.0
	00470	Anesthesia for partial rib resection; not otherwise specified	6.0
	00472	thoracoplasty (any type)	10.0
	00474	radical procedures (eg, pectus excavatum)	13.0

Intrathoracic

UPD	Code	Description	Units
	00500	Anesthesia for all procedures on esophagus	15.0
	00520	Anesthesia for closed chest procedures (including esophagoscopy, bronchoscopy, diagnostic thoracoscopy); not otherwise specified	6.0
	00522	needle biopsy of pleura	4.0
	00524	pneumocentesis	4.0
	00528	mediastinoscopy	8.0

UPD	Code	Description	Units
	00530	Anesthesia for transvenous pacemaker insertion	4.0
	00532	Anesthesia for access to central venous circulation	4.0
	00534	Anesthesia for transvenous insertion or replacement of cardioverter/defibrillator	7.0
	00540	Anesthesia for thoracotomy procedures involving lungs, pleura, diaphragm, and mediastinum (including surgical thoracoscopy); not otherwise specified	13.0
	00542	decortication	15.0
	00544	pleurectomy	15.0
	00546	pulmonary resection with thoracoplasty	15.0
97.2	00548	intrathoracic procedures on the trachea and bronchi	15.0
	00560	Anesthesia for procedures on heart, pericardium, and great vessels of chest; without pump oxygenator	15.0
	00562	with pump oxygenator	20.0
	00580	Anesthesia for heart transplant or heart/lung transplant	20.0

Spine and Spinal Cord

UPD	Code	Description	Units
	00600	Anesthesia for procedures on cervical spine and cord; not otherwise specified	10.0
	00604	posterior cervical laminectomy in sitting position	13.0
	00620	Anesthesia for procedures on thoracic spine and cord; not otherwise specified	10.0
	00622	thoracolumbar sympathectomy	13.0
	00630	Anesthesia for procedures in lumbar region; not otherwise specified	8.0
	00632	lumbar sympathectomy	7.0
	00634	chemonucleolysis	10.0
	00670	Anesthesia for extensive spine and spinal cord procedures (eg, Harrington rod technique)	13.0

Upper Abdomen

UPD	Code	Description	Units
	00700	Anesthesia for procedures on upper anterior abdominal wall; not otherwise specified	3.0
	00702	percutaneous liver biopsy	4.0
	00730	Anesthesia for procedures on upper posterior abdominal wall	5.0
	00740	Anesthesia for upper gastrointestinal endoscopic procedures	5.0
	00750	Anesthesia for hernia repairs in upper abdomen; not otherwise specified	4.0
	00752	lumbar and ventral (incisional) hernias and/or wound dehiscence	6.0
	00754	omphalocele	7.0
	00756	transabdominal repair of diaphragmatic hernia	7.0

UPD	Code	Description	Units
	00770	Anesthesia for all procedures on major abdominal blood vessels	15.0
	00790	Anesthesia for intraperitoneal procedures in upper abdomen including laparoscopy; not otherwise specified	7.0
	00792	partial hepatectomy (excluding liver biopsy)	13.0
	00794	pancreatectomy, partial or total (eg, Whipple procedure)	8.0
	00796	liver transplant (recipient)	30.0

Lower Abdomen

UPD	Code	Description	Units
	00800	Anesthesia for procedures on lower anterior abdominal wall; not otherwise specified	3.0
	00802	panniculectomy	5.0
97.1	00810	Anesthesia for intestinal endoscopic procedures	5.0
	00820	Anesthesia for procedures on lower posterior abdominal wall	5.0
	00830	Anesthesia for hernia repairs in lower abdomen; not otherwise specified	4.0
	00832	ventral and incisional hernias	6.0
	00840	Anesthesia for intraperitoneal procedures in lower abdomen including laparoscopy; not otherwise specified	6.0
	00842	amniocentesis	4.0
	00844	abdominoperineal resection	7.0
	00846	radical hysterectomy	8.0
	00848	pelvic exenteration	8.0
	00850	cesarean section	7.0
	00855	cesarean hysterectomy	8.0
	00857	Continuous epidural analgesia, for labor and cesarean section	7.0
	00860	Anesthesia for extraperitoneal procedures in lower abdomen, including urinary tract; not otherwise specified	6.0
	00862	renal procedures, including upper 1/3 of ureter, or donor nephrectomy	7.0
	00864	total cystectomy	8.0
	00865	radical prostatectomy (suprapubic, retropubic)	8.0
	00866	adrenalectomy	10.0
	00868	renal transplant (recipient)	10.0
	00870	cystolithotomy	5.0
	00872	Anesthesia for lithotripsy, extracorporeal shock wave; with water bath	7.0
	00873	without water bath	5.0

UPD	Code	Description	Units
	00880	Anesthesia for procedures on major lower abdominal vessels; not otherwise specified	15.0
	00882	inferior vena cava ligation	10.0
	00884	transvenous umbrella insertion	5.0

Perineum

UPD	Code	Description	Units
	00900	Anesthesia for procedures on perineal integumentary system (including biopsy of male genital system); not otherwise specified	3.0
	00902	anorectal procedure (including endoscopy and/or biopsy)	4.0
	00904	radical perineal procedure	7.0
	00906	vulvectomy	4.0
	00908	perineal prostatectomy	6.0
	00910	Anesthesia for transurethral procedures (including urethrocystoscopy); not otherwise specified	3.0
	00912	transurethral resection of bladder tumor(s)	5.0
	00914	transurethral resection of prostate	5.0
	00916	post-transurethral resection bleeding	5.0
	00918	with fragmentation and/or removal of ureteral calculus	5.0
	00920	Anesthesia for procedures on male external genitalia; not otherwise specified	3.0
	00922	seminal vesicles	6.0
	00924	undescended testis, unilateral or bilateral	4.0
	00926	radical orchiectomy, inguinal	4.0
	00928	radical orchiectomy, abdominal	6.0
	00930	orchiopexy, unilateral or bilateral	4.0
	00932	complete amputation of penis	4.0
	00934	radical amputation of penis with bilateral inguinal lymphadenectomy	6.0
	00936	radical amputation of penis with bilateral inguinal and iliac lymphadenectomy	8.0
	00938	insertion of penile prosthesis (perineal approach)	4.0
	00940	Anesthesia for vaginal procedures (including biopsy of labia, vagina, cervix or endometrium); not otherwise specified	3.0
	00942	colpotomy, colpectomy, colporrhaphy	4.0
	00944	vaginal hysterectomy	6.0
	00946	vaginal delivery	5.0
	00948	cervical cerclage	4.0

UPD	Code	Description	Units
	00950	culdoscopy	5.0
	00952	hysteroscopy	4.0
	00955	Continuous epidural analgesia, for labor and vaginal delivery	5.0

Pelvis (Except Hip)

UPD	Code	Description	Units
	01000	Anesthesia for procedures on anterior integumentary system of pelvis (anterior to iliac crest), except external genitalia	3.0
	01110	Anesthesia for procedures on posterior integumentary system of pelvis (posterior to iliac crest), except perineum	5.0
	01120	Anesthesia for procedures on bony pelvis	6.0
	01130	Anesthesia for body cast application or revision	3.0
	01140	Anesthesia for interpelviabdominal (hindquarter) amputation	15.0
	01150	Anesthesia for radical procedures for tumor of pelvis, except hindquarter amputation	8.0
	01160	Anesthesia for closed procedures involving symphysis pubis or sacroiliac joint	4.0
	01170	Anesthesia for open procedures involving symphysis pubis or sacroiliac joint	8.0
	01180	Anesthesia for obturator neurectomy; extrapelvic	3.0
	01190	intrapelvic	4.0

Upper Leg (Except Knee)

UPD	Code	Description	Units
	01200	Anesthesia for all closed procedures involving hip joint	4.0
	01202	Anesthesia for arthroscopic procedures of hip joint	4.0
	01210	Anesthesia for open procedures involving hip joint; not otherwise specified	6.0
	01212	hip disarticulation	10.0
97.1	01214	total hip replacement or revision	8.0
	01220	Anesthesia for all closed procedures involving upper 2/3 of femur	4.0
	01230	Anesthesia for open procedures involving upper 2/3 of femur; not otherwise specified	6.0
	01232	amputation	5.0
	01234	radical resection	8.0
	01240	Anesthesia for all procedures on integumentary system of upper leg	3.0
	01250	Anesthesia for all procedures on nerves, muscles, tendons, fascia, and bursa of upper leg	4.0
	01260	Anesthesia for all procedures involving veins of upper leg, including exploration	3.0
	01270	Anesthesia for procedures involving arteries of upper leg, including bypass graft; not otherwise specified	8.0

UPD	Code	Description	Units
	01272	femoral artery ligation	4.0
	01274	femoral artery embolectomy	6.0

Knee and Popliteal Area

UPD	Code	Description	Units
	01300	Anesthesia for all procedures on integumentary system of knee and/or popliteal area	3.0
	01320	Anesthesia for all procedures on nerves, muscles, tendons, fascia, and bursa of knee and/or popliteal area	4.0
	01340	Anesthesia for all closed procedures on lower 1/3 of femur	4.0
	01360	Anesthesia for all open procedures on lower 1/3 of femur	5.0
	01380	Anesthesia for all closed procedures on knee joint	3.0
	01382	Anesthesia for arthroscopic procedures of knee joint	3.0
	01390	Anesthesia for all closed procedures on upper ends of tibia, fibula, and/or patella	3.0
	01392	Anesthesia for all open procedures on upper ends of tibia, fibula, and/or patella	4.0
	01400	Anesthesia for open procedures on knee joint; not otherwise specified	4.0
	01402	total knee replacement	7.0
	01404	disarticulation at knee	5.0
	01420	Anesthesia for all cast applications, removal, or repair involving knee joint	3.0
	01430	Anesthesia for procedures on veins of knee and popliteal area; not otherwise specified	3.0
97.1	01432	arteriovenous fistula	6.0
	01440	Anesthesia for procedures on arteries of knee and popliteal area; not otherwise specified	5.0
	01442	popliteal thromboendarterectomy, with or without patch graft	8.0
	01444	popliteal excision and graft or repair for occlusion or aneurysm	8.0

Lower Leg (Below Knee)

UPD	Code	Description	Units
	01460	Anesthesia for all procedures on integumentary system of lower leg, ankle, and foot	3.0
	01462	Anesthesia for all closed procedures on lower leg, ankle, and foot	3.0
	01464	Anesthesia for arthroscopic procedures of ankle joint	3.0
	01470	Anesthesia for procedures on nerves, muscles, tendons, and fascia of lower leg, ankle, and foot; not otherwise specified	3.0
	01472	repair of ruptured Achilles tendon, with or without graft	5.0
	01474	gastrocnemius recession (eg, Strayer procedure)	5.0
	01480	Anesthesia for open procedures on bones of lower leg, ankle, and foot; not otherwise specified	3.0

UPD	Code	Description	Units
	01482	radical resection	4.0
	01484	osteotomy or osteoplasty of tibia and/or fibula	4.0
	01486	total ankle replacement	7.0
	01490	Anesthesia for lower leg cast application, removal, or repair	3.0
	01500	Anesthesia for procedures on arteries of lower leg, including bypass graft; not otherwise specified	8.0
	01502	embolectomy, direct or catheter	6.0
	01520	Anesthesia for procedures on veins of lower leg; not otherwise specified	3.0
	01522	venous thrombectomy, direct or catheter	5.0

Shoulder and Axilla

UPD	Code	Description	Units
	01600	Anesthesia for all procedures on integumentary system of shoulder and axilla	3.0
	01610	Anesthesia for all procedures on nerves, muscles, tendons, fascia, and bursa of shoulder and axilla	5.0
	01620	Anesthesia for all closed procedures on humeral head and neck, sternoclavicular joint, acromioclavicular joint, and shoulder joint	4.0
	01622	Anesthesia for arthroscopic procedures of shoulder joint	4.0
	01630	Anesthesia for open procedures on humeral head and neck, sternoclavicular joint, acromioclavicular joint, and shoulder joint; not otherwise specified	5.0
	01632	radical resection	6.0
	01634	shoulder disarticulation	9.0
	01636	interthoracoscapular (forequarter) amputation	15.0
	01638	total shoulder replacement	10.0
	01650	Anesthesia for procedures on arteries of shoulder and axilla; not otherwise specified	6.0
	01652	axillary-brachial aneurysm	10.0
	01654	bypass graft	8.0
	01656	axillary-femoral bypass graft	10.0
	01670	Anesthesia for all procedures on veins of shoulder and axilla	4.0
	01680	Anesthesia for shoulder cast application, removal or repair; not otherwise specified	3.0
	01682	shoulder spica	4.0

Upper Arm and Elbow

UPD	Code	Description	Units
	01700	Anesthesia for all procedures on integumentary system of upper arm and elbow	3.0
	01710	Anesthesia for procedures on nerves, muscles, tendons, fascia, and bursa of upper arm and elbow; not otherwise specified	3.0

UPD	Code	Description	Units
	01712	tenotomy, elbow to shoulder, open	5.0
	01714	tenoplasty, elbow to shoulder	5.0
	01716	tenodesis, rupture of long tendon of biceps	5.0
	01730	Anesthesia for all closed procedures on humerus and elbow	3.0
	01732	Anesthesia for arthroscopic procedures of elbow joint	3.0
	01740	Anesthesia for open procedures on humerus and elbow; not otherwise specified	4.0
	01742	osteotomy of humerus	5.0
	01744	repair of nonunion or malunion of humerus	5.0
	01756	radical procedures	6.0
	01758	excision of cyst or tumor of humerus	5.0
	01760	otal elbow replacement	7.0
97.1	01770	Anesthesia for procedures on arteries of upper arm and elbow; not otherwise specified	6.0
	01772	embolectomy	6.0
	01780	Anesthesia for procedures on veins of upper arm and elbow; not otherwise specified	3.0
	01782	phleborrhaphy	4.0
	01784	Anesthesia for repair of arterio-venous (A-V) fistula, congenital or acquired	6.0

Forearm, Wrist, and Hand

UPD	Code	Description	Units
	01800	Anesthesia for all procedures on integumentary system of forearm, wrist, and hand	3.0
	01810	Anesthesia for all procedures on nerves, muscles, tendons, fascia, and bursa of forearm, wrist, and hand	3.0
	01820	Anesthesia for all closed procedures on radius, ulna, wrist, or hand bones	3.0
	01830	Anesthesia for open procedures on radius, ulna, wrist, or hand bones; not otherwise specified	3.0
	01832	total wrist replacement	6.0
	01840	Anesthesia for procedures on arteries of forearm, wrist, and hand; not otherwise specified	6.0
	01842	embolectomy	6.0
	01844	Anesthesia for vascular shunt, or shunt revision, any type (eg, dialysis)	6.0
	01850	Anesthesia for procedures on veins of forearm, wrist, and hand; not otherwise specified	3.0
	01852	phleborrhaphy	4.0
	01860	Anesthesia for forearm, wrist, or hand cast application, removal, or repair	3.0

UPD			Code	Description	Units

Radiological Procedures

UPD			Code	Description	Units
			01900	Anesthesia for injection procedure for hysterosalpingography	3.0
			01902	Anesthesia for burr hole(s) for ventriculography	9.0
			01904	Anesthesia for injection procedure for pneumoencephalography	7.0
			01906	Anesthesia for injection procedure for myelography; lumbar	5.0
			01908	cervical	5.0
			01910	posterior fossa	9.0
			01912	Anesthesia for injection procedure for diskography; lumbar	5.0
			01914	cervical	6.0
			01916	Anesthesia for arteriograms, needle; carotid, or vertebral	5.0
			01918	retrograde, brachial or femoral	5.0
			01920	Anesthesia for cardiac catheterization including coronary arteriography and ventriculography (not to include Swan-Ganz catheter)	7.0
			01921	Anesthesia for angioplasty	7.0
			01922	Anesthesia for non-invasive imaging or radiation therapy	7.0

Other Procedures

UPD			Code	Description	Units
			01990	Physiological support for harvesting of organ(s) from brain-dead patient	7.0
97.2			01995	Regional IV administration of local anesthetic agent or other medication (upper or lower extremity)	5.0
			01996	Daily management of epidural or subarachnoid drug administration	3.0
			01999	Unlisted anesthesia procedure(s)	BR

Qualifying Circumstances for Anesthesia

UPD			Code	Description	Units
98.2	▲	+	99100	Anesthesia for patient of extreme age, under one year and over seventy (List separately in addition to code for primary anesthesia procedure)	1.0
98.2	▲	+	99116	Anesthesia complicated by utilization of total body hypothermia (List separately in addition to code for primary anesthesia procedure)	5.0
98.2	▲	+	99135	Anesthesia complicated by utilization of controlled hypotension (List separately in addition to code for primary anesthesia procedure)	5.0
98.2	▲	+	99140	Anesthesia complicated by emergency conditions (specify) (List separately in addition to code for primary anesthesia procedure)	2.0

Surgery

Guidelines

I. **Global Values:**

   A. The relative values for **therapeutic surgical procedures** are considered global and include:

      1. The immediate preoperative care that starts after the decision for surgery has been made in which there are no complications requiring extra stabilizing care.

         a. Additional value is warranted for preoperative services under the following circumstances:

            (1) Evaluation and Management services unrelated to the primary procedure.

            (2) Services required to stabilize the patient for the primary procedure.

            (3) When procedures not usually part of the basic surgical procedure (e.g., bronchoscopy prior to chest surgery) are provided during the immediate preoperative period.

      2. The surgical procedure, including local infiltration, digital block, or topical anesthesia, when used.

      3. Normal uncomplicated follow-up care for the period indicated: "FUD" (follow-up days).

         a. Additional value is warranted for care rendered during the follow-up period caused by an unusual circumstance or complication.

   B. Care for diagnostic procedures (e.g., endoscopy, injection procedures for radiography, etc.) includes only that care related to the diagnostic procedure itself. Care of the condition for which the diagnostic procedure was performed or other concomitant conditions is not included, and may be listed separately. Follow-up care related to the diagnostic procedure is included for the period listed under "FUD."

   C. When an additional surgical procedure(s) is carried out within the listed period of follow-up care for a previous surgery, the follow-up periods will continue concurrently to their normal terminations.

II. **Starred (*) Procedures:** Global values do not apply to starred (*) procedure codes. Use the following rules:

The service as listed includes the surgical procedure only. Associated pre- and postoperative services are not included in the service as listed.

Examples:

   A. When the procedure constitutes the only service at the initial visit, procedure number 99025 is to be used in conjunction with the starred procedure code.

   B. When the procedure is carried out at the time of other significant identifiable services, the appropriate service code is listed in addition to the starred (*) procedure.

   C. When the procedure is the only service provided on an established patient, a service visit is not appropriate.

III.   **Separate Procedures:** Procedures identified as "(separate procedures)" are frequently included in the global value of other procedures. Listing of separate codes is not appropriate when a procedure is included in the global value of another (e.g., 29870 is not appropriate to list in conjunction with 29874).

IV.   **Unusual Service Or Procedure:** A service may necessitate use of the skills and time of the physician over and above listed services and values. If substantiated "by report" (BR), additional values may be warranted. Use modifier -22 to indicate these procedures.

V.   **Unlisted Service Or Procedure:** When a service or procedure provided is not adequately identified, use of the unlisted procedure code for the related anatomical area is appropriate. Most codes of this nature have 99 for the last two digits. Value should be substantiated "by report" (BR).

VI.   **Procedures Without Specified Unit Values:** Procedures which have RNE or BR in the units column, should be substantiated "by report". RNE means that the relativity for the procedures has not been established.

VII.   **By Report (BR):** Value of a procedure should be established for any "by report" circumstance by identifying a similar service and justifying value difference. When a report is indicated, the report should include the following:

   A.   Accurate procedure definition or description;

   B.   Operative report;

   C.   Justification for procedural variance, when appropriate;

   D.   Similar procedure and value comparisons; and

   E.   Justification for value difference.

VIII.   **Reduced Values:** Under some circumstances, value for a procedure may be reduced or eliminated. Use the modifier (-52) to identify reduced value services.

IX.   **Operating Microscope:** When an operating microscope is used to perform a procedure, report 69990 in addition to the code.

X.   **Anesthesia By Surgeon:** Regional or general anesthesia provided by a surgeon should be indicated using modifier -47. The surgeon may receive a value for the procedure equal to the base anesthesia value listed in the column of ANES. Anesthesia and surgery relative value units are based on different scales. Note: Customary conversion factors for anesthesia are approximately 25% of surgery conversion factors.

XI.   **Preoperative, Surgery, And/or Postoperative Care Provided By Different Physicians:**

   A.   Surgical care only: When a physician provides only the surgical care and another physician provides preoperative and postoperative care, this circumstance should be indicated by the use of modifier -54. A customary 70% of the listed value is allowed for this circumstance.

   B.   Postoperative management only: If a physician provides the postoperative care only, the use of modifier -55 is warranted. A customary value of 30% of the listed value is appropriate.

   C.   Preoperative management only: If a physician provides the preoperative care only, the use of modifier -56 is warranted. A customary value of 10% of the listed value is appropriate.

XII.   **Two Surgeons:** Under certain circumstances, the skills of two surgeons (usually with different skills) may be required in the management of a specific surgical problem (e.g., a urologist and a general surgeon in the creation of an ideal conduit, etc.) The procedure should be valued at the customary value of 125% of the value listed. The total value (125%) may be apportioned in relation to the responsibility and work done, provided the patient is made aware of the arrangement. Such procedures should be marked using modifier -62.

XIII.   **Surgical Team:** Under some circumstances, a highly complex procedure(s) identified by a single code requires the services of several physicians, often of different specialties. These circumstances should be identified by adding modifier -66. The value should be supported by a report to include itemization of the services and personnel included in a "global" value. See CONCURRENT CARE and MULTIPLE PROCEDURES for help in determining the "global" value.

XIV.   **Surgical Assistants:** An assistant surgeon, regardless of "type," can provide other services on the same date. These services warrant a value of 100% of the values listed.

A. Assistant Surgeon: When surgical assistance is provided by a qualified physician, the use of modifier -80 is appropriate. The use of this modifier customarily warrants 20% of the listed values.

B. Minimum Assistant Surgeon: When minimal surgical assistance is provided, the use of modifier -81 is appropriate. The use of this modifier customarily warrants 10% of the listed values.

C. Assistant Surgeon (when a qualified resident surgeon is not available): When a qualified resident surgeon is unavailable and a qualified nonresident surgeon provides surgical assistance, use of modifier -82 is appropriate. The use of this modifier customarily warrants 20% of the listed values.

XV. **Concurrent Care:** When separate procedures or services are provided by two or more physicians on the same date, each physician should indicate his or her service(s) by appropriate procedure code(s). This circumstance does not warrant any increase or reduction in value. It is important to note that this circumstance can be used only if the procedures performed do not qualify for the use of modifiers -62 or -66. See Medicine Value Guidelines for appropriate modifier and use for evaluation and management codes.

Example: A general surgeon performs 49505 (herniorrhaphy) on the same patient on the same day as an urologist performs 52601 (TURP). Both bill at 100% of listed value with no modifier and are governed separately by the global value rules.

XVI. **Multiple Procedures, Same Surgeon:** Procedures performed at the same operative setting that significantly increase time and skill warrant the use of modifier -51. Modifier -51 should be added to the secondary, tertiary, etc. procedure(s) code(s). Multiple procedures should be listed according to value. (Multiple Procedure Guidelines do not apply to codes specifically identified as Add-on/Additional Procedures.) The primary procedure should reflect the greatest value and should not add modifier -51. All other procedures should be listed using modifier -51 in decreasing value. The values appropriate for each procedure are as follows:

1. Primary procedure   100% of listed value

2. Secondary procedure and each additional   50% of listed value

   Example: A general surgeon performs a 39502 (hiatal hernia repair) RVU 17.2 and 47600 (cholecystectomy) RVU 14.2 at the same operative setting. The correct billing:

		RVU
39502		17.20
47600-51	(14.2) (50%)	= 7.1

XVII. **Bilateral Procedures:** Some procedures that are performed on both the left and right (bilateral procedures) warrant the use of modifier -50 for the second procedure. Follow appropriate rules of evaluation listed under MULTIPLE PROCEDURES, dependent upon the number of incisions required.

XVIII. **Distinct Procedural Service:** Under certain circumstances, the physician may need to indicate that a procedure or service was distinct or independent from other services performed on the same day. Modifier '-59' is used to identify procedures/services that are not normally reported together, but are appropriate under the circumstances. This may represent a different session or patient encounter, different procedure or surgery, different site or organ system, separate incision/excision, separate lesion, or separate injury (or area of injury in extensive injuries) not ordinarily encountered or performed on the same day by the same physician. However, when another already established modifier is appropriate, it should be used rather than modifier '-59'. Only if no more descriptive modifier is available, and the use of modifier '-59' best explains the circumstances, should modifier '-59' be used. Payment for codes that qualify for this modifier should be 100% of listed value, if performed at a separate patient encounter. Some payers may require the listing of this modifier in addition to other appropriate modifiers for electronic processing of claims. If the circumstance warrants the use of a second modifier in conjunction with -59, the level of payment is determined by the guideline for the second modifier.

XIX. **Multiple Modifiers:** If circumstances require the use of more than one modifier with any one procedure code, modifier -99 should be added to the procedure code. Other modifiers are then attached to the procedure code and listed separately with appropriate values for each.

XX. **Add-on Procedures:** Procedures which are indicated by an editors note following the code as an add-on procedure are not subject to multiple procedure guideline reductions. RVP has added modifier -60 to indicate such procedures. This procedure is non-CPT compatable. Some payers require reporting of these procedures with no modifier.

Surgical Section

UPD			Code	Description	Units	FUD	Anes

Integumentary System

UPD			Code	Description	Units	FUD	Anes
			10040*	Acne surgery (eg, marsupialization, opening or removal of multiple milia, comedones, cysts, pustules)	0.5	0	3
			10060*	Incision and drainage of abscess (eg, carbuncle, suppurative hidradenitis, cutaneous or subcutaneous abscess, cyst, furuncle, or paronychia); simple or single	0.8	0	3
			10061	complicated or multiple	1.6	0	3
98.2			10080*	Incision and drainage of pilonidal cyst; simple	0.8	0	3
98.2			10081	complicated	1.2	0	3
			10120*	Incision and removal of foreign body, subcutaneous tissues; simple	1.0	0	3
			10121	complicated	2.3	0	3
			10140*	Incision and drainage of hematoma, seroma or fluid collection	0.8	0	3
			10160*	Puncture aspiration of abscess, hematoma, bulla, or cyst	0.6	0	3
			10180	Incision and drainage, complex, postoperative wound infection	2.6	0	3
96.2			11000*	Debridement of extensive eczematous or infected skin; up to 10% of body surface	0.8	0	3
98.2	▲	+	11001	each additional 10% of the body surface (List separately in addition to code for primary procedure) Note: This code is an add-on procedure and as such is valued appropriately. Multiple procedure guidelines for reduction of value are not applicable.	0.4	0	0
96.2			11010	Debridement including removal of foreign material associated with open fracture(s) and/or dislocation(s); skin and subcutaneous tissues	(I) 6.2	0	3
98.2			11011	skin, subcutaneous tissue, muscle fascia, and muscle	(I) 7.3	0	3
98.2			11012	skin, subcutaneous tissue, muscle fascia, muscle, and bone	(I) 10.0	0	3
96.2			11040	Debridement; skin, partial thickness	1.0	0	3
96.2			11041	skin, full thickness	1.5	0	3
96.2			11042	skin, and subcutaneous tissue	2.2	0	3
96.2			11043	skin, subcutaneous tissue, and muscle	3.0	0	3
96.2			11044	subcutaneous tissue, muscle, and bone	4.0	0	3
97.2	M		11050	Paring or curettement of benign hyperkeratotic skin lesion with or without chemical To report paring, see 11055-11057, or to report destruction, see 17000-17004	0.5	0	3

UPD			Code	Description	Units	FUD	Anes
97.2	**M**		**11051**	two to four lesions To report paring, see 11055-11057, or to report destruction, see 17000-17004	0.7	0	3
97.2	**M**		**11052**	more than four lesions To report paring, see 11055-11057, or to report destruction, see 17000-17004	0.9	0	3
97.2			**11055**	Paring or cutting of benign hyperkeratotic lesion (eg, corn or callus); single lesion	(I) 0.5	0	3
97.2			**11056**	Paring or cutting of benign hyperkeratotic lesion (eg, corn or callus); two to four lesions	(I) 0.7	0	3
97.2			**11057**	Paring or cutting of benign hyperkeratotic lesion (eg, corn or callus); more than four lesions	(I) 0.9	0	3
			11100	Biopsy of skin, subcutaneous tissue and/or mucous membrane (including simple closure), unless otherwise listed (separate procedure); single lesion	1.0	7	3
98.2	▲ +		**11101**	each separate/additional lesion (List separately in addition to code for primary procedure) Note: This code is an add-on procedure and as such is valued appropriately. Multiple procedure guidelines for reduction of value are not applicable.	0.7	0	0
			11200*	Removal of skin tags, multiple fibrocutaneous tags, any area; up to and including 15 lesions	0.7	0	3
98.2	▲ +		**11201**	each additional ten lesions (List separately in addition to code for primary procedure)	0.4	7	0
			11300*	Shaving of epidermal or dermal lesion, single lesion, trunk, arms or legs; lesion diameter 0.5 cm or less	(I) 1.0	0	3
			11301	lesion diameter 0.6 to 1.0 cm	(I) 1.5	0	3
			11302	lesion diameter 1.1 to 2.0 cm	(I) 1.8	0	3
			11303	lesion diameter over 2.0 cm	(I) 2.2	0	3
			11305*	Shaving of epidermal or dermal lesion, single lesion, scalp, neck, hands, feet, genitalia; lesion diameter 0.5 cm or less	(I) 1.2	0	3
			11306	lesion diameter 0.6 to 1.0 cm	(I) 1.7	0	3
			11307	lesion diameter 1.1 to 2.0 cm	(I) 2.0	0	3
			11308	lesion diameter over 2.0 cm	(I) 2.4	0	3
98.2			**11310***	Shaving of epidermal or dermal lesion, single lesion, face, ears, eyelids, nose, lips, mucous membrane; lesion diameter 0.5 cm or less	(I) 1.3	0	5
98.2			**11311**	lesion diameter 0.6 to 1.0 cm	(I) 1.8	0	5
98.2			**11312**	lesion diameter 1.1 to 2.0 cm	(I) 2.1	0	5
98.2			**11313**	lesion diameter over 2.0 cm	(I) 2.8	0	5
97.1			**11400**	Excision, benign lesion, except skin tag (unless listed elsewhere), trunk, arms or legs; lesion diameter 0.5 cm or less	0.8	15	3

UPD	Code	Description	Units	FUD	Anes
97.1	**11401**	lesion diameter 0.6 to 1.0 cm	1.0	15	3
97.1	**11402**	lesion diameter 1.1 to 2.0 cm	1.2	15	3
97.1	**11403**	lesion diameter 2.1 to 3.0 cm	1.5	15	3
97.1	**11404**	lesion diameter 3.1 to 4.0 cm	1.8	15	3
97.1	**11406**	lesion diameter over 4.0 cm	2.1	15	3
98.2	**11420**	Excision, benign lesion, except skin tag (unless listed elsewhere), scalp, neck, hands, feet, genitalia; lesion diameter 0.5 cm or less	0.9	15	5
98.2	**11421**	lesion diameter 0.6 to 1.0 cm	1.1	15	5
98.2	**11422**	lesion diameter 1.1 to 2.0 cm	1.5	15	5
98.2	**11423**	lesion diameter 2.1 to 3.0 cm	2.0	15	5
98.2	**11424**	lesion diameter 3.1 to 4.0 cm	2.5	15	5
98.2	**11426**	lesion diameter over 4.0 cm	2.9	15	5
97.1	**11440**	Excision, other benign lesion (unless listed elsewhere), face, ears, eyelids, nose, lips, mucous membrane; lesion diameter 0.5 cm or less	1.2	15	5
97.1	**11441**	lesion diameter 0.6 to 1.0 cm	1.6	15	5
97.1	**11442**	lesion diameter 1.1 to 2.0 cm	1.9	15	5
97.1	**11443**	lesion diameter 2.1 to 3.0 cm	2.4	15	5
97.1	**11444**	lesion diameter 3.1 to 4.0 cm	2.9	15	5
97.1	**11446**	lesion diameter over 4.0 cm	3.3	15	5
98.2	**11450**	Excision of skin and subcutaneous tissue for hidradenitis, axillary; with simple or intermediate repair	4.5	15	3
98.2	**11451**	with complex repair	5.5	15	3
98.2	**11462**	Excision of skin and subcutaneous tissue for hidradenitis, inguinal; with simple or intermediate repair	5.0	15	3
98.2	**11463**	with complex repair	5.5	15	3
98.2	**11470**	Excision of skin and subcutaneous tissue for hidradenitis, perianal, perineal, or umbilical; with simple or intermediate repair	5.5	15	3
98.2	**11471**	with complex repair	6.2	15	3
	11600	Excision, malignant lesion, trunk, arms, or legs; lesion diameter 0.5 cm or less	1.5	90	3
	11601	lesion diameter 0.6 to 1.0 cm	1.9	90	3
	11602	lesion diameter 1.1 to 2.0 cm	2.3	90	3
	11603	lesion diameter 2.1 to 3.0 cm	2.5	90	3

UPD			Code	Description	Units	FUD	Anes
			11604	lesion diameter 3.1 to 4.0 cm	3.0	90	3
			11606	lesion diameter over 4.0 cm	3.4	90	3
98.2			11620	Excision, malignant lesion, scalp, neck, hands, feet, genitalia; lesion diameter 0.5 cm or less	2.0	90	5
98.2			11621	lesion diameter 0.6 to 1.0 cm	2.8	90	5
98.2			11622	lesion diameter 1.1 to 2.0 cm	3.6	90	5
98.2			11623	lesion diameter 2.1 to 3.0 cm	4.4	90	5
98.2			11624	lesion diameter 3.1 to 4.0 cm	5.2	90	5
98.2			11626	lesion diameter over 4.0 cm	6.0	90	5
			11640	Excision, malignant lesion, face, ears, eyelids, nose, lips; lesion diameter 0.5 cm or less	3.0	90	5
			11641	diameter 0.6 to 1.0 cm	4.0	90	5
			11642	lesion diameter 1.1 to 2.0 cm	5.0	90	5
			11643	lesion diameter 2.1 to 3.0 cm	6.0	90	5
			11644	lesion diameter 3.1 to 4.0 cm	7.0	90	5
			11646	lesion diameter over 4.0 cm	8.0	90	5
96.2	M		11700*	Debridement of nails, manual; five or less To report, use 11720, 11721	0.4	0	3
96.2	M		11701	each additional, five or less To report, use 11720, 11721	0.4	0	3
96.2	M		11710*	Debridement of nails, electric grinder; five or less To report, use 11720, 11721	0.6	0	3
96.2	M		11711	each additional, five or less To report, use 11720, 11721	0.6	0	3
97.2			11719	Trimming of nondystrophic nails, any number	(I) 0.3	0	3
96.2			11720	Debridement of nail(s) by any method(s); one to five	0.5	0	3
96.2			11721	six or more	0.9	0	3
			11730*	Avulsion of nail plate, partial or complete, simple; single	1.0	0	3
98.2	M		11731	second nail plate To report, use 11732	0.8	0	3
98.2	▲ +		11732	each additional nail plate (List separately in addition to code for primary procedure) Note: This code is an add-on procedure and as such is valued appropriately. Multiple procedure guidelines for reduction of value are not applicable.	0.7	0	0
			11740	Evacuation of subungual hematoma	0.6	0	3

UPD			Code	Description	Units	FUD	Anes
			11750	Excision of nail and nail matrix, partial or complete, (eg, ingrown or deformed nail) for permanent removal;	2.5	0	3
			11752	with amputation of tuft of distal phalanx	3.8	0	3
			11755	Biopsy of nail unit, any method (eg, plate, bed, matrix, hyponychium, proximal and lateral nail folds) (separate procedure)	(I) 1.8	0	3
			11760	Repair of nail bed	3.5	60	3
			11762	Reconstruction of nail bed with graft	5.0	90	3
			11765	Wedge excision of skin of nail fold (eg, for ingrown toenail)	1.2	60	3
			11770	Excision of pilonidal cyst or sinus; simple	2.2	30	5
			11771	extensive	6.5	60	5
			11772	complicated	8.0	60	5
			11900*	Injection, intralesional; up to and including seven lesions	0.5	0	3
			11901*	more than seven lesions	0.6	0	3
			11920	Tattooing, intradermal introduction of insoluble opaque pigments to correct color defects of skin, including micropigmentation; 6.0 sq cm or less	5.0	90	3
			11921	6.1 to 20.0 sq cm	10.0	90	3
98.2	▲	+	11922	each additional 20.0 sq cm (List separately in addition to code for primary procedure) Note: This code is an add-on procedure and as such is valued appropriately. Multiple procedure guidelines for reduction of value are not applicable.	5.0	90	0
			11950	Subcutaneous injection of "filling" material (eg, collagen); 1 cc or less	2.0	30	3
			11951	1.1 to 5.0 cc	4.0	30	3
			11952	5.1 to 10.0 cc	8.0	30	3
			11954	over 10.0 cc	BR	30	3
			11960	Insertion of tissue expander(s) for other than breast, including subsequent expansion	13.5	90	3
98.2			11970	Replacement of tissue expander with permanent prosthesis	15.0	90	3
			11971	Removal of tissue expander(s) without insertion of prosthesis	3.0	30	3
			11975	Insertion, implantable contraceptive capsules	1.5	15	3
			11976	Removal, implantable contraceptive capsules	2.0	15	3
			11977	Removal with reinsertion, implantable contraceptive capsules	(I) 4.0	15	3
98.2			12001*	Simple repair of superficial wounds of scalp, neck, axillae, external genitalia, trunk and/or extremities (including hands and feet); 2.5 cm or less	1.0	0	5

UPD	Code	Description	Units	FUD	Anes
98.2	**12002***	2.6 cm to 7.5 cm	1.4	0	5
98.2	**12004***	7.6 cm to 12.5 cm	1.8	0	5
98.2	**12005**	12.6 cm to 20.0 cm	2.2	7	5
98.2	**12006**	20.1 cm to 30.0 cm	2.6	7	5
98.2	**12007**	over 30.0 cm	3.0	7	5
	12011*	Simple repair of superficial wounds of face, ears, eyelids, nose, lips and/or mucous membranes; 2.5 cm or less	1.1	0	5
	12013*	2.6 cm to 5.0 cm	1.5	0	5
	12014	5.1 cm to 7.5 cm	1.9	7	5
	12015	7.6 cm to 12.5 cm	2.3	7	5
	12016	12.6 cm to 20.0 cm	2.7	7	5
	12017	20.1 cm to 30.0 cm	3.1	7	5
	12018	over 30.0 cm	3.5	7	5
98.2	**12020**	Treatment of superficial wound dehiscence; simple closure	1.6	7	3
98.2	**12021**	Treatment of superficial wound dehiscence; with packing	1.8	7	3
98.2	**12031***	Layer closure of wounds of scalp, axillae, trunk and/or extremities (excluding hands and feet); 2.5 cm or less	1.4	0	5
98.2	**12032***	2.6 cm to 7.5 cm	1.9	0	5
98.2	**12034**	7.6 cm to 12.5 cm	2.4	15	5
98.2	**12035**	12.6 cm to 20.0 cm	2.9	15	5
98.2	**12036**	20.1 cm to 30.0 cm	3.4	15	5
98.2	**12037**	over 30.0 cm	3.9	15	5
98.2	**12041***	Layer closure of wounds of neck, hands, feet and/or external genitalia; 2.5 cm or less	1.7	0	5
98.2	**12042**	2.6 cm to 7.5 cm	2.2	15	5
98.2	**12044**	7.6 cm to 12.5 cm	2.7	15	5
98.2	**12045**	12.6 cm to 20.0 cm	3.2	15	5
98.2	**12046**	20.1 cm to 30.0 cm	3.7	15	5
98.2	**12047**	over 30.0 cm	4.2	15	5
	12051*	Layer closure of wounds of face, ears, eyelids, nose, lips and/or mucous membranes; 2.5 cm or less	1.8	0	5
	12052	2.6 cm to 5.0 cm	2.4	15	5
	12053	5.1 cm to 7.5 cm	3.0	15	5
	12054	7.6 cm to 12.5 cm	3.6	15	5

UPD		Code	Description	Units	FUD	Anes
		12055	12.6 cm to 20.0 cm	4.2	15	5
		12056	20.1 cm to 30.0 cm	4.8	15	5
		12057	over 30.0 cm	5.4	15	5
		13100	Repair, complex, trunk; 1.1 cm to 2.5 cm	1.3	30	3
		13101	2.6 cm to 7.5 cm	3.0	30	3
98.2		13120	Repair, complex, scalp, arms, and/or legs; 1.1 cm to 2.5 cm	2.5	30	5
98.2		13121	2.6 cm to 7.5 cm	4.0	30	5
		13131	Repair, complex, forehead, cheeks, chin, mouth, neck, axillae, genitalia, hands and/or feet; 1.1 cm to 2.5 cm	3.2	30	5
		13132	2.6 cm to 7.5 cm	5.2	30	5
		13150	Repair, complex, eyelids, nose, ears and/or lips; 1.0 cm or less	2.5	30	5
		13151	1.1 cm to 2.5 cm	4.0	30	5
		13152	2.6 cm to 7.5 cm	6.5	30	5
98.2		13160	Secondary closure of surgical wound or dehiscence, extensive or complicated	3.5	30	3
98.2		13300	Repair, unusual, complicated, over 7.5 cm, any area	BR	0	3
		14000	Adjacent tissue transfer or rearrangement, trunk; defect 10 sq cm or less	6.5	60	3
		14001	defect 10.1 sq cm to 30.0 sq cm	7.5	60	3
98.2		14020	Adjacent tissue transfer or rearrangement, scalp, arms and/or legs; defect 10 sq cm or less	7.5	90	5
98.2		14021	defect 10.1 sq cm to 30.0 sq cm	9.5	90	5
		14040	Adjacent tissue transfer or rearrangement, forehead, cheeks, chin, mouth, neck, axillae, genitalia, hands and/or feet; defect 10 sq cm or less	9.5	60	5
		14041	defect 10.1 sq cm to 30.0 sq cm	12.0	60	5
		14060	Adjacent tissue transfer or rearrangement, eyelids, nose, ears and/or lips; defect 10 sq cm or less	13.0	60	5
		14061	defect 10.1 sq cm to 30.0 sq cm	15.5	90	5
		14300	Adjacent tissue transfer or rearrangement, more than 30 sq cm, unusual or complicated, any area	16.5	90	5
		14350	Filleted finger or toe flap, including preparation of recipient site	8.0	60	3
98.2	▲	15000	Surgical preparation or creation of recipient site by excision of open wounds, burn eschar, or scar (including subcutaneous tissues); first 100 sq cm or one percent of body area of infants and children	3.5	0	3

UPD			Code	Description	Units	FUD	Anes
98.2	●	+	**15001**	each additional 100 sq cm or each additional one percent of body area of infants and children (List separately in addition to code for primary procedure) Note: This code is an add-on procedure and as such is valued appropriately. Multiple procedure guidelines for reduction of value are not applicable.	1.8	0	0
			15050	Pinch graft, single or multiple, to cover small ulcer, tip of digit, or other minimal open area (except on face), up to defect size 2 cm diameter	3.5	30	3
98.2	▲		**15100**	Split graft, trunk, arms, legs; first 100 sq cm or less, or one percent of body area of infants and children (except 15050)	6.1	45	3
98.2	▲	+	**15101**	each additional 100 sq cm, or each additional one percent of body area of infants and children, or part thereof (List separately in addition to code for primary procedure) Note: This code is an add-on procedure and as such is valued appropriately. Multiple procedure guidelines for reduction of value are not applicable.	2.2	45	0
98.2	▲		**15120**	Split graft, face, scalp, eyelids, mouth, neck, ears, orbits, genitalia, hands, feet and/or multiple digits; first 100 sq cm or less, or one percent of body area of infants and children (except 15050)	11.0	45	5
98.2	▲	+	**15121**	each additional 100 sq cm, or each additional one percent of body area of infants and children, or part thereof (List separately in addition to code for primary procedure) Note: This code is an add-on procedure and as such is valued appropriately. Multiple procedure guidelines for reduction of value are not applicable.	4.1	45	0
			15200	Full thickness graft, free, including direct closure of donor site, trunk; 20 sq cm or less	4.8	45	3
98.2	▲	+	**15201**	each additional 20 sq cm (List separately in addition to code for primary procedure) Note: This code is an add-on procedure and as such is valued appropriately. Multiple procedure guidelines for reduction of value are not applicable.	2.0	45	0
98.2			**15220**	Full thickness graft, free, including direct closure of donor site, scalp, arms, and/or legs; 20 sq cm or less	6.3	45	5
98.2	▲	+	**15221**	each additional 20 sq cm (List separately in addition to code for primary procedure) Note: This code is an add-on procedure and as such is valued appropriately. Multiple procedure guidelines for reduction of value are not applicable.	3.0	45	0
98.2			**15240**	Full thickness graft, free, including direct closure of donor site, forehead, cheeks, chin, mouth, neck, axillae, genitalia, hands, and/or feet; 20 sq cm or less	9.5	45	5

UPD			Code	Description	Units	FUD	Anes
98.2	▲	+	15241	each additional 20 sq cm (List separately in addition to code for primary procedure)	4.0	45	0
				Note: This code is an add-on procedure and as such is valued appropriately. Multiple procedure guidelines for reduction of value are not applicable.			
			15260	Full thickness graft, free, including direct closure of donor site, nose, ears, eyelids, and/or lips; 20 sq cm or less	12.0	45	5
98.2	▲	+	15261	each additional 20 sq cm (List separately in addition to code for primary procedure)	6.0	45	0
				Note: This code is an add-on procedure and as such is valued appropriately. Multiple procedure guidelines for reduction of value are not applicable.			
98.2	▲		15350	Application of allograft, skin; 100 sq cm or less	(I) 3.5	0	3
98.2	●	+	15351	each additional 100 sq cm (List separately in addition to code for primary procedure)	1.6	0	0
				Note: This code is an add-on procedure and as such is valued appropriately. Multiple procedure guidelines for reduction of value are not applicable.			
98.2	▲		15400	Application of xenograft, skin; 100 sq cm or less	(I) 3.2	0	3
98.2	●	+	15401	each additional 100 sq cm (List separately in addition to code for primary procedure)	1.4	0	0
				Note: This code is an add-on procedure and as such is valued appropriately. Multiple procedure guidelines for reduction of value are not applicable.			
			15570	Formation of direct or tubed pedicle, with or without transfer; trunk	10.0	90	3
98.2			15572	scalp, arms, or legs	13.0	90	5
			15574	forehead, cheeks, chin, mouth, neck, axillae, genitalia, hands or feet	13.0	90	5
			15576	eyelids, nose, ears, lips, or intraoral	11.0	90	5
			15580	Cross finger flap, including free graft to donor site	10.0	45	3
			15600	Delay of flap or sectioning of flap (division and inset); at trunk	5.0	45	3
98.2			15610	at scalp, arms, or legs	5.0	45	5
98.2			15620	at forehead, cheeks, chin, neck, axillae, genitalia, hands (except 15625), or feet	5.5	45	5
			15625	section pedicle of cross finger flap	5.0	45	3
98.2			15630	at eyelids, nose, ears, or lips	6.5	45	5
			15650	Transfer, intermediate, of any pedicle flap (eg, abdomen to wrist, "Walking" tube), any location	8.0	45	3

UPD			Code	Description	Units	FUD	Anes
98.2			**15732**	Muscle, myocutaneous, or fasciocutaneous flap; head and neck (eg, temporalis, masseter, sternocleidomastoid, levator scapulae)	21.0	90	5
			15734	trunk	19.0	90	3
98.2			**15736**	upper extremity	19.0	90	5
98.2			**15738**	lower extremity	19.0	90	4
98.2			**15740**	Flap; island pedicle	11.0	90	3
98.2			**15750**	neurovascular pedicle	12.0	90	3
96.2	M		**15755**	Free flap (microvascular transfer) To report, see 15756-15758	45.0	90	4
98.2			**15756**	Free muscle flap with or without skin with microvascular anastomosis	(I) 45.0	90	3
98.2			**15757**	Free skin flap with microvascular anastomosis	(I) 45.0	90	3
96.2			**15758**	Free fascial flap with microvascular anastomosis	(I) 45.0	90	4
98.2			**15760**	Graft; composite (eg, full thickness of external ear or nasal ala), including primary closure, donor area	9.0	45	5
98.2			**15770**	derma-fat-fascia	12.0	60	5
98.2			**15775**	Punch graft for hair transplant; 1 to 15 punch grafts	0.5	90	5
98.2			**15776**	more than 15 punch grafts	0.8	90	5
			15780	Dermabrasion; total face (eg, for acne scarring, fine wrinkling, rhytids, general keratosis)	10.0	90	5
			15781	segmental, face	5.0	90	5
98.2			**15782**	regional, other than face	4.0	90	3
			15783	superficial, any site, (eg, tattoo removal)	2.0	60	3
			15786*	Abrasion; single lesion (eg, keratosis, scar)	0.4	0	5
98.2	▲ +		**15787**	each additional four lesions or less (List separately in addition to code for primary procedure) Note: This code is an add-on procedure and as such is valued appropriately. Multiple procedure guidelines for reduction of value are not applicable.	0.8	30	0
			15788	Chemical peel, facial; epidermal	(I) 7.0	60	5
			15789	dermal	(I) 9.0	60	5
98.2			**15792**	Chemical peel, nonfacial; epidermal	(I) 5.0	60	3
98.2			**15793**	dermal	(I) 7.0	60	3
98.2			**15810**	Salabrasion; 20 sq cm or less	0.8	30	3
98.2			**15811**	over 20 sq cm	2.0	30	3

UPD	Code	Description	Units	FUD	Anes
	15819	Cervicoplasty	18.7	60	5
98.2	**15820**	Blepharoplasty, lower eyelid;	10.0	60	5
98.2	**15821**	with extensive herniated fat pad	10.5	60	5
	15822	Blepharoplasty, upper eyelid;	8.5	30	5
98.2	**15823**	with excessive skin weighting down lid	9.0	60	5
	15824	Rhytidectomy; forehead	11.8	30	5
	15825	neck with platysmal tightening (platysmal flap, "P-flap")	10.2	30	5
	15826	glabellar frown lines	8.5	30	5
	15828	cheek, chin, and neck	29.0	60	5
98.2	**15829**	superficial musculoaponeurotic system (SMAS) flap	29.0	60	3
98.2	**15831**	Excision, excessive skin and subcutaneous tissue (including lipectomy); abdomen (abdominoplasty)	20.0	60	5
	15832	thigh	16.6	60	3
	15833	leg	16.6	60	3
	15834	hip	16.6	60	3
	15835	buttock	16.6	60	3
	15836	arm	10.0	60	3
	15837	forearm or hand	8.3	60	3
98.2	**15838**	submental fat pad	8.0	60	5
	15839	other area	BR	60	3
	15840	Graft for facial nerve paralysis; free fascia graft (including obtaining fascia)	24.0	90	5
	15841	free muscle graft (including obtaining graft)	28.0	90	5
	15842	free muscle graft by microsurgical technique	35.0	90	5
98.2	**15845**	regional muscle transfer	25.0	90	3
	15850	Removal of sutures under anesthesia (other than local), same surgeon	3.5	30	3
	15851	Removal of sutures under anesthesia (other than local), other surgeon	5.0	30	3
	15852	Dressing change (for other than burns) under anesthesia (other than local)	2.5	30	3
	15860	Intravenous injection of agent (eg, fluorescein) to test blood flow in flap or graft	2.5	0	3
98.2	**15876**	Suction assisted lipectomy; head and neck	7.0	60	5
	15877	trunk	12.5	60	3

UPD		Code	Description	Units	FUD	Anes
		15878	upper extremity	7.0	60	3
		15879	lower extremity	12.5	60	3
98.2		**15920**	Excision, coccygeal pressure ulcer, with coccygectomy; with primary suture	6.5	90	6
98.2		**15922**	with flap closure	8.5	90	6
98.2		**15931**	Excision, sacral pressure ulcer, with primary suture;	6.5	90	3
98.2		**15933**	with ostectomy	11.0	90	6
98.2		**15934**	Excision, sacral pressure ulcer, with skin flap closure;	8.5	90	3
98.2		**15935**	with ostectomy	13.0	90	6
98.2	▲	**15936**	Excision, sacral pressure ulcer, in preparation for muscle or myocutaneous flap or skin graft closure;	10.0	90	3
98.2		**15937**	with ostectomy	14.5	90	6
98.2		**15940**	Excision, ischial pressure ulcer, with primary suture;	8.0	90	3
98.2		**15941**	with ostectomy (ischiectomy)	11.0	90	6
98.2		**15944**	Excision, ischial pressure ulcer, with skin flap closure;	10.0	90	3
98.2		**15945**	with ostectomy	12.0	90	6
98.2	▲	**15946**	Excision, ischial pressure ulcer, with ostectomy, in preparation for muscle or myocutaneous flap or skin graft closure	(I) 20.0	90	6
		15950	Excision, trochanteric pressure ulcer, with primary suture;	2.1	60	5
98.2		**15951**	with ostectomy	6.0	60	6
		15952	Excision, trochanteric pressure ulcer, with skin flap closure;	8.0	90	5
98.2		**15953**	with ostectomy	10.0	90	6
98.2	▲	**15956**	Excision, trochanteric pressure ulcer, in preparation for muscle or myocutaneous flap or skin graft closure;	11.5	90	5
98.2		**15958**	with ostectomy	13.5	90	6
98.2		**15999**	Unlisted procedure, excision pressure ulcer	BR	0	5
98.2		**16000**	Initial treatment, first degree burn, when no more than local treatment is required	0.5	0	3
98.2		**16010**	Dressings and/or debridement, initial or subsequent; under anesthesia, small	1.0	0	3
98.2		**16015**	under anesthesia, medium or large, or with major debridement	2.0	0	3
		16020*	without anesthesia, office or hospital, small	0.6	0	0
		16025*	without anesthesia, medium (eg, whole face or whole extremity)	1.0	0	0

UPD			Code	Description	Units	FUD	Anes
			16030	without anesthesia, large (eg, more than one extremity)	2.0	0	0
			16035	Escharotomy	5.0	0	3
98.2	M		16040	Excision burn wound, without skin grafting, employing alloplastic dressing (eg, synthetic mesh), any anatomic site; up to one percent total body surface To report, use 15000	(I) 1.3	0	3
98.2	M		16041	greater than one percent and up to nine percent total body surface area To report, use 15000	(I) 3.4	0	3
98.2	M		16042	each additional nine percent total body surface area, or part thereof To report, use 15000	(I) 3.4	0	3
97.2			17000*	Destruction by any method, including laser, with or without surgical curettement, all benign or premalignant lesions (eg, actinic keratoses) other than skin tags or cutaneous vascular proliferative lesions, including local anesthesia; first lesion	0.9	0	3
97.2	M		17001	second and third lesions, each To report, use 17003, 17004	0.5	0	3
97.2	M		17002	over three lesions, each additional lesion To report, use 17003, 17004	0.2	0	3
98.2		+	17003	second through 14 lesions, each (List separately in addition to code for first lesion) Note: This code is an add-on procedure and as such is valued appropriately. Multiple procedure guidelines for reduction of value are not applicable.	(I) 0.2	0	3
98.2	▲ ⊘		17004	Destruction by any method, including laser, with or without surgical curettement, all benign or premalignant lesions (eg, actinic keratoses) other than skin tags or cutaneous vascular proliferative lesions, including local anesthesia, 15 or more lesions Note: Procedure listed may be considered a necessary part of and/or procedure and in such cases, not billable. If the procedure is distinct by encounter or performed in conjunction with a procedure for which the listed service is not considered a necessary component, then multiple procedure guidelines for reduction of value do not apply for this code.	(I) 3.2	0	3
97.2	M		17010	complicated lesion(s) To report, see specific anatomic site code	2.7	0	3
97.2	M		17100	Destruction by any method, including laser, of benign skin lesions other than cutaneous vascular proliferative lesions on any area other than the face, including local anesthesia; one lesion To report, see 17000, 17003, 17004	0.6	0	3
97.2	M		17101	second lesion To report, see 17000, 17003, 17004	0.4	0	3

UPD		Code	Description	Units	FUD	Anes
97.2	**M**	**17102**	over two lesions, each additional lesion up to 15 lesions To report, see 17000, 17003, 17004	0.2	0	3
97.2	**M**	**17104**	15 or more lesions To report, see 17000, 17003, 17004	3.8	0	3
97.2	**M**	**17105**	complicated or extensive lesions To report, see 17000, 17003, 17004	2.5	0	3
		17106	Destruction of cutaneous vascular proliferative lesions (eg, laser technique); less than 10 sq cm	(I) 4.2	0	3
		17107	10.0 - 50.0 sq cm	(I) 8.0	0	3
		17108	over 50.0 sq cm	(I) 12.0	0	3
97.2		**17110***	Destruction by any method of flat warts, molluscum contagiosum, or milia; up to 14 lesions	0.6	0	3
97.2		**17111**	15 or more lesions	(I) 1.0	0	3
97.2	**M**	**17200***	Electrosurgical destruction of multiple fibrocutaneous tags; up to 15 lesions To report, see 11200, 11201	0.6	0	3
97.2	**M**	**17201**	each additional ten lesions To report, see 11200, 11201	0.5	0	3
		17250*	Chemical cauterization of granulation tissue (proud flesh, sinus or fistula)	0.8	0	3
		17260*	Destruction, malignant lesion, any method, trunk, arms or legs; lesion diameter 0.5 cm or less	(I) 1.3	15	3
		17261	lesion diameter 0.6 to 1.0 cm	(I) 1.7	15	3
		17262	lesion diameter 1.1 to 2.0 cm	(I) 2.3	15	3
		17263	lesion diameter 2.1 to 3.0 cm	(I) 2.6	15	3
		17264	lesion diameter 3.1 to 4.0 cm	(I) 2.8	15	3
		17266	lesion diameter over 4.0 cm	(I) 3.4	15	3
98.2		**17270***	Destruction, malignant lesion, any method, scalp, neck, hands, feet, genitalia; lesion diameter 0.5 cm or less	(I) 1.4	15	5
98.2		**17271**	lesion diameter 0.6 to 1.0 cm	(I) 2.1	15	5
98.2		**17272**	lesion diameter 1.1 to 2.0 cm	(I) 2.5	15	5
98.2		**17273**	lesion diameter 2.1 to 3.0 cm	(I) 3.0	15	5
98.2		**17274**	lesion diameter 3.1 to 4.0 cm	(I) 3.7	15	5
98.2		**17276**	lesion diameter over 4.0 cm	(I) 4.6	15	5
98.2		**17280***	Destruction, malignant lesion, any method, face, ears, eyelids, nose, lips, mucous membrane; lesion diameter 0.5 cm or less	(I) 1.6	15	5
98.2		**17281**	lesion diameter 0.6 to 1.0 cm	(I) 2.5	15	5

UPD		Code	Description	Units	FUD	Anes
98.2		**17282**	lesion diameter 1.1 to 2.0 cm	(I) 2.9	15	5
98.2		**17283**	lesion diameter 2.1 to 3.0 cm	(I) 3.8	15	5
98.2		**17284**	lesion diameter 3.1 to 4.0 cm	(I) 4.9	15	5
98.2		**17286**	lesion diameter over 4.0 cm	(I) 6.4	15	5
98.2		**17304**	Chemosurgery (Mohs' micrographic technique), including removal of all gross tumor, surgical excision of tissue specimens, mapping, color coding of specimens, microscopic examination of specimens by the surgeon, and complete histopathologic preparation; first stage, fresh tissue technique, up to 5 specimens	(I) 9.2	0	5
98.2	⊘	**17305**	second stage, fixed or fresh tissue, up to 5 specimens Note: Procedure listed may be considered a necessary part of and/or procedure and in such cases, not billable. If the procedure is distinct by encounter or performed in conjunction with a procedure for which the listed service is not considered a necessary component, then multiple procedure guidelines for reduction of value do not apply for this code.	(I) 3.5	0	5
98.2	⊘	**17306**	third stage, fixed or fresh tissue, up to 5 specimens Note: Procedure listed may be considered a necessary part of and/or procedure and in such cases, not billable. If the procedure is distinct by encounter or performed in conjunction with a procedure for which the listed service is not considered a necessary component, then multiple procedure guidelines for reduction of value do not apply for this code.	(I) 3.5	0	5
98.2	⊘	**17307**	additional stage(s), up to 5 specimens, each stage Note: Multiple procedure guidelines for reduction of value are not applicable for this code.	(I) 3.5	0	5
98.2	⊘	**17310**	more than 5 specimens, fixed or fresh tissue, any stage Note: Procedure listed may be considered a necessary part of and/or procedure and in such cases, not billable. If the procedure is distinct by encounter or performed in conjunction with a procedure for which the listed service is not considered a necessary component, then multiple procedure guidelines for reduction of value do not apply for this code.	BR	0	5
98.2		**17340***	Cryotherapy (CO2 slush, liquid N2) for acne	0.5	0	5
98.2		**17360***	Chemical exfoliation for acne (eg, acne paste, acid)	0.4	0	5
98.2		**17380***	Electrolysis epilation, each 1/2 hour	0.7	0	5
98.2		**17999**	Unlisted procedure, skin, mucous membrane and subcutaneous tissue	BR	0	5
96.1		**19000***	Puncture aspiration of cyst of breast;	1.2	0	3

UPD			Code	Description	Units	FUD	Anes
98.2	▲	+	19001	each additional cyst (List separately in addition to code for primary procedure)	0.3	0	0
				Note: This code is an add-on procedure and as such is valued appropriately. Multiple procedure guidelines for reduction of value are not applicable.			
			19020	Mastotomy with exploration or drainage of abscess, deep	3.0	0	3
			19030	Injection procedure only for mammary ductogram or galactogram	0.7	0	3
			19100*	Biopsy of breast; needle core (separate procedure)	1.1	0	3
			19101	incisional	3.5	30	3
96.1			19110	Nipple exploration, with or without excision of a solitary lactiferous duct or a papilloma lactiferous duct	(I) 4.3	30	3
			19112	Excision of lactiferous duct fistula	(I) 4.2	30	3
97.2			19120	Excision of cyst, fibroadenoma, or other benign or malignant tumor aberrant breast tissue, duct lesion, nipple or areolar lesion (except 19140), male or female, one or more lesions	5.0	30	3
			19125	Excision of breast lesion identified by pre-operative placement of radiological marker; single lesion	7.0	30	3
98.2	▲	+	19126	each additional lesion separately identified by a radiological marker (List separately in addition to code for primary procedure)	3.5	30	0
				Note: This code is an add-on procedure and as such is valued appropriately. Multiple procedure guidelines for reduction of value are not applicable.			
			19140	Mastectomy for gynecomastia	7.0	60	3
			19160	Mastectomy, partial;	6.0	60	3
98.2			19162	with axillary lymphadenectomy	17.0	60	5
			19180	Mastectomy, simple, complete	10.4	60	3
			19182	Mastectomy, subcutaneous	10.0	60	3
			19200	Mastectomy, radical, including pectoral muscles, axillary lymph nodes	19.0	90	5
			19220	Mastectomy, radical, including pectoral muscles, axillary and internal mammary lymph nodes (Urban type operation)	26.0	120	13
			19240	Mastectomy, modified radical, including axillary lymph nodes, with or without pectoralis minor muscle, but excluding pectoralis major muscle	19.0	60	5
98.2			19260	Excision of chest wall tumor including ribs	17.0	90	6
			19271	Excision of chest wall tumor involving ribs, with plastic reconstruction; without mediastinal lymphadenectomy	28.0	120	13
			19272	with mediastinal lymphadenectomy	35.0	120	13
98.2			19290	Preoperative placement of needle localization wire, breast;	(I) 1.7	0	3

UPD	Code	Description	Units	FUD	Anes
98.2 ▲ +	19291	each additional lesion (List separately in addition to code for primary procedure)	0.9	0	0
		Note: This code is an add-on procedure and as such is valued appropriately. Multiple procedure guidelines for reduction of value are not applicable.			
	19316	Mastopexy	13.0	90	5
	19318	Reduction mammaplasty	18.0	90	5
	19324	Mammaplasty, augmentation; without prosthetic implant	5.0	90	5
	19325	with prosthetic implant	11.0	90	5
	19328	Removal of intact mammary implant	4.5	90	5
	19330	Removal of mammary implant material	6.5	90	5
	19340	Immediate insertion of breast prosthesis following mastopexy, mastectomy or in reconstruction	14.5	90	5
	19342	Delayed insertion of breast prosthesis following mastopexy, mastectomy or in reconstruction	16.0	90	5
	19350	Nipple/areola reconstruction	8.0	90	5
	19355	Correction of inverted nipples	7.0	90	5
	19357	Breast reconstruction, immediate or delayed, with tissue expander, including subsequent expansion	(I) 24.0	90	5
	19361	Breast reconstruction with latissimus dorsi flap, with or without prosthetic implant	35.0	90	5
	19364	Breast reconstruction with free flap	36.0	90	5
	19366	Breast reconstruction with other technique	36.0	90	5
	19367	Breast reconstruction with transverse rectus abdominis myocutaneous flap (TRAM), single pedicle, including closure of donor site;	(I) 36.0	90	5
	19368	with microvascular anastomosis (supercharging)	(I) 45.0	90	5
	19369	Breast reconstruction with transverse rectus abdominis myocutaneous flap (TRAM), double pedicle, including closure of donor site	(I) 43.0	90	5
	19370	Open periprosthetic capsulotomy, breast	7.0	90	5
	19371	Periprosthetic capsulectomy, breast	8.0	90	5
	19380	Revision of reconstructed breast	BR	90	5
	19396	Preparation of moulage for custom breast implant	2.2	90	5
98.2	19499	Unlisted procedure, breast	BR	0	5

UPD		Code	Description	Units	FUD	Anes

Musculoskeletal System

UPD		Code	Description	Units	FUD	Anes
		20000*	Incision of soft tissue abscess (eg, secondary to osteomyelitis); superficial	1.0	0	3
		20005	deep or complicated	4.0	21	3
		20100	Exploration of penetrating wound (separate procedure); neck	(I) 13.5	90	5
98.2		20101	chest	(I) 4.2	90	3
98.2		20102	abdomen/flank/back	(I) 5.3	90	3
98.2		20103	extremity	(I) 7.0	90	3
98.2		20150	Excision of epiphyseal bar, with or without autogenous soft tissue graft obtained through same fascial incision	(I) 20.0	90	6
		20200	Biopsy, muscle; superficial	1.1	7	3
		20205	deep	2.4	15	3
		20206*	Biopsy, muscle, percutaneous needle	1.1	0	3
		20220	Biopsy, bone, trocar, or needle; superficial (eg, ilium, sternum, spinous process, ribs)	1.4	15	3
98.2		20225	deep (vertebral body, femur)	4.4	15	10
98.2	▲	20240	Biopsy, bone, excisional; superficial (eg, ilium, sternum, spinous process, ribs, trochanter of femur)	4.0	21	6
98.2		20245	deep (eg, humerus, ischium, femur)	5.0	30	5
		20250	Biopsy, vertebral body, open; thoracic	19.5	45	10
98.2		20251	lumbar or cervical	16.0	45	8
		20500*	Injection of sinus tract; therapeutic (separate procedure)	0.4	0	3
		20501*	diagnostic (sinogram)	1.0	0	3
		20520*	Removal of foreign body in muscle or tendon sheath; simple	1.7	0	3
		20525	deep or complicated	4.0	30	3
98.2		20550*	Injection, tendon sheath, ligament, trigger points or ganglion cyst	0.4	0	3
		20600*	Arthrocentesis, aspiration and/or injection; small joint, bursa or ganglion cyst (eg, fingers, toes)	0.4	0	3
		20605*	intermediate joint, bursa or ganglion cyst (eg, temporomandibular, acromioclavicular, wrist, elbow or ankle, olecranon bursa)	0.5	0	3
98.2		20610*	major joint or bursa (eg, shoulder, hip, knee joint, subacromial bursa)	0.6	0	4
		20615	Aspiration and injection for treatment of bone cyst	4.0	60	3

UPD		Code	Description	Units	FUD	Anes
98.2		**20650***	Insertion of wire or pin with application of skeletal traction, including removal (separate procedure)	1.5	0	4
98.2	⊘	**20660**	Application of cranial tongs, caliper, or stereotactic frame, including removal (separate procedure) Note: Procedure listed may be considered a necessary part of and/or procedure and in such cases, not billable. If the procedure is distinct by encounter or performed in conjunction with a procedure for which the listed service is not considered a necessary component, then multiple procedure guidelines for reduction of value do not apply for this code.	3.0	21	5
		20661	Application of halo, including removal; cranial	3.6	21	5
		20662	pelvic	5.0	21	6
		20663	femoral	5.0	21	4
98.1		**20664**	Application of halo, including removal, cranial, 6 or more pins placed, for thin skull osteology (eg, pediatric patients, hydrocephalus, osteogenesis imperfecta), requiring general anesthesia	(I) 8.5	21	5
		20665*	Removal of tongs or halo applied by another physician	0.4	0	5
		20670*	Removal of implant; superficial, (eg, buried wire, pin or rod) (separate procedure)	1.5	0	3
98.2		**20680**	deep (eg, buried wire, pin, screw, metal band, nail, rod or plate)	4.0	21	5
98.2	⊘	**20690**	Application of a uniplane (pins or wires in one plane), unilateral, external fixation system Note: Multiple procedure guidelines for reduction of value are not applicable for this code.	5.0	21	3
98.2	⊘	**20692**	Application of a multiplane (pins or wires in more than one plane), unilateral, external fixation system (eg, Ilizarov, Monticelli type) Note: Multiple procedure guidelines for reduction of value are not applicable for this code.	(I) 9.0	21	3
		20693	Adjustment or revision of external fixation system requiring anesthesia (eg, new pin(s) or wire(s) and/or new ring(s) or bar(s))	4.5	21	3
		20694	Removal, under anesthesia, of external fixation system	2.0	21	3
98.2		**20802**	Replantation, arm (includes surgical neck of humerus through elbow joint), complete amputation	65.0	180	6
98.2		**20805**	Replantation, forearm (includes radius and ulna to radial carpal joint), complete amputation	65.0	180	6
98.2		**20808**	Replantation, hand (includes hand through metacarpophalangeal joints), complete amputation	60.0	180	6
98.2		**20816**	Replantation, digit, excluding thumb (includes metacarpophalangeal joint to insertion of flexor sublimis tendon), complete amputation	28.0	180	6

UPD	Code	Description	Units	FUD	Anes
98.2	**20822**	Replantation, digit, excluding thumb (includes distal tip to sublimis tendon insertion), complete amputation	20.0	180	6
98.2	**20824**	Replantation, thumb (includes carpometacarpal joint to MP joint), complete amputation	32.0	180	6
98.2	**20827**	Replantation, thumb (includes distal tip to MP joint), complete amputation	27.5	180	6
	20838	Replantation, foot, complete amputation	65.0	180	8
98.2	⊘ **20900**	Bone graft, any donor area; minor or small (eg, dowel or button) Note: Procedure listed may be considered a necessary part of and/or procedure and in such cases, not billable. If the procedure is distinct by encounter or performed in conjunction with a procedure for which the listed service is not considered a necessary component, then multiple procedure guidelines for reduction of value do not apply for this code.	2.4	0	3
98.2	⊘ **20902**	major or large Note: Procedure listed may be considered a necessary part of and/or procedure and in such cases, not billable. If the procedure is distinct by encounter or performed in conjunction with a procedure for which the listed service is not considered a necessary component, then multiple procedure guidelines for reduction of value do not apply for this code.	5.2	0	6
98.2	⊘ **20910**	Cartilage graft; costochondral Note: Procedure listed may be considered a necessary part of and/or procedure and in such cases, not billable. If the procedure is distinct by encounter or performed in conjunction with a procedure for which the listed service is not considered a necessary component, then multiple procedure guidelines for reduction of value do not apply for this code.	4.8	0	6
98.2	⊘ **20912**	nasal septum Note: Procedure listed may be considered a necessary part of and/or procedure and in such cases, not billable. If the procedure is distinct by encounter or performed in conjunction with a procedure for which the listed service is not considered a necessary component, then multiple procedure guidelines for reduction of value do not apply for this code.	4.8	0	5
98.2	⊘ **20920**	Fascia lata graft; by stripper Note: Procedure listed may be considered a necessary part of and/or procedure and in such cases, not billable. If the procedure is distinct by encounter or performed in conjunction with a procedure for which the listed service is not considered a necessary component, then multiple procedure guidelines for reduction of value do not apply for this code.	2.0	0	4

UPD	Code	Description	Units	FUD	Anes
98.2	⊘ 20922	by incision and area exposure, complex or sheet	4.0	0	4
		Note: Procedure listed may be considered a necessary part of and/or procedure and in such cases, not billable. If the procedure is distinct by encounter or performed in conjunction with a procedure for which the listed service is not considered a necessary component, then multiple procedure guidelines for reduction of value do not apply for this code.			
98.2	⊘ 20924	Tendon graft, from a distance (eg, palmaris, toe extensor, plantaris)	2.0	15	4
		Note: Procedure listed may be considered a necessary part of and/or procedure and in such cases, not billable. If the procedure is distinct by encounter or performed in conjunction with a procedure for which the listed service is not considered a necessary component, then multiple procedure guidelines for reduction of value do not apply for this code.			
98.2	⊘ 20926	Tissue grafts, other (eg, paratenon, fat, dermis)	2.0	15	3
		Note: Procedure listed may be considered a necessary part of and/or procedure and in such cases, not billable. If the procedure is distinct by encounter or performed in conjunction with a procedure for which the listed service is not considered a necessary component, then multiple procedure guidelines for reduction of value do not apply for this code.			
98.2	⊘ 20930	Allograft for spine surgery only; morselized	0.0	0	0
		Note: Multiple procedure guidelines for reduction of value are not applicable for this code.			
98.2	⊘ 20931	structural	(I) 2.8	0	0
		Note: Multiple procedure guidelines for reduction of value are not applicable for this code.			
98.2	⊘ 20936	Autograft for spine surgery only (includes harvesting the graft); local (eg, ribs, spinous process, or laminar fragments) obtained from same incision	0.0	0	0
		Note: Multiple procedure guidelines for reduction of value are not applicable for this code.			
98.2	⊘ 20937	morselized (through separate skin or fascial incision)	(I) 4.1	0	0
		Note: Multiple procedure guidelines for reduction of value are not applicable for this code.			
98.2	⊘ 20938	structural, bicortical or tricortical (through separate skin or fascial incision)	4.5	0	0
		Note: Multiple procedure guidelines for reduction of value are not applicable for this code.			
	20950	Monitoring of interstitial fluid pressure (includes insertion of device, eg, wick catheter technique, needle manometer technique) in detection of muscle compartment syndrome	1.5	0	3
96.2	20955	Bone graft with microvascular anastomosis; fibula	61.0	90	8

UPD		Code	Description	Units	FUD	Anes
96.2		**20956**	iliac crest	(I) 61.0	90	6
98.2		**20957**	metatarsal	(I) 61.0	90	8
96.2	**M**	**20960**	rib To report, see 20962	61.0	90	8
96.2		**20962**	other than fibula, iliac crest, or metatarsal	BR	90	8
96.2		**20969**	Free osteocutaneous flap with microvascular anastomosis; other than iliac crest, metatarsal, or great toe	BR	90	8
98.2		**20970**	iliac crest	61.0	90	6
96.2	**M**	**20971**	rib To report, see 20969	61.0	90	8
		20972	metatarsal	61.0	90	8
		20973	great toe with web space	61.0	90	8
98.2	⊘	**20974**	Electrical stimulation to aid bone healing; noninvasive (nonoperative) Note: Multiple procedure guidelines for reduction of value are not applicable for this code.	3.0	0	5
98.2	⊘	**20975**	invasive (operative) Note: Multiple procedure guidelines for reduction of value are not applicable for this code.	4.5	90	3
		20999	Unlisted procedure, musculoskeletal system, general	BR	0	0
		21010	Arthrotomy, temporomandibular joint	13.0	90	5
98.2		**21015**	Radical resection of tumor (eg, malignant neoplasm), soft tissue of face or scalp	8.0	90	5
		21025	Excision of bone (eg, for osteomyelitis or bone abscess); mandible	9.0	90	5
		21026	facial bone(s)	10.0	90	5
		21029	Removal by contouring of benign tumor of facial bone (eg, fibrous dysplasia)	11.0	90	5
		21030	Excision of benign tumor or cyst of facial bone other than mandible	13.0	90	5
		21031	Excision of torus mandibularis	6.8	90	5
		21032	Excision of maxillary torus palatinus	6.0	90	5
		21034	Excision of malignant tumor of facial bone other than mandible	16.0	90	5
		21040	Excision of benign cyst or tumor of mandible; simple	8.0	90	5
		21041	complex	12.5	90	5
98.2		**21044**	Excision of malignant tumor of mandible;	15.9	90	5

UPD	Code	Description	Units	FUD	Anes
	21045	radical resection	39.0	90	7
	21050	Condylectomy, temporomandibular joint (separate procedure)	18.5	90	5
	21060	Meniscectomy, partial or complete, temporomandibular joint (separate procedure)	15.0	90	5
	21070	Coronoidectomy (separate procedure)	19.0	90	5
98.2	21076	Impression and custom preparation; surgical obturator prosthesis	21.0	90	5
98.2	21077	orbital prosthesis	76.0	90	5
98.2	21079	interim obturator prosthesis	32.0	90	5
98.2	21080	definitive obturator prosthesis	46.0	90	5
98.2	21081	mandibular resection prosthesis	50.0	90	5
98.2	21082	palatal augmentation prosthesis	35.5	90	5
98.2	21083	palatal lift prosthesis	34.0	90	5
98.2	21084	speech aid prosthesis	41.0	90	5
98.2	21085	oral surgical splint	18.0	90	5
98.2	21086	auricular prosthesis	36.0	90	5
98.2	21087	nasal prosthesis	53.0	90	5
98.2	21088	facial prosthesis	(I) 9.2	90	5
98.2	21089	Unlisted maxillofacial prosthetic procedure	BR	90	5
	21100*	Application of halo type appliance for maxillofacial fixation, includes removal (separate procedure)	2.9	0	5
	21110	Application of interdental fixation device for conditions other than fracture or dislocation, includes removal	6.5	30	5
98.2	21116	Injection procedure for temporomandibular joint arthrography	1.3	0	5
	21120	Genioplasty; augmentation (autograft, allograft, prosthetic material)	(I) 12.0	90	5
	21121	sliding osteotomy, single piece	(I) 15.0	90	5
	21122	sliding osteotomies, two or more osteotomies (eg, wedge excision or bone wedge reversal for asymmetrical chin)	(I) 19.5	90	5
	21123	sliding, augmentation with interpositional bone grafts (includesobtaining autografts)	(I) 22.5	90	5
	21125	Augmentation, mandibular body or angle; prosthetic material	(I) 13.0	90	5
	21127	with bone graft, onlay or interpositional (includes obtaining autograft)	(I) 17.2	90	5
	21137	Reduction forehead; contouring only	(I) 17.2	90	5

UPD	Code	Description	Units	FUD	Anes
98.2	**21138**	contouring and application of prosthetic material or bone graft (includes obtaining autograft)	(I) 22.5	90	7
98.2	**21139**	contouring and setback of anterior frontal sinus wall	(I) 24.0	90	7
	21141	Reconstruction midface, LeFort 1; single piece, segment movement in any direction (eg, for Long Face Syndrome), without bone graft	(I) 28.3	90	5
98.2	**21142**	two pieces, segment movement in any direction, without bone graft	(I) 29.0	90	7
98.2	**21143**	three or more pieces, segment movement in any direction, without bone graft	(I) 30.5	90	7
98.2	**21145**	single piece, segment movement in any direction, requiring bone grafts (includes obtaining autografts)	(I) 32.5	90	7
98.2	**21146**	two pieces, segment movement in any direction, requiring bone grafts (includes obtaining autografts) (eg, ungrafted unilateral alveolar cleft)	(I) 37.5	90	7
98.2	**21147**	three or more pieces, segment movement in any direction, requiring bone grafts (includes obtaining autografts) (eg, ungrafted bilateral alveolar cleft or multiple osteotomies)	(I) 41.0	90	7
98.2	**21150**	Reconstruction midface, LeFort II; anterior intrusion (eg, Treacher-Collins Syndrome)	(I) 44.0	90	7
98.2	**21151**	any direction, requiring bone grafts (includes obtaining autografts)	(I) 49.0	90	7
98.2	**21154**	Reconstruction midface, LeFort III (extracranial), any type, requiring bone grafts (includes obtaining autografts); without LeFort I	(I) 53.0	90	7
98.2	**21155**	with LeFort I	(I) 61.0	90	7
98.2	**21159**	Reconstruction midface, LeFort III (extra and intracranial) with forehead advancement (eg, mono bloc), requiring bone grafts (includes obtaining autografts); without LeFort I	(I) 72.0	90	7
98.2	**21160**	with LeFort I	(I) 80.0	90	7
98.2	**21172**	Reconstruction superior-lateral orbital rim and lower forehead, advancement or alteration, with or without grafts (includes obtaining autografts)	(I) 48.5	90	7
98.2	**21175**	Reconstruction, bifrontal, superior-lateral orbital rims and lower forehead, advancement or alteration (eg, plagiocephaly, trigonocephaly, brachycephaly), with or without grafts (includes obtaining autografts)	(I) 58.0	90	7
98.2	**21179**	Reconstruction, entire or majority of forehead and/or supraorbital rims; with grafts (allograft or prosthetic material)	(I) 35.0	90	7
98.2	**21180**	with autograft (includes obtaining grafts)	(I) 41.0	90	7
98.2	**21181**	Reconstruction by contouring of benign tumor of cranial bones (eg, fibrous dysplasia), extracranial	(I) 13.0	90	7

UPD	Code	Description	Units	FUD	Anes
98.2	21182	Reconstruction of orbital walls, rims, forehead, nasoethmoid complex following intra- and extracranial excision of benign tumor of cranial bone (eg, fibrous dysplasia), with multiple autografts (includes obtaining grafts); total area of bone grafting less than 40 cm2	(I) 42.0	90	7
98.2	21183	total area of bone grafting greater than 40 cm2 but less than 80 cm2	(I) 45.0	90	7
98.2	21184	total area of bone grafting greater than 80 cm2	(I) 47.3	90	7
98.2	21188	Reconstruction midface, osteotomies (other than LeFort type) and bone grafts (includes obtaining autografts)	(I) 35.0	90	7
	21193	Reconstruction of mandibular rami, horizontal, vertical, "C", or "L" osteotomy; without bone graft	(I) 30.0	90	7
	21194	with bone graft (includes obtaining graft)	(I) 42.2	90	7
	21195	Reconstruction of mandibular rami and/or body, sagittal split; without internal rigid fixation	(I) 36.0	90	7
	21196	with internal rigid fixation	(I) 38.0	90	7
	21198	Osteotomy, mandible, segmental	(I) 19.0	90	7
	21206	Osteotomy, maxilla, segmental (eg, Wassmund or Schuchard)	23.0	90	7
98.2	21208	Osteoplasty, facial bones; augmentation (autograft, allograft, or prosthetic implant)	13.0	90	7
98.2	21209	reduction	19.0	90	7
	21210	Graft, bone; nasal, maxillary or malar areas (includes obtaining graft)	20.0	90	5
	21215	mandible (includes obtaining graft)	25.0	90	5
	21230	Graft; rib cartilage, autogenous, to face, chin, nose or ear (includes obtaining graft)	19.0	90	5
	21235	ear cartilage, autogenous, to nose or ear (includes obtaining graft)	14.0	90	5
	21240	Arthroplasty, temporomandibular joint, with or without autograft (includes obtaining graft)	(I) 26.5	90	5
	21242	Arthroplasty, temporomandibular joint, with allograft	28.0	90	5
	21243	Arthroplasty, temporomandibular joint, with prosthetic joint replacement	28.0	90	5
	21244	Reconstruction of mandible, extraoral, with transosteal bone plate (eg, mandibular staple bone plate)	(I) 26.0	90	5
98.2	21245	Reconstruction of mandible or maxilla, subperiosteal implant; partial	(I) 19.0	90	7
98.2	21246	complete	(I) 37.0	90	7
98.2	21247	Reconstruction of mandibular condyle with bone and cartilage autografts (includes obtaining grafts) (eg, for hemifacial microsomia)	(I) 39.0	90	7

UPD	Code	Description	Units	FUD	Anes
98.2	**21248**	Reconstruction of mandible or maxilla, endosteal implant (eg, blade, cylinder); partial	(I) 15.0	90	7
98.2	**21249**	complete	(I) 18.0	90	7
98.2	**21255**	Reconstruction of zygomatic arch and glenoid fossa with bone and cartilage (includes obtaining autografts)	24.0	90	7
98.2	**21256**	Reconstruction of orbit with osteotomies (extracranial) and with bone grafts (includes obtaining autografts) (eg, micro-ophthalmia)	(I) 55.0	90	7
98.2	**21260**	Periorbital osteotomies for orbital hypertelorism, with bone grafts; extracranial approach	39.0	90	7
	21261	combined intra- and extracranial approach	65.0	90	11
98.2	**21263**	with forehead advancement	65.0	90	7
98.2	**21267**	Orbital repositioning, periorbital osteotomies, unilateral, with bone grafts; extracranial approach	39.0	90	7
	21268	combined intra- and extracranial approach	65.0	90	11
	21270	Malar augmentation, prosthetic material	17.0	90	5
98.2	**21275**	Secondary revision of orbitocraniofacial reconstruction	BR	90	7
	21280	Medial canthopexy (separate procedure)	(I) 17.0	90	5
	21282	Lateral canthopexy	(I) 13.5	90	5
	21295	Reduction of masseter muscle and bone (eg, for treatment of benign masseteric hypertrophy); extraoral approach	(I) 11.0	90	5
	21296	intraoral approach	(I) 15.0	90	5
	21299	Unlisted craniofacial and maxillofacial procedure	BR	90	5
98.2	**21300**	Closed treatment of skull fracture without operation	1.3	0	7
	21310	Closed treatment of nasal bone fracture without manipulation	1.1	0	5
	21315*	Closed treatment of nasal bone fracture; without stabilization	1.5	0	5
	21320	with stabilization	4.5	90	5
	21325	Open treatment of nasal fracture; uncomplicated	5.0	90	5
	21330	complicated, with internal and/or external skeletal fixation	10.0	90	5
	21335	with concomitant open treatment of fractured septum	18.0	90	5
	21336	Open treatment of nasal septal fracture, with or without stabilization	(I) 8.2	90	5
	21337	Closed treatment of nasal septal fracture, with or without stabilization	1.7	90	5
	21338	Open treatment of nasoethmoid fracture; without external fixation	15.0	90	5

UPD	Code	Description	Units	FUD	Anes
	21339	with external fixation	17.2	90	5
	21340	Percutaneous treatment of nasoethmoid complex fracture, with splint, wire or headcap fixation, including repair of canthal ligaments and/or the nasolacrimal apparatus	17.0	90	5
	21343	Open treatment of depressed frontal sinus fracture	14.0	90	5
	21344	Open treatment of complicated (eg, comminuted or involving posterior wall) frontal sinus fracture, via coronal or multiple approaches	(I) 26.7	90	5
98.2	**21345**	Closed treatment of nasomaxillary complex fracture (LeFort II type), with interdental wire fixation or fixation of denture or splint	10.0	90	7
98.2	**21346**	Open treatment of nasomaxillary complex fracture (LeFort II type); with wiring and/or local fixation	15.0	90	7
98.2	**21347**	requiring multiple open approaches	17.2	90	7
98.2	**21348**	with bone grafting (includes obtaining graft)	(I) 27.4	90	7
	21355*	Percutaneous treatment of fracture of malar area, including zygomatic arch and malar tripod, with manipulation	7.5	0	5
	21356	Open treatment of depressed zygomatic arch fracture (eg, Gilles approach)	(I) 7.4	0	5
98.2	**21360**	Open treatment of depressed malar fracture, including zygomatic arch and malar tripod	13.3	90	7
98.2	**21365**	Open treatment of complicated (eg, comminuted or involving cranial nerve foramina) fracture(s) of malar area, including zygomatic arch and malar tripod; with internal fixation and multiple surgical approaches	15.0	90	7
98.2	**21366**	with bone grafting (includes obtaining graft)	(I) 24.0	90	7
98.2	**21385**	Open treatment of orbital floor "blowout" fracture; transantral approach (Caldwell-Luc type operation)	13.6	90	7
98.2	**21386**	periorbital approach	18.0	90	7
98.2	**21387**	combined approach	18.0	90	7
98.2	**21390**	periorbital approach, with alloplastic or other implant	19.0	90	7
98.2	**21395**	periorbital approach with bone graft (includes obtaining graft)	25.8	90	7
	21400	Closed treatment of fracture of orbit, except "blowout"; without manipulation	1.3	0	5
	21401	with manipulation	14.0	90	5
98.2	**21406**	Open treatment of fracture of orbit, except "blowout"; without implant	16.0	90	7
98.2	**21407**	with implant	18.0	90	7
98.2	**21408**	with bone grafting (includes obtaining graft)	(I) 20.6	90	7

UPD	Code	Description	Units	FUD	Anes
	21421	Closed treatment of palatal or maxillary fracture (LeFort I type), with interdental wire fixation or fixation of denture or splint	12.5	90	5
98.2	21422	Open treatment of palatal or maxillary fracture (LeFort I type);	15.0	90	7
98.2	21423	complicated (comminuted or involving cranial nerve foramina), multiple approaches	(I) 21.3	90	7
	21431	Closed treatment of craniofacial separation (LeFort III type) using interdental wire fixation of denture or splint	16.0	90	5
98.2	21432	Open treatment of craniofacial separation (LeFort III type); with wiring and/or internal fixation	19.0	90	7
98.2	21433	complicated (eg, comminuted or involving cranial nerve foramina), multiple surgical approaches	22.0	90	7
98.2	21435	complicated, utilizing internal and/or external fixation techniques (eg, head cap, halo device, and/or intermaxillary fixation)	24.0	90	7
98.2	21436	complicated, multiple surgical approaches, internal fixation, with bone grafting (includes obtaining graft)	(I) 32.9	90	7
98.2	21440	Closed treatment of mandibular or maxillary alveolar ridge fracture (separate procedure)	13.0	30	7
98.2	21445	Open treatment of mandibular or maxillary alveolar ridge fracture (separate procedure)	16.0	30	7
	21450	Closed treatment of mandibular fracture; without manipulation	1.2	90	5
	21451	with manipulation	(I) 8.0	90	5
	21452	Percutaneous treatment of mandibular fracture, with external fixation	1.2	90	5
	21453	Closed treatment of mandibular fracture with interdental fixation	(I) 8.7	90	5
	21454	Open treatment of mandibular fracture with external fixation	15.0	90	5
	21461	Open treatment of mandibular fracture; without interdental fixation	14.5	90	5
	21462	with interdental fixation	17.2	90	5
	21465	Open treatment of mandibular condylar fracture	14.5	90	5
	21470	Open treatment of complicated mandibular fracture by multiple surgical approaches including internal fixation, interdental fixation, and/or wiring of dentures or splints	19.0	90	5
	21480	Closed treatment of temporomandibular dislocation; initial or subsequent	4.0	30	5
	21485	complicated (eg, recurrent requiring intermaxillary fixation or splinting), initial or subsequent	(I) 8.7	90	5
	21490	Open treatment of temporomandibular dislocation	13.0	90	5

UPD	Code	Description	Units	FUD	Anes
	21493	Closed treatment of hyoid fracture; without manipulation	1.3	0	5
	21494	with manipulation	14.0	90	5
	21495	Open treatment of hyoid fracture	19.0	90	5
	21497	Interdental wiring, for condition other than fracture	13.0	90	5
	21499	Unlisted musculoskeletal procedure, head	BR	90	5
	21501	Incision and drainage, deep abscess or hematoma, soft tissues of neck or thorax;	4.5	21	5
98.2	21502	with partial rib ostectomy	6.3	30	6
98.2	21510	Incision, deep, with opening of bone cortex (eg, for osteomyelitis or bone abscess), thorax	4.0	21	10
98.2	21550	Biopsy, soft tissue of neck or thorax	1.3	0	5
98.2	21555	Excision tumor, soft tissue of neck or thorax; subcutaneous	3.0	15	5
98.2	21556	deep, subfascial, intramuscular	5.0	15	5
98.2	21557	Radical resection of tumor (eg, malignant neoplasm), soft tissue of neck or thorax	15.0	180	6
	21600	Excision of rib, partial	5.5	60	6
	21610	Costotransversectomy (separate procedure)	20.0	60	6
	21615	Excision first and/or cervical rib;	16.0	60	6
	21616	with sympathectomy	20.4	60	6
98.2	21620	Ostectomy of sternum, partial	20.0	60	6
98.2	21627	Sternal debridement	(I) 8.0	60	10
	21630	Radical resection of sternum;	25.0	60	13
	21632	with mediastinal lymphadenectomy	40.0	60	13
98.2	21700	Division of scalenus anticus; without resection of cervical rib	6.5	60	5
	21705	with resection of cervical rib	12.5	60	6
98.2	21720	Division of sternocleidomastoid for torticollis, open operation; without cast application	6.5	60	5
98.2	21725	with cast application	8.5	60	5
	21740	Reconstructive repair of pectus excavatum or carinatum	24.0	90	13
98.2	21750	Closure of sternotomy separation with or without debridement (separate procedure)	(I) 20.0	90	10
	21800	Closed treatment of rib fracture, uncomplicated, each	1.0	30	6
	21805	Open treatment of rib fracture without fixation, each	10.0	60	6
98.2	21810	Treatment of rib fracture requiring external fixation ("flail chest")	24.0	60	10

UPD		Code	Description	Units	FUD	Anes
		21820	Closed treatment of sternum fracture	2.5	30	6
98.2		21825	Open treatment of sternum fracture with or without skeletal fixation	10.0	60	10
		21899	Unlisted procedure, neck or thorax	BR	30	6
		21920	Biopsy, soft tissue of back or flank; superficial	1.3	30	5
		21925	deep	3.0	60	5
		21930	Excision, tumor, soft tissue of back or flank	3.0	60	5
98.2		21935	Radical resection of tumor (eg, malignant neoplasm), soft tissue of back or flank	15.0	90	5
		22100	Partial excision of posterior vertebral component (eg, spinous process, lamina or facet) for intrinsic bony lesion, single vertebral segment; cervical	(I) 12.0	90	10
		22101	thoracic	(I) 11.8	90	10
		22102	lumbar	(I) 11.0	90	8
98.2	+	22103	each additional segment (List separately in addition to code for primary procedure) Note: This code is an add-on procedure and as such is valued appropriately. Multiple procedure guidelines for reduction of value are not applicable.	(I) 3.4	0	0
		22110	Partial excision of vertebral body for intrinsic bony lesion, without decompression of spinal cord or nerve root(s), single vertebral segment; cervical	(I) 16.5	90	10
		22112	thoracic	(I) 16.5	90	10
		22114	lumbar	(I) 14.0	90	8
	+	22116	each additional vertebral segment (List separately in addition to code for primary procedure) Note: This code is an add-on procedure and as such is valued appropriately. Multiple procedure guidelines for reduction of value are not applicable.	(I) 3.4	0	0
98.2		22210	Osteotomy of spine, posterior or posterolateral approach, one vertebral segment; cervical	(I) 32.5	90	13
98.2		22212	thoracic	(I) 28.0	90	13
98.2		22214	lumbar	(I) 27.0	90	13
98.2	+	22216	each additional vertebral segment (List separately in addition to primary procedure) Note: This code is an add-on procedure and as such is valued appropriately. Multiple procedure guidelines for reduction of value are not applicable.	(I) 9.0	0	0
		22220	Osteotomy of spine, including diskectomy, anterior approach, single vertebral segment; cervical	31.0	90	10
		22222	thoracic	31.0	90	10

UPD		Code	Description	Units	FUD	Anes
		22224	lumbar	31.0	90	8
98.2	+	22226	each additional vertebral segment (List separately in addition to code for primary procedure) Note: This code is an add-on procedure and as such is valued appropriately. Multiple procedure guidelines for reduction of value are not applicable.	(I) 9.0	0	0
		22305	Closed treatment of vertebral process fracture(s)	2.5	90	8
		22310	Closed treatment of vertebral body fracture(s), without manipulation, requiring and including casting or bracing	3.5	90	8
98.2		22315	Closed treatment of vertebral fracture(s) and/or dislocations(s) requiring casting or bracing, with and including casting and/or bracing, with or without anesthesia, by manipulation or traction	(I) 10.0	90	0
		22325	Open treatment and/or reduction of vertebral fracture(s) and/or dislocation(s); posterior approach, one fractured vertebrae or dislocated segment; lumbar	(I) 18.0	90	8
		22326	cervical	(I) 26.0	90	10
		22327	thoracic	24.0	90	10
98.2	+	22328	each additional fractured vertebrae or dislocated segment (List separately in addition to code for primary procedure) Note: This code is an add-on procedure and as such is valued appropriately. Multiple procedure guidelines for reduction of value are not applicable.	(I) 7.0	0	0
98.2		22505	Manipulation of spine requiring anesthesia, any region	1.5	0	3
98.2		22548	Arthrodesis, anterior transoral or extraoral technique, clivus-C1-C2 (atlas-axis), with or without excision of odontoid process	(I) 34.5	90	13
		22554	Arthrodesis, anterior interbody technique, including minimal diskectomy to prepare interspace (other than for decompression); cervical below C2	(I) 26.0	90	10
		22556	thoracic	30.0	90	10
		22558	lumbar	(I) 28.0	90	8
98.2	+	22585	each additional interspace (List separately in addition to code for primary procedure) Note: This code is an add-on procedure and as such is valued appropriately. Multiple procedure guidelines for reduction of value are not applicable.	(I) 8.0	0	0
		22590	Arthrodesis, posterior technique, craniocervical (occiput-C2)	(I) 32.0	90	10
		22595	Arthrodesis, posterior technique, atlas-axis (C1-C2)	(I) 32.0	90	10
		22600	Arthrodesis, posterior or posterolateral technique, single level; cervical below C2 segment	(I) 26.0	90	10
		22610	thoracic (with or without lateral transverse technique)	25.0	90	10

UPD		Code	Description	Units	FUD	Anes
		22612	lumbar (with or without lateral transverse technique)	(I) 30.0	90	8
98.2	**+**	**22614**	each additional vertebral segment (List separately in addition to code for primary procedure)	(I) 9.0	0	0
			Note: This code is an add-on procedure and as such is valued appropriately. Multiple procedure guidelines for reduction of value are not applicable.			
		22630	Arthrodesis, posterior interbody technique, single interspace; lumbar	25.0	90	8
98.2	**+**	**22632**	each additional interspace (List separately in addition to code for primary procedure)	(I) 7.5	0	0
			Note: This code is an add-on procedure and as such is valued appropriately. Multiple procedure guidelines for reduction of value are not applicable.			
		22800	Arthrodesis, posterior, for spinal deformity, with or without cast; up to 6 vertebral segments	30.0	90	13
		22802	7 to 12 vertebral segments	(I) 42.0	90	13
		22804	13 or more vertebral segments	(I) 50.0	90	13
		22808	Arthrodesis, anterior, for spinal deformity, with or without cast; 2 to 3 vertebral segments	(I) 35.0	90	13
		22810	4 to 7 vertebral segments	(I) 41.0	90	13
		22812	8 or more vertebral segments	(I) 44.0	90	13
97.2		**22818**	Kyphectomy, circumferential exposure of spine and resection of vertebral segment(s) (including body and posterior elements); single or 2 segments	(I) 36.0	90	13
97.2		**22819**	3 or more segments	(I) 41.5	90	13
		22830	Exploration of spinal fusion	18.0	90	13
98.2	⊘	**22840**	Posterior non-segmental instrumentation (eg, single Harrington rod technique)	(I) 9.0	0	13
			Note: Multiple procedure guidelines for reduction of value are not applicable for this code.			
98.2	⊘	**22841**	Internal spinal fixation by wiring of spinous processes	0.0	0	10
			Note: Procedure listed may be considered a necessary part of and/or procedure and in such cases, not billable. If the procedure is distinct by encounter or performed in conjunction with a procedure for which the listed service is not considered a necessary component, then multiple procedure guidelines for reduction of value do not apply for this code.			
98.2	⊘	**22842**	Posterior segmental instrumentation (eg, pedicle fixation, dual rods with multiple hooks and sublaminal wires); 3 to 6 vertebral segments	(I) 18.0	0	13
			Note: Multiple procedure guidelines for reduction of value are not applicable for this code.			

UPD		Code	Description	Units	FUD	Anes
98.2	⊘	22843	7 to 12 vertebral segments	(I) 19.5	0	13
			Note: Multiple procedure guidelines for reduction of value are not applicable for this code.			
98.2	⊘	22844	13 or more vertebral segments	(I) 22.0	0	13
			Note: Multiple procedure guidelines for reduction of value are not applicable for this code.			
98.2	⊘•	22845	Anterior instrumentation; 2 to 3 vertebral segments	(I) 17.0	0	13
			Note: Multiple procedure guidelines for reduction of value are not applicable for this code.			
98.2	⊘	22846	4 to 7 vertebral segments	(I) 18.0	0	13
			Note: Multiple procedure guidelines for reduction of value are not applicable for this code.			
98.2	⊘	22847	8 or more vertebral segments	(I) 20.0	0	13
			Note: Multiple procedure guidelines for reduction of value are not applicable for this code.			
98.2	⊘	22848	Pelvic fixation (attachment of caudal end of instrumentation to pelvic bony structures) other than sacrum	(I) 8.5	0	13
			Note: Multiple procedure guidelines for reduction of value are not applicable for this code.			
98.2		22849	Reinsertion of spinal fixation device	(I) 25.0	0	13
96.1		22850	Removal of posterior nonsegmental instrumentation (eg, Harrington rod)	10.0	90	13
98.2	⊘	22851	Application of prosthetic device (eg, metal cages, methylmethacrylate) to vertebral defect or interspace	(I) 9.5	0	13
			Note: Multiple procedure guidelines for reduction of value are not applicable for this code.			
96.1		22852	Removal of posterior segmental instrumentation	14.0	90	13
96.1		22855	Removal of anterior instrumentation	12.0	90	13
98.2		22899	Unlisted procedure, spine	BR	90	3
		22900	Excision, abdominal wall tumor, subfascial (eg, desmoid)	5.0	30	3
98.2		22999	Unlisted procedure, abdomen, musculoskeletal system	BR	0	3
98.2	▲	23000	Removal of subdeltoid (or intratendinous) calcareous deposits, any method	6.2	60	5
98.2	▲	23020	Capsular contracture release (eg, Sever type procedure)	11.4	60	5
		23030	Incision and drainage, shoulder area; deep abscess or hematoma	4.0	15	5
		23031	infected bursa	3.5	15	5
98.2	▲	23035	Incision, bone cortex (eg, osteomyelitis or bone abscess), shoulder area	12.0	30	5

UPD		Code	Description	Units	FUD	Anes
98.2	▲	23040	Arthrotomy, glenohumeral joint, including exploration, drainage, or removal of foreign body	11.4	60	5
98.2	▲	23044	Arthrotomy, acromioclavicular, sternoclavicular joint, including exploration, drainage, or removal of foreign body	7.0	45	5
		23065	Biopsy, soft tissue of shoulder area; superficial	2.0	0	3
		23066	deep	3.2	0	5
98.2	▲	23075	Excision, soft tissue tumor, shoulder area; subcutaneous	3.0	7	3
		23076	deep, subfascial or intramuscular	5.0	15	5
98.2		23077	Radical resection of tumor (eg, malignant neoplasm), soft tissue of shoulder area	15.0	90	5
98.2	▲	23100	Arthrotomy, glenohumeral joint, including biopsy	11.4	60	5
98.2	▲	23101	Arthrotomy, acromioclavicular joint or sternoclavicular joint, including biopsy and/or excision of torn cartilage	11.4	60	5
98.2	▲	23105	Arthrotomy; glenohumeral joint, with synovectomy, with or without biopsy	15.0	90	5
98.2	▲	23106	sternoclavicular joint, with synovectomy, with or without biopsy	12.0	90	5
		23107	Arthrotomy, glenohumeral joint, with joint exploration, with or without removal of loose or foreign body	12.0	90	5
		23120	Claviculectomy; partial	8.0	60	5
98.2		23125	total	16.0	60	6
98.2	▲	23130	Acromioplasty or acromionectomy, partial, with or without coracoacromial ligament release	8.0	60	5
		23140	Excision or curettage of bone cyst or benign tumor of clavicle or scapula;	6.2	60	5
		23145	with autograft (includes obtaining graft)	9.3	90	5
		23146	with allograft	7.5	90	5
		23150	Excision or curettage of bone cyst or benign tumor of proximal humerus;	12.0	30	5
		23155	with autograft (includes obtaining graft)	15.0	90	5
		23156	with allograft	13.0	90	5
		23170	Sequestrectomy (eg, for osteomyelitis or bone abscess), clavicle	6.0	90	5
		23172	Sequestrectomy (eg, for osteomyelitis or bone abscess), scapula	6.0	30	5
		23174	Sequestrectomy (eg, for osteomyelitis or bone abscess), humeral head to surgical neck	12.2	90	5
98.2	▲	23180	Partial excision (craterization, saucerization, or diaphysectomy) bone (eg, osteomyelitis), clavicle	7.5	90	5

UPD		Code	Description	Units	FUD	Anes
98.2	▲	23182	Partial excision (craterization, saucerization, or diaphysectomy) bone (eg, osteomyelitis), scapula	6.0	30	5
98.2	▲	23184	Partial excision (craterization, saucerization, or diaphysectomy) bone (eg, osteomyelitis), proximal humerus	10.0	30	5
		23190	Ostectomy of scapula, partial (eg, superior medial angle)	6.5	60	5
		23195	Resection humeral head	15.0	30	5
		23200	Radical resection for tumor; clavicle	12.0	30	6
		23210	scapula	16.0	30	6
98.2	▲	23220	Radical resection of bone tumor, proximal humerus;	16.0	30	6
		23221	with autograft (includes obtaining graft)	18.0	90	6
		23222	with prosthetic replacement	18.0	90	6
98.2		23330	Removal of foreign body, shoulder; subcutaneous	9.0	60	3
98.2	▲	23331	deep (eg, Neer hemiarthroplasty removal)	11.0	60	5
98.2	▲	23332	complicated (eg, total shoulder)	BR	60	10
98.2		23350	Injection procedure for shoulder arthrography	0.8	0	4
		23395	Muscle transfer, any type, shoulder or upper arm; single	10.5	60	5
		23397	multiple	12.5	60	5
		23400	Scapulopexy (eg, Sprengel's deformity or for paralysis)	15.0	60	5
98.2	▲	23405	Tenotomy, shoulder area; single tendon	8.5	60	5
98.2	▲	23406	multiple tendons through same incision	11.7	60	5
		23410	Repair of ruptured musculotendinous cuff (eg, rotator cuff); acute	14.0	90	5
		23412	chronic	15.2	60	5
		23415	Coracoacromial ligament release, with or without acromioplasty	10.0	60	5
98.2	▲	23420	Reconstruction of complete shoulder (rotator) cuff avulsion, chronic (includes acromioplasty)	19.0	120	5
		23430	Tenodesis of long tendon of biceps	12.0	90	5
		23440	Resection or transplantation of long tendon of biceps	12.0	90	5
		23450	Capsulorrhaphy, anterior; Putti-Platt procedure or Magnuson type operation	16.8	90	5
98.2	▲	23455	with labral repair (eg, Bankart procedure)	18.9	90	5
		23460	Capsulorrhaphy, anterior, any type; with bone block	20.2	90	5
		23462	with coracoid process transfer	19.0	90	5

UPD		Code	Description	Units	FUD	Anes
98.2	▲	23465	Capsulorrhaphy, glenohumeral joint, posterior, with or without bone block	19.0	90	5
98.2	▲	23466	Capsulorrhaphy, glenohumeral joint, any type multi-directional instability	20.0	90	5
98.2	▲	23470	Arthroplasty, glenohumeral joint; hemiarthroplasty	20.0	90	5
98.2	▲	23472	total shoulder (glenoid and proximal humeral replacement (eg, total shoulder))	35.0	90	10
		23480	Osteotomy, clavicle, with or without internal fixation;	10.0	90	5
		23485	with bone graft for nonunion or malunion (includes obtaining graft and/or necessary fixation)	13.0	90	5
		23490	Prophylactic treatment (nailing, pinning, plating or wiring) with or without methylmethacrylate; clavicle	7.0	90	5
98.2	▲	23491	proximal humerus	9.0	90	5
		23500	Closed treatment of clavicular fracture; without manipulation	2.2	0	5
		23505	with manipulation	3.5	90	5
		23515	Open treatment of clavicular fracture, with or without internal or external fixation	9.0	90	5
		23520	Closed treatment of sternoclavicular dislocation; without manipulation	2.0	0	4
		23525	with manipulation	2.4	90	4
		23530	Open treatment of sternoclavicular dislocation, acute or chronic;	8.0	90	5
		23532	with fascial graft (includes obtaining graft)	11.0	90	5
98.2		23540	Closed treatment of acromioclavicular dislocation; without manipulation	1.3	0	4
98.2		23545	with manipulation	2.4	60	4
		23550	Open treatment of acromioclavicular dislocation, acute or chronic;	11.5	60	5
		23552	with fascial graft (includes obtaining graft)	13.0	90	5
		23570	Closed treatment of scapular fracture; without manipulation	1.6	90	5
		23575	with manipulation, with or without skeletal traction (with or without shoulder joint involvement)	2.8	90	5
		23585	Open treatment of scapular fracture (body, glenoid or acromion) with or without internal fixation	11.5	90	5
		23600	Closed treatment of proximal humeral (surgical or anatomical neck) fracture; without manipulation	2.0	90	4
		23605	with manipulation, with or without skeletal traction	5.0	90	4
		23615	Open treatment of proximal humeral (surgical or anatomical neck) fracture, with or without internal or external fixation, with or without repair of tuberosity(-ies);	12.0	90	5

UPD		Code	Description	Units	FUD	Anes
		23616	with proximal humeral prosthetic replacement	(I) 28.7	90	5
98.2	▲	23620	Closed treatment of greater humeral tuberosity fracture; without manipulation	1.3	90	4
		23625	with manipulation	2.6	90	4
98.2	▲	23630	Open treatment of greater humeral tuberosity fracture, with or without internal or external fixation	9.1	90	5
		23650	Closed treatment of shoulder dislocation, with manipulation; without anesthesia	2.7	30	0
		23655	requiring anesthesia	3.9	30	4
		23660	Open treatment of acute shoulder dislocation	11.5	90	5
98.2	▲	23665	Closed treatment of shoulder dislocation, with fracture of greater humeral tuberosity, with manipulation	3.0	90	4
98.2	▲	23670	Open treatment of shoulder dislocation, with fracture of greater humeral tuberosity, with or without internal or external fixation	11.5	90	5
		23675	Closed treatment of shoulder dislocation, with surgical or anatomical neck fracture, with manipulation	4.5	90	4
		23680	Open treatment of shoulder dislocation, with surgical or anatomical neck fracture, with or without internal or external fixation	14.5	90	5
		23700*	Manipulation under anesthesia, shoulder joint, including application of fixation apparatus (dislocation excluded)	3.0	0	4
98.2	▲	23800	Arthrodesis, glenohumeral joint;	20.0	90	5
98.2	▲	23802	with autogenous graft (includes obtaining graft)	21.0	90	5
		23900	Interthoracoscapular amputation (forequarter)	27.0	90	15
		23920	Disarticulation of shoulder;	19.0	90	9
		23921	secondary closure or scar revision	5.0	30	5
98.2		23929	Unlisted procedure, shoulder	BR	0	5
		23930	Incision and drainage, upper arm or elbow area; deep abscess or hematoma	3.5	30	3
98.2	▲	23931	bursa	2.5	0	3
98.2		23935	Incision, deep, with opening of bone cortex (eg, for osteomyelitis or bone abscess), humerus or elbow	6.0	0	4
98.2	▲	24000	Arthrotomy, elbow, including exploration, drainage, or removal of foreign body	11.0	60	4
98.2		24006	Arthrotomy of the elbow, with capsular excision for capsular release (separate procedure)	(I) 14.2	60	4
		24065	Biopsy, soft tissue of upper arm or elbow area; superficial	1.2	0	3
98.2	▲	24066	deep (subfascial or intramuscular)	4.0	0	3

UPD		Code	Description	Units	FUD	Anes
		24075	Excision, tumor, upper arm or elbow area; subcutaneous	3.0	21	3
		24076	deep, subfascial or intramuscular	5.0	30	3
		24077	Radical resection of tumor (eg, malignant neoplasm), soft tissue of upper arm or elbow area	12.0	90	6
98.2		**24100**	Arthrotomy, elbow; with synovial biopsy only	6.9	60	4
98.2		**24101**	with joint exploration, with or without biopsy, with or without removal of loose or foreign body	11.0	60	4
98.2		**24102**	with synovectomy	14.5	90	4
98.2		**24105**	Excision, olecranon bursa	5.0	60	3
		24110	Excision or curettage of bone cyst or benign tumor, humerus;	10.0	60	5
		24115	with autograft (includes obtaining graft)	13.5	90	5
		24116	with allograft	11.0	90	5
98.2		**24120**	Excision or curettage of bone cyst or benign tumor of head or neck of radius or olecranon process;	8.2	60	4
98.2		**24125**	with autograft (includes obtaining graft)	10.3	90	4
98.2		**24126**	with allograft	9.0	90	4
98.2		**24130**	Excision, radial head	8.5	60	3
		24134	Sequestrectomy (eg, for osteomyelitis or bone abscess), shaft or distal humerus	12.0	30	4
98.2		**24136**	Sequestrectomy (eg, for osteomyelitis or bone abscess), radial head or neck	12.0	30	3
98.2		**24138**	Sequestrectomy (eg, for osteomyelitis or bone abscess), olecranon process	12.0	30	3
98.2	▲	**24140**	Partial excision (craterization, saucerization, or diaphysectomy) bone (eg, osteomyelitis), humerus	12.0	60	4
98.2	▲	**24145**	Partial excision (craterization, saucerization, or diaphysectomy) bone (eg, osteomyelitis), radial head or neck	8.0	30	3
98.2	▲	**24147**	Partial excision (craterization, saucerization, or diaphysectomy) bone (eg, osteomyelitis), olecranon process	7.5	60	3
98.2		**24149**	Radical resection of capsule, soft tissue, and heterotopic bone, elbow, with contracture release (separate procedure)	(I) 20.0	90	6
		24150	Radical resection for tumor, shaft or distal humerus;	17.0	90	6
		24151	with autograft (includes obtaining graft)	19.0	90	6
		24152	Radical resection for tumor, radial head or neck;	15.0	90	6
		24153	with autograft (includes obtaining graft)	20.0	90	6
98.2		**24155**	Resection of elbow joint (arthrectomy)	12.4	60	4
98.2		**24160**	Implant removal; elbow joint	9.7	60	4

UPD		Code	Description	Units	FUD	Anes
98.2		**24164**	radial head	8.5	30	4
		24200	Removal of foreign body, upper arm or elbow area; subcutaneous	2.2	30	3
98.2	▲	**24201**	deep (subfascial or intramuscular)	3.9	30	3
		24220	Injection procedure for elbow arthrography	1.0	0	3
		24301	Muscle or tendon transfer, any type, upper arm or elbow, single (excluding 24320-24331)	14.0	30	3
98.2	▲	**24305**	Tendon lengthening, upper arm or elbow, each tendon	5.8	60	3
98.2	▲	**24310**	Tenotomy, open, elbow to shoulder, each tendon	5.0	30	5
		24320	Tenoplasty, with muscle transfer, with or without free graft, elbow to shoulder, single (Seddon-Brookes type procedure)	17.0	90	5
		24330	Flexor-plasty, elbow (eg, Steindler type advancement);	11.0	90	3
		24331	with extensor advancement	14.3	90	3
		24340	Tenodesis of biceps tendon at elbow (separate procedure)	14.0	90	5
96.2		**24341**	Repair, tendon or muscle, upper arm or elbow, each tendon or muscle, primary or secondary (excludes rotator cuff)	(I) 13.0	90	3
96.2		**24342**	Reinsertion of ruptured biceps or triceps tendon, distal, with or without tendon graft	14.0	90	3
		24350	Fasciotomy, lateral or medial (eg, "tennis elbow" or epicondylitis);	5.0	30	3
		24351	with extensor origin detachment	6.0	30	3
		24352	with annular ligament resection	8.0	30	3
		24354	with stripping	7.0	30	3
		24356	with partial ostectomy	8.0	30	3
98.2	▲	**24360**	Arthroplasty, elbow; with membrane (eg, fascial)	22.0	90	4
98.2		**24361**	with distal humeral prosthetic replacement	22.0	90	4
98.2		**24362**	with implant and fascia lata ligament reconstruction	23.0	90	4
98.2	▲	**24363**	with distal humerus and proximal ulnar prosthetic replacement (eg, total elbow)	28.0	90	7
98.2		**24365**	Arthroplasty, radial head;	10.0	60	4
98.2		**24366**	with implant	11.0	60	4
		24400	Osteotomy, humerus, with or without internal fixation	13.6	90	5
		24410	Multiple osteotomies with realignment on intramedullary rod, humeral shaft (Sofield type procedure)	15.5	90	5
		24420	Osteoplasty, humerus (eg, shortening or lengthening) (excluding 64876)	15.5	90	5

UPD		Code	Description	Units	FUD	Anes
		24430	Repair of nonunion or malunion, humerus; without graft (eg, compression technique)	17.0	90	5
		24435	with iliac or other autograft (includes obtaining graft)	20.0	90	5
98.2	▲	24470	Hemiepiphyseal arrest (eg, cubitus varus or valgus, distal humerus)	8.5	90	4
98.2		24495	Decompression fasciotomy, forearm, with brachial artery exploration	12.0	60	3
98.2	▲	24498	Prophylactic treatment (nailing, pinning, plating or wiring), with or without methylmethacrylate, humeral shaft	10.0	90	5
		24500	Closed treatment of humeral shaft fracture; without manipulation	1.3	90	3
		24505	with manipulation, with or without skeletal traction	6.3	90	3
		24515	Open treatment of humeral shaft fracture with plate/screws, with or without cerclage	(I) 15.8	90	4
		24516	Open treatment of humeral shaft fracture, with insertion of intramedullary implant, with or without cerclage and/or locking screws	(I) 15.8	90	4
		24530	Closed treatment of supracondylar or transcondylar humeral fracture, with or without intercondylar extension; without manipulation	2.5	90	3
		24535	with manipulation, with or without skin or skeletal traction	5.3	90	3
		24538	Percutaneous skeletal fixation of supracondylar or transcondylar humeral fracture, with or without intercondylar extension	9.0	90	3
		24545	Open treatment of humeral supracondylar or transcondylar fracture, with or without internal or external fixation; without intercondylar extension	(I) 13.9	90	4
		24546	with intercondylar extension	(I) 21.2	90	4
		24560	Closed treatment of humeral epicondylar fracture, medial or lateral; without manipulation	2.2	90	3
		24565	with manipulation	4.0	90	3
		24566	Percutaneous skeletal fixation of humeral epicondylar fracture, medial or lateral, with manipulation	(I) 7.3	90	3
		24575	Open treatment of humeral epicondylar fracture, medial or lateral, with or without internal or external fixation	10.0	90	4
		24576	Closed treatment of humeral condylar fracture, medial or lateral; without manipulation	1.3	60	3
		24577	with manipulation	4.0	60	3
		24579	Open treatment of humeral condylar fracture, medial or lateral, with or without internal or external fixation	10.0	90	4
		24582	Percutaneous skeletal fixation of humeral condylar fracture, medial or lateral, with manipulation	(I) 8.0	90	3

+ Add-on Code   ⊘ Modifier -51 Exempt   ▲ Revised code   ● New code   **M** RVSI code or deleted from CPT   **(I)** Interim Value

UPD		Code	Description	Units	FUD	Anes
		24586	Open treatment of periarticular fracture and/or dislocation of the elbow (fracture distal humerus and proximal ulna and/or proximal radius);	15.4	90	4
98.2		24587	with implant arthroplasty	22.0	90	4
		24600	Treatment of closed elbow dislocation; without anesthesia	2.5	60	0
		24605	requiring anesthesia	3.2	60	3
98.2		24615	Open treatment of acute or chronic elbow dislocation	10.6	90	3
		24620	Closed treatment of Monteggia type of fracture dislocation at elbow (fracture proximal end of ulna with dislocation of radial head), with manipulation	6.0	90	3
		24635	Open treatment of Monteggia type of fracture dislocation at elbow (fracture proximal end of ulna with dislocation of radial head), with or without internal or external fixation	12.0	90	4
		24640*	Closed treatment of radial head subluxation in child, "nursemaid elbow", with manipulation	2.0	0	3
		24650	Closed treatment of radial head or neck fracture; without manipulation	2.0	60	3
		24655	with manipulation	3.5	90	3
98.2		24665	Open treatment of radial head or neck fracture, with or without internal fixation or radial head excision;	8.0	90	3
98.2		24666	with radial head prosthetic replacement	9.3	90	3
		24670	Closed treatment of ulnar fracture, proximal end (olecranon process); without manipulation	2.0	60	3
		24675	with manipulation	4.5	90	3
98.2		24685	Open treatment of ulnar fracture proximal end (olecranon process), with or without internal or external fixation	8.3	90	3
98.2	▲	24800	Arthrodesis, elbow joint; local	16.5	90	3
98.2	▲	24802	with autogenous graft (includes obtaining graft)	20.0	90	3
		24900	Amputation, arm through humerus; with primary closure	10.0	90	6
		24920	open, circular (guillotine)	9.1	90	6
		24925	secondary closure or scar revision	3.1	30	6
		24930	re-amputation	9.0	90	6
		24931	with implant	11.5	90	6
		24935	Stump elongation, upper extremity	15.0	90	6
98.2		24940	Cineplasty, upper extremity, complete procedure	15.0	90	4
98.2		24999	Unlisted procedure, humerus or elbow	BR	0	4
98.2	▲	25000	Incision, extensor tendon sheath, wrist (eg, deQuervain's disease)	4.5	30	3

UPD		Code	Description	Units	FUD	Anes
		25020	Decompression fasciotomy, forearm and/or wrist; flexor or extensor compartment	5.5	30	3
		25023	with debridement of nonviable muscle and/or nerve	6.0	30	3
		25028	Incision and drainage, forearm and/or wrist; deep abscess or hematoma	4.0	30	3
98.2	▲	25031	bursa	2.0	30	3
98.2	▲	25035	Incision, deep, bone cortex, forearm and/or wrist (eg, osteomyelitis or bone abscess)	5.0	60	3
		25040	Arthrotomy, radiocarpal or midcarpal joint, with exploration, drainage, or removal of foreign body	5.5	60	3
		25065	Biopsy, soft tissue of forearm and/or wrist; superficial	1.3	0	3
98.2	▲	25066	deep (subfascial or intramuscular)	3.1	0	3
		25075	Excision, tumor, forearm and/or wrist area; subcutaneous	3.0	30	3
		25076	deep, subfascial or intramuscular	5.0	60	3
		25077	Radical resection of tumor (eg, malignant neoplasm), soft tissue of forearm and/or wrist area	12.0	90	3
98.2	▲	25085	Capsulotomy, wrist (eg, contracture)	5.4	60	3
		25100	Arthrotomy, wrist joint; with biopsy	5.0	60	3
		25101	with joint exploration, with or without biopsy, with or without removal of loose or foreign body	5.9	60	3
		25105	with synovectomy	8.0	60	3
98.2	▲	25107	Arthrotomy, distal radioulnar joint including repair of triangular cartilage, complex	7.0	60	3
		25110	Excision, lesion of tendon sheath, forearm and/or wrist	3.5	30	3
		25111	Excision of ganglion, wrist (dorsal or volar); primary	4.5	30	3
		25112	recurrent	5.7	30	3
		25115	Radical excision of bursa, synovia of wrist, or forearm tendon sheaths (eg, tenosynovitis, fungus, Tbc, or other granulomas, rheumatoid arthritis); flexors	10.0	60	3
		25116	extensors, with or without transposition of dorsal retinaculum	10.0	60	3
		25118	Synovectomy, extensor tendon sheath, wrist, single compartment;	7.0	60	3
		25119	with resection of distal ulna	10.0	60	3
		25120	Excision or curettage of bone cyst or benign tumor of radius or ulna (excluding head or neck of radius and olecranon process);	8.3	60	3
		25125	with autograft (includes obtaining graft)	10.5	90	3

UPD	Code	Description	Units	FUD	Anes
	25126	with allograft	9.5	90	3
	25130	Excision or curettage of bone cyst or benign tumor of carpal bones;	6.0	60	3
	25135	with autograft (includes obtaining graft)	8.0	90	3
	25136	with allograft	6.0	90	3
	25145	Sequestrectomy (eg, for osteomyelitis or bone abscess), forearm and/or wrist	12.0	90	3
	25150	Partial excision (craterization, saucerization or diaphysectomy) of bone (eg, for osteomyelitis); ulna	6.4	60	3
	25151	radius	7.5	60	3
	25170	Radical resection for tumor, radius or ulna	15.0	60	3
	25210	Carpectomy; one bone	7.0	60	3
	25215	all bones of proximal row	10.0	60	3
	25230	Radial styloidectomy (separate procedure)	5.4	60	3
	25240	Excision distal ulna partial or complete (eg, Darrach type or matched resection)	5.4	60	3
	25246	Injection procedure for wrist arthrography	1.3	0	3
	25248	Exploration with removal of deep foreign body, forearm or wrist	5.0	60	3
98.2	25250	Removal of wrist prosthesis; (separate procedure)	10.0	30	3
	25251	complicated, including "total wrist"	15.0	30	6
	25260	Repair, tendon or muscle, flexor, forearm and/or wrist; primary, single, each tendon or muscle	8.0	60	3
	25263	secondary, single, each tendon or muscle	8.5	60	3
	25265	secondary, with free graft (includes obtaining graft), each tendon or muscle	10.0	90	3
	25270	Repair, tendon or muscle, extensor, forearm and/or wrist; primary, single, each tendon or muscle	5.0	60	3
	25272	secondary, single, each tendon or muscle	6.0	60	3
	25274	Repair, tendon or muscle, extensor, secondary, with tendon graft (includes obtaining graft), forearm and/or wrist, each tendon or muscle	8.4	90	3
	25280	Lengthening or shortening of flexor or extensor tendon, forearm and/or wrist, single, each tendon	7.2	60	3
	25290	Tenotomy, open, flexor or extensor tendon, forearm and/or wrist, single, each tendon	4.3	60	3
	25295	Tenolysis, flexor or extensor tendon, forearm and/or wrist, single, each tendon	5.3	60	3
	25300	Tenodesis at wrist; flexors of fingers	9.5	90	3

UPD		Code	Description	Units	FUD	Anes
		25301	extensors of fingers	8.5	90	3
		25310	Tendon transplantation or transfer, flexor or extensor, forearm and/or wrist, single; each tendon	9.8	90	3
		25312	with tendon graft(s) (includes obtaining graft), each tendon	12.0	90	3
		25315	Flexor origin slide (eg, for cerebral palsy, Volkmann contracture), forearm and/or wrist;	11.0	90	3
		25316	with tendon(s) transfer	13.0	90	3
		25320	Capsulorrhaphy or reconstruction, wrist, any method (eg, capsulodesis, ligament repair, tendon transfer or graft) (includes synovectomy, capsulotomy and open reduction) for carpal instability	15.0	90	3
96.2	M	25330	Arthroplasty, wrist; To report, see 25332 and 25441-25446	15.0	90	3
96.2	M	25331	with implant To report, see 25332 and 25441-25446	16.0	90	3
96.2		25332	Arthroplasty, wrist, with or without interposition, with or without external or internal fixation	15.0	90	3
		25335	Centralization of wrist on ulna (eg, radial club hand)	18.0	90	3
		25337	Reconstruction for stabilization of unstable distal ulna or distal radioulnar joint, secondary by soft tissue stabilization (eg, tendon transfer, tendon graft or weave, or tenodesis) with or without open reduction of distal radioulnar joint	(I) 13.5	90	3
		25350	Osteotomy, radius; distal third	10.3	90	3
		25355	middle or proximal third	12.3	90	3
		25360	Osteotomy; ulna	10.3	90	3
		25365	radius and ulna	14.4	90	3
		25370	Multiple osteotomies, with realignment on intramedullary rod (Sofield type procedure); radius OR ulna	12.0	90	3
		25375	radius AND ulna	18.0	90	3
		25390	Osteoplasty, radius OR ulna; shortening	11.1	90	3
98.2		25391	lengthening with autograft	14.6	90	3
		25392	Osteoplasty, radius AND ulna; shortening (excluding 64876)	15.0	90	3
98.2		25393	lengthening with autograft	18.0	90	3
		25400	Repair of nonunion or malunion, radius OR ulna; without graft (eg, compression technique)	12.0	90	3
98.2		25405	with iliac or other autograft (includes obtaining graft)	14.5	90	3
		25415	Repair of nonunion or malunion, radius AND ulna; without graft (eg, compression technique)	17.0	90	3

UPD		Code	Description	Units	FUD	Anes
		25420	with iliac or other autograft (includes obtaining graft)	19.8	90	3
		25425	Repair of defect with autograft; radius OR ulna	13.6	90	3
		25426	radius AND ulna	19.0	90	3
		25440	Repair of nonunion, scaphoid (navicular) bone, with or without radial styloidectomy (includes obtaining graft and necessary fixation)	13.5	90	3
98.2		25441	Arthroplasty with prosthetic replacement; distal radius	14.0	90	3
98.2		25442	distal ulna	9.0	90	3
98.2		25443	scaphoid (navicular)	11.0	90	3
98.2		25444	lunate	11.0	90	3
98.2		25445	trapezium	11.0	90	3
98.2		25446	distal radius and partial or entire carpus ("total wrist")	22.5	90	6
98.2	▲	25447	Arthroplasty, interposition, intercarpal or carpometacarpal joints	15.0	90	3
98.2		25449	Revision of arthroplasty, including removal of implant, wrist joint	10.0	90	3
		25450	Epiphyseal arrest by epiphysiodesis or stapling; distal radius OR ulna	6.1	90	3
		25455	distal radius AND ulna	8.5	90	3
		25490	Prophylactic treatment (nailing, pinning, plating or wiring) with or without methylmethacrylate; radius	6.0	90	3
		25491	ulna	6.0	90	3
		25492	radius AND ulna	6.0	90	3
		25500	Closed treatment of radial shaft fracture; without manipulation	2.2	60	3
		25505	with manipulation	4.3	90	3
		25515	Open treatment of radial shaft fracture, with or without internal or external fixation	9.1	90	3
		25520	Closed treatment of radial shaft fracture, with dislocation of distal radio-ulnar joint (Galeazzi fracture/dislocation)	(I) 8.7	90	3
98.2		25525	Open treatment of radial shaft fracture, with internal and/or external fixation and closed treatment of dislocation of distal radio-ulnar joint (Galeazzi fracture/dislocation), with or without percutaneous skeletal fixation	(I) 16.9	90	3
98.2		25526	Open treatment of radial shaft fracture, with internal and/or external fixation and open treatment, with or without internal or external fixation of distal radio-ulnar joint (Galeazzi fracture/dislocation), includes repair of triangular cartilage	(I) 25.8	90	3
		25530	Closed treatment of ulnar shaft fracture; without manipulation	3.3	60	3

UPD	Code	Description	Units	FUD	Anes
	25535	with manipulation	4.0	90	3
98.2	**25545**	Open treatment of ulnar shaft fracture, with or without internal or external fixation	9.0	90	3
	25560	Closed treatment of radial and ulnar shaft fractures; without manipulation	2.9	60	3
	25565	with manipulation	5.9	60	3
	25574	Open treatment of radial AND ulnar shaft fractures, with internal or external fixation; of radius or ulna	(I) 8.7	90	3
	25575	of radius AND ulna	13.7	90	3
	25600	Closed treatment of distal radial fracture (eg, Colles or Smith type) or epiphyseal separation, with or without fracture of ulnar styloid; without manipulation	3.0	60	3
	25605	with manipulation	4.5	90	3
	25611	Percutaneous skeletal fixation of distal radial fracture (eg, Colles or Smith type) or epiphyseal separation, with or without fracture of ulnar styloid, requiring manipulation, with or without external fixation	8.5	90	3
	25620	Open treatment of distal radial fracture (eg, Colles or Smith type) or epiphyseal separation, with or without fracture of ulnar styloid, with or without internal or external fixation	9.0	90	3
	25622	Closed treatment of carpal scaphoid (navicular) fracture; without manipulation	3.5	60	3
	25624	with manipulation	4.0	90	3
	25628	Open treatment of carpal scaphoid (navicular) fracture, with or without internal or external fixation	7.0	90	3
	25630	Closed treatment of carpal bone fracture (excluding carpal scaphoid (navicular)); without manipulation, each bone	3.5	60	3
	25635	with manipulation, each bone	4.2	60	3
	25645	Open treatment of carpal bone fracture (excluding carpal scaphoid (navicular)), each bone	6.3	90	3
	25650	Closed treatment of ulnar styloid fracture	5.8	90	3
	25660	Closed treatment of radiocarpal or intercarpal dislocation, one or more bones, with manipulation	3.0	90	3
	25670	Open treatment of radiocarpal or intercarpal dislocation, one or more bones	7.9	90	3
	25675	Closed treatment of distal radioulnar dislocation with manipulation	3.1	60	3
	25676	Open treatment of distal radioulnar dislocation, acute or chronic	8.0	90	3
	25680	Closed treatment of trans-scaphoperilunar type of fracture dislocation, with manipulation	3.0	60	3

UPD		Code	Description	Units	FUD	Anes
		25685	Open treatment of trans-scaphoperilunar type of fracture dislocation	11.0	90	3
		25690	Closed treatment of lunate dislocation, with manipulation	5.1	90	3
		25695	Open treatment of lunate dislocation	10.0	60	3
98.2	▲	25800	Arthrodesis, wrist; complete, without bone graft (includes radiocarpal and/or intercarpal and/or carpometacarpal joints)	12.5	90	3
		25805	with sliding graft	15.7	90	3
		25810	with iliac or other autograft (includes obtaining graft)	14.0	90	3
98.2	▲	25820	Arthrodesis, wrist; limited, without bone graft (eg, intercarpal or radiocarpal)	11.5	90	3
		25825	with autograft (includes obtaining graft)	13.0	90	3
98.2	▲	25830	Arthrodesis, distal radioulnar joint with segmental resection of ulna, with or without bone graft (eg, Sauve-Kapandji procedure)	(I) 13.5	90	3
98.2		25900	Amputation, forearm, through radius and ulna;	9.3	90	3
		25905	open, circular (guillotine)	8.0	90	3
		25907	secondary closure or scar revision	3.1	30	3
		25909	re-amputation	9.3	90	3
		25915	Krukenberg procedure	10.5	60	3
		25920	Disarticulation through wrist;	8.3	90	3
		25922	secondary closure or scar revision	3.2	30	3
		25924	re-amputation	8.4	90	3
		25927	Transmetacarpal amputation;	10.0	90	3
		25929	secondary closure or scar revision	3.1	30	3
		25931	re-amputation	10.0	90	3
98.2		25999	Unlisted procedure, forearm or wrist	BR	0	3
		26010*	Drainage of finger abscess; simple	0.8	0	3
		26011*	complicated (eg, felon)	3.0	0	3
98.2	▲	26020	Drainage of tendon sheath, digit and/or palm, each	5.1	30	3
98.2	▲	26025	Drainage of palmar bursa; single, bursa	5.5	30	3
98.2	▲	26030	multiple bursa	9.0	30	3
98.2	▲	26034	Incision, bone cortex, hand or finger (eg, osteomyelitis or bone abscess)	6.0	30	3
		26035	Decompression fingers and/or hand, injection injury (eg, grease gun)	14.5	60	3

UPD		Code	Description	Units	FUD	Anes
		26037	Decompressive fasciotomy, hand (excludes 26035)	12.0	30	3
98.2	▲	26040	Fasciotomy, palmar (eg, Dupuytrens contracture); percutaneous	3.0	30	3
		26045	open, partial	5.0	60	3
		26055	Tendon sheath incision (eg, for trigger finger)	4.5	30	3
96.2		26060	Tenotomy, percutaneous, single, each digit	2.5	15	3
98.2	▲	26070	Arthrotomy, with exploration, drainage, or removal of loose or foreign body; carpometacarpal joint	5.1	30	3
98.2	▲	26075	metacarpophalangeal joint, each	5.0	30	3
		26080	interphalangeal joint, each	4.5	30	3
98.2	▲	26100	Arthrotomy with biopsy; carpometacarpal joint, each	5.1	30	3
98.2	▲	26105	metacarpophalangeal joint, each	5.0	30	3
		26110	interphalangeal joint, each	4.5	30	3
		26115	Excision, tumor or vascular malformation, hand or finger; subcutaneous	3.0	30	3
		26116	deep, subfascial, intramuscular	5.0	30	3
		26117	Radical resection of tumor (eg, malignant neoplasm), soft tissue of hand or finger	12.0	90	3
96.2		26121	Fasciectomy, palm only, with or without Z-plasty, other local tissue rearrangement, or skin grafting (includes obtaining graft)	12.0	90	3
96.2		26123	Fasciectomy, partial palmar with release of single digit including proximal interphalangeal joint, with or without Z-plasty, other local tissue rearrangement, or skin grafting (includes obtaining graft);	14.0	90	3
98.2	+	26125	each additional digit (List separately in addition to code for primary procedure) Note: This code is an add-on procedure and as such is valued appropriately. Multiple procedure guidelines for reduction of value are not applicable.	6.0	90	0
		26130	Synovectomy, carpometacarpal joint	8.0	90	3
		26135	Synovectomy, metacarpophalangeal joint including intrinsic release and extensor hood reconstruction, each digit	9.0	90	3
		26140	Synovectomy, proximal interphalangeal joint, including extensor reconstruction, each interphalangeal joint	8.0	90	3
98.2	▲	26145	Synovectomy, tendon sheath, radical (tenosynovectomy), flexor tendon, palm and/or finger, each tendon	9.0	90	3
		26160	Excision of lesion of tendon sheath or capsule (eg, cyst, mucous cyst, or ganglion), hand or finger	4.0	30	3
		26170	Excision of tendon, palm, flexor, single (separate procedure), each	4.5	30	3

UPD		Code	Description	Units	FUD	Anes
98.2	▲	26180	Excision of tendon, finger, flexor (separate procedure), each tendon	5.0	30	3
96.2		26185	Sesamoidectomy, thumb or finger (separate procedure)	(I) 5.8	90	3
		26200	Excision or curettage of bone cyst or benign tumor of metacarpal;	6.2	60	3
		26205	with autograft (includes obtaining graft)	7.5	90	3
		26210	Excision or curettage of bone cyst or benign tumor of proximal, middle or distal phalanx of finger;	5.4	60	3
		26215	with autograft (includes obtaining graft)	6.5	90	3
98.2	▲	26230	Partial excision (craterization, saucerization, or diaphysectomy) bone (eg, osteomyelitis); metacarpal	5.5	60	3
		26235	proximal or middle phalanx of finger	5.0	60	3
		26236	distal phalanx of finger	5.0	60	3
98.2	▲	26250	Radical resection, metacarpal; (eg, tumor)	10.0	90	3
		26255	with autograft (includes obtaining graft)	13.0	90	3
98.2	▲	26260	Radical resection, proximal or middle phalanx of finger (eg, tumor);	10.5	90	3
		26261	with autograft (includes obtaining graft)	12.5	90	3
98.2	▲	26262	Radical resection, distal phalanx of finger (eg, tumor)	10.0	90	3
		26320	Removal of implant from finger or hand	5.0	30	3
98.2	▲	26350	Repair or advancement, flexor tendon, not in digital flexor tendon sheath (eg, no man's land); primary or secondary without free graft, 2635003 each tendon	8.0	90	3
		26352	secondary with free graft (includes obtaining graft), each tendon	11.5	90	3
98.2	▲	26356	Repair or advancement, flexor tendon, in digital flexor tendon sheath (eg, no man's land); primary, each tendon	10.5	90	3
		26357	secondary, each tendon	10.0	90	3
		26358	secondary with free graft (includes obtaining graft), each tendon	12.5	90	3
98.2	▲	26370	Repair or advancement of profundus tendon, with intact superficialis tendon; primary, each tendon	8.0	60	3
98.2	▲	26372	secondary with free graft (includes obtaining graft), each tendon	11.3	60	3
98.2	▲	26373	secondary without free graft, each tendon	8.8	90	3
98.2	▲	26390	Excision flexor tendon, implantation of prosthetic rod for delayed tendon graft, hand or finger, each tendon	8.5	90	3
98.2	▲	26392	Removal of prosthetic rod and insertion of flexor tendon graft, hand or finger (includes obtaining graft), each tendon	11.0	60	3

UPD		Code	Description	Units	FUD	Anes
98.2	▲	26410	Repair, extensor tendon, hand, primary or secondary; without free graft, each tendon	4.6	60	3
		26412	with free graft (includes obtaining graft), each tendon	7.0	60	3
98.2	▲	26415	Excision of extensor tendon, implantation of prosthetic rod for delayed tendon graft, hand or finger	8.5	60	3
98.2	▲	26416	Removal of prosthetic rod and insertion of extensor tendon graft (includes obtaining graft), hand or finger, each rod	10.0	60	3
98.2	▲	26418	Repair, extensor tendon, finger, primary or secondary; without free graft, each tendon	5.0	90	3
98.2		26420	with free graft (includes obtaining graft) each tendon	7.0	90	3
98.2	▲	26426	Repair of extensor tendon, central slip, secondary (eg, boutonniere deformity); using local tissue(s), including lateral band(s), each tendon	7.3	90	3
98.2	▲	26428	with free graft (includes obtaining graft), each tendon	9.0	90	3
98.2	▲	26432	Closed treatment of distal extensor tendon insertion, with or without percutaneous pinning (eg, mallet finger)	6.0	30	3
98.2	▲	26433	Repair of extensor tendon, distal insertion, primary or secondary; without graft (eg, mallet finger)	6.0	30	3
		26434	with free graft (includes obtaining graft)	8.0	90	3
98.2	▲	26437	Realignment of extensor tendon, hand, each tendon	6.0	60	3
98.2	▲	26440	Tenolysis, flexor tendon; palm OR finger; each tendon	5.8	60	3
		26442	palm AND finger, each tendon	7.0	60	3
98.2	▲	26445	Tenolysis, extensor tendon, hand or finger; each tendon	6.0	60	3
98.2	▲	26449	Tenolysis, complex, extensor tendon, finger, including forearm, each tendon	8.0	60	3
98.2	▲	26450	Tenotomy, flexor, palm, open, each tendon	4.0	30	3
98.2	▲	26455	Tenotomy, flexor, finger, open, each tendon	5.0	30	3
98.2	▲	26460	Tenotomy, extensor, hand or finger, open, each tendon	3.5	30	3
98.2	▲	26471	Tenodesis; of proximal interphalangeal joint, each joint	7.1	90	3
98.2	▲	26474	of distal joint, each joint	5.2	90	3
98.2	▲	26476	Lengthening of tendon, extensor, hand or finger, each tendon	5.0	90	3
98.2	▲	26477	Shortening of tendon, extensor, hand or finger, each tendon	5.0	90	3
98.2	▲	26478	Lengthening of tendon, flexor, hand or finger, each tendon	6.0	90	3
98.2	▲	26479	Shortening of tendon, flexor, hand or finger, each tendon	6.0	90	3
98.2	▲	26480	Transfer or transplant of tendon, carpometacarpal area or dorsum of hand; without free graft, each tendon	9.0	90	3

UPD		Code	Description	Units	FUD	Anes
		26483	with free tendon graft (includes obtaining graft), each tendon	12.0	90	3
98.2	▲	26485	Transfer or transplant of tendon, palmar; without free tendon graft, each tendon	10.3	90	3
		26489	with free tendon graft (includes obtaining graft), each tendon	13.3	90	3
98.2	▲	26490	Opponensplasty; superficialis tendon transfer type, each tendon	10.2	90	3
98.2	▲	26492	tendon transfer with graft (includes obtaining graft), each tendon	13.2	90	3
		26494	hypothenar muscle transfer	12.0	90	3
		26496	other methods	14.0	90	3
98.2	▲	26497	Transfer of tendon to restore intrinsic function; ring and small finger	12.0	90	3
		26498	all four fingers	16.5	90	3
		26499	Correction claw finger, other methods	16.5	90	3
98.2	▲	26500	Reconstruction of tendon pulley, each tendon; with local tissues (separate procedure)	6.3	90	3
98.2		26502	with tendon or fascial graft (includes obtaining graft) (separate procedure)	8.0	90	3
		26504	with tendon prosthesis (separate procedure)	8.0	90	3
98.2	▲	26508	Release of thenar muscle(s) (eg, thumb contracture)	8.0	90	3
		26510	Cross intrinsic transfer	8.0	90	3
98.2	▲	26516	Capsulodesis, metacarpophalangeal joint; single digit	7.5	90	3
		26517	two digits	9.0	90	3
		26518	three or four digits	11.2	90	3
98.2	▲	26520	Capsulectomy or capsulotomy; metacarpophalangeal joint, each joint	7.5	90	3
98.2	▲	26525	interphalangeal joint, each joint	7.0	90	3
98.2	▲	26530	Arthroplasty, metacarpophalangeal joint; each joint	8.0	90	3
98.2	▲	26531	with prosthetic implant, each joint	10.0	90	3
98.2	▲	26535	Arthroplasty, interphalangeal joint; each joint	8.0	90	3
98.2	▲	26536	with prosthetic implant, each joint	10.0	90	3
96.2		26540	Repair of collateral ligament, metacarpophalangeal or interphalangeal joint	10.5	90	3
96.2		26541	Reconstruction, collateral ligament, metacarpophalangeal joint, single, with tendon or fascial graft (includes obtaining graft)	11.5	90	3

UPD			Code	Description	Units	FUD	Anes
			26542	with local tissue (eg, adductor advancement)	10.0	90	3
			26545	Reconstruction, collateral ligament, interphalangeal joint, single, including graft, each joint	7.5	90	3
96.2			26546	Repair non-union, metacarpal or phalanx, (includes obtaining bone graft with or without external or internal fixation)	(I) 10.4	90	3
			26548	Repair and reconstruction, finger, volar plate, interphalangeal joint	8.0	90	3
			26550	Pollicization of a digit	22.0	90	3
98.2	▲		26551	Transfer, toe-to-hand with microvascular anastomosis; great toe "wrap-around" with bone graft	(I) 55.0	90	6
96.2	M		26552	Reconstruction thumb with toe To report, see 20973 or 26551, 26553, 26554	28.0	90	3
98.2			26553	other than great toe, single	(I) 55.0	90	6
98.2			26554	other than great toe, double	(I) 65.0	90	6
98.2	▲		26555	Transfer, finger to another position without microvascular anastomosis	12.0	90	3
98.2	▲		26556	Transfer, free toe joint, with microvascular anastomosis	(I) 55.0	90	6
96.2	M		26557	Toe to finger transfer; first stage To report, see 20973, or 26551, 26553, 26554	8.0	90	3
96.2	M		26558	each delay To report, see 20973, or 26551, 26553, 26554	5.0	90	3
96.2	M		26559	second stage To report, see 20973, or 26551, 26553, 26554	10.0	90	3
			26560	Repair of syndactyly (web finger) each web space; with skin flaps	10.0	45	3
			26561	with skin flaps and grafts	14.2	45	3
			26562	complex (eg, involving bone, nails)	16.0	90	3
98.2	▲		26565	Osteotomy; metacarpal, each	8.5	90	3
98.2	▲		26567	phalanx of finger, each	7.0	90	3
98.2	▲		26568	Osteoplasty, lengthening, metacarpal or phalanx	9.2	90	3
			26580	Repair cleft hand	20.0	90	3
			26585	Repair bifid digit	15.0	90	3
			26587	Reconstruction of supernumerary digit, soft tissue and bone	6.5	90	3
			26590	Repair macrodactylia	8.0	90	3
98.2	▲		26591	Repair, intrinsic muscles of hand, each muscle	7.0	90	3
98.2	▲		26593	Release, intrinsic muscles of hand, each muscle	6.0	90	3
			26596	Excision of constricting ring of finger, with multiple Z-plasties	12.0	90	3

UPD	Code	Description	Units	FUD	Anes
	26597	Release of scar contracture, flexor or extensor, with skin grafts, rearrangement flaps, or Z-plasties, hand and/or finger	13.0	90	3
	26600	Closed treatment of metacarpal fracture, single; without manipulation, each bone	1.5	60	3
	26605	with manipulation, each bone	2.5	60	3
	26607	Closed treatment of metacarpal fracture, with manipulation, with internal or external fixation, each bone	5.0	60	3
	26608	Percutaneous skeletal fixation of metacarpal fracture, each bone	(I) 7.4	60	3
	26615	Open treatment of metacarpal fracture, single, with or without internal or external fixation, each bone	7.0	60	3
	26641	Closed treatment of carpometacarpal dislocation, thumb, with manipulation	2.0	60	3
	26645	Closed treatment of carpometacarpal fracture dislocation, thumb (Bennett fracture), with manipulation	4.0	45	3
	26650	Percutaneous skeletal fixation of carpometacarpal fracture dislocation, thumb (Bennett fracture), with manipulation, with or without external fixation	7.5	45	3
	26665	Open treatment of carpometacarpal fracture dislocation, thumb (Bennett fracture), with or without internal or external fixation	10.5	60	3
	26670	Closed treatment of carpometacarpal dislocation, other than thumb (Bennett fracture), single, with manipulation; without anesthesia	1.5	30	0
	26675	requiring anesthesia	2.5	45	3
	26676	Percutaneous skeletal fixation of carpometacarpal dislocation, other than thumb (Bennett fracture), single, with manipulation	2.5	45	3
	26685	Open treatment of carpometacarpal dislocation, other than thumb (Bennett fracture); single, with or without internal or external fixation	6.0	60	3
	26686	complex, multiple or delayed reduction	8.0	60	3
	26700	Closed treatment of metacarpophalangeal dislocation, single, with manipulation; without anesthesia	1.9	30	0
	26705	requiring anesthesia	2.2	45	3
	26706	Percutaneous skeletal fixation of metacarpophalangeal dislocation, single, with manipulation	4.0	45	3
	26715	Open treatment of metacarpophalangeal dislocation, single, with or without internal or external fixation	7.0	45	3
	26720	Closed treatment of phalangeal shaft fracture, proximal or middle phalanx, finger or thumb; without manipulation, each	1.5	45	3
	26725	with manipulation, with or without skin or skeletal traction, each	2.1	45	3

UPD			Code	Description	Units	FUD	Anes
			26727	Percutaneous skeletal fixation of unstable phalangeal shaft fracture, proximal or middle phalanx, finger or thumb, with manipulation, each	3.2	45	3
			26735	Open treatment of phalangeal shaft fracture, proximal or middle phalanx, finger or thumb, with or without internal or external fixation, each	6.0	60	3
			26740	Closed treatment of articular fracture, involving metacarpophalangeal or interphalangeal joint; without manipulation, each	2.5	60	3
			26742	with manipulation, each	3.5	60	3
			26746	Open treatment of articular fracture, involving metacarpophalangeal or interphalangeal joint, with or without internal or external fixation, each	6.0	60	3
			26750	Closed treatment of distal phalangeal fracture, finger or thumb; without manipulation, each	0.8	45	3
			26755	with manipulation, each	1.0	30	3
			26756	Percutaneous skeletal fixation of distal phalangeal fracture, finger or thumb, each	1.6	60	3
			26765	Open treatment of distal phalangeal fracture, finger or thumb, with or without internal or external fixation, each	4.0	60	3
			26770	Closed treatment of interphalangeal joint dislocation, single, with manipulation; without anesthesia	1.0	30	0
			26775	requiring anesthesia	1.5	45	3
			26776	Percutaneous skeletal fixation of interphalangeal joint dislocation, single, with manipulation	1.6	60	3
			26785	Open treatment of interphalangeal joint dislocation, with or without internal or external fixation, single	3.0	60	3
			26820	Fusion in opposition, thumb, with autogenous graft (includes obtaining graft)	11.8	90	3
			26841	Arthrodesis, carpometacarpal joint, thumb, with or without internal fixation;	8.0	90	3
			26842	with autograft (includes obtaining graft)	10.1	90	3
			26843	Arthrodesis, carpometacarpal joint, digits, other than thumb;	8.0	90	3
			26844	with autograft (includes obtaining graft)	10.1	90	3
			26850	Arthrodesis, metacarpophalangeal joint, with or without internal fixation;	7.7	90	3
			26852	with autograft (includes obtaining graft)	9.0	90	3
			26860	Arthrodesis, interphalangeal joint, with or without internal fixation;	5.8	90	3
98.2	▲	+	26861	each additional interphalangeal joint (List separately in addition to code for primary procedure)	2.0	90	0

UPD			Code	Description	Units	FUD	Anes
				Note: This code is an add-on procedure and as such is valued appropriately. Multiple procedure guidelines for reduction of value are not applicable.			
			26862	with autograft (includes obtaining graft)	7.7	90	3
98.2	▲	+	26863	with autograft (includes obtaining graft), each additional joint (List separately in addition to code for primary procedure)	3.0	90	0
				Note: This code is an add-on procedure and as such is valued appropriately. Multiple procedure guidelines for reduction of value are not applicable.			
			26910	Amputation, metacarpal, with finger or thumb (ray amputation), single, with or without interosseous transfer	8.0	90	3
			26951	Amputation, finger or thumb, primary or secondary, any joint or phalanx, single, including neurectomies; with direct closure	5.5	45	3
			26952	with local advancement flaps (V-Y, hood)	7.0	45	3
98.2			26989	Unlisted procedure, hands or fingers	BR	0	3
98.2			26990	Incision and drainage, pelvis or hip joint area; deep abscess or hematoma	4.0	30	6
98.2			26991	infected bursa	1.1	30	6
98.2	▲		26992	Incision, bone cortex, pelvis and/or hip joint (eg, osteomyelitis or bone abscess)	5.0	30	6
98.2	▲		27000	Tenotomy, adductor of hip, percutaneous (separate procedure)	2.0	30	4
98.2	▲		27001	Tenotomy, adductor of hip, open	3.0	30	4
			27003	Tenotomy, adductor, subcutaneous, open, with obturator neurectomy	7.0	45	4
98.2	▲		27005	Tenotomy, hip flexor(s), open (separate procedure)	6.0	60	4
	▲		27006	Tenotomy, abductors and/or extensor(s) of hip, open (separate procedure)	7.0	60	4
			27025	Fasciotomy, hip or thigh, any type	10.1	90	4
98.2	▲		27030	Arthrotomy, hip, with drainage (eg, infection)	14.0	90	6
98.2	▲		27033	Arthrotomy, hip, including exploration or removal of loose or foreign body	14.1	90	6
98.2	▲		27035	Denervation, hip joint, intrapelvic or extrapelvic intra-articular branches of sciatic, femoral, or obturator nerves	17.2	90	6
98.2	▲		27036	Capsulectomy or capsulotomy, hip, with or without excision of heterotopic bone, with release of hip flexor muscles (ie, gluteus medius, gluteus minimus, tensor fascia latae, rectus femoris, sartorius, iliopsoas)	(I) 16.5	90	6
			27040	Biopsy, soft tissue of pelvis and hip area; superficial	1.2	0	3
98.2	▲		27041	deep, subfascial or intramuscular	2.4	0	3

+ Add-on Code   ⊘ Modifier -51 Exempt   ▲ Revised code   ● New code   **M** RVSI code or deleted from CPT   **(I)** Interim Value

Copyright © 1999 St. Anthony Publishing

UPD		Code	Description	Units	FUD	Anes
98.2	▲	27047	Excision, tumor, pelvis and hip area; subcutaneous tissue	3.0	7	3
98.2		27048	deep, subfascial, intramuscular	5.0	15	6
98.2	▲	27049	Radical resection of tumor, soft tissue of pelvis and hip area (eg, malignant neoplasm)	15.0	90	10
98.2		27050	Arthrotomy, with biopsy; sacroiliac joint	6.0	90	8
		27052	hip joint	13.5	90	6
		27054	Arthrotomy with synovectomy, hip joint	20.2	90	6
		27060	Excision; ischial bursa	5.5	60	4
		27062	trochanteric bursa or calcification	4.0	60	4
		27065	Excision of bone cyst or benign tumor; superficial (wing of ilium, symphysis pubis, or greater trochanter of femur) with or without autograft	5.0	60	6
		27066	deep, with or without autograft	9.5	90	6
		27067	with autograft requiring separate incision	12.0	90	6
98.2	▲	27070	Partial excision (craterization, saucerization) (eg, osteomyelitis or bone abscess); superficial (eg, wing of ilium, symphysis pubis, or greater trochanter of femur)	6.0	60	8
98.2	▲	27071	deep (subfascial or intramuscular)	12.0	60	6
		27075	Radical resection of tumor or infection; wing of ilium, one pubic or ischial ramus or symphysis pubis	18.0	60	8
98.2		27076	ilium, including acetabulum, both pubic rami, or ischium and acetabulum	32.0	90	10
98.2		27077	innominate bone, total	45.0	90	10
98.2		27078	ischial tuberosity and greater trochanter of femur	12.0	90	10
98.2		27079	ischial tuberosity and greater trochanter of femur, with skin flaps	14.0	90	10
		27080	Coccygectomy, primary	6.0	90	6
98.2		27086*	Removal of foreign body, pelvis or hip; subcutaneous tissue	1.2	0	6
98.2	▲	27087	deep (subfascial or intramuscular)	2.3	30	6
98.2		27090	Removal of hip prosthesis; (separate procedure)	14.0	90	6
98.2	▲	27091	complicated, including total hip prosthesis, methylmethacrylate with or without insertion of spacer	40.0	90	10
		27093	Injection procedure for hip arthrography; without anesthesia	1.3	0	0
		27095	with anesthesia	4.0	0	4
98.2	▲	27097	Release or recession, hamstring, proximal	6.0	90	4
98.2	▲	27098	Transfer, adductor to ischium	12.0	90	4

UPD		Code	Description	Units	FUD	Anes
		27100	Transfer external oblique muscle to greater trochanter including fascial or tendon extension (graft)	14.5	90	4
		27105	Transfer paraspinal muscle to hip (includes fascial or tendon extension graft)	15.5	90	4
		27110	Transfer iliopsoas; to greater trochanter	18.5	90	4
		27111	to femoral neck	19.0	90	4
		27120	Acetabuloplasty; (eg, Whitman, Colonna, Haygroves, or cup type)	24.0	120	6
98.2	▲	27122	resection, femoral head (eg, Girdlestone procedure)	25.0	120	6
98.2	▲	27125	Hemiarthroplasty, hip, partial (eg, femoral stem prosthesis, bipolar arthroplasty)	27.0	90	8
98.2		27130	Arthroplasty, acetabular and proximal femoral prosthetic replacement (total hip replacement), with or without autograft or allograft	32.5	90	8
98.2		27132	Conversion of previous hip surgery to total hip replacement, with or without autograft or allograft	36.0	90	8
		27134	Revision of total hip arthroplasty; both components, with or without autograft or allograft	38.0	90	10
		27137	acetabular component only, with or without autograft or allograft	32.0	90	10
		27138	femoral component only, with or without allograft	32.0	90	10
		27140	Osteotomy and transfer of greater trochanter (separate procedure)	12.2	90	6
		27146	Osteotomy, iliac, acetabular or innominate bone;	23.0	90	6
		27147	with open reduction of hip	26.0	90	6
		27151	with femoral osteotomy	26.0	90	6
		27156	with femoral osteotomy and with open reduction of hip	29.0	90	6
98.2	▲	27158	Osteotomy, pelvis, bilateral (eg, congenital malformation)	23.0	90	6
		27161	Osteotomy, femoral neck (separate procedure)	18.0	90	6
		27165	Osteotomy, intertrochanteric or subtrochanteric including internal or external fixation and/or cast	23.2	90	6
		27170	Bone graft, femoral head, neck, intertrochanteric or subtrochanteric area (includes obtaining bone graft)	24.3	90	6
		27175	Treatment of slipped femoral epiphysis; by traction, without reduction	11.0	90	4
		27176	by single or multiple pinning, in situ	21.5	90	6
		27177	Open treatment of slipped femoral epiphysis; single or multiple pinning or bone graft (includes obtaining graft)	22.5	90	6
		27178	closed manipulation with single or multiple pinning	22.8	90	6

UPD	Code	Description	Units	FUD	Anes
	27179	osteoplasty of femoral neck (Heyman type procedure)	16.5	90	6
	27181	osteotomy and internal fixation	24.2	90	6
	27185	Epiphyseal arrest by epiphysiodesis or stapling, greater trochanter	5.5	90	6
98.2	27187	Prophylactic treatment (nailing, pinning, plating or wiring) with or without methylmethacrylate, femoral neck and proximal femur	35.0	120	6
	27193	Closed treatment of pelvic ring fracture, dislocation, diastasis or subluxation; without manipulation	(I) 7.3	90	4
	27194	with manipulation, requiring more than local anesthesia	(I) 8.3	90	4
98.2	27200	Closed treatment of coccygeal fracture	1.6	60	6
	27202	Open treatment of coccygeal fracture	3.0	90	6
	27215	Open treatment of iliac spine(s), tuberosity avulsion, or iliac wing fracture(s) (eg, pelvic fracture(s) which do not disrupt the pelvic ring), with internal fixation	(I) 13.5	90	6
98.2	27216	Percutaneous skeletal fixation of posterior pelvic ring fracture and/or dislocation (includes ilium, sacroiliac joint and/or sacrum)	(I) 31.3	90	4
98.2	27217	Open treatment of anterior ring fracture and/or dislocation with internal fixation, (includes pubic symphysis and/or rami)	(I) 25.0	90	8
98.2	27218	Open treatment of posterior ring fracture and/or dislocation with internal fixation (includes ilium, sacroiliac joint and/or sacrum)	(I) 35.8	90	8
	27220	Closed treatment of acetabulum (hip socket) fracture(s); without manipulation	3.0	90	4
	27222	with manipulation, with or without skeletal traction	8.0	90	4
98.2	27226	Open treatment of posterior or anterior acetabular wall fracture, with internal fixation	(I) 27.1	90	10
98.2	27227	Open treatment of acetabular fracture(s) involving anterior or posterior (one) column, or a fracture running transversely across the acetabulum, with internal fixation	(I) 52.1	90	10
98.2	27228	Open treatment of acetabular fracture(s) involving anterior and posterior (two) columns, includes T-fracture and both column fracture with complete articular detachment, or single column or transverse fracture with associated acetabular wall fracture, with internal fixation	(I) 83.3	90	10
	27230	Closed treatment of femoral fracture, proximal end, neck; without manipulation	2.0	90	4
	27232	with manipulation, with or without skeletal traction	10.0	90	4
98.2	27235	Percutaneous skeletal fixation of femoral fracture, proximal end, neck, undisplaced, mildly displaced, or impacted fracture	21.0	90	4

UPD		Code	Description	Units	FUD	Anes
		27236	Open treatment of femoral fracture, proximal end, neck, internal fixation or prosthetic replacement (direct fracture exposure)	27.0	90	6
		27238	Closed treatment of intertrochanteric, pertrochanteric, or subtrochanteric femoral fracture; without manipulation	2.0	90	4
		27240	with manipulation, with or without skin or skeletal traction	11.0	90	4
		27244	Open treatment of intertrochanteric, pertrochanteric or subtrochanteric femoral fracture; with plate/screw type implant, with or without cerclage	19.7	90	6
		27245	with intramedullary implant, with or without interlocking screws and/or cerclage	(I) 25.6	90	6
		27246	Closed treatment of greater trochanteric fracture, without manipulation	2.0	0	4
		27248	Open treatment of greater trochanteric fracture, with or without internal or external fixation	7.1	90	6
		27250	Closed treatment of hip dislocation, traumatic; without anesthesia	3.5	60	0
		27252	requiring anesthesia	4.8	90	4
		27253	Open treatment of hip dislocation, traumatic, without internal fixation	17.0	90	6
		27254	Open treatment of hip dislocation, traumatic, with acetabular wall and femoral head fracture, with or without internal or external fixation	25.0	90	6
98.2		27256*	Treatment of spontaneous hip dislocation (developmental, including congenital or pathological), by abduction, splint or traction; without anesthesia, without manipulation	6.8	0	0
		27257*	with manipulation, requiring anesthesia	12.0	0	4
		27258	Open treatment of spontaneous hip dislocation (developmental, including congenital or pathological), replacement of femoral head in acetabulum (including tenotomy, etc);	18.0	90	6
		27259	with femoral shaft shortening	19.0	90	6
		27265	Closed treatment of post hip arthroplasty dislocation; without anesthesia	(I) 4.0	90	0
		27266	requiring regional or general anesthesia	(I) 5.5	90	4
		27275*	Manipulation, hip joint, requiring general anesthesia	3.0	0	4
		27280	Arthrodesis, sacroiliac joint (including obtaining graft)	14.0	90	8
		27282	Arthrodesis, symphysis pubis (including obtaining graft)	18.0	90	8
98.2	▲	27284	Arthrodesis, hip joint (including obtaining graft);	27.0	120	6
		27286	with subtrochanteric osteotomy	30.0	120	6
		27290	Interpelviabdominal amputation (hindquarter amputation)	40.0	120	15

UPD		Code	Description	Units	FUD	Anes
98.2		**27295**	Disarticulation of hip	27.0	120	10
98.2		**27299**	Unlisted procedure, pelvis or hip joint	BR	0	6
98.2	▲	**27301**	Incision and drainage, deep abscess, bursa, or hematoma, thigh or knee region	3.0	30	4
98.2	▲	**27303**	Incision, deep, with opening of bone cortex, femur or knee (eg, osteomyelitis or bone abscess)	5.5	30	6
		27305	Fasciotomy, iliotibial (tenotomy), open	6.0	45	4
98.2	▲	**27306**	Tenotomy, percutaneous, adductor or hamstring; single tendon (separate procedure)	2.4	30	4
98.2	▲	**27307**	multiple tendons	3.0	30	4
98.2	▲	**27310**	Arthrotomy, knee, with exploration, drainage, or removal of foreign body (eg, infection)	12.5	90	4
		27315	Neurectomy, hamstring muscle	11.0	30	4
		27320	Neurectomy, popliteal (gastrocnemius)	11.0	30	4
		27323	Biopsy, soft tissue of thigh or knee area; superficial	1.2	0	3
98.2	▲	**27324**	deep (subfascial or intramuscular)	2.4	0	4
		27327	Excision, tumor, thigh or knee area; subcutaneous	3.0	15	3
		27328	deep, subfascial, or intramuscular	5.0	15	4
98.2		**27329**	Radical resection of tumor (eg, malignant neoplasm), soft tissue of thigh or knee area	14.0	90	4
		27330	Arthrotomy, knee; with synovial biopsy only	12.5	90	4
98.2	▲	**27331**	including joint exploration, biopsy, or removal of loose or foreign bodies	13.5	90	4
98.2	▲	**27332**	Arthrotomy, with excision of semilunar cartilage (meniscectomy) knee; medial OR lateral	16.0	90	4
		27333	medial AND lateral	16.1	90	4
98.2	▲	**27334**	Arthrotomy, with synovectomy knee; anterior OR posterior	18.0	90	4
		27335	anterior AND posterior including popliteal area	19.0	90	4
		27340	Excision, prepatellar bursa	8.0	60	4
98.2	▲	**27345**	Excision of synovial cyst of popliteal space (eg, Bakers cyst)	9.0	60	4
98.2	●	**27347**	Excision of lesion of meniscus or capsule (eg, cyst, ganglion), knee	(I) 7.5	90	4
		27350	Patellectomy or hemipatellectomy	12.0	60	4
98.2		**27355**	Excision or curettage of bone cyst or benign tumor of femur;	11.0	60	5
98.2		**27356**	with allograft	14.0	90	5
98.2		**27357**	with autograft (includes obtaining graft)	15.0	90	5

UPD			Code	Description	Units	FUD	Anes
98.2	▲	+	27358	Excision or curettage of bone cyst or benign tumor of femur; with internal fixation (List in addition to code for primary procedure) Note: This code is an add-on procedure and as such is valued appropriately. Multiple procedure guidelines for reduction of value are not applicable.	16.0	90	0
98.2	▲		27360	Partial excision (craterization, saucerization, or diaphysectomy) bone, femur, proximal tibia and/or fibula (eg, osteomyelitis or bone abscess)	12.0	90	5
98.2			27365	Radical resection of tumor, bone, femur or knee	18.0	90	5
			27370	Injection procedure for knee arthrography	0.7	0	3
98.2			27372	Removal of foreign body, deep, thigh region or knee area	5.2	30	4
			27380	Suture of infrapatellar tendon; primary	11.0	90	4
			27381	secondary reconstruction, including fascial or tendon graft	13.0	90	4
			27385	Suture of quadriceps or hamstring muscle rupture; primary	13.1	90	4
			27386	reconstruction, including fascial or tendon graft	16.0	90	4
98.2	▲		27390	Tenotomy, open, hamstring, knee to hip; single tendon	6.0	30	4
98.2	▲		27391	multiple tendons, one leg	8.0	45	4
98.2	▲		27392	multiple tendons, bilateral	12.0	45	4
98.2	▲		27393	Lengthening of hamstring tendon; single tendon	7.0	30	4
98.2	▲		27394	multiple tendons, one leg	9.0	30	4
98.2	▲		27395	multiple tendons, bilateral	13.0	30	4
98.2	▲		27396	Transplant, hamstring tendon to patella; single tendon	16.2	90	4
98.2	▲		27397	multiple tendons	17.9	90	4
98.2	▲		27400	Transfer, tendon or muscle, hamstrings to femur (eg, Egger's type procedure)	15.0	90	4
98.2	▲		27403	Arthrotomy with meniscus repair, knee	17.0	90	4
			27405	Repair, primary, torn ligament and/or capsule, knee; collateral	14.0	90	4
			27407	cruciate	17.0	90	4
			27409	collateral and cruciate ligaments	20.0	90	4
98.2	▲		27418	Anterior tibial tubercleplasty (eg, Maquet type procedure)	21.0	90	4
98.2	▲		27420	Reconstruction of dislocating patella; (eg, Hauser type procedure)	15.5	90	4
98.2	▲		27422	with extensor realignment and/or muscle advancement or release (eg, Campbell, Goldwaite type procedure)	15.5	90	4
			27424	with patellectomy	16.5	90	4

UPD		Code	Description	Units	FUD	Anes
		27425	Lateral retinacular release (any method)	16.0	90	4
		27427	Ligamentous reconstruction (augmentation), knee; extra-articular	19.0	90	4
		27428	intra-articular (open)	27.0	90	4
		27429	intra-articular (open) and extra-articular	30.0	90	4
98.2	▲	**27430**	Quadricepsplasty (eg, Bennett or Thompson type)	15.5	90	4
98.2	▲	**27435**	Capsulotomy, posterior capsular release, knee	14.4	90	4
		27437	Arthroplasty, patella; without prosthesis	15.0	90	4
		27438	with prosthesis	20.0	90	4
		27440	Arthroplasty, knee, tibial plateau;	21.0	90	4
		27441	with debridement and partial synovectomy	22.0	90	4
98.2	▲	**27442**	Arthroplasty, femoral condyles or tibial plateau(s), knee;	23.0	90	4
98.2		**27443**	with debridement and partial synovectomy	22.0	90	4
98.2	▲	**27445**	Arthroplasty, knee, hinge prosthesis (eg, Walldius type)	30.0	90	4
98.2		**27446**	Arthroplasty, knee, condyle and plateau; medial OR lateral compartment	28.0	90	4
		27447	medial AND lateral compartments with or without patella resurfacing ("total knee replacement")	38.0	120	7
98.2		**27448**	Osteotomy, femur, shaft or supracondylar; without fixation	18.5	90	6
98.2		**27450**	with fixation	21.0	90	6
98.2	▲	**27454**	Osteotomy, multiple, with realignment on intramedullary rod, femoral shaft (eg, Sofield type procedure)	20.5	90	6
		27455	Osteotomy, proximal tibia, including fibular excision or osteotomy (includes correction of genu varus (bowleg) or genu valgus (knock-knee)); before epiphyseal closure	13.0	90	4
		27457	after epiphyseal closure	15.5	90	4
		27465	Osteoplasty, femur; shortening (excluding 64876)	20.5	90	5
		27466	lengthening	26.5	90	5
		27468	combined, lengthening and shortening with femoral segment transfer	38.5	90	5
98.2		**27470**	Repair, nonunion or malunion, femur, distal to head and neck; without graft (eg, compression technique)	20.5	90	6
98.2		**27472**	with iliac or other autogenous bone graft (includes obtaining graft)	23.0	90	6
98.2	▲	**27475**	Arrest, epiphyseal, any method (eg, epiphydiodesis); distal femur	14.1	90	5
		27477	tibia and fibula, proximal	16.1	90	4

UPD		Code	Description	Units	FUD	Anes
		27479	combined distal femur, proximal tibia and fibula	20.5	90	5
98.2	▲	27485	Arrest, hemiepiphyseal, distal femur or proximal tibia or fibula (eg, genu varus or valgus)	11.1	90	5
98.2		27486	Revision of total knee arthroplasty, with or without allograft; one component	BR	90	7
98.2	▲	27487	femoral and entire tibial component	45.0	90	7
98.2	▲	27488	Removal of prosthesis, including total knee prosthesis, methylmethacrylate with or without insertion of spacer, knee	12.5	90	7
98.2		27495	Prophylactic treatment (nailing, pinning, plating or wiring) with or without methylmethacrylate, femur	14.0	90	6
98.2		27496	Decompression fasciotomy, thigh and/or knee, one compartment (flexor or extensor or adductor);	(I) 7.2	90	4
98.2		27497	with debridement of nonviable muscle and/or nerve	(I) 12.7	90	4
98.2		27498	Decompression fasciotomy, thigh and/or knee, multiple compartments;	(I) 14.5	90	4
98.2		27499	with debridement of nonviable muscle and/or nerve	(I) 19.9	90	4
		27500	Closed treatment of femoral shaft fracture, without manipulation	(I) 8.1	90	4
		27501	Closed treatment of supracondylar or transcondylar femoral fracture with or without intercondylar extension, without manipulation	(I) 8.1	90	4
		27502	Closed treatment of femoral shaft fracture, with manipulation, with or without skin or skeletal traction	7.5	90	4
		27503	Closed treatment of supracondylar or transcondylar femoral fracture with or without intercondylar extension, with manipulation, with or without skin or skeletal traction	(I) 12.8	90	4
98.2		27506	Open treatment of femoral shaft fracture, with or without external fixation, with insertion of intramedullary implant, with or without cerclage and/or locking screws	(I) 23.0	90	6
98.2		27507	Open treatment of femoral shaft fracture with plate/screws, with or without cerclage	(I) 18.6	90	6
		27508	Closed treatment of femoral fracture, distal end, medial or lateral condyle, without manipulation	6.0	90	4
98.2		27509	Percutaneous skeletal fixation of femoral fracture, distal end, medial or lateral condyle, or supracondylar or transcondylar, with or without intercondylar extension, or distal femoral epiphyseal separation	9.8	90	4
		27510	Closed treatment of femoral fracture, distal end, medial or lateral condyle, with manipulation	8.4	90	4
		27511	Open treatment of femoral supracondylar or transcondylar fracture without intercondylar extension, with or without internal or external fixation	(I) 18.1	90	5

UPD		Code	Description	Units	FUD	Anes
		27513	Open treatment of femoral supracondylar or transcondylar fracture with intercondylar extension, with or without internal or external fixation	(I) 24.3	90	5
		27514	Open treatment of femoral fracture, distal end, medial or lateral condyle, with or without internal or external fixation	20.0	90	5
		27516	Closed treatment of distal femoral epiphyseal separation; without manipulation	7.0	90	4
		27517	with manipulation, with or without skin or skeletal traction	9.4	90	4
		27519	Open treatment of distal femoral epiphyseal separation, with or without internal or external fixation	23.0	90	5
		27520	Closed treatment of patellar fracture, without manipulation	2.6	60	3
		27524	Open treatment of patellar fracture, with internal fixation and/ or partial or complete patellectomy and soft tissue repair	12.0	90	4
		27530	Closed treatment of tibial fracture, proximal (plateau); without manipulation	3.0	90	3
		27532	with or without manipulation, with skeletal traction	5.2	90	3
		27535	Open treatment of tibial fracture, proximal (plateau); unicondylar, with or without internal or external fixation	(I) 12.7	90	4
		27536	bicondylar, with or without internal fixation	(I) 18.3	90	4
		27538	Closed treatment of intercondylar spine(s) and/or tuberosity fracture(s) of knee, with or without manipulation	(I) 6.5	90	3
		27540	Open treatment of intercondylar spine(s) and/or tuberosity fracture(s) of the knee, with or without internal or external fixation	14.3	90	4
		27550	Closed treatment of knee dislocation; without anesthesia	2.3	45	0
		27552	requiring anesthesia	3.3	45	3
		27556	Open treatment of knee dislocation, with or without internal or external fixation; without primary ligamentous repair or augmentation/reconstruction	15.5	90	4
		27557	with primary ligamentous repair	17.0	90	4
96.2		27558	with primary ligamentous repair, with augmentation/ reconstruction	(I) 20.0	90	4
		27560	Closed treatment of patellar dislocation; without anesthesia	2.3	45	0
		27562	requiring anesthesia	3.5	45	3
98.2		27566	Open treatment of patellar dislocation, with or without partial or total patellectomy	12.1	90	4
		27570*	Manipulation of knee joint under general anesthesia (includes application of traction or other fixation devices)	3.0	0	3
98.2	▲	27580	Arthrodesis, knee, any technique	21.0	90	4
		27590	Amputation, thigh, through femur, any level;	14.5	90	5

UPD		Code	Description	Units	FUD	Anes
		27591	immediate fitting technique including first cast	15.0	90	5
		27592	open, circular (guillotine)	16.0	90	5
98.2		27594	secondary closure or scar revision	5.0	90	4
		27596	re-amputation	14.0	90	5
		27598	Disarticulation at knee	14.0	120	5
98.2		27599	Unlisted procedure, femur or knee	BR	0	4
98.2		27600	Decompression fasciotomy, leg; anterior and/or lateral compartments only	6.0	30	3
98.2		27601	posterior compartment(s) only	8.0	30	3
98.2		27602	anterior and/or lateral, and posterior compartment(s)	11.0	30	3
		27603	Incision and drainage, leg or ankle; deep abscess or hematoma	5.0	60	3
		27604	infected bursa	1.1	30	3
98.2	▲	27605*	Tenotomy, percutaneous, Achilles tendon (separate procedure); local anesthesia	2.5	0	3
		27606	general anesthesia	3.0	30	3
98.2	▲	27607	Incision (eg, osteomyelitis or bone abscess), leg or ankle	4.0	30	3
98.2	▲	27610	Arthrotomy, ankle, including exploration, drainage, or removal of foreign body	9.1	60	3
98.2	▲	27612	Arthrotomy, posterior capsular release, ankle, with or without Achilles tendon lengthening	10.0	60	3
		27613	Biopsy, soft tissue of leg or ankle area; superficial	3.0	0	3
98.2	▲	27614	deep (subfascial or intramuscular)	5.0	0	3
98.2		27615	Radical resection of tumor (eg, malignant neoplasm), soft tissue of leg or ankle area	12.5	90	3
98.2	▲	27618	Excision, tumor, leg or ankle area; subcutaneous tissue	3.0	21	3
		27619	deep (subfascial or intramuscular)	5.0	30	3
		27620	Arthrotomy, ankle, with joint exploration, with or without biopsy, with or without removal of loose or foreign body	9.1	60	3
		27625	Arthrotomy, ankle, with synovectomy;	12.0	90	3
		27626	including tenosynovectomy	13.0	90	3
		27630	Excision of lesion of tendon sheath or capsule (eg, cyst or ganglion), leg and/or ankle	4.0	45	3
		27635	Excision or curettage of bone cyst or benign tumor, tibia or fibula;	10.5	60	3
		27637	with autograft (includes obtaining graft)	13.0	90	3
		27638	with allograft	13.0	90	3

UPD			Code	Description	Units	FUD	Anes
98.2	▲		27640	Partial excision (craterization, saucerization, or diaphysectomy) bone (eg, osteomyelitis or exostosis); tibia	12.0	90	3
			27641	fibula	12.0	90	3
			27645	Radical resection of tumor, bone; tibia	19.0	90	4
			27646	fibula	13.0	90	4
			27647	talus or calcaneus	18.0	90	4
			27648	Injection procedure for ankle arthrography	1.3	0	3
			27650	Repair, primary, open or percutaneous, ruptured Achilles tendon;	11.0	90	5
			27652	with graft (includes obtaining graft)	14.0	90	5
98.2	▲		27654	Repair, secondary, Achilles tendon, with or without graft	16.0	90	5
			27656	Repair, fascial defect of leg	6.0	45	3
98.2	▲		27658	Repair, flexor tendon, leg; primary, without graft, each tendon	6.5	90	3
98.2	▲		27659	secondary, with or without graft, each tendon	8.0	90	3
98.2	▲		27664	Repair, extensor tendon, leg; primary, without graft, each tendon	4.3	90	3
98.2	▲		27665	secondary, with or without graft, each tendon	6.0	90	3
98.2	▲		27675	Repair, dislocating peroneal tendons; without fibular osteotomy	5.5	30	3
			27676	with fibular osteotomy	6.5	60	3
98.2	▲		27680	Tenolysis, flexor or extensor tendon, leg and/or ankle; single, each tendon	5.0	60	3
98.2	▲		27681	multiple tendons (through separate incision(s))	6.0	60	3
98.2	▲		27685	Lengthening or shortening of tendon, leg or ankle; single tendon (separate procedure)	7.1	90	3
98.2	▲		27686	multiple tendons (through same incision), each	8.0	90	3
			27687	Gastrocnemius recession (eg, Strayer procedure)	7.6	90	5
			27690	Transfer or transplant of single tendon (with muscle redirection or rerouting); superficial (eg, anterior tibial extensors into midfoot)	8.0	90	3
			27691	deep (eg, anterior tibial or posterior tibial through interosseous space, flexor digitorum longus, flexor hallucis longus, or peroneal tendon to midfoot or hindfoot)	10.0	90	3
98.2	▲	+	27692	each additional tendon (List in addition to code for primary procedure)	2.0	90	3
				Note: This code is an add-on procedure and as such is valued appropriately. Multiple procedure guidelines for reduction of value are not applicable.			

UPD		Code	Description	Units	FUD	Anes
98.2	▲	27695	Repair, primary, disrupted ligament, ankle; collateral	10.0	90	3
		27696	both collateral ligaments	14.0	90	3
98.2	▲	27698	Repair, secondary disrupted ligament, ankle, collateral (eg, Watson-Jones procedure)	15.5	90	3
		27700	Arthroplasty, ankle;	20.0	90	3
		27702	with implant ("total ankle")	31.0	120	7
98.2	▲	27703	revision, total ankle	29.5	90	7
		27704	Removal of ankle implant	11.0	30	3
		27705	Osteotomy; tibia	12.5	90	4
		27707	fibula	7.0	90	4
		27709	tibia and fibula	15.0	90	4
98.2	▲	27712	multiple, with realignment on intramedullary rod (eg, Sofield type procedure)	18.2	90	4
98.2	▲	27715	Osteoplasty, tibia and fibula, lengthening or shortening	24.5	90	4
		27720	Repair of nonunion or malunion, tibia; without graft, (eg, compression technique)	18.0	90	3
98.2		27722	with sliding graft	19.5	90	3
98.2		27724	with iliac or other autograft (includes obtaining graft)	21.0	90	3
		27725	by synostosis, with fibula, any method	28.0	90	3
		27727	Repair of congenital pseudarthrosis, tibia	22.0	90	3
98.2	▲	27730	Arrest, epiphyseal (epiphysiodesis), any method; distal tibia	11.5	90	3
		27732	distal fibula	6.2	90	3
		27734	distal tibia and fibula	13.6	90	3
98.2	▲	27740	Arrest, epiphyseal (epiphysiodesis), any method, combined, proximal and distal tibia and fibula;	18.5	90	3
98.2		27742	and distal femur	22.5	90	4
98.2		27745	Prophylactic treatment (nailing, pinning, plating or wiring) with or without methylmethacrylate, tibia	15.2	90	3
		27750	Closed treatment of tibial shaft fracture (with or without fibular fracture); without manipulation	(I) 5.6	90	3
		27752	with manipulation, with or without skeletal traction	(I) 7.0	90	3
		27756	Percutaneous skeletal fixation of tibial shaft fracture (with or without fibular fracture) (eg, pins or screws)	(I) 8.5	90	3
		27758	Open treatment of tibial shaft fracture, (with or without fibular fracture) with plate/screws, with or without cerclage	(I) 12.7	90	3

UPD	Code	Description	Units	FUD	Anes
98.2	27759	Open treatment of tibial shaft fracture (with or without fibular fracture) by intramedullary implant, with or without interlocking screws and/or cerclage	(I) 12.7	90	4
	27760	Closed treatment of medial malleolus fracture; without manipulation	2.7	90	3
	27762	with manipulation, with or without skin or skeletal traction	3.5	90	3
	27766	Open treatment of medial malleolus fracture, with or without internal or external fixation	9.4	90	3
	27780	Closed treatment of proximal fibula or shaft fracture; without manipulation	2.0	90	3
	27781	with manipulation	3.0	90	3
	27784	Open treatment of proximal fibula or shaft fracture, with or without internal or external fixation	8.3	90	3
	27786	Closed treatment of distal fibular fracture (lateral malleolus); without manipulation	3.0	90	3
	27788	with manipulation	4.0	90	3
	27792	Open treatment of distal fibular fracture (lateral malleolus), with or without internal or external fixation	9.0	90	3
	27808	Closed treatment of bimalleolar ankle fracture, (including Potts); without manipulation	3.0	90	3
	27810	with manipulation	5.0	90	3
	27814	Open treatment of bimalleolar ankle fracture, with or without internal or external fixation	12.5	90	3
	27816	Closed treatment of trimalleolar ankle fracture; without manipulation	3.0	90	3
	27818	with manipulation	6.5	90	3
	27822	Open treatment of trimalleolar ankle fracture, with or without internal or external fixation, medial and/or lateral malleolus; without fixation of posterior lip	14.5	90	3
	27823	with fixation of posterior lip	15.6	90	3
	27824	Closed treatment of fracture of weight bearing articular portion of distal tibia (eg, pilon or tibial plafond), with or without anesthesia; without manipulation	(I) 3.9	90	3
	27825	with skeletal traction and/or requiring manipulation	(I) 7.8	90	3
	27826	Open treatment of fracture of weight bearing articular surface/ portion of distal tibia (eg, pilon or tibial plafond), with internal or external fixation; of fibula only	(I) 11.7	90	3
	27827	of tibia only	(I) 18.7	90	3
	27828	of both tibia and fibula	(I) 21.7	90	3
	27829	Open treatment of distal tibiofibular joint (syndesmosis) disruption, with or without internal or external fixation	(I) 7.0	90	3

UPD		Code	Description	Units	FUD	Anes
		27830	Closed treatment of proximal tibiofibular joint dislocation; without anesthesia	2.5	90	0
		27831	requiring anesthesia	3.0	30	3
		27832	Open treatment of proximal tibiofibular joint dislocation, with or without internal or external fixation, or with excision of proximal fibula	8.1	90	3
		27840	Closed treatment of ankle dislocation; without anesthesia	1.8	45	0
		27842	requiring anesthesia, with or without percutaneous skeletal fixation	2.7	45	3
		27846	Open treatment of ankle dislocation, with or without percutaneous skeletal fixation; without repair or internal fixation	11.0	90	3
		27848	with repair or internal or external fixation	12.2	90	3
		27860*	Manipulation of ankle under general anesthesia (includes application of traction or other fixation apparatus)	1.4	0	3
		27870	Arthrodesis, ankle, any method	17.4	120	3
		27871	Arthrodesis, tibiofibular joint, proximal or distal	4.5	120	3
		27880	Amputation, leg, through tibia and fibula;	14.5	90	3
		27881	with immediate fitting technique including application of first cast	16.0	90	3
		27882	open, circular (guillotine)	10.5	90	3
		27884	secondary closure or scar revision	5.0	45	3
		27886	re-amputation	15.0	45	3
98.2	▲	27888	Amputation, ankle, through malleoli of tibia and fibula (eg, Syme, Pirogoff type procedures), with plastic closure and resection of nerves	11.5	90	3
		27889	Ankle disarticulation	11.5	90	3
		27892	Decompression fasciotomy, leg; anterior and/or lateral compartments only, with debridement of nonviable muscle and/or nerve	(I) 12.7	90	3
		27893	posterior compartment(s) only, with debridement of nonviable muscle and/or nerve	(I) 12.7	90	3
		27894	anterior and/or lateral, and posterior compartment(s), with debridement of nonviable muscle and/or nerve	(I) 19.9	90	3
98.2		27899	Unlisted procedure, leg or ankle	BR	0	3
98.2	▲	28001*	Incision and drainage, bursa, foot	1.0	0	3
98.2	▲	28002*	Incision and drainage below fascia, with or without tendon sheath involvement, foot; single bursal space	1.8	0	3
		28003	multiple areas	2.0	21	3

UPD		Code	Description	Units	FUD	Anes
98.2	▲	28005	Incision, bone cortex (eg, osteomyelitis or bone abscess), foot	5.0	45	3
		28008	Fasciotomy, foot and/or toe	3.2	60	3
98.2	▲	28010	Tenotomy, percutaneous, toe; single tendon	1.0	30	3
98.2	▲	28011	multiple tendons	1.5	30	3
98.2	▲	28020	Arthrotomy, including exploration, drainage, or removal of loose or foreign body; intertarsal or tarsometatarsal joint	6.2	60	3
		28022	metatarsophalangeal joint	4.0	60	3
		28024	interphalangeal joint	3.0	60	3
98.2	▲	28030	Neurectomy, intrinsic musculature of foot	12.0	60	3
98.2	▲	28035	Release, tarsal tunnel (posterior tibial nerve decompression)	10.0	30	3
98.2	▲	28043	Excision, tumor, foot; subcutaneous tissue	3.0	21	3
		28045	deep, subfascial, intramuscular	5.0	21	3
98.2		28046	Radical resection of tumor (eg, malignant neoplasm), soft tissue of foot	12.0	180	3
98.2	▲	28050	Arthrotomy with biopsy; intertarsal or tarsometatarsal joint	6.2	60	3
		28052	metatarsophalangeal joint	4.0	60	3
		28054	interphalangeal joint	3.0	60	3
98.2	▲	28060	Fasciectomy, plantar fascia; partial (separate procedure)	5.5	60	3
		28062	radical (separate procedure)	11.5	90	3
		28070	Synovectomy; intertarsal or tarsometatarsal joint, each	6.2	90	3
		28072	metatarsophalangeal joint, each	4.0	90	3
98.2	▲	28080	Excision, interdigital (Morton) neuroma, single, each	4.5	30	3
		28086	Synovectomy, tendon sheath, foot; flexor	10.0	60	3
		28088	extensor	6.5	60	3
98.2	▲	28090	Excision of lesion, tendon, tendon sheath, or capsule (including synovectomy) (eg, cyst or ganglion); foot	4.0	45	3
98.2	▲	28092	toe(s), each	2.5	30	3
		28100	Excision or curettage of bone cyst or benign tumor, talus or calcaneus;	6.2	60	3
		28102	with iliac or other autograft (includes obtaining graft)	7.0	120	3
		28103	with allograft	6.0	120	3
		28104	Excision or curettage of bone cyst or benign tumor, tarsal or metatarsal bones, except talus or calcaneus;	4.9	60	3
		28106	with iliac or other autograft (includes obtaining graft)	6.0	120	3

UPD		Code	Description	Units	FUD	Anes
		28107	with allograft	5.0	120	3
		28108	Excision or curettage of bone cyst or benign tumor, phalanges of foot	4.0	60	3
		28110	Ostectomy, partial excision, fifth metatarsal head (bunionette) (separate procedure)	3.0	60	3
		28111	Ostectomy, complete excision; first metatarsal head	4.5	30	3
		28112	other metatarsal head (second, third or fourth)	4.0	60	3
		28113	fifth metatarsal head	5.0	30	3
98.2	▲	28114	all metatarsal heads, with partial proximal phalangectomy, excluding first metatarsal (eg, Clayton type procedure)	12.0	60	3
		28116	Ostectomy, excision of tarsal coalition	7.0	60	3
		28118	Ostectomy, calcaneus;	7.0	60	3
		28119	for spur, with or without plantar fascial release	5.0	60	3
98.2	▲	28120	Partial excision (craterization, saucerization, sequestrectomy, or diaphysectomy) bone (eg, osteomyelitis or bossing); talus or calcaneus	6.0	60	3
98.2	▲	28122	tarsal or metatarsal bone, except talus or calcaneus	4.8	60	3
98.2	▲	28124	phalanx of toe	3.6	60	3
98.2	▲	28126	Resection, partial or complete, phalangeal base, each toe	3.5	60	3
		28130	Talectomy (astragalectomy)	10.0	90	3
		28140	Metatarsectomy	6.0	60	3
98.2	▲	28150	Phalangectomy, toe, each toe	3.5	30	3
98.2	▲	28153	Resection, condyle(s), distal end of phalanx, each toe	4.0	30	3
98.2	▲	28160	Hemiphalangectomy or interphalangeal joint excision, toe, proximal end of phalanx, each	4.0	30	3
		28171	Radical resection of tumor, bone; tarsal (except talus or calcaneus)	10.0	90	4
		28173	metatarsal	10.0	90	4
		28175	phalanx of toe	6.5	90	4
		28190*	Removal of foreign body, foot; subcutaneous	1.3	0	3
		28192	deep	3.0	30	3
		28193	complicated	4.5	30	3
98.2	▲	28200	Repair, tendon, flexor, foot; primary or secondary, without free graft, each tendon	6.0	90	3
		28202	secondary with free graft, each tendon (includes obtaining graft)	8.0	90	3

UPD		Code	Description	Units	FUD	Anes
98.2	▲	28208	Repair, tendon, extensor, foot; primary or secondary, each tendon	3.0	90	3
		28210	secondary with free graft, each tendon (includes obtaining graft)	4.4	90	3
98.2	▲	28220	Tenolysis, flexor, foot; single tendon	5.0	60	3
98.2	▲	28222	multiple tendons	6.0	60	3
98.2	▲	28225	Tenolysis, extensor, foot; single tendon	2.8	60	3
98.2	▲	28226	multiple tendons	3.6	60	3
98.2	▲	28230	Tenotomy, open, tendon flexor; foot, single or multiple tendon(s) (separate procedure)	3.0	30	3
98.2	▲	28232	toe, single tendon (separate procedure)	1.4	30	3
	▲	28234	Tenotomy, open, extensor, foot or toe, each tendon	1.0	30	3
98.2	▲	28238	Reconstruction (advancement), posterior tibial tendon with excision of accessory navicular bone (eg, Kidner type procedure)	6.9	60	3
		28240	Tenotomy, lengthening, or release, abductor hallucis muscle	3.6	60	3
98.2	▲	28250	Division of plantar fascia and muscle (eg, Steindler stripping) (separate procedure)	6.0	60	3
		28260	Capsulotomy, midfoot; medial release only (separate procedure)	9.4	60	3
		28261	with tendon lengthening	10.7	60	3
98.2	▲	28262	extensive, including posterior talotibial capsulotomy and tendon(s) lengthening (eg, resistant clubfoot deformity)	20.0	90	3
98.2	▲	28264	Capsulotomy, midtarsal (eg, Heyman type procedure)	12.1	90	3
98.2	▲	28270	Capsulotomy; metatarsophalangeal joint, with or without tenorrhaphy, each joint (separate procedure)	2.4	60	3
98.2	▲	28272	interphalangeal joint, each joint (separate procedure)	1.7	60	3
98.2	▲	28280	Syndactylization, toes (eg, webbing or Kelikian type procedure)	3.4	45	3
98.2	▲	28285	Correction, hammertoe (eg, interphalangeal fusion, partial or total phalangectomy)	4.8	60	3
98.2	▲	28286	Correction, cock-up fifth toe, with plastic skin closure (eg, Ruiz-Mora type procedure)	4.8	60	3
98.2	▲	28288	Ostectomy, partial, exostectomy or condylectomy, metatarsal head, each metatarsal head	4.8	60	3
98.2	●	28289	Hallux rigidus correction with cheilectomy, debridement and capsular release of the first metatarsophalangeal joint	(I) 5.5	90	3
98.2	▲	28290	Correction, hallux valgus (bunion), with or without sesamoidectomy; simple exostectomy (eg, Silver type procedure)	6.5	90	3

UPD		Code	Description	Units	FUD	Anes
		28292	Keller, McBride or Mayo type procedure	7.6	90	3
		28293	resection of joint with implant	8.5	90	3
98.2	▲	28294	with tendon transplants (eg, Joplin type procedure)	9.5	90	3
		28296	with metatarsal osteotomy (eg, Mitchell, Chevron, or concentric type procedures)	12.5	90	3
		28297	Lapidus type procedure	9.5	90	3
		28298	by phalanx osteotomy	7.0	90	3
		28299	by other methods (eg, double osteotomy)	12.5	90	3
98.2	▲	28300	Osteotomy; calcaneus (eg, Dwyer or Chambers type procedure), with or without internal fixation	9.6	90	3
		28302	talus	9.0	90	3
98.2	▲	28304	Osteotomy, tarsal bones, other than calcaneus or talus;	8.1	90	3
98.2	▲	28305	with autograft (includes obtaining graft) (eg, Fowler type)	10.0	90	3
98.2	▲	28306	Osteotomy, with or without lengthening, shortening or angular correction, metatarsal; first metatarsal	7.2	90	3
98.2	▲	28307	first metatarsal with autograft (other than first toe)	8.2	90	3
98.2	▲	28308	other than first metatarsal, each	5.6	90	3
98.2	▲	28309	multiple (eg, Swanson type cavus foot procedure)	7.0	60	3
98.2	▲	28310	Osteotomy, shortening, angular or rotational correction; proximal phalanx, first toe (separate procedure)	3.1	90	3
		28312	other phalanges, any toe	2.0	90	3
98.2	▲	28313	Reconstruction, angular deformity of toe, soft tissue procedures only (eg, overlapping second toe, fifth toe, curly toes)	4.2	90	3
		28315	Sesamoidectomy, first toe (separate procedure)	4.0	90	3
98.2	▲	28320	Repair, nonunion or malunion; tarsal bones	8.0	120	3
		28322	metatarsal, with or without bone graft (includes obtaining graft)	4.9	120	3
		28340	Reconstruction, toe, macrodactyly; soft tissue resection	10.0	90	3
		28341	requiring bone resection	12.0	90	3
		28344	Reconstruction, toe(s); polydactyly	6.0	90	3
		28345	syndactyly, with or without skin graft(s), each web	8.0	90	3
		28360	Reconstruction, cleft foot	BR	90	3
		28400	Closed treatment of calcaneal fracture; without manipulation	2.6	90	3
		28405	with manipulation	4.0	90	3

+ Add-on Code   ⊘ Modifier -51 Exempt   ▲ Revised code   ● New code   **M** RVSI code or deleted from CPT   **(I)** Interim Value

UPD	Code	Description	Units	FUD	Anes
	28406	Percutaneous skeletal fixation of calcaneal fracture, with manipulation	5.5	90	3
	28415	Open treatment of calcaneal fracture, with or without internal or external fixation;	10.2	90	3
	28420	with primary iliac or other autogenous bone graft (includes obtaining graft)	14.0	90	3
	28430	Closed treatment of talus fracture; without manipulation	2.7	90	3
	28435	with manipulation	3.7	90	3
	28436	Percutaneous skeletal fixation of talus fracture, with manipulation	4.4	90	3
	28445	Open treatment of talus fracture, with or without internal or external fixation	10.2	90	3
	28450	Treatment of tarsal bone fracture (except talus and calcaneus); without manipulation, each	2.6	90	3
	28455	with manipulation, each	3.2	90	3
	28456	Percutaneous skeletal fixation of tarsal bone fracture (except talus and calcaneus), with manipulation, each	3.9	90	3
	28465	Open treatment of tarsal bone fracture (except talus and calcaneus), with or without internal or external fixation, each	6.1	90	3
	28470	Closed treatment of metatarsal fracture; without manipulation, each	2.2	60	3
	28475	with manipulation, each	2.5	60	3
	28476	Percutaneous skeletal fixation of metatarsal fracture, with manipulation, each	3.2	60	3
	28485	Open treatment of metatarsal fracture, with or without internal or external fixation, each	6.1	90	3
	28490	Closed treatment of fracture great toe, phalanx or phalanges; without manipulation	1.0	30	3
	28495	with manipulation	1.1	30	3
	28496	Percutaneous skeletal fixation of fracture great toe, phalanx or phalanges, with manipulation	1.8	30	3
	28505	Open treatment of fracture great toe, phalanx or phalanges, with or without internal or external fixation	4.2	60	3
	28510	Closed treatment of fracture, phalanx or phalanges, other than great toe; without manipulation, each	0.7	30	3
	28515	with manipulation, each	1.1	30	3
	28525	Open treatment of fracture, phalanx or phalanges, other than great toe, with or without internal or external fixation, each	3.3	60	3
	28530	Closed treatment of sesamoid fracture	2.0	60	3
	28531	Open treatment of sesamoid fracture, with or without internal fixation	(I) 2.9	60	3

UPD		Code	Description	Units	FUD	Anes
		28540	Closed treatment of tarsal bone dislocation, other than talotarsal; without anesthesia	3.0	45	0
		28545	requiring anesthesia	4.5	45	3
		28546	Percutaneous skeletal fixation of tarsal bone dislocation, other than talotarsal, with manipulation	5.5	45	3
		28555	Open treatment of tarsal bone dislocation, with or without internal or external fixation	8.5	90	3
		28570	Closed treatment of talotarsal joint dislocation; without anesthesia	2.4	45	0
		28575	requiring anesthesia	3.9	45	3
		28576	Percutaneous skeletal fixation of talotarsal joint dislocation, with manipulation	(I) 5.4	45	3
		28585	Open treatment of talotarsal joint dislocation, with or without internal or external fixation	10.0	90	3
		28600	Closed treatment of tarsometatarsal joint dislocation; without anesthesia	2.0	45	0
		28605	requiring anesthesia	2.6	45	3
		28606	Percutaneous skeletal fixation of tarsometatarsal joint dislocation, with manipulation	3.6	45	3
		28615	Open treatment of tarsometatarsal joint dislocation, with or without internal or external fixation	6.2	90	3
		28630*	Closed treatment of metatarsophalangeal joint dislocation; without anesthesia	1.8	7	0
		28635*	requiring anesthesia	2.8	0	3
		28636	Percutaneous skeletal fixation of metatarsophalangeal joint dislocation, with manipulation	(I) 3.9	7	3
		28645	Open treatment of metatarsophalangeal joint dislocation, with or without internal or external fixation	4.2	90	3
		28660*	Closed treatment of interphalangeal joint dislocation; without anesthesia	1.2	0	0
		28665*	requiring anesthesia	2.2	0	3
		28666	Percutaneous skeletal fixation of interphalangeal joint dislocation, with manipulation	(I) 3.7	45	3
		28675	Open treatment of interphalangeal joint dislocation, with or without internal or external fixation	4.2	60	3
98.2	▲	28705	Arthrodesis; pantalar	18.0	120	3
98.2	▲	28715	triple	15.0	120	3
98.2	▲	28725	subtalar	12.0	120	3
		28730	Arthrodesis, midtarsal or tarsometatarsal, multiple or transverse;	11.0	120	3

UPD		Code	Description	Units	FUD	Anes
98.2	▲	28735	with osteotomy (eg, flatfoot correction)	14.0	120	3
98.2	▲	28737	Arthrodesis, with tendon lengthening and advancement, midtarsal navicular-cuneiform (eg, Miller type procedure)	12.0	120	3
		28740	Arthrodesis, midtarsal or tarsometatarsal, single joint	9.0	120	3
		28750	Arthrodesis, great toe; metatarsophalangeal joint	7.1	120	3
		28755	interphalangeal joint	4.8	120	3
98.2	▲	28760	Arthrodesis, with extensor hallucis longus transfer to first metatarsal neck, great toe, interphalangeal joint (eg, Jones type procedure)	6.2	120	3
98.2	▲	28800	Amputation, foot; midtarsal (eg, Chopart type procedure)	10.5	90	3
		28805	transmetatarsal	10.5	90	3
		28810	Amputation, metatarsal, with toe, single	5.8	90	3
		28820	Amputation, toe; metatarsophalangeal joint	3.1	45	3
		28825	interphalangeal joint	2.4	45	3
98.2		28899	Unlisted procedure, foot or toes	BR	0	3
		29000	Application of halo type body cast (see 20661-20663 for insertion)	5.0	2	3
		29010	Application of Risser jacket, localizer, body; only	3.2	2	3
		29015	including head	3.9	2	3
		29020	Application of turnbuckle jacket, body; only	3.2	2	3
		29025	including head	3.9	2	3
		29035	Application of body cast, shoulder to hips;	1.8	2	3
		29040	including head, Minerva type	2.8	2	3
		29044	including one thigh	2.2	2	3
		29046	including both thighs	2.4	2	3
98.2		29049	Application; plaster figure-of-eight	1.3	2	4
98.2		29055	shoulder spica	2.0	2	4
98.2		29058	plaster Velpeau	1.3	2	4
		29065	shoulder to hand (long arm)	0.8	2	3
		29075	elbow to finger (short arm)	0.6	2	3
		29085	hand and lower forearm (gauntlet)	0.6	2	3
		29105	Application of long arm splint (shoulder to hand)	0.6	2	3
		29125	Application of short arm splint (forearm to hand); static	0.5	2	3
		29126	dynamic	1.3	2	3

UPD	Code	Description	Units	FUD	Anes
	29130	Application of finger splint; static	0.5	2	3
	29131	dynamic	1.3	2	3
	29200	Strapping; thorax	0.4	0	3
	29220	low back	0.5	0	3
98.2	29240	shoulder (eg, Velpeau)	0.6	0	4
	29260	elbow or wrist	0.3	0	3
	29280	hand or finger	0.3	0	3
	29305	Application of hip spica cast; one leg	2.0	2	3
	29325	one and one-half spica or both legs	2.2	2	3
	29345	Application of long leg cast (thigh to toes);	1.1	2	3
	29355	walker or ambulatory type	1.3	2	3
	29358	Application of long leg cast brace	1.0	2	3
	29365	Application of cylinder cast (thigh to ankle)	1.0	2	3
	29405	Application of short leg cast (below knee to toes);	0.8	2	3
	29425	walking or ambulatory type	1.0	2	3
	29435	Application of patellar tendon bearing (PTB) cast	1.5	2	3
	29440	Adding walker to previously applied cast	0.3	2	3
	29445	Application of rigid total contact leg cast	(I) 1.6	2	3
	29450	Application of clubfoot cast with molding or manipulation, long or short leg	0.4	2	3
	29505	Application of long leg splint (thigh to ankle or toes)	0.7	2	3
	29515	Application of short leg splint (calf to foot)	0.6	2	3
98.2	29520	Strapping; hip	0.5	0	4
	29530	knee	0.4	0	3
	29540	ankle	0.3	0	3
	29550	toes	0.3	0	3
	29580	Unna boot	0.5	0	3
	29590	Denis-Browne splint strapping	1.3	0	3
	29700	Removal or bivalving; gauntlet, boot or body cast	0.4	0	3
	29705	full arm or full leg cast	0.4	0	3
	29710	shoulder or hip spica, Minerva, or Risser jacket, etc.	0.6	0	3
	29715	turnbuckle jacket	0.7	0	3

UPD	Code	Description	Units	FUD	Anes
	29720	Repair of spica, body cast or jacket	0.3	0	3
	29730	Windowing of cast	0.3	0	3
	29740	Wedging of cast (except clubfoot casts)	0.3	0	3
	29750	Wedging of clubfoot cast	0.3	0	3
98.2	29799	Unlisted procedure, casting or strapping	BR	0	3
98.2	29800	Arthroscopy, temporomandibular joint, diagnostic, with or without synovial biopsy (separate procedure)	6.5	0	5
98.2	29804	Arthroscopy, temporomandibular joint, surgical	13.0	60	5
98.2	29815	Arthroscopy, shoulder, diagnostic, with or without synovial biopsy (separate procedure)	5.0	0	4
98.2	29819	Arthroscopy, shoulder, surgical; with removal of loose body or foreign body	12.0	60	4
98.2	29820	synovectomy, partial	13.0	60	4
98.2	29821	synovectomy, complete	16.0	60	4
98.2	29822	debridement, limited	15.0	60	4
98.2	29823	debridement, extensive	15.5	60	4
98.2	29825	with lysis and resection of adhesions, with or without manipulation	7.0	60	4
98.2	29826	decompression of subacromial space with partial acromioplasty, with or without coracoacromial release	14.0	60	4
	29830	Arthroscopy, elbow, diagnostic, with or without synovial biopsy (separate procedure)	5.0	0	3
	29834	Arthroscopy, elbow, surgical; with removal of loose body or foreign body	10.0	60	3
	29835	synovectomy, partial	12.0	60	3
	29836	synovectomy, complete	16.0	60	3
	29837	debridement, limited	10.0	60	3
	29838	debridement, extensive	10.5	60	3
	29840	Arthroscopy, wrist, diagnostic, with or without synovial biopsy (separate procedure)	7.2	0	3
	29843	Arthroscopy, wrist, surgical; for infection, lavage and drainage	7.5	60	3
	29844	synovectomy, partial	7.6	60	3
	29845	synovectomy, complete	9.0	60	3
	29846	excision and/or repair of triangular fibrocartilage and/or joint debridement	9.8	60	3
	29847	internal fixation for fracture or instability	9.8	60	3

UPD		Code	Description	Units	FUD	Anes
	▲	29848	Endoscopy, wrist, surgical, with release of transverse carpal ligament	(I) 8.5	90	3
		29850	Arthroscopically aided treatment of intercondylar spine(s) and/or tuberosity fracture(s) of the knee, with or without manipulation; without internal or external fixation (includes arthroscopy)	(I) 11.5	90	3
		29851	with internal or external fixation (includes arthroscopy)	(I) 17.9	90	3
		29855	Arthroscopically aided treatment of tibial fracture, proximal (plateau); unicondylar, with or without internal or external fixation (includes arthroscopy)	(I) 12.7	90	3
		29856	bicondylar, with or without internal or external fixation (includes arthroscopy)	(I) 13.7	90	3
97.2		29860	Arthroscopy, hip, diagnostic with or without synovial biopsy (separate procedure)	(I) 10.4	0	4
97.2		29861	Arthroscopy, hip, surgical; with removal of loose body or foreign body	(I) 13.6	90	4
97.2		29862	Arthroscopy, hip, surgical; with debridement/shaving of articular cartilage (chondroplasty), abrasion arthroplasty, and/or resection of labrum	(I) 17.6	90	4
97.2		29863	Arthroscopy, hip, surgical; with synovectomy	(I) 17.6	90	4
		29870	Arthroscopy, knee, diagnostic, with or without synovial biopsy (separate procedure)	6.8	0	3
		29871	Arthroscopy, knee, surgical; for infection, lavage and drainage	7.5	60	3
		29874	for removal of loose body or foreign body (eg, osteochondritis dissecans fragmentation, chondral fragmentation)	10.0	60	3
		29875	synovectomy, limited (eg, plica or shelf resection) (separate procedure)	14.0	60	3
		29876	synovectomy, major, two or more compartments (eg, medial or lateral)	16.0	60	3
		29877	debridement/shaving of articular cartilage (chondroplasty)	14.0	60	3
		29879	abrasion arthroplasty (includes chondroplasty where necessary) or multiple drilling	14.0	60	3
		29880	with meniscectomy (medial AND lateral, including any meniscal shaving)	18.1	60	3
		29881	with meniscectomy (medial OR lateral, including any meniscal shaving)	14.0	60	3
		29882	with meniscus repair (medial OR lateral)	17.5	60	3
		29883	with meniscus repair (medial AND lateral)	21.0	60	3
		29884	with lysis of adhesions, with or without manipulation (separate procedure)	16.0	60	3

+ Add-on Code   ⊘ Modifier -51 Exempt   ▲ Revised code   ● New code   M RVSI code or deleted from CPT   (I) Interim Value

UPD	Code	Description	Units	FUD	Anes
	29885	drilling for osteochondritis dissecans with bone grafting, with or without internal fixation (including debridement of base of lesion)	16.0	60	3
	29886	drilling for intact osteochondritis dissecans lesion	16.0	60	3
	29887	drilling for intact osteochondritis dissecans lesion with internal fixation	17.5	60	3
98.2	**29888**	Arthroscopically aided anterior cruciate ligament repair/augmentation or reconstruction	31.0	60	3
98.2	**29889**	Arthroscopically aided posterior cruciate ligament repair/augmentation or reconstruction	31.0	60	3
97.2	**29891**	Arthroscopy, ankle, surgical; excision of osteochondral defect of talus and/or tibia, including drilling of the defect	(I) 11.5	90	3
97.2	**29892**	Arthroscopically aided repair of large osteochondritis dissecans lesion, talar dome fracture, or tibial plafond fracture, with or without internal fixation (includes arthroscopy)	(I) 11.0	90	3
97.2	**29893**	Endoscopic plantar fasciotomy	(I) 6.0	90	3
	29894	Arthroscopy, ankle (tibiotalar and fibulotalar joints), surgical; with removal of loose body or foreign body	9.0	60	3
	29895	synovectomy, partial	9.0	60	3
	29897	debridement, limited	9.0	60	3
	29898	debridement, extensive	10.0	60	3
98.2	**29909**	Unlisted procedure, arthroscopy	BR	0	4

UPD		Code	Description	Units	FUD	Anes
Respiratory System						
98.2		**30000***	Drainage abscess or hematoma, nasal, internal approach	1.3	0	5
		30020*	Drainage abscess or hematoma, nasal septum	1.4	0	5
		30100	Biopsy, intranasal	0.7	0	4
		30110	Excision, nasal polyp(s), simple	2.4	7	5
		30115	Excision, nasal polyp(s), extensive	5.1	15	5
		30117	Excision or destruction, any method (including laser), intranasal lesion; internal approach	2.0	7	5
		30118	external approach (lateral rhinotomy)	7.5	30	5
		30120	Excision or surgical planing of skin of nose for rhinophyma	9.0	60	5
		30124	Excision dermoid cyst, nose; simple, skin, subcutaneous	1.7	30	5
		30125	complex, under bone or cartilage	8.5	30	5
98.2	▲	**30130**	Excision turbinate, partial or complete, any method	2.0	30	5
98.2	▲	**30140**	Submucous resection turbinate, partial or complete, any method	5.7	90	5
98.2		**30150**	Rhinectomy; partial	6.2	90	7
98.2		**30160**	total	13.9	90	7
		30200*	Injection into turbinate(s), therapeutic	0.6	0	5
		30210*	Displacement therapy (Proetz type)	1.1	0	5
		30220	Insertion, nasal septal prosthesis (button)	1.0	30	5
98.2		**30300***	Removal foreign body, intranasal; office type procedure	1.0	0	5
98.2		**30310**	requiring general anesthesia	2.6	7	5
		30320	by lateral rhinotomy	6.2	30	5
		30400	Rhinoplasty, primary; lateral and alar cartilages and/or elevation of nasal tip	15.7	90	5
		30410	complete, external parts including bony pyramid, lateral and alar cartilages, and/or elevation of nasal tip	21.6	90	5
		30420	including major septal repair	26.2	90	5
		30430	Rhinoplasty, secondary; minor revision (small amount of nasal tip work)	6.5	45	5
		30435	intermediate revision (bony work with osteotomies)	12.5	45	5
		30450	major revision (nasal tip work and osteotomies)	16.0	45	5

UPD	Code	Description	Units	FUD	Anes
	30460	Rhinoplasty for nasal deformity secondary to congenital cleft lip and/or palate, including columellar lengthening; tip only	(I) 13.7	45	5
96.2	30462	tip, septum, osteotomies	(I) 25.0	45	5
	30520	Septoplasty or submucous resection, with or without cartilage scoring, contouring or replacement with graft	11.0	90	5
	30540	Repair choanal atresia; intranasal	13.7	60	5
	30545	transpalatine	17.4	60	5
	30560*	Lysis intranasal synechia	0.9	7	5
	30580	Repair fistula; oromaxillary (combine with 31030 if antrotomy is included)	10.0	90	5
	30600	oronasal	10.0	90	5
	30620	Septal or other intranasal dermatoplasty (does not include obtaining graft)	10.0	90	5
	30630	Repair nasal septal perforations	11.0	90	5
	30801*	Cauterization and/or ablation, mucosa of turbinates, unilateral or bilateral, any method, (separate procedure); superficial	(I) 0.8	0	5
	30802	intramural	(I) 1.6	15	5
	30901*	Control nasal hemorrhage, anterior, simple (limited cautery and/or packing) any method	1.0	0	5
	30903*	Control nasal hemorrhage, anterior, complex (extensive cautery and/or packing) any method	1.5	0	5
	30905*	Control nasal hemorrhage, posterior, with posterior nasal packs and/or cauterization, any method; initial	2.9	0	5
	30906*	subsequent	2.3	0	5
	30915	Ligation arteries; ethmoidal	12.5	30	5
	30920	internal maxillary artery, transantral	15.0	30	5
	30930	Fracture nasal turbinate(s), therapeutic	1.0	30	5
98.2	30999	Unlisted procedure, nose	BR	0	5
	31000*	Lavage by cannulation; maxillary sinus (antrum puncture or natural ostium)	1.0	0	5
	31002*	sphenoid sinus	1.0	0	5
	31020	Sinusotomy, maxillary (antrotomy); intranasal	5.5	90	5
	31030	radical (Caldwell-Luc) without removal of antrochoanal polyps	13.5	90	7
	31032	radical (Caldwell-Luc) with removal of antrochoanal polyps	14.0	90	7
	31040	Pterygomaxillary fossa surgery, any approach	20.0	90	5

UPD		Code	Description	Units	FUD	Anes
		31050	Sinusotomy, sphenoid, with or without biopsy;	8.5	90	5
		31051	with mucosal stripping or removal of polyp(s)	10.0	90	5
		31070	Sinusotomy frontal; external, simple (trephine operation)	10.5	90	5
		31075	transorbital, unilateral (for mucocele or osteoma, Lynch type)	16.0	120	5
		31080	obliterative without osteoplastic flap, brow incision (includes ablation)	16.5	120	5
		31081	obliterative, without osteoplastic flap, coronal incision (includes ablation)	16.5	120	5
		31084	obliterative, with osteoplastic flap, brow incision	24.0	120	5
		31085	obliterative, with osteoplastic flap, coronal incision	24.0	120	5
		31086	nonobliterative, with osteoplastic flap, brow incision	18.0	90	5
		31087	nonobliterative, with osteoplastic flap, coronal incision	18.0	90	5
98.2	▲	31090	Sinusotomy, unilateral, three or more paranasal sinuses (frontal, maxillary, ethmoid, sphenoid)	25.0	120	5
		31200	Ethmoidectomy; intranasal, anterior	7.0	90	5
		31201	intranasal, total	11.5	90	5
		31205	extranasal, total	14.5	90	5
98.2		31225	Maxillectomy; without orbital exenteration	22.5	120	5
		31230	with orbital exenteration (en bloc)	28.0	120	7
		31231	Nasal endoscopy, diagnostic, unilateral or bilateral (separate procedure)	1.2	0	5
		31233	Nasal/sinus endoscopy, diagnostic with maxillary sinusoscopy (via inferior meatus or canine fossa puncture)	2.6	0	5
		31235	Nasal/sinus endoscopy, diagnostic with sphenoid sinusoscopy (via puncture of sphenoidal face or cannulation of ostium)	4.5	0	5
98.1		31237	Nasal/sinus endoscopy, surgical; with biopsy, polypectomy or debridement (separate procedure)	3.2	0	5
98.1		31238	with control of epistaxis	5.4	0	5
		31239	with dacryocystorhinostomy	(I) 12.0	15	5
98.1		31240	with concha bullosa resection	4.3	0	5
98.1		31254	Nasal/sinus endoscopy, surgical; with ethmoidectomy, partial (anterior)	(I) 6.8	0	5
98.1		31255	with ethmoidectomy, total (anterior and posterior)	(I) 10.5	0	5
98.1		31256	Nasal/sinus endoscopy, surgical, with maxillary antrostomy;	(I) 5.0	0	5
98.1		31267	with removal of tissue from maxillary sinus	(I) 9.0	0	5

UPD	Code	Description	Units	FUD	Anes
98.1	31276	Nasal/sinus endoscopy, surgical with frontal sinus exploration, with or without removal of tissue from frontal sinus	(I) 13.0	0	5
98.1	31287	Nasal/sinus endoscopy, surgical, with sphenoidotomy;	7.6	0	5
98.1	31288	with removal of tissue from the sphenoid sinus	9.0	0	5
98.1	31290	Nasal/sinus endoscopy, surgical, with repair of cerebrospinal fluid leak; ethmoid region	(I) 19.0	15	5
98.1	31291	sphenoid region	(I) 20.0	15	5
98.1	31292	Nasal/sinus endoscopy, surgical; with medial or inferior orbital wall decompression	(I) 15.0	15	5
98.1	31293	with medial orbital wall and inferior orbital wall decompression	(I) 17.0	15	5
98.1	31294	with optic nerve decompression	(I) 19.0	15	5
	31299	Unlisted procedure, accessory sinuses	BR	90	5
	31300	Laryngotomy (thyrotomy, laryngofissure); with removal of tumor or laryngocele, cordectomy	14.5	90	6
	31320	diagnostic	8.0	60	6
	31360	Laryngectomy; total, without radical neck dissection	25.0	120	6
	31365	total, with radical neck dissection	36.0	120	6
	31367	subtotal supraglottic, without radical neck dissection	25.0	90	6
	31368	subtotal supraglottic, with radical neck dissection	36.0	90	6
	31370	Partial laryngectomy (hemilaryngectomy); horizontal	29.0	120	6
	31375	laterovertical	23.0	120	6
	31380	anterovertical	23.0	120	6
	31382	antero-latero-vertical	23.0	120	6
	31390	Pharyngolaryngectomy, with radical neck dissection; without reconstruction	31.0	90	6
	31395	with reconstruction	38.5	90	6
	31400	Arytenoidectomy or arytenoidopexy, external approach	20.0	120	6
	31420	Epiglottidectomy	16.0	90	6
98.2	⊘ 31500	Intubation, endotracheal, emergency procedure	1.5	0	6
		Note: Procedure listed may be considered a necessary part of and/or procedure and in such cases, not billable. If the procedure is distinct by encounter or performed in conjunction with a procedure for which the listed service is not considered a necessary component, then multiple procedure guidelines for reduction of value do not apply for this code.			

UPD	Code	Description	Units	FUD	Anes
	31502	Tracheotomy tube change prior to establishment of fistula tract	1.0	0	6
	31505	Laryngoscopy, indirect (separate procedure); diagnostic	1.0	0	6
	31510	with biopsy	1.5	14	6
	31511	with removal of foreign body	1.6	14	6
	31512	with removal of lesion	1.5	14	6
	31513	with vocal cord injection	1.0	14	6
	31515	Laryngoscopy direct, with or without tracheoscopy; for aspiration	0.7	14	6
	31520	diagnostic, newborn	2.4	0	6
	31525	diagnostic, except newborn	3.4	0	6
	31526	diagnostic, with operating microscope	4.4	0	6
	31527	with insertion of obturator	7.5	30	6
	31528	with dilatation, initial	4.5	14	6
	31529	with dilatation, subsequent	2.5	14	6
	31530	Laryngoscopy, direct, operative, with foreign body removal;	6.0	30	6
	31531	with operating microscope	7.5	30	6
	31535	Laryngoscopy, direct, operative, with biopsy;	6.0	30	6
	31536	with operating microscope	7.5	30	6
	31540	Laryngoscopy, direct, operative, with excision of tumor and/or stripping of vocal cords or epiglottis;	6.2	30	6
	31541	with operating microscope	7.7	30	6
	31560	Laryngoscopy, direct, operative, with arytenoidectomy;	15.5	60	6
	31561	with operating microscope	19.0	60	6
	31570	Laryngoscopy, direct, with injection into vocal cord(s), therapeutic;	8.0	30	6
	31571	with operating microscope	10.0	60	6
	31575	Laryngoscopy, flexible fiberoptic; diagnostic	1.8	0	6
	31576	with biopsy	2.9	14	6
	31577	with removal of foreign body	7.0	30	6
	31578	with removal of lesion	7.8	30	6
	31579	Laryngoscopy, flexible or rigid fiberoptic, with stroboscopy	(I) 3.0	14	6
	31580	Laryngoplasty; for laryngeal web, two stage, with keel insertion and removal	25.0	90	6

UPD		Code	Description	Units	FUD	Anes
		31582	for laryngeal stenosis, with graft or core mold, including tracheotomy	24.5	90	6
		31584	with open reduction of fracture	24.5	90	6
		31585	Treatment of closed laryngeal fracture; without manipulation	2.0	0	6
		31586	with closed manipulative reduction	4.0	0	6
		31587	Laryngoplasty, cricoid split	29.0	90	6
		31588	Laryngoplasty, not otherwise specified (eg, for burns, reconstruction after partial laryngectomy)	BR	90	6
		31590	Laryngeal reinnervation by neuromuscular pedicle	20.0	120	6
		31595	Section recurrent laryngeal nerve, therapeutic (separate procedure), unilateral	16.0	120	6
98.2		31599	Unlisted procedure, larynx	BR	0	6
		31600	Tracheostomy, planned (separate procedure);	5.4	14	6
		31601	under two years	6.5	14	6
		31603	Tracheostomy, emergency procedure; transtracheal	6.5	14	6
		31605	cricothyroid membrane	6.5	14	6
		31610	Tracheostomy, fenestration procedure with skin flaps	7.0	14	6
		31611	Construction of tracheoesophageal fistula and subsequent insertion of an alaryngeal speech prosthesis (eg, voice button, Blom-Singer prosthesis)	3.0	14	6
		31612	Tracheal puncture, percutaneous with transtracheal aspiration and/or injection	0.3	0	6
		31613	Tracheostoma revision; simple, without flap rotation	4.8	60	6
		31614	complex, with flap rotation	10.8	60	6
		31615	Tracheobronchoscopy through established tracheostomy incision	2.5	0	6
98.2	▲	31622	Bronchoscopy; diagnostic, (flexible or rigid), with or without cell washing	4.7	0	6
98.2	●	31623	with brushing or protected brushings	(I) 4.7	0	6
98.2	●	31624	with bronchial alveolar lavage	(I) 4.7	0	6
		31625	with biopsy	5.8	14	6
		31628	with transbronchial lung biopsy, with or without fluoroscopic guidance	6.0	14	6
		31629	with transbronchial needle aspiration biopsy	5.8	14	6
		31630	with tracheal or bronchial dilation or closed reduction of fracture	6.5	14	6
		31631	with tracheal dilation and placement of tracheal stent	5.5	14	6

UPD		Code	Description	Units	FUD	Anes
		31635	with removal of foreign body	6.5	14	6
		31640	with excision of tumor	6.8	14	6
		31641	with destruction of tumor or relief of stenosis by any method other than excision (eg, laser)	10.0	30	6
98.2	●	31643	with placement of catheter(s) for intracavitary radioelement application	(I) 5.0	0	6
		31645	with therapeutic aspiration of tracheobronchial tree, initial (eg, drainage of lung abscess)	5.5	0	6
		31646	with therapeutic aspiration of tracheobronchial tree, subsequent	4.7	0	6
		31656	with injection of contrast material for segmental bronchography (fiberscope only)	4.4	0	6
		31700	Catheterization, transglottic (separate procedure)	2.5	0	6
		31708	Instillation of contrast material for laryngography or bronchography, without catheterization	1.0	0	6
		31710	Catheterization for bronchography, with or without instillation of contrast material	1.4	0	6
		31715	Transtracheal injection for bronchography	0.9	0	6
		31717	Catheterization with bronchial brush biopsy	1.2	0	6
		31720	Catheter aspiration (separate procedure); nasotracheal	0.3	0	6
		31725	tracheobronchial with fiberscope, bedside	3.5	0	6
		31730	Transtracheal (percutaneous) introduction of needle wire dilator/stent or indwelling tube for oxygen therapy	(I) 4.1	0	6
	M	31731	Percutaneous insertion of catheter for transtracheal oxygen administration	(I) 3.0	0	6
		31750	Tracheoplasty; cervical	23.0	90	6
		31755	tracheopharyngeal fistulization, each stage	25.0	90	6
		31760	intrathoracic	25.0	90	15
		31766	Carinal reconstruction	25.0	90	15
		31770	Bronchoplasty; graft repair	25.0	90	15
		31775	excision stenosis and anastomosis	25.0	90	15
		31780	Excision tracheal stenosis and anastomosis; cervical	25.0	90	6
		31781	cervicothoracic	28.0	90	15
		31785	Excision of tracheal tumor or carcinoma; cervical	25.0	90	6
		31786	thoracic	32.0	90	15
		31800	Suture of tracheal wound or injury; cervical	20.0	30	6

UPD		Code	Description	Units	FUD	Anes
		31805	intrathoracic	22.0	30	15
		31820	Surgical closure tracheostomy or fistula; without plastic repair	3.0	0	6
		31825	with plastic repair	4.9	0	6
		31830	Revision of tracheostomy scar	3.0	0	6
98.2		31899	Unlisted procedure, trachea, bronchi	BR	0	15
98.2	⊘	32000*	Thoracentesis, puncture of pleural cavity for aspiration, initial or subsequent Note: Procedure listed may be considered a necessary part of and/or procedure and in such cases, not billable. If the procedure is distinct by encounter or performed in conjunction with a procedure for which the listed service is not considered a necessary component, then multiple procedure guidelines for reduction of value do not apply for this code.	2.0	0	4
98.2	●	32001	Total lung lavage (unilateral)	(I) 5.0	0	6
98.2	⊘	32002	Thoracentesis with insertion of tube with or without water seal (eg, for pneumothorax) (separate procedure) Note: Procedure listed may be considered a necessary part of and/or procedure and in such cases, not billable. If the procedure is distinct by encounter or performed in conjunction with a procedure for which the listed service is not considered a necessary component, then multiple procedure guidelines for reduction of value do not apply for this code.	2.5	0	6
98.2		32005	Chemical pleurodesis (eg, for recurrent or persistent pneumothorax)	2.2	0	4
98.2	⊘	32020	Tube thoracostomy with or without water seal (eg, for abscess, hemothorax, empyema) (separate procedure) Note: Procedure listed may be considered a necessary part of and/or procedure and in such cases, not billable. If the procedure is distinct by encounter or performed in conjunction with a procedure for which the listed service is not considered a necessary component, then multiple procedure guidelines for reduction of value do not apply for this code.	2.5	0	6
98.2		32035	Thoracostomy; with rib resection for empyema	9.0	90	6
98.2		32036	with open flap drainage for empyema	10.0	90	6
	M	32050	Insertion Pluralperitoneal Shunt (Denver Shunt)	(I) 20.0	90	15
		32095	Thoracotomy, limited, for biopsy of lung or pleura	9.0	90	13
		32100	Thoracotomy, major; with exploration and biopsy	14.0	90	13
		32110	with control of traumatic hemorrhage and/or repair of lung tear	16.0	90	13
		32120	for postoperative complications	15.0	90	13

UPD		Code	Description	Units	FUD	Anes
		32124	with open intrapleural pneumonolysis	16.0	90	13
		32140	with cyst(s) removal, with or without a pleural procedure	16.0	90	13
		32141	with excision-plication of bullae, with or without any pleural procedure	16.0	90	13
		32150	with removal of intrapleural foreign body or fibrin deposit	14.0	90	13
		32151	with removal of intrapulmonary foreign body	14.0	90	13
98.2		32160	with cardiac massage	15.0	90	15
		32200	Pneumonostomy; with open drainage of abscess or cyst	14.0	90	13
98.2		32201	Pneumonostomy; with percutaneous drainage of abscess or cyst	(I) 5.0	10	13
		32215	Pleural scarification for repeat pneumothorax	14.0	90	13
		32220	Decortication, pulmonary, (separate procedure); total	20.0	90	15
		32225	Decortication, pulmonary (separate procedure); partial	14.0	90	15
		32310	Pleurectomy, parietal (separate procedure)	27.0	90	15
		32320	Decortication and parietal pleurectomy	24.0	90	15
		32400*	Biopsy, pleura; percutaneous needle	1.2	0	4
		32402	open	10.0	0	13
98.2		32405	Biopsy, lung or mediastinum, percutaneous needle	3.5	0	4
		32420*	Pneumonocentesis, puncture of lung for aspiration	1.5	0	4
98.2		32440	Removal of lung, total pneumonectomy;	27.0	90	13
	M	32441	donor pneumectomy	(I) 32.0	0	7
		32442	Removal of lung, total pneumonectomy; with resection of segment of trachea followed by broncho-tracheal anastomosis (sleeve pneumonectomy)	(I) 34.0	90	15
98.2		32445	Removal of lung, total pneumonectomy; extrapleural	(I) 30.0	90	13
98.2		32480	Removal of lung, other than total pneumonectomy; single lobe (lobectomy)	25.0	90	13
98.2		32482	two lobes (bilobectomy)	26.5	90	13
98.2		32484	single segment (segmentectomy)	28.0	90	13
		32486	with circumferential resection of segment of bronchus followed by broncho-bronchial anastomosis (sleeve lobectomy)	29.0	90	15
98.2		32488	all remaining lung following previous removal of a portion of lung (completion pneumonectomy)	33.5	90	13

UPD		Code	Description	Units	FUD	Anes
98.2		**32491**	excision-plication of emphysematous lung(s) (bullous or non-bullous) for lung volume reduction, sternal split or transthoracic approach, with or without any pleural procedure	(I) 29.0	90	13
98.2		**32500**	wedge resection, single or multiple	19.0	90	13
98.2	**+**	**32501**	Resection and repair of portion of bronchus (bronchoplasty) when performed at time of lobectomy or segmentectomy (List separately in addition to code for primary procedure) Note: This code is an add-on procedure and as such is valued appropriately. Multiple procedure guidelines for reduction of value are not applicable.	(I) 7.0	0	0
98.2		**32520**	Resection of lung; with resection of chest wall	30.0	90	15
98.2		**32522**	with reconstruction of chest wall, without prosthesis	34.0	90	15
98.2		**32525**	with major reconstruction of chest wall, with prosthesis	36.0	90	15
		32540	Extrapleural enucleation of empyema (empyemectomy)	20.0	90	13
96.1		**32601**	Thoracoscopy, diagnostic (separate procedure); lungs and pleural space, without biopsy	(I) 7.0	0	13
96.1		**32602**	lungs and pleural space, with biopsy	(I) 7.5	15	13
96.1		**32603**	pericardial sac, without biopsy	(I) 13.0	15	13
96.1		**32604**	pericardial sac, with biopsy	(I) 14.4	15	13
96.1		**32605**	mediastinal space, without biopsy	(I) 8.8	15	13
96.1		**32606**	mediastinal space, with biopsy	(I) 13.7	15	13
98.2		**32650**	Thoracoscopy, surgical; with pleurodesis, any method	(I) 13.4	15	15
98.2		**32651**	with partial pulmonary decortication	(I) 18.4	15	15
98.2		**32652**	with total pulmonary decortication, including intrapleural pneumonolysis	(I) 23.6	15	15
96.1		**32653**	with removal of intrapleural foreign body or fibrin deposit	(I) 10.2	15	13
96.1		**32654**	with control of traumatic hemorrhage	(I) 15.4	15	13
96.1		**32655**	with excision-plication of bullae, including any pleural procedure	(I) 16.0	15	13
96.1		**32656**	with parietal pleurectomy	(I) 14.3	15	13
96.1		**32657**	with wedge resection of lung, single or multiple	(I) 17.3	15	13
98.2		**32658**	with removal of clot or foreign body from pericardial sac	(I) 16.6	15	15
98.2		**32659**	with creation of pericardial window or partial resection of pericardial sac for drainage	(I) 15.0	15	15
98.2		**32660**	with total pericardiectomy	(I) 22.3	15	15
98.2		**32661**	with excision of pericardial cyst, tumor, or mass	(I) 16.0	15	15

+ Add-on Code   ⊘ Modifier -51 Exempt   ▲ Revised code   ● New code   **M** RVSI code or deleted from CPT   **(I)** Interim Value

UPD	Code	Description	Units	FUD	Anes
96.1	**32662**	with excision of mediastinal cyst, tumor, or mass	(I) 16.2	15	13
96.1	**32663**	with lobectomy, total or segmental	(I) 26.2	15	13
96.1	**32664**	with thoracic sympathectomy	(I) 18.3	15	13
96.1	**32665**	with esophagomyotomy (Heller type)	(I) 19.5	15	13
	32800	Repair lung hernia through chest wall	12.0	30	13
	32810	Closure of chest wall following open flap drainage for empyema (Clagett type procedure)	20.0	60	13
98.2	**32815**	Open closure of major bronchial fistula	30.0	60	15
98.2	**32820**	Major reconstruction, chest wall (post-traumatic)	30.0	60	10
	32850	Donor pneumonectomy(ies) with preparation and maintenance of allograft (cadaver)	(I) 17.0	0	7
98.2	**32851**	Lung transplant, single; without cardiopulmonary bypass	(I) 50.0	90	20
98.2	**32852**	with cardiopulmonary bypass	(I) 56.0	90	20
98.2	**32853**	Lung transplant, double (bilateral sequential or en bloc); without cardiopulmonary bypass	(I) 60.0	90	20
98.2	**32854**	with cardiopulmonary bypass	(I) 65.0	90	20
M	**32855**	with bronchoplasty	(I) 144.0	90	15
98.2	**32900**	Resection of ribs, extrapleural, all stages	14.0	90	6
	32905	Thoracoplasty, Schede type or extrapleural (all stages);	14.0	90	10
	32906	with closure of bronchopleural fistula	20.0	90	10
98.2	**32940**	Pneumonolysis, extraperiosteal, including filling or packing procedures	14.0	90	13
	32960*	Pneumothorax, therapeutic, intrapleural injection of air	1.2	0	4
98.2	**32999**	Unlisted procedure, lungs and pleura	BR	90	13

Cardiovascular System

UPD	Code	Description	Units	FUD	Anes
	33010*	Pericardiocentesis; initial	2.2	0	15
	33011*	subsequent	2.2	0	15
	33015	Tube pericardiostomy	3.0	10	15
	33020	Pericardiotomy for removal of clot or foreign body (primary procedure)	16.0	90	15
	33025	Creation of pericardial window or partial resection for drainage	17.0	90	15
	33030	Pericardiectomy, subtotal or complete; without cardiopulmonary bypass	20.0	90	15
98.2	**33031**	with cardiopulmonary bypass	29.0	90	20

UPD		Code	Description	Units	FUD	Anes
		33050	Excision of pericardial cyst or tumor	19.0	90	15
98.2		**33120**	Excision of intracardiac tumor, resection with cardiopulmonary bypass	50.0	90	20
		33130	Resection of external cardiac tumor	30.0	90	15
		33200	Insertion of permanent pacemaker with epicardial electrode(s); by thoracotomy	19.5	90	15
		33201	by xiphoid approach	15.0	90	15
96.1		**33206**	Insertion or replacement of permanent pacemaker with transvenous electrode(s); atrial	10.5	90	4
		33207	ventricular	12.5	90	4
96.1		**33208**	atrial and ventricular	13.0	90	4
96.1		**33210**	Insertion or replacement of temporary transvenous single chamber cardiac electrode or pacemaker catheter (separate procedure)	5.5	7	4
96.1		**33211**	Insertion or replacement of temporary transvenous dual chamber pacing electrodes (separate procedure)	(I) 6.0	7	4
98.2		**33212**	Insertion or replacement of pacemaker pulse generator only; single chamber, atrial or ventricular	9.0	7	4
98.2		**33213**	dual chamber	(I) 10.5	7	4
96.1		**33214**	Upgrade of implanted pacemaker system, conversion of single chamber system to dual chamber system (includes removal of previously placed pulse generator, testing of existing lead, insertion of new lead, insertion of new pulse generator)	(I) 13.0	15	4
96.1		**33216**	Insertion, replacement or repositioning of permanent transvenous electrode(s) only (15 days or more after initial insertion); single chamber, atrial or ventricular	8.5	15	4
96.1		**33217**	dual chamber	(I) 9.5	15	4
96.1		**33218**	Repair of pacemaker electrode(s) only; single chamber, atrial or ventricular	7.0	15	4
96.1	M	**33219**	with replacement of pulse generator	8.1	15	4
96.1		**33220**	dual chamber	(I) 9.0	15	4
96.1		**33222**	Revision or relocation of skin pocket for pacemaker	8.0	15	3
96.1		**33223**	Revision or relocation of skin pocket for implantable cardioverter-defibrillator	(I) 11.0	15	3
98.2		**33233**	Removal of permanent pacemaker pulse generator	(I) 3.2	15	4
98.2		**33234**	Removal of transvenous pacemaker electrode(s); single lead system, atrial or ventricular	(I) 15.3	15	6
98.2		**33235**	dual lead system	(I) 17.0	15	6
		33236	Removal of permanent epicardial pacemaker and electrodes by thoracotomy; single lead system, atrial or ventricular	(I) 20.5	90	15

UPD	Code	Description	Units	FUD	Anes
	33237	dual lead system	(I) 22.0	90	15
98.2	33238	Removal of permanent transvenous electrode(s) by thoracotomy	(I) 24.0	90	13
98.2	33240	Insertion or replacement of implantable cardioverter-defibrillator pulse generator only	(I) 12.0	15	7
98.2	33241	Removal of implantable cardioverter-defibrillator pulse generator only	(I) 8.5	15	7
	33242	Repair of implantable cardioverter-defibrillator pulse generator and/or leads	(I) 18.7	15	7
	33243	Removal of implantable cardioverter-defibrillator pulse generator and/or lead system; by thoracotomy	(I) 42.5	90	15
	33244	by other than thoracotomy	(I) 24.0	15	7
96.1	33245	Implantation or replacement of implantable cardioverter-defibrillator pads by thoracotomy, with or without sensing electrodes;	19.0	15	15
	33246	with insertion of implantable cardioverter-defibrillator pulse generator	27.5	90	15
96.1	33247	Insertion or replacement of implantable cardioverter-defibrillator lead(s), by other than thoracotomy;	(I) 17.0	90	7
96.1	33249	with insertion of cardio-defibrillator pulse generator	(I) 27.0	90	7
	33250	Operative ablation of supraventricular arrhythmogenic focus or pathway (eg, Wolff-Parkinson-White, A-V node re-entry), tract(s) and/or focus (foci); without cardiopulmonary bypass	(I) 25.0	90	15
	33251	with cardiopulmonary bypass	(I) 32.0	90	20
98.2	33253	Operative incisions and reconstruction of atria for treatment of atrial fibrillation or atrial flutter (eg, maze procedure)	(I) 43.0	90	20
	33261	Operative ablation of ventricular arrhythmogenic focus with cardiopulmonary bypass	(I) 28.5	90	20
	33300	Repair of cardiac wound; without bypass	24.0	90	15
	33305	with cardiopulmonary bypass	33.0	90	20
	33310	Cardiotomy, exploratory (includes removal of foreign body); without bypass	24.0	90	15
	33315	with cardiopulmonary bypass	40.0	90	20
	33320	Suture repair of aorta or great vessels; without shunt or cardiopulmonary bypass	36.0	90	15
98.2	33321	with shunt bypass	(I) 40.0	90	15
	33322	with cardiopulmonary bypass	45.0	90	20
	33330	Insertion of graft, aorta or great vessels; without shunt, or cardiopulmonary bypass	45.0	90	15
98.2	33332	with shunt bypass	(I) 47.0	90	15

UPD	Code	Description	Units	FUD	Anes
	33335	with cardiopulmonary bypass	56.0	90	20
	33400	Valvuloplasty, aortic valve; open, with cardiopulmonary bypass	40.0	90	20
98.2	33401	open, with inflow occlusion	38.0	90	20
	33403	using transventricular dilation, with cardiopulmonary bypass	41.0	90	20
98.2	33404	Construction of apical-aortic conduit	BR	90	20
	33405	Replacement, aortic valve, with cardiopulmonary bypass; with prosthetic valve other than homograft	43.0	90	20
	33406	with homograft valve (freehand)	(I) 47.0	90	20
	33411	Replacement, aortic valve; with aortic annulus enlargement, noncoronary cusp	(I) 46.0	90	20
	33412	with transventricular aortic annulus enlargement (Konno procedure)	(I) 46.0	90	20
98.2	33413	by translocation of autologous pulmonary valve with homograft replacement of pulmonary valve (Ross procedure)	(I) 51.0	90	20
98.2	33414	Repair of left ventricular outflow tract obstruction by patch enlargement of the outflow tract	(I) 44.0	90	20
	33415	Resection or incision of subvalvular tissue for discrete subvalvular aortic stenosis	42.0	90	20
	33416	Ventriculomyotomy (-myectomy) for idiopathic hypertrophic subaortic stenosis (eg, asymmetric septal hypertrophy)	(I) 42.0	90	20
	33417	Aortoplasty (gusset) for supravalvular stenosis	43.0	90	20
	33420	Valvotomy, mitral valve; closed heart	32.0	90	15
	33422	open heart, with cardiopulmonary bypass	43.0	90	20
	33425	Valvuloplasty, mitral valve, with cardiopulmonary bypass;	45.0	90	20
	33426	with prosthetic ring	(I) 45.0	90	20
	33427	radical reconstruction, with or without ring	45.0	90	20
	33430	Replacement, mitral valve, with cardiopulmonary bypass	45.0	90	20
	33460	Valvectomy, tricuspid valve, with cardiopulmonary bypass	40.0	90	20
98.2	33463	Valvuloplasty, tricuspid valve; without ring insertion	43.0	90	20
98.2	33464	with ring insertion	45.5	90	20
	33465	Replacement, tricuspid valve, with cardiopulmonary bypass	41.0	90	20
	33468	Tricuspid valve repositioning and plication for Ebstein anomaly	40.0	90	20
	33470	Valvotomy, pulmonary valve, closed heart; transventricular	30.0	90	15

UPD	Code	Description	Units	FUD	Anes
	33471	via pulmonary artery	32.5	90	15
98.2	**33472**	Valvotomy, pulmonary valve, open heart; with inflow occlusion	34.0	90	20
	33474	with cardiopulmonary bypass	37.0	90	20
98.2	**33475**	Replacement, pulmonary valve	(I) 43.0	90	20
	33476	Right ventricular resection for infundibular stenosis, with or without commissurotomy	42.0	90	20
	33478	Outflow tract augmentation (gusset), with or without commissurotomy or infundibular resection	42.0	90	20
97.2	**33496**	Repair of non-structural prosthetic valve dysfunction with cardiopulmonary bypass (separate procedure)	(I) 42.5	90	20
	33500	Repair of coronary arteriovenous or arteriocardiac chamber fistula; with cardiopulmonary bypass	35.0	90	20
98.2	**33501**	without cardiopulmonary bypass	23.3	90	15
	33502	Repair of anomalous coronary artery; by ligation	28.0	90	15
	33503	by graft, without cardiopulmonary bypass	31.0	90	15
	33504	by graft, with cardiopulmonary bypass	40.0	90	20
98.2	**33505**	with construction of intrapulmonary artery tunnel (Takeuchi procedure)	(I) 43.0	90	20
98.2	**33506**	by translocation from pulmonary artery to aorta	(I) 43.0	90	20
	33510	Coronary artery bypass, vein only; single coronary venous graft	42.0	90	20
	33511	two coronary venous grafts	45.0	90	20
	33512	three coronary venous grafts	48.0	90	20
	33513	four coronary venous grafts	51.0	90	20
	33514	five coronary venous grafts	54.0	90	20
	33516	six or more coronary venous grafts	56.0	90	20
98.2	⊘ **33517**	Coronary artery bypass, using venous graft(s) and arterial graft(s); single vein graft (list separately in addition to code for arterial graft) Note: Multiple procedure guidelines for reduction of value are not applicable for this code.	(I) 2.7	0	20
98.2	⊘ **33518**	two venous grafts (list separately in addition to code for arterial graft) Note: Multiple procedure guidelines for reduction of value are not applicable for this code.	(I) 5.5	0	20

UPD		Code	Description	Units	FUD	Anes
98.2	⊘	33519	three venous grafts (list separately in addition to code for arterial graft)	(I) 8.2	0	20
			Note: Multiple procedure guidelines for reduction of value are not applicable for this code.			
98.2	⊘	33521	four venous grafts (list separately in addition to code for arterial graft)	(I) 11.0	0	20
			Note: Multiple procedure guidelines for reduction of value are not applicable for this code.			
98.2	⊘	33522	five venous grafts (list separately in addition to code for arterial graft)	(I) 13.7	0	20
			Note: Multiple procedure guidelines for reduction of value are not applicable for this code.			
98.2	⊘	33523	six or more venous grafts (list separately in addition to code for arterial graft)	(I) 16.5	0	20
			Note: Multiple procedure guidelines for reduction of value are not applicable for this code.			
98.2	+	33530	Reoperation, coronary artery bypass procedure or valve procedure, more than one month after original operation (list separately in addition to code for primary procedure)	(I) 8.0	0	0
			Note: This code is an add-on procedure and as such is valued appropriately. Multiple procedure guidelines for reduction of value are not applicable.			
		33533	Coronary artery bypass, using arterial graft(s); single arterial graft	(I) 44.0	90	20
		33534	two coronary arterial grafts	(I) 47.0	90	20
		33535	three coronary arterial grafts	(I) 50.0	90	20
		33536	four or more coronary arterial grafts	(I) 53.0	90	20
		33542	Myocardial resection (eg, ventricular aneurysmectomy)	46.0	90	20
		33545	Repair of postinfarction ventricular septal defect, with or without myocardial resection	(I) 53.0	90	20
98.2	+	33572	Coronary endarterectomy, open, any method, of left anterior descending, circumflex, or right coronary artery performed in conjunction with coronary artery bypass graft procedure, each vessel (list separately in addition to primary procedure)	(I) 7.0	0	0
			Note: This code is an add-on procedure and as such is valued appropriately. Multiple procedure guidelines for reduction of value are not applicable.			
		33600	Closure of atrioventricular valve (mitral or tricuspid) by suture or patch	44.0	90	20
		33602	Closure of semilunar valve (aortic or pulmonary) by suture or patch	43.0	90	20
		33606	Anastomosis of pulmonary artery to aorta (Damus-Kaye-Stansel procedure)	45.0	90	20

+ Add-on Code   ⊘ Modifier -51 Exempt   ▲ Revised code   ● New code   **M** RVSI code or deleted from CPT   **(I)** Interim Value

UPD	Code	Description	Units	FUD	Anes
	33608	Repair of complex cardiac anomaly other than pulmonary atresia with ventricular septal defect by construction or replacement of conduit from right or left ventricle to pulmonary artery	46.0	90	20
	33610	Repair of complex cardiac anomalies (eg, single ventricle with subaortic obstruction) by surgical enlargement of interventricular septal defect	45.0	90	20
	33611	Repair of double outlet right ventricle with intraventricular tunnel repair;	48.0	90	20
	33612	with repair of right ventricular outflow tract obstruction	49.0	90	20
	33615	Repair of complex cardiac anomalies (eg, tricuspid atresia) by closure of atrial septal defect and anastomosis of atria or vena cava to pulmonary artery (simple Fontan procedure)	47.0	90	20
	33617	Repair of complex cardiac anomalies (eg, single ventricle) by modified Fontan procedure	49.5	90	20
	33619	Repair of single ventricle with aortic outflow obstruction and aortic arch hypoplasia (hypoplastic left heart syndrome) (eg, Norwood procedure)	54.0	90	20
	33641	Repair atrial septal defect, secundum, with cardiopulmonary bypass, with or without patch	34.0	90	20
98.2	33645	Direct or patch closure, sinus venosus, with or without anomalous pulmonary venous drainage	37.0	90	15
	33647	Repair of atrial septal defect and ventricular septal defect, with direct or patch closure	37.0	90	20
	33660	Repair of incomplete or partial atrioventricular canal (ostium primum atrial septal defect), with or without atrioventricular valve repair	43.5	90	20
	33665	Repair of intermediate or transitional atrioventricular canal, with or without atrioventricular valve repair	47.0	90	20
	33670	Repair of complete atrioventricular canal, with or without prosthetic valve	48.0	90	20
	33681	Closure of ventricular septal defect, with or without patch	37.5	90	20
	33684	with or without patch with pulmonary valvotomy or infundibular resection (acyanotic)	44.0	90	20
	33688	with or without patch with removal of pulmonary artery band, with or without gusset	44.0	90	20
	33690	Banding of pulmonary artery	24.0	90	15
98.2	33692	Complete repair tetralogy of Fallot without pulmonary atresia;	44.0	90	20
98.2	33694	with transannular patch	45.0	90	20
98.2	33697	Complete repair tetralogy of Fallot with pulmonary atresia including construction of conduit from right ventricle to pulmonary artery and closure of ventricular septal defect	49.5	90	20
	33702	Repair sinus of Valsalva fistula, with cardiopulmonary bypass;	40.5	90	20

UPD	Code	Description	Units	FUD	Anes
	33710	with repair of ventricular septal defect	44.0	90	20
	33720	Repair sinus of Valsalva aneurysm, with cardiopulmonary bypass	41.0	90	20
98.2	33722	Closure of aortico-left ventricular tunnel	43.0	90	20
	33730	Complete repair of anomalous venous return (supracardiac, intracardiac, or infracardiac types)	41.0	90	20
98.2	33732	Repair of cor triatriatum or supravalvular mitral ring by resection of left atrial membrane	40.0	90	20
98.2	33735	Atrial septectomy or septostomy; closed heart (Blalock-Hanlon type operation)	26.0	90	15
	33736	open heart with cardiopulmonary bypass	31.0	90	20
	33737	open heart, with inflow occlusion	28.0	90	20
	33750	Shunt; subclavian to pulmonary artery (Blalock-Taussig type operation)	30.0	90	15
	33755	ascending aorta to pulmonary artery (Waterston type operation)	30.0	90	15
	33762	descending aorta to pulmonary artery (Potts-Smith type operation)	30.0	90	15
	33764	central, with prosthetic graft	26.0	90	15
	33766	superior vena cava to pulmonary artery for flow to one lung (classical Glenn procedure)	30.0	90	15
	33767	superior vena cava to pulmonary artery for flow to both lungs (bidirectional Glenn procedure)	32.6	90	15
98.2	33770	Repair of transposition of the great arteries with ventricular septal defect and subpulmonary stenosis; without surgical enlargement of ventricular septal defect	47.0	90	20
98.2	33771	with surgical enlargement of ventricular septal defect	49.0	90	20
	33774	Repair of transposition of the great arteries, atrial baffle procedure (eg, Mustard or Senning type) with cardiopulmonary bypass;	44.0	90	20
	33775	with removal of pulmonary band	45.5	90	20
	33776	with closure of ventricular septal defect	47.5	90	20
	33777	with repair of subpulmonic obstruction	46.8	90	20
98.2	33778	Repair of transposition of the great arteries, aortic pulmonary artery reconstruction (eg, Jatene type);	50.5	90	20
98.2	33779	with removal of pulmonary band	50.8	90	20
98.2	33780	with closure of ventricular septal defect	51.8	90	20
98.2	33781	with repair of subpulmonic obstruction	51.2	90	20
98.2	33786	Total repair, truncus arteriosus (Rastelli type operation)	50.0	90	20

UPD		Code	Description	Units	FUD	Anes
98.2		**33788**	Reimplantation of an anomalous pulmonary artery	30.0	90	20
98.2		**33800**	Aortic suspension (aortopexy) for tracheal decompression (eg, for tracheomalacia) (separate procedure)	(I) 22.0	90	15
98.2		**33802**	Division of aberrant vessel (vascular ring);	24.0	90	20
		33803	with reanastomosis	28.0	90	20
		33813	Obliteration of aortopulmonary septal defect; without cardiopulmonary bypass	28.0	90	15
		33814	with cardiopulmonary bypass	39.0	90	20
		33820	Repair of patent ductus arteriosus; by ligation	20.0	90	15
		33822	by division, under 18 years	20.0	90	15
		33824	by division, 18 years and older	25.0	90	15
	M	**33826**	28 years and older, with bypass	38.0	90	20
98.2		**33840**	Excision of coarctation of aorta, with or without associated patent ductus arteriosus; with direct anastomosis	30.0	90	20
98.2		**33845**	with graft	33.0	90	20
98.2		**33851**	repair using either left subclavian artery or prosthetic material as gusset for enlargement	33.0	90	20
		33852	Repair of hypoplastic or interrupted aortic arch using autogenous or prosthetic material; without cardiopulmonary bypass	35.0	90	15
		33853	with cardiopulmonary bypass	45.0	90	20
98.2		**33860**	Ascending aorta graft, with cardiopulmonary bypass, with or without valve suspension;	(I) 51.0	90	20
98.2		**33861**	with coronary reconstruction	(I) 51.5	90	20
98.2		**33863**	with aortic root replacement using composite prosthesis and coronary reconstruction	(I) 54.0	90	20
		33870	Transverse arch graft, with cardiopulmonary bypass	56.0	90	20
		33875	Descending thoracic aorta graft, with or without bypass	(I) 50.5	90	20
		33877	Repair of thoracoabdominal aortic aneurysm with graft, with or without cardiopulmonary bypass	(I) 53.0	90	20
		33910	Pulmonary artery embolectomy; with cardiopulmonary bypass	38.0	90	20
		33915	without cardiopulmonary bypass	27.0	90	15
		33916	Pulmonary endarterectomy, with or without embolectomy, with cardiopulmonary bypass	39.0	90	20
98.2		**33917**	Repair of pulmonary artery stenosis by reconstruction with patch or graft	38.0	90	20

UPD			Code	Description	Units	FUD	Anes
			33918	Repair of pulmonary atresia with ventricular septal defect, by unifocalization of pulmonary arteries; without cardiopulmonary bypass	40.5	90	15
			33919	with cardiopulmonary bypass	47.0	90	20
98.2			33920	Repair of pulmonary atresia with ventricular septal defect, by construction or replacement of conduit from right or left ventricle to pulmonary artery	(I) 46.5	90	20
			33922	Transection of pulmonary artery with cardiopulmonary bypass	37.0	90	20
98.2		+	33924	Ligation and takedown of a systemic-to-pulmonary artery shunt, performed in conjunction with a congenital heart procedure (List separately in addition to code for primary procedure) Note: This code is an add-on procedure and as such is valued appropriately. Multiple procedure guidelines for reduction of value are not applicable.	(I) 8.0	0	0
			33930	Donor cardiectomy-pneumonectomy, with preparation and maintenance of allograft	24.0	0	7
			33935	Heart-lung transplant with recipient cardiectomy-pneumonectomy	(I) 160.0	0	20
			33940	Donor cardiectomy, with preparation and maintenance of allograft	21.0	0	7
			33945	Heart transplant, with or without recipient cardiectomy	(I) 128.0	0	20
			33960	Prolonged extracorporeal circulation for cardiopulmonary insufficiency; initial 24 hours	(I) 36.0	0	0
98.2	▲	+	33961	each additional 24 hours (List separately in addition to code for primary procedure) Note: This code is an add-on procedure and as such is valued appropriately. Multiple procedure guidelines for reduction of value are not applicable.	(I) 18.0	0	0
			33970	Insertion of intra-aortic balloon assist device through the femoral artery, open approach	(I) 10.0	15	8
			33971	Removal of intra-aortic balloon assist device including repair of femoral artery, with or without graft	(I) 5.0	15	8
98.2			33973	Insertion of intra-aortic balloon assist device through the ascending aorta	(I) 13.0	15	15
98.2			33974	Removal of intra-aortic balloon assist device from the ascending aorta, including repair of the ascending aorta, with or without graft	(I) 17.0	15	15
98.2			33975	Implantation of ventricular assist device; single ventricle support	(I) 24.0	15	15
98.2			33976	biventricular support	(I) 34.0	15	15
98.2			33977	Removal of ventricular assist device; single ventricle support	(I) 21.0	15	15
98.2			33978	biventricular support	(I) 24.0	15	15

UPD	Code	Description	Units	FUD	Anes
98.2	**33999**	Unlisted procedure, cardiac surgery	BR	0	20
	34001	Embolectomy or thrombectomy, with or without catheter; carotid, subclavian or innominate artery, by neck incision	10.0	60	10
	34051	innominate, subclavian artery, by thoracic incision	20.0	60	15
98.2	**34101**	axillary, brachial, innominate, subclavian artery, by arm incision	8.0	60	6
	34111	radial or ulnar artery, by arm incision	8.0	60	6
98.2	**34151**	renal, celiac, mesentery, aortoiliac artery, by abdominal incision	15.0	60	15
98.2	**34201**	femoropopliteal, aortoiliac artery, by leg incision	12.0	60	6
98.2	**34203**	popliteal-tibio-peroneal artery, by leg incision	12.0	60	6
98.2	**34401**	Thrombectomy, direct or with catheter; vena cava, iliac vein, by abdominal incision	12.0	90	15
98.2	**34421**	vena cava, iliac, femoropopliteal vein, by leg incision	8.0	90	5
98.2	**34451**	vena cava, iliac, femoropopliteal vein, by abdominal and leg incision	15.0	90	15
	34471	subclavian vein, by neck incision	10.0	90	10
98.2	**34490**	axillary and subclavian vein, by arm incision	7.0	90	3
	34501	Valvuloplasty, femoral vein	(I) 12.0	90	8
	34502	Reconstruction of vena cava, any method	(I) 37.0	90	15
98.2	**34510**	Venous valve transposition, any vein donor	(I) 15.0	90	3
98.2	**34520**	Cross-over vein graft to venous system	25.0	90	3
98.2	**34530**	Saphenopopliteal vein anastomosis	(I) 17.0	90	3
	35001	Direct repair of aneurysm, false aneurysm, or excision (partial or total) and graft insertion, with or without patch graft; for aneurysm and associated occlusive disease, carotid, subclavian artery, by neck incision	20.0	90	10
	35002	for ruptured aneurysm, carotid, subclavian artery, by neck incision	25.0	90	10
	35005	for aneurysm, false aneurysm, and associated occlusive disease, vertebral artery	BR	90	10
98.2	**35011**	for aneurysm and associated occlusive disease, axillary-brachial artery, by arm incision	18.0	90	10
98.2	**35013**	for ruptured aneurysm, axillary-brachial artery, by arm incision	23.0	90	10
	35021	for aneurysm, false aneurysm, and associated occlusive disease, innominate, subclavian artery, by thoracic incision	18.0	90	15
	35022	for ruptured aneurysm, innominate, subclavian artery, by thoracic incision	23.0	90	15

UPD	Code	Description	Units	FUD	Anes
	35045	for aneurysm, false aneurysm, and associated occlusive disease, radial or ulnar artery	18.0	90	6
	35081	for aneurysm, false aneurysm, and associated occlusive disease, abdominal aorta	25.0	90	15
	35082	for ruptured aneurysm, abdominal aorta	35.0	90	15
	35091	for aneurysm, false aneurysm, and associated occlusive disease, abdominal aorta involving visceral vessels (mesenteric, celiac, renal)	28.0	90	15
	35092	for ruptured aneurysm, abdominal aorta involving visceral vessels (mesenteric, celiac, renal)	38.0	90	15
	35102	for aneurysm, false aneurysm, and associated occlusive disease, abdominal aorta involving iliac vessels (common, hypogastric, external)	30.0	90	15
	35103	for ruptured aneurysm, abdominal aorta involving iliac vessels (common, hypogastric, external)	35.0	90	15
	35111	for aneurysm, false aneurysm, and associated occlusive disease, splenic artery	20.0	90	15
	35112	for ruptured aneurysm, splenic artery	30.0	90	15
	35121	for aneurysm, false aneurysm, and associated occlusive disease, hepatic, celiac, renal, or mesenteric artery	25.0	90	15
	35122	for ruptured aneurysm, hepatic, celiac, renal, or mesenteric artery	30.0	90	15
	35131	for aneurysm, false aneurysm, and associated occlusive disease, iliac artery (common, hypogastric, external)	20.0	90	15
	35132	for ruptured aneurysm, iliac artery (common, hypogastric, external)	28.0	90	15
	35141	for aneurysm, false aneurysm, and associated occlusive disease, common femoral artery (profunda femoris, superficial femoral)	18.0	90	8
	35142	for ruptured aneurysm, common femoral artery (profunda femoris, superficial femoral)	22.0	90	8
	35151	for aneurysm, false aneurysm, and associated occlusive disease, popliteal artery	20.0	90	8
	35152	for ruptured aneurysm, popliteal artery	25.0	90	8
98.2	35161	for aneurysm, false aneurysm, and associated occlusive disease, other arteries	(I) 18.0	90	6
98.2	35162	for ruptured aneurysm, other arteries	(I) 18.0	90	6
	35180	Repair, congenital arteriovenous fistula; head and neck	20.0	90	10
	35182	thorax and abdomen	26.0	90	15
98.2	35184	extremities	20.0	90	6
	35188	Repair, acquired or traumatic arteriovenous fistula; head and neck	22.0	90	10

UPD	Code	Description	Units	FUD	Anes
	35189	thorax and abdomen	32.0	90	15
98.2	**35190**	extremities	22.0	90	6
	35201	Repair blood vessel, direct; neck	21.0	60	10
98.2	**35206**	upper extremity	21.0	60	4
	35207	hand, finger	21.0	60	6
	35211	intrathoracic, with bypass	33.0	90	20
	35216	intrathoracic, without bypass	24.0	90	15
	35221	intra-abdominal	27.0	90	15
	35226	lower extremity	16.2	90	8
	35231	Repair blood vessel with vein graft; neck	26.0	90	10
98.2	**35236**	upper extremity	26.0	90	6
	35241	intrathoracic, with bypass	37.0	90	20
	35246	intrathoracic, without bypass	25.0	90	15
	35251	intra-abdominal	32.5	90	15
	35256	lower extremity	22.2	90	8
	35261	Repair blood vessel with graft other than vein; neck	16.0	90	10
98.2	**35266**	upper extremity	16.0	90	6
	35271	intrathoracic, with bypass	32.0	90	20
	35276	intrathoracic, without bypass	22.0	90	15
	35281	intra-abdominal	20.0	90	15
	35286	lower extremity	19.0	90	8
	35301	Thromboendarterectomy, with or without patch graft; carotid, vertebral, subclavian, by neck incision	20.0	60	10
	35311	subclavian, innominate, by thoracic incision	25.0	90	15
98.2	**35321**	axillary-brachial	18.0	60	6
	35331	abdominal aorta	24.0	90	15
	35341	mesenteric, celiac, or renal	22.0	90	15
	35351	iliac	22.0	90	15
98.2	**35355**	iliofemoral	23.0	90	15
	35361	combined aortoiliac	24.0	90	15
	35363	combined aortoiliofemoral	26.0	90	15
98.2	**35371**	common femoral	18.0	90	6

UPD		Code	Description	Units	FUD	Anes
98.2		**35372**	deep (profunda) femoral	19.0	90	6
		35381	femoral and/or popliteal, and/or tibioperoneal	20.0	90	8
98.2 ▲ +		**35390**	Reoperation, carotid, thromboendarterectomy, more than one month after original operation (List separately in addition to code for primary procedure) Note: This code is an add-on procedure and as such is valued appropriately. Multiple procedure guidelines for reduction of value are not applicable.	(I) 6.0	0	0
98.2 +		**35400**	Angioscopy (non-coronary vessels or grafts) during therapeutic intervention (List separately in addition to code for primary procedure) Note: This code is an add-on procedure and as such is valued appropriately. Multiple procedure guidelines for reduction of value are not applicable.	(I) 6.0	0	0
		35450	Transluminal balloon angioplasty, open; renal or other visceral artery	14.0	90	7
98.2		**35452**	aortic	10.0	90	15
98.2		**35454**	iliac	(I) 12.0	90	15
98.2		**35456**	femoral-popliteal	(I) 12.0	90	8
98.2		**35458**	brachiocephalic trunk or branches, each vessel	(I) 12.0	90	6
		35459	tibioperoneal trunk and branches	(I) 12.0	90	8
98.2		**35460**	venous	(I) 12.0	90	3
98.2		**35470**	Transluminal balloon angioplasty, percutaneous; tibioperoneal trunk or branches, each vessel	(I) 12.0	90	8
98.2		**35471**	renal or visceral artery	(I) 14.0	90	8
98.2		**35472**	aortic	(I) 10.0	90	8
98.2		**35473**	iliac	(I) 9.0	90	8
98.2		**35474**	femoral-popliteal	(I) 11.0	90	8
98.2		**35475**	brachiocephalic trunk or branches, each vessel	(I) 13.5	90	8
98.2		**35476**	venous	(I) 9.5	90	8
98.2		**35480**	Transluminal peripheral atherectomy, open; renal or other visceral artery	(I) 16.0	90	15
98.2		**35481**	aortic	(I) 11.0	90	15
		35482	iliac	(I) 9.6	90	8
		35483	femoral-popliteal	(I) 11.7	90	8
98.2		**35484**	brachiocephalic trunk or branches, each vessel	(I) 15.1	90	6
		35485	tibioperoneal trunk and branches	(I) 13.7	90	8

UPD		Code	Description	Units	FUD	Anes
98.2		**35490**	Transluminal peripheral atherectomy, percutaneous; renal or other visceral artery	(I) 15.9	90	8
98.2		**35491**	aortic	(I) 11.0	90	7
98.2		**35492**	iliac	(I) 9.2	90	8
98.2		**35493**	femoral-popliteal	(I) 11.7	90	8
98.2		**35494**	brachiocephalic trunk or branches, each vessel	(I) 15.1	90	8
98.2		**35495**	tibioperoneal trunk and branches	(I) 13.7	90	8
98.2	● +	**35500**	Harvest of upper extremity vein, one segment, for lower extremity bypass procedure (List separately in addition to code for primary procedure) Note: This code is an add-on procedure and as such is valued appropriately. Multiple procedure guidelines for reduction of value are not applicable.	(I) 3.0	0	0
		35501	Bypass graft, with vein; carotid	15.0	90	10
		35506	carotid-subclavian	20.0	90	10
		35507	subclavian-carotid	20.0	90	10
		35508	carotid-vertebral	20.0	90	10
		35509	carotid-carotid	20.0	90	10
98.2		**35511**	subclavian-subclavian	22.0	90	8
		35515	subclavian-vertebral	22.0	90	10
98.2		**35516**	subclavian-axillary	22.0	90	8
		35518	axillary-axillary	22.0	90	8
98.2		**35521**	axillary-femoral	25.0	90	10
		35526	aortosubclavian or carotid	32.0	90	15
		35531	aortoceliac or aortomesenteric	26.0	90	15
98.2		**35533**	axillary-femoral-femoral	26.0	90	10
		35536	splenorenal	26.0	90	15
		35541	aortoiliac or bi-iliac	24.0	90	15
		35546	aortofemoral or bifemoral	26.0	90	15
		35548	aortoiliofemoral, unilateral	26.0	90	15
		35549	aortoiliofemoral, bilateral	28.0	90	15
		35551	aortofemoral-popliteal	29.0	90	15
		35556	femoral-popliteal	26.0	90	8
		35558	femoral-femoral	22.0	90	8

UPD	Code	Description	Units	FUD	Anes
	35560	aortorenal	26.0	90	15
	35563	ilioiliac	24.0	90	15
	35565	iliofemoral	26.0	90	15
	35566	femoral-anterior tibial, posterior tibial, peroneal artery or other distal vessels	26.0	90	8
	35571	popliteal-tibial, -peroneal artery or other distal vessels	25.0	90	8
	35582	In-situ vein bypass; aortofemoral-popliteal (only femoral-popliteal portion in-situ)	24.0	90	8
	35583	femoral-popliteal	23.0	90	8
	35585	femoral-anterior tibial, posterior tibial, or peroneal artery	24.0	90	8
	35587	popliteal-tibial, peroneal	24.0	90	8
	35601	Bypass graft, with other than vein; carotid	24.0	90	10
	35606	carotid-subclavian	24.0	90	10
98.2	35612	subclavian-subclavian	24.0	90	8
98.2	35616	subclavian-axillary	24.0	90	8
98.2	35621	axillary-femoral	24.0	90	10
98.2	35623	axillary-popliteal or -tibial	(I) 23.0	90	10
	35626	aortosubclavian or carotid	28.0	90	15
	35631	aortoceliac, aortomesenteric, aortorenal	28.0	90	15
	35636	splenorenal (splenic to renal arterial anastomosis)	28.0	90	15
	35641	aortoiliac or bi-iliac	32.0	90	15
	35642	carotid-vertebral	32.0	90	10
	35645	subclavian-vertebral	32.0	90	10
	35646	aortofemoral or bifemoral	32.0	90	15
98.2	35650	axillary-axillary	22.0	90	4
	35651	aortofemoral-popliteal	30.0	90	15
98.2	35654	axillary-femoral-femoral	28.0	90	10
	35656	femoral-popliteal	25.0	90	8
	35661	femoral-femoral	20.0	90	8
	35663	ilioiliac	24.0	90	15
	35665	iliofemoral	24.0	90	15
	35666	femoral-anterior tibial, posterior tibial, or peroneal artery	26.0	90	8
	35671	popliteal-tibial or -peroneal artery	24.0	90	8

UPD			Code	Description	Units	FUD	Anes
98.2	▲	+	35681	Bypass graft; composite, prosthetic and vein (List separately in addition to code for primary procedure) Note: This code is an add-on procedure and as such is valued appropriately. Multiple procedure guidelines for reduction of value are not applicable.	(I) 6.0	0	0
98.2	●	+	35682	autogenous composite, two segments of veins from two locations (List separately in addition to code for primary procedure) Note: This code is an add-on procedure and as such is valued appropriately. Multiple procedure guidelines for reduction of value are not applicable.	(I) 7.0	0	0
98.2	●	+	35683	autogenous composite, three or more segments of vein from two or more locations (List separately in addition to code for primary procedure) Note: This code is an add-on procedure and as such is valued appropriately. Multiple procedure guidelines for reduction of value are not applicable.	(I) 8.0	0	0
98.2			35691	Transposition and/or reimplantation; vertebral to carotid artery	(I) 24.0	90	10
98.2			35693	vertebral to subclavian artery	(I) 24.0	90	10
98.2			35694	subclavian to carotid artery	(I) 26.5	90	10
98.2			35695	carotid to subclavian artery	(I) 26.5	90	10
98.2		+	35700	Reoperation, femoral-popliteal or femoral (popliteal) - anterior tibial, posterior tibial, peroneal artery or other distal vessels, more than one month after original operation (List separately in addition to code for primary procedure) Note: This code is an add-on procedure and as such is valued appropriately. Multiple procedure guidelines for reduction of value are not applicable.	(I) 6.5	0	0
			35701	Exploration (not followed by surgical repair), with or without lysis of artery; carotid artery	9.1	90	10
			35721	femoral artery	7.1	90	8
			35741	popliteal artery	7.1	90	8
			35761	other vessels	8.1	90	0
			35800	Exploration for postoperative hemorrhage, thrombosis or infection; neck	10.0	90	10
			35820	chest	20.0	90	15
			35840	abdomen	15.0	90	15
98.2			35860	extremity	9.0	90	6
98.2			35870	Repair of graft-enteric fistula	35.0	90	6
98.2	▲		35875	Thrombectomy of arterial or venous graft (other than hemodialysis graft or fistula);	13.5	90	5

UPD	Code	Description	Units	FUD	Anes
98.2	35876	with revision of arterial or venous graft	(I) 19.0	90	5
98.2	35901	Excision of infected graft; neck	(I) 14.0	90	10
	35903	extremity	(I) 16.0	90	8
98.2	35905	thorax	(I) 32.5	90	8
	35907	abdomen	(I) 33.5	90	15
98.2	36000*	Introduction of needle or intracatheter, vein	1.0	0	5
98.2	36005	Injection procedure for contrast venography (including introduction of needle or intracatheter)	(I) 2.5	0	5
98.2	36010	Introduction of catheter, superior or inferior vena cava	2.0	0	5
98.2	36011	Selective catheter placement, venous system; first order branch (eg, renal vein, jugular vein)	(I) 3.0	0	5
98.2	36012	second order, or more selective, branch (eg, left adrenal vein, petrosal sinus)	(I) 4.5	0	5
98.2	36013	Introduction of catheter, right heart or main pulmonary artery	(I) 3.0	0	7
98.2	36014	Selective catheter placement, left or right pulmonary artery	(I) 4.5	0	7
98.2	36015	Selective catheter placement, segmental or subsegmental pulmonary artery	(I) 4.5	0	7
	36100	Introduction of needle or intracatheter, carotid or vertebral artery	4.0	0	5
	36120	Introduction of needle or intracatheter; retrograde brachial artery	4.0	0	5
	36140	extremity artery	3.0	0	5
96.1	36145	arteriovenous shunt created for dialysis (cannula, fistula, or graft)	5.0	0	6
	36160	Introduction of needle or intracatheter, aortic, translumbar	3.0	0	5
98.2	36200	Introduction of catheter, aorta	4.0	0	3
	36215	Selective catheter placement, arterial system; each first order thoracic or brachiocephalic branch, within a vascular family	6.2	0	5
	36216	initial second order thoracic or brachiocephalic branch, within a vascular family	(I) 7.5	0	5
	36217	initial third order or more selective thoracic or brachiocephalic branch, within a vascular family	(I) 9.0	0	5
98.2 ▲ +	36218	additional second order, third order, and beyond, thoracic or brachiocephalic branch, within a vascular family (List in addition to code for initial second or third order vessel as appropriate) Note: This code is an add-on procedure and as such is valued appropriately. Multiple procedure guidelines for reduction of value are not applicable.	(I) 1.5	0	0

UPD			Code	Description	Units	FUD	Anes
			36245	Selective catheter placement, arterial system; each first order abdominal, pelvic, or lower extremity artery branch, within a vascular family	(I) 7.0	0	5
			36246	initial second order abdominal, pelvic, or lower extremity artery branch, within a vascular family	(I) 7.5	0	5
			36247	initial third order or more selective abdominal, pelvic, or lower extremity artery branch, within a vascular family	(I) 9.2	0	5
98.2	▲	+	36248	additional second order, third order, and beyond, abdominal, pelvic, or lower extremity artery branch, within a vascular family (List in addition to code for initial second or third order vessel as appropriate) Note: This code is an add-on procedure and as such is valued appropriately. Multiple procedure guidelines for reduction of value are not applicable.	(I) 1.5	0	0
98.2			36260	Insertion of implantable intra-arterial infusion pump (eg, for chemotherapy of liver)	6.5	45	4
98.2			36261	Revision of implanted intra-arterial infusion pump	6.5	45	4
98.2			36262	Removal of implanted intra-arterial infusion pump	4.5	45	3
98.2			36299	Unlisted procedure, vascular injection	BR	0	4
98.2			36400	Venipuncture, under age 3 years; femoral, jugular or sagittal sinus	0.4	0	3
98.2			36405*	scalp vein	0.6	0	3
98.2			36406	other vein	0.7	0	3
98.2			36410*	Venipuncture, child over age 3 years or adult, necessitating physician's skill (separate procedure), for diagnostic or therapeutic purposes. Not to be used for routine venipuncture.	0.3	0	3
			36415*	Routine venipuncture or finger/heel/ear stick for collection of specimen(s)	0.2	0	0
	M		36417	Phlebotomy, therapeutic (independent procedure)	0.4	0	0
98.2			36420	Venipuncture, cutdown; under age 1 year	1.0	0	3
			36425	age 1 or over	0.8	0	3
			36430	Transfusion, blood or blood components	0.4	0	0
			36440*	Push transfusion, blood, 2 years or under	1.2	0	0
			36450	Exchange transfusion, blood; newborn	7.0	0	0
			36455	other than newborn	10.0	0	0
98.2			36460	Transfusion, intrauterine, fetal	10.0	0	6
98.2			36468	Single or multiple injections of sclerosing solutions, spider veins (telangiectasia); limb or trunk	0.9	0	3
98.2			36469	face	1.1	0	5

UPD		Code	Description	Units	FUD	Anes
98.2		**36470***	Injection of sclerosing solution; single vein	0.6	0	3
98.2		**36471***	multiple veins, same leg	0.9	0	3
98.2		**36481**	Percutaneous portal vein catheterization by any method	(I) 9.5	0	4
98.2	⊘	**36488***	Placement of central venous catheter (subclavian, jugular, or other vein) (eg, for central venous pressure, hyperalimentation, hemodialysis, or chemotherapy); percutaneous, age 2 years or under Note: Procedure listed may be considered a necessary part of and/or procedure and in such cases, not billable. If the procedure is distinct by encounter or performed in conjunction with a procedure for which the listed service is not considered a necessary component, then multiple procedure guidelines for reduction of value do not apply for this code.	1.5	0	4
98.2	⊘	**36489***	percutaneous, over age 2 Note: Procedure listed may be considered a necessary part of and/or procedure and in such cases, not billable. If the procedure is distinct by encounter or performed in conjunction with a procedure for which the listed service is not considered a necessary component, then multiple procedure guidelines for reduction of value do not apply for this code.	1.4	0	4
98.2	⊘	**36490***	cutdown, age 2 years or under Note: Procedure listed may be considered a necessary part of and/or procedure and in such cases, not billable. If the procedure is distinct by encounter or performed in conjunction with a procedure for which the listed service is not considered a necessary component, then multiple procedure guidelines for reduction of value do not apply for this code.	2.3	0	4
98.2	⊘	**36491***	cutdown, over age 2 Note: Procedure listed may be considered a necessary part of and/or procedure and in such cases, not billable. If the procedure is distinct by encounter or performed in conjunction with a procedure for which the listed service is not considered a necessary component, then multiple procedure guidelines for reduction of value do not apply for this code.	2.5	0	4
98.2		**36493**	Repositioning of previously placed central venous catheter under fluoroscopic guidance	(I) 1.8	0	4
98.2		**36500**	Venous catheterization for selective organ blood sampling	3.5	0	4
98.2		**36510***	Catheterization of umbilical vein for diagnosis or therapy, newborn	1.0	0	4
		36520	Therapeutic apheresis (plasma and/or cell exchange)	3.0	0	0
		36522	Photopheresis, extracorporeal	(I) 2.5	0	0
98.2		**36530**	Insertion of implantable intravenous infusion pump	(I) 8.0	15	4

UPD		Code	Description	Units	FUD	Anes
98.2		**36531**	Revision of implantable intravenous infusion pump	(I) 8.0	15	4
98.2		**36532**	Removal of implantable intravenous infusion pump	(I) 6.0	15	4
98.2		**36533**	Insertion of implantable venous access port, with or without subcutaneous reservoir	(I) 7.0	15	4
98.2		**36534**	Revision of implantable venous access port and/or subcutaneous reservoir	(I) 7.0	15	4
98.2		**36535**	Removal of implantable venous access port and/or subcutaneous reservoir	(I) 4.0	15	4
		36600*	Arterial puncture, withdrawal of blood for diagnosis	0.4	0	1
98.2	⊘	**36620**	Arterial catheterization or cannulation for sampling, monitoring or transfusion (separate procedure); percutaneous	1.1	0	3
98.2		**36625**	cutdown	1.5	0	6
98.2		**36640**	Arterial catheterization for prolonged infusion therapy (chemotherapy), cutdown	1.4	0	4
98.2	⊘	**36660***	Catheterization, umbilical artery, newborn, for diagnosis or therapy	1.4	0	5
98.2		**36680**	Placement of needle for intraosseous infusion	1.5	7	3
98.2		**36800**	Insertion of cannula for hemodialysis, other purpose (separate procedure); vein to vein	3.0	7	3
98.2		**36810**	arteriovenous, external (Scribner type)	9.0	14	6
98.2		**36815**	arteriovenous, external revision, or closure	6.0	14	6
98.2		**36821**	Arteriovenous anastomosis, direct, any site (eg, Cimino type) (separate procedure)	13.0	30	6
98.2		**36822**	Insertion of cannula(s) for prolonged extracorporeal circulation for cardiopulmonary insufficiency (ECMO) (separate procedure)	11.0	30	6
98.2	●	**36823**	Insertion of arterial and venous cannula(s) for isolated extracorporeal circulation and regional chemotherapy perfusion to an extremity, with or without hyperthermia, with removal of cannula(s) and repair of arteriotomy and venotomy sites	(I) 11.0	30	6
98.2		**36825**	Creation of arteriovenous fistula by other than direct arteriovenous anastomosis (separate procedure); autogenous graft	14.5	30	6
98.2		**36830**	nonautogenous graft	13.0	30	6
98.2	●	**36831**	Thrombectomy, arteriovenous fistula without revision, autogenous or nonautogenous dialysis graft (separate procedure)	(I) 6.0	30	6
98.2	▲	**36832**	Revision, arteriovenous fistula; without thrombectomy, autogenous or nonautogenous, dialysis graft (separate procedure)	9.0	30	6
98.2	●	**36833**	with thrombectomy, autogenous or nonautogenous dialysis graft (separate procedure)	(I) 9.5	30	6

UPD			Code	Description	Units	FUD	Anes
98.2			**36834**	Plastic repair of arteriovenous aneurysm (separate procedure)	(I) 14.5	30	6
98.2			**36835**	Insertion of Thomas shunt (separate procedure)	13.0	30	6
98.2	▲		**36860**	External cannula declotting (separate procedure); without balloon catheter	1.0	0	6
98.2			**36861**	with balloon catheter	2.0	0	6
			37140	Venous anastomosis; portocaval	31.0	90	15
			37145	renoportal	30.0	90	15
			37160	caval-mesenteric	31.0	90	15
			37180	splenorenal, proximal	31.0	90	15
			37181	splenorenal, distal (selective decompression of esophagogastric varices, any technique)	40.0	90	15
98.2			**37195**	Thrombolysis, cerebral, by intravenous infusion	(I) 7.0	0	11
98.2			**37200**	Transcatheter biopsy	(I) 8.0	0	6
98.2			**37201**	Transcatheter therapy, infusion for thrombolysis other than coronary	(I) 12.0	0	6
98.2			**37202**	Transcatheter therapy, infusion other than for thrombolysis, any type (eg, spasmolytic, vasoconstrictive)	(I) 8.6	0	6
98.2			**37203**	Transcatheter retrieval, percutaneous, of intravascular foreign body (eg, fractured venous or arterial catheter)	(I) 7.8	0	6
98.2			**37204**	Transcatheter occlusion or embolization (eg, for tumor destruction, to achieve hemostasis, to occlude a vascular malformation), percutaneous, any method, non-central nervous system, non-head or neck	(I) 26.0	0	6
98.2			**37205**	Transcatheter placement of an intravascular stent(s), (non-coronary vessel), percutaneous; initial vessel	(I) 17.2	0	6
98.2	▲	+	**37206**	each additional vessel (List separately in addition to code for primary procedure) Note: This code is an add-on procedure and as such is valued appropriately. Multiple procedure guidelines for reduction of value are not applicable.	(I) 8.6	0	0
98.2			**37207**	Transcatheter placement of an intravascular stent(s), (non-coronary vessel), open; initial vessel	(I) 17.2	0	6
98.2	▲	+	**37208**	each additional vessel (List separately in addition to code for primary procedure) Note: This code is an add-on procedure and as such is valued appropriately. Multiple procedure guidelines for reduction of value are not applicable.	(I) 8.9	0	0
98.2			**37209**	Exchange of a previously placed arterial catheter during thrombolytic therapy	(I) 6.5	0	6

+ Add-on Code   ⊘ Modifier -51 Exempt   ▲ Revised code   ● New code   **M** RVSI code or deleted from CPT   **(I)** Interim Value

CPT codes and descriptions only copyright © 1998 American Medical Association   Copyright © 1999 St. Anthony Publishing

UPD		Code	Description	Units	FUD	Anes
98.2	+	37250	Intravascular ultrasound (non-coronary vessel) during therapeutic intervention; initial vessel (List separately in addition to code for primary procedure) Note: This code is an add-on procedure and as such is valued appropriately. Multiple procedure guidelines for reduction of value are not applicable.	(I) 2.3	0	0
98.2	+	37251	Intravascular ultrasound (non-coronary vessel) during therapeutic intervention; each additional vessel (List separately in addition to code for primary procedure) Note: This code is an add-on procedure and as such is valued appropriately. Multiple procedure guidelines for reduction of value are not applicable.	(I) 1.5	0	0
		37565	Ligation, internal jugular vein	10.0	30	5
		37600	Ligation; external carotid artery	7.5	30	5
		37605	internal or common carotid artery	8.0	30	5
		37606	internal or common carotid artery, with gradual occlusion, as with Selverstone or Crutchfield clamp	10.0	60	5
		37607	Ligation or banding of angioaccess arteriovenous fistula	(I) 8.0	30	5
		37609	Ligation or biopsy, temporal artery	1.5	0	5
98.2		37615	Ligation, major artery (eg, post-traumatic, rupture); neck	8.0	30	5
		37616	chest	20.0	60	15
98.2		37617	abdomen	15.0	60	15
		37618	extremity	10.0	30	4
		37620	Interruption, partial or complete, of inferior vena cava by suture, ligation, plication, clip, extravascular, intravascular (umbrella device)	15.0	90	10
		37650	Ligation of femoral vein	7.0	30	3
98.2		37660	Ligation of common iliac vein	10.0	90	10
		37700	Ligation and division of long saphenous vein at saphenofemoral junction, or distal interruptions	4.0	30	3
		37720	Ligation and division and complete stripping of long or short saphenous veins	7.0	30	3
		37730	Ligation and division and complete stripping of long and short saphenous veins	10.0	30	3
		37735	Ligation and division and complete stripping of long or short saphenous veins with radical excision of ulcer and skin graft and/or interruption of communicating veins of lower leg, with excision of deep fascia	17.5	60	3
		37760	Ligation of perforators, subfascial, radical (Linton type), with or without skin graft	20.0	120	3
		37780	Ligation and division of short saphenous vein at saphenopopliteal junction (separate procedure)	2.0	30	3

UPD	Code	Description	Units	FUD	Anes
	37785	Ligation, division, and/or excision of recurrent or secondary varicose veins (clusters), one leg	1.2	30	3
	37788	Penile revascularization, artery, with or without vein graft	(I) 10.0	90	3
	37790	Penile venous occlusive procedure	(I) 20.0	90	3
98.2	37799	Unlisted procedure, vascular surgery	BR	0	10

Hemic and Lymphatic Systems

UPD	Code	Description	Units	FUD	Anes
	38100	Splenectomy; total (separate procedure)	16.0	45	7
	38101	partial (separate procedure)	16.0	45	7
98.2 ▲ +	38102	total, en bloc for extensive disease, in conjunction with other procedure (List in addition to code for primary procedure) Note: This code is an add-on procedure and as such is valued appropriately. Multiple procedure guidelines for reduction of value are not applicable.	(I) 9.5	0	0
	38115	Repair of ruptured spleen (splenorrhaphy) with or without partial splenectomy	16.0	45	7
	38200	Injection procedure for splenoportography	2.0	0	5
	38230	Bone marrow harvesting for transplantation	7.5	30	5
98.2	38231	Blood-derived peripheral stem cell harvesting for transplantation, per collection	(I) 2.5	0	3
	38240	Bone marrow or blood-derived peripheral stem cell transplantation; allogenic	6.5	30	5
	38241	autologous	6.5	30	5
98.2	38300*	Drainage of lymph node abscess or lymphadenitis; simple	1.0	0	6
98.2	38305	extensive	2.0	30	6
98.2	38308	Lymphangiotomy or other operations on lymphatic channels	5.0	30	5
	38380	Suture and/or ligation of thoracic duct; cervical approach	5.0	45	6
98.2	38381	thoracic approach	14.0	60	13
98.2	38382	abdominal approach	14.0	60	6
98.2	38500	Biopsy or excision of lymph node(s); superficial (separate procedure)	1.5	0	6
98.2	38505	by needle, superficial (eg, cervical, inguinal, axillary)	1.5	0	6
	38510	deep cervical node(s)	3.4	0	6
	38520	deep cervical node(s) with excision	5.0	0	6
98.2	38525	deep axillary node(s)	4.0	0	5
	38530	internal mammary node(s) (separate procedure)	6.9	0	13

UPD			Code	Description	Units	FUD	Anes
98.2			38542	Dissection, deep jugular node(s)	6.0	60	6
			38550	Excision of cystic hygroma, axillary or cervical; without deep neurovascular dissection	6.0	60	6
			38555	with deep neurovascular dissection	10.0	60	6
97.1			38562	Limited lymphadenectomy for staging (separate procedure); pelvic and para-aortic	10.0	60	6
	M		38562 -10	Laparoscopic limited lymphadenectomy for staging (separate procedure); pelvic and para-aortic	10.0	15	6
			38564	retroperitoneal (aortic and/or splenic)	(I) 12.0	60	6
			38700	Suprahyoid lymphadenectomy	12.0	60	6
			38720	Cervical lymphadenectomy (complete)	21.0	60	6
			38724	Cervical lymphadenectomy (modified radical neck dissection)	21.0	60	6
98.2			38740	Axillary lymphadenectomy; superficial	8.0	60	5
98.2			38745	complete	14.0	60	5
98.2	▲	+	38746	Thoracic lymphadenectomy, regional, including mediastinal and peritracheal nodes (List in addition to code for primary procedure) Note: This code is an add-on procedure and as such is valued appropriately. Multiple procedure guidelines for reduction of value are not applicable.	(I) 6.1	0	0
98.2	▲	+	38747	Abdominal lymphadenectomy, regional, including celiac, gastric, portal, peripancreatic, with or without para-aortic and vena caval nodes (List separately in addition to code for primary procedure) Note: This code is an add-on procedure and as such is valued appropriately. Multiple procedure guidelines for reduction of value are not applicable.	(I) 6.7	0	0
98.2			38760	Inguinofemoral lymphadenectomy, superficial, including Cloquet's node (separate procedure)	8.0	60	3
98.2			38765	Inguinofemoral lymphadenectomy, superficial, in continuity with pelvic lymphadenectomy, including external iliac, hypogastric, and obturator nodes (separate procedure)	18.0	60	6
98.2			38770	Pelvic lymphadenectomy, including external iliac, hypogastric, and obturator nodes (separate procedure)	18.0	60	6
98.2			38780	Retroperitoneal transabdominal lymphadenectomy, extensive, including pelvic, aortic, and renal nodes (separate procedure)	27.0	60	6
98.2	▲		38790	Injection procedure; lymphangiography	3.0	0	3
98.2	● ⊘		38792	for identification of sentinel node	(I) 2.0	0	3
98.2			38794	Cannulation, thoracic duct	4.0	0	6
			38999	Unlisted procedure, hemic or lymphatic system	BR	0	0

UPD	Code	Description	Units	FUD	Anes

Mediastinum and Diaphragm

UPD	Code	Description	Units	FUD	Anes
98.2	**39000**	Mediastinotomy with exploration, drainage, removal of foreign body, or biopsy; cervical approach	6.0	0	8
	39010	transthoracic approach, including either transthoracic or median sternotomy	12.0	90	13
	39200	Excision of mediastinal cyst	18.2	90	13
	39220	Excision of mediastinal tumor	18.2	90	13
	39400	Mediastinoscopy, with or without biopsy	6.5	0	8
98.2	**39499**	Unlisted procedure, mediastinum	BR	0	13
	39501	Repair, laceration of diaphragm, any approach	18.7	90	13
98.2	**39502**	Repair, paraesophageal hiatus hernia, transabdominal, with or without fundoplasty, vagotomy, and/or pyloroplasty, except neonatal	17.2	90	7
98.2	**39503**	Repair, neonatal diaphragmatic hernia, with or without chest tube insertion and with or without creation of ventral hernia	22.0	90	7
98.2	**39520**	Repair, diaphragmatic hernia (esophageal hiatal); transthoracic	17.0	90	13
	39530	combined, thoracoabdominal	19.0	90	13
	39531	combined, thoracoabdominal, with dilation of stricture (with or without gastroplasty)	19.0	90	13
98.2	**39540**	Repair, diaphragmatic hernia (other than neonatal), traumatic; acute	19.0	90	7
98.2	**39541**	chronic	19.0	90	7
	39545	Imbrication of diaphragm for eventration, transthoracic or transabdominal, paralytic or nonparalytic	12.0	90	13
98.2	**39599**	Unlisted procedure, diaphragm	BR	0	13

UPD	Code	Description	Units	FUD	Anes
Digestive System					
	40490	Biopsy of lip	0.6	0	5
	40500	Vermilionectomy (lip shave), with mucosal advancement	8.2	30	5
	40510	Excision of lip; transverse wedge excision with primary closure	7.5	30	5
	40520	V-excision with primary direct linear closure	6.9	30	5
	40525	full thickness, reconstruction with local flap (eg, Estlander or fan)	7.9	30	5
98.2	40527	full thickness, reconstruction with cross lip flap (Abbe-Estlander)	20.0	90	5
	40530	Resection of lip, more than one-fourth, without reconstruction	7.2	30	5
	40650	Repair lip, full thickness; vermilion only	3.0	30	5
	40652	up to half vertical height	4.0	30	5
	40654	over one-half vertical height, or complex	6.0	30	5
	40700	Plastic repair of cleft lip/nasal deformity; primary, partial or complete, unilateral	16.0	90	6
	40701	primary bilateral, one stage procedure	24.0	90	6
	40702	primary bilateral, one of two stages	14.0	90	6
	40720	secondary, by recreation of defect and reclosure	16.0	90	6
	40761	with cross lip pedicle flap (Abbe-Estlander type), including sectioning and inserting of pedicle	25.0	90	6
	40799	Unlisted procedure, lips	BR	0	5
	40800*	Drainage of abscess, cyst, hematoma, vestibule of mouth; simple	0.8	0	5
	40801	complicated	1.5	0	5
	40804*	Removal of embedded foreign body, vestibule of mouth; simple	0.8	0	5
	40805	complicated	1.5	0	5
	40806	Incision of labial frenum (frenotomy)	1.5	0	5
	40808	Biopsy, vestibule of mouth	0.7	0	5
	40810	Excision of lesion of mucosa and submucosa, vestibule of mouth; without repair	0.6	0	5
	40812	with simple repair	1.5	30	5
	40814	with complex repair	2.0	30	5

UPD	Code	Description	Units	FUD	Anes
	40816	complex, with excision of underlying muscle	3.0	60	5
	40818	Excision of mucosa of vestibule of mouth as donor graft	2.0	60	5
	40819	Excision of frenum, labial or buccal (frenumectomy, frenulectomy, frenectomy)	1.5	0	5
	40820	Destruction of lesion or scar of vestibule of mouth by physical methods (eg, laser, thermal, cryo, chemical)	0.5	0	5
	40830	Closure of laceration, vestibule of mouth; 2.5 cm or less	1.0	7	5
	40831	over 2.5 cm or complex	1.9	30	5
	40840	Vestibuloplasty; anterior	8.0	90	5
	40842	posterior, unilateral	8.0	90	5
	40843	posterior, bilateral	10.0	90	5
	40844	entire arch	12.0	90	5
	40845	complex (including ridge extension, muscle repositioning)	14.0	120	5
98.2	**40899**	Unlisted procedure, vestibule of mouth	BR	0	5
	41000*	Intraoral incision and drainage of abscess, cyst, or hematoma of tongue or floor of mouth; lingual	0.8	0	5
	41005*	sublingual, superficial	0.8	0	5
	41006	sublingual, deep, supramylohyoid	0.8	0	5
	41007	submental space	0.8	0	5
	41008	submandibular space	0.8	0	5
	41009	Intraoral incision and drainage of abscess, cyst, or hematoma of tongue or floor of mouth; masticator space	0.8	0	5
	41010	Incision of lingual frenum (frenotomy)	1.4	0	5
	41015	Extraoral incision and drainage of abscess, cyst, or hematoma of floor of mouth; sublingual	0.7	0	5
	41016	submental	1.0	0	5
	41017	submandibular	1.3	0	5
	41018	masticator space	1.8	0	5
	41100	Biopsy of tongue; anterior two-thirds	0.7	0	5
	41105	posterior one-third	1.0	0	5
	41108	Biopsy of floor of mouth	0.7	0	5
	41110	Excision of lesion of tongue without closure	0.9	7	5
	41112	Excision of lesion of tongue with closure; anterior two-thirds	1.4	7	5
	41113	posterior one-third	1.4	7	5

UPD	Code	Description	Units	FUD	Anes
	41114	with local tongue flap	(I) 5.0	7	5
	41115	Excision of lingual frenum (frenectomy)	0.5	7	5
	41116	Excision, lesion of floor of mouth	(I) 4.0	7	5
	41120	Glossectomy; less than one-half tongue	9.0	120	5
	41130	hemiglossectomy	11.0	120	5
	41135	partial, with unilateral radical neck dissection	22.0	120	7
98.2	**41140**	complete or total, with or without tracheostomy, without radical neck dissection	17.5	120	7
	41145	complete or total, with or without tracheostomy, with unilateral radical neck dissection	28.0	120	7
	41150	composite procedure with resection floor of mouth and mandibular resection, without radical neck dissection	22.0	120	7
	41153	composite procedure with resection floor of mouth, with suprahyoid neck dissection	28.0	120	7
	41155	composite procedure with resection floor of mouth, mandibular resection, and radical neck dissection (Commando type)	30.0	120	7
	41250*	Repair of laceration 2.5 cm or less; floor of mouth and/or anterior two-thirds of tongue	1.1	0	5
	41251*	posterior one-third of tongue	1.5	0	5
	41252*	Repair of laceration of tongue, floor of mouth, over 2.6 cm or complex	3.0	0	5
	41500	Fixation of tongue, mechanical, other than suture (eg, K-wire)	5.0	30	5
	41510	Suture of tongue to lip for micrognathia (Douglas type procedure)	10.0	30	5
	41520	Frenoplasty (surgical revision of frenum, eg, with Z-plasty)	2.0	30	5
	41599	Unlisted procedure, tongue, floor of mouth	BR	0	5
	41800*	Drainage of abscess, cyst, hematoma from dentoalveolar structures	0.9	0	5
	41805	Removal of embedded foreign body from dentoalveolar structures; soft tissues	0.8	0	5
	41806	bone	1.0	0	5
	41820	Gingivectomy, excision gingiva, each quadrant	4.0	0	5
	41821	Operculectomy, excision pericoronal tissues	0.8	0	5
	41822	Excision of fibrous tuberosities, dentoalveolar structures	1.0	0	5
	41823	Excision of osseous tuberosities, dentoalveolar structures	2.0	0	5
	41825	Excision of lesion or tumor (except listed above), dentoalveolar structures; without repair	0.6	0	5

UPD	Code	Description	Units	FUD	Anes
	41826	with simple repair	1.0	0	5
	41827	with complex repair	2.0	7	5
	41828	Excision of hyperplastic alveolar mucosa, each quadrant (specify)	1.5	0	5
	41830	Alveolectomy, including curettage of osteitis or sequestrectomy	(I) 1.5	0	5
	41850	Destruction of lesion (except excision), dentoalveolar structures	0.6	0	5
	41870	Periodontal mucosal grafting	3.8	90	5
	41872	Gingivoplasty, each quadrant (specify)	2.9	90	5
	41874	Alveoloplasty, each quadrant (specify)	2.9	90	5
	41899	Unlisted procedure, dentoalveolar structures	BR	0	5
	42000*	Drainage of abscess of palate, uvula	0.8	0	5
	42100	Biopsy of palate, uvula	0.6	0	5
	42104	Excision, lesion of palate, uvula; without closure	0.8	0	5
	42106	with simple primary closure	1.4	0	5
	42107	with local flap closure	16.0	90	5
	42120	Resection of palate or extensive resection of lesion	15.0	90	5
	42140	Uvulectomy, excision of uvula	1.0	15	5
	42145	Palatopharyngoplasty (eg, uvulopalatopharyngoplasty, uvulopharyngoplasty)	13.6	90	5
	42160	Destruction of lesion, palate or uvula (thermal, cryo or chemical)	0.9	0	5
	42180	Repair, laceration of palate; up to 2 cm	1.6	15	5
	42182	over 2 cm or complex	3.0	15	5
	42200	Palatoplasty for cleft palate, soft and/or hard palate only	16.2	90	6
	42205	Palatoplasty for cleft palate, with closure of alveolar ridge; soft tissue only	20.0	90	6
	42210	with bone graft to alveolar ridge (includes obtaining graft)	22.5	90	6
	42215	Palatoplasty for cleft palate; major revision	16.2	90	6
	42220	secondary lengthening procedure	17.1	90	6
	42225	attachment pharyngeal flap	17.1	90	6
98.2	42226	Lengthening of palate, and pharyngeal flap	17.5	90	5
98.2	42227	Lengthening of palate, with island flap	17.5	90	5

UPD	Code	Description	Units	FUD	Anes
	42235	Repair of anterior palate, including vomer flap	5.5	90	5
	42260	Repair of nasolabial fistula	6.0	90	5
	42280	Maxillary impression for palatal prosthesis	0.8	90	5
	42281	Insertion of pin-retained palatal prosthesis	0.4	90	5
	42299	Unlisted procedure, palate, uvula	BR	0	5
	42300*	Drainage of abscess; parotid, simple	1.8	0	5
	42305	parotid, complicated	3.0	0	5
	42310*	Drainage of abscess; submaxillary or sublingual, intraoral	1.2	0	5
	42320*	submaxillary, external	2.5	0	5
	42325	Fistulization of sublingual salivary cyst (ranula);	1.0	30	5
	42326	with prosthesis	1.2	30	5
	42330	Sialolithotomy; submandibular (submaxillary), sublingual or parotid, uncomplicated, intraoral	0.9	15	5
	42335	submandibular (submaxillary), complicated, intraoral	2.4	30	5
	42340	parotid, extraoral or complicated intraoral	6.0	30	5
	42400*	Biopsy of salivary gland; needle	1.0	0	5
	42405	incisional	2.1	0	5
	42408	Excision of sublingual salivary cyst (ranula)	3.0	15	5
	42409	Marsupialization of sublingual salivary cyst (ranula)	2.5	15	5
	42410	Excision of parotid tumor or parotid gland; lateral lobe, without nerve dissection	6.2	60	5
	42415	lateral lobe, with dissection and preservation of facial nerve	16.5	60	5
	42420	total, with dissection and preservation of facial nerve	20.4	60	5
	42425	total, en bloc removal with sacrifice of facial nerve	13.6	60	5
98.2	42426	total, with unilateral radical neck dissection	28.0	60	6
	42440	Excision of submandibular (submaxillary) gland	10.5	60	5
	42450	Excision of sublingual gland	10.5	60	5
	42500	Plastic repair of salivary duct, sialodochoplasty; primary or simple	7.1	60	5
	42505	secondary or complicated	10.5	60	5
	42507	Parotid duct diversion, bilateral (Wilke type procedure);	13.0	60	5
	42508	with excision of one submandibular gland	13.0	60	5
	42509	with excision of both submandibular glands	22.0	60	5

UPD	Code	Description	Units	FUD	Anes
	42510	with ligation of both submandibular (Wharton's) ducts	13.5	60	5
	42550	Injection procedure for sialography	0.7	0	5
	42600	Closure salivary fistula	10.0	60	5
	42650*	Dilation salivary duct	0.5	0	5
	42660*	Dilation and catheterization of salivary duct, with or without injection	0.6	0	5
	42665	Ligation salivary duct, intraoral	1.2	0	5
	42699	Unlisted procedure, salivary glands or ducts	BR	0	5
	42700*	Incision and drainage abscess; peritonsillar	1.3	0	5
	42720	retropharyngeal or parapharyngeal, intraoral approach	2.0	0	5
	42725	retropharyngeal or parapharyngeal, external approach	5.0	15	5
	42800	Biopsy; oropharynx	0.9	7	5
	42802	hypopharynx	1.5	7	5
	42804	nasopharynx, visible lesion, simple	1.1	7	5
	42806	nasopharynx, survey for unknown primary lesion	1.2	7	5
	42808	Excision or destruction of lesion of pharynx, any method	3.0	30	5
	42809	Removal of foreign body from pharynx	1.0	0	5
	42810	Excision branchial cleft cyst or vestige, confined to skin and subcutaneous tissues	3.8	30	5
	42815	Excision branchial cleft cyst, vestige, or fistula, extending beneath subcutaneous tissues and/or into pharynx	10.3	30	5
	42820	Tonsillectomy and adenoidectomy; under age 12	5.1	30	5
	42821	age 12 or over	5.5	30	5
	42825	Tonsillectomy, primary or secondary; under age 12	4.9	30	5
	42826	age 12 or over	5.3	30	5
	42830	Adenoidectomy, primary; under age 12	2.9	30	5
	42831	age 12 or over	3.2	30	5
	42835	Adenoidectomy, secondary; under age 12	2.7	30	5
	42836	age 12 or over	2.9	30	5
	42842	Radical resection of tonsil, tonsillar pillars, and/or retromolar trigone; without closure	15.2	30	7
	42844	closure with local flap (eg, tongue, buccal)	18.2	30	7
	42845	closure with other flap	18.2	30	7
	42860	Excision of tonsil tags	3.0	30	5

UPD		Code	Description	Units	FUD	Anes
		42870	Excision or destruction lingual tonsil, any method (separate procedure)	5.2	30	5
96.2	M	42880	Excision nasopharyngeal lesion (eg, fibroma) For resection of the nasopharynx (eg, juvenile angiofibroma) by bicoronal and/or transzygomatic approach, see 61586 and 61600	7.0	30	5
		42890	Limited pharyngectomy	12.0	60	7
		42892	Resection of lateral pharyngeal wall or pyriform sinus, direct closure by advancement of lateral and posterior pharyngeal walls	16.0	60	7
		42894	Resection of pharyngeal wall requiring closure with myocutaneous flap	19.0	60	7
		42900	Suture pharynx for wound or injury	5.0	30	5
		42950	Pharyngoplasty (plastic or reconstructive operation on pharynx)	12.5	60	5
98.2		42953	Pharyngoesophageal repair	12.5	60	7
		42955	Pharyngostomy (fistulization of pharynx, external for feeding)	4.5	0	5
		42960	Control oropharyngeal hemorrhage, primary or secondary (eg, post-tonsillectomy); simple	1.3	0	5
		42961	complicated, requiring hospitalization	1.5	0	5
		42962	with secondary surgical intervention	2.8	0	5
		42970	Control of nasopharyngeal hemorrhage, primary or secondary (eg, postadenoidectomy); simple, with posterior nasal packs, with or without anterior packs and/or cauterization	2.5	0	5
		42971	complicated, requiring hospitalization	3.0	0	5
		42972	with secondary surgical intervention	3.7	0	5
		42999	Unlisted procedure, pharynx, adenoids, or tonsils	BR	0	5
		43020	Esophagotomy, cervical approach, with removal of foreign body	14.0	90	6
		43030	Cricopharyngeal myotomy	13.0	90	6
		43045	Cricopharyngeal myotomy esophagotomy, thoracic approach, with removal of foreign body	19.0	90	15
		43100	Excision of lesion, esophagus, with primary repair; cervical approach	15.0	90	6
		43101	thoracic or abdominal approach	22.0	90	15
98.2		43107	Total or near total esophagectomy, without thoracotomy; with pharyngogastrostomy or cervical esophagogastrostomy, with or without pyloroplasty (transhiatal)	(I) 46.0	90	15

UPD	Code	Description	Units	FUD	Anes
98.2	**43108**	with colon interposition or small bowel reconstruction, including bowel mobilization, preparation and anastomosis(es)	(I) 53.0	90	15
	43112	Total or near total esophagectomy, with thoracotomy; with pharyngogastrostomy or cervical esophagogastrostomy, with or without pyloroplasty	(I) 48.0	90	15
	43113	with colon interposition or small bowel reconstruction, including bowel mobilization, preparation, and anastomosis(es)	(I) 55.0	90	15
98.2	**43116**	Partial esophagectomy, cervical, with free intestinal graft, including microvascular anastomosis, obtaining the graft and intestinal reconstruction	(I) 48.0	90	15
	43117	Partial esophagectomy, distal two-thirds, with thoracotomy and separate abdominal incision, with or without proximal gastrectomy; with thoracic esophagogastrostomy, with or without pyloroplasty (Ivor Lewis)	(I) 47.0	90	15
	43118	with colon interposition or small bowel reconstruction, including bowel mobilization, preparation, and anastomosis(es)	(I) 50.0	90	15
	43121	Partial esophagectomy, distal two-thirds, with thoracotomy only, with or without proximal gastrectomy, with thoracic esophagogastrostomy, with or without pyloroplasty	(I) 46.5	90	15
	43122	Partial esophagectomy, thoracoabdominal or abdominal approach, with or without proximal gastrectomy; with esophagogastrostomy, with or without pyloroplasty	(I) 46.5	90	15
	43123	with colon interposition or small bowel reconstruction, including bowel mobilization, preparation, and anastomosis(es)	(I) 50.0	90	15
	43124	Total or partial esophagectomy, without reconstruction (any approach), with cervical esophagostomy	(I) 42.0	90	15
	43130	Diverticulectomy of hypopharynx or esophagus, with or without myotomy; cervical approach	13.5	90	6
	43135	thoracic approach	20.0	90	15
	43200	Esophagoscopy, rigid or flexible; diagnostic, with or without collection of specimen(s) by brushing or washing (separate procedure)	3.0	0	5
	43202	with biopsy, single or multiple	3.5	0	5
	43204	with injection sclerosis of esophageal varices	5.7	0	5
	43205	with band ligation of esophageal varices	(I) 6.1	0	5
	43215	with removal of foreign body	4.2	0	5
	43216	with removal of tumor(s), polyp(s), or other lesion(s) by hot biopsy forceps or bipolar cautery	(I) 4.3	0	5
	43217	with removal of tumor(s), polyp(s), or other lesion(s) by snare technique	4.4	0	5
	43219	with insertion of plastic tube or stent	4.5	0	5

UPD	Code	Description	Units	FUD	Anes
	43220	with balloon dilation (less than 30 mm diameter)	4.0	0	5
	43226	with insertion of guide wire followed by dilation over guide wire	4.1	0	5
	43227	with control of bleeding, any method	5.7	0	5
	43228	with ablation of tumor(s), polyp(s), or other lesion(s), not amenable to removal by hot biopsy forceps, bipolar cautery or snare technique	5.7	0	5
	43234	Upper gastrointestinal endoscopy, simple primary examination (eg, with small diameter flexible endoscope) (separate procedure)	3.1	0	5
	43235	Upper gastrointestinal endoscopy including esophagus, stomach, and either the duodenum and/or jejunum as appropriate; diagnostic, with or without collection of specimen(s) by brushing or washing (separate procedure)	4.2	0	5
	43239	with biopsy, single or multiple	4.3	0	5
	43241	with transendoscopic tube or catheter placement	4.2	0	5
	43243	with injection sclerosis of esophageal and/or gastric varices	7.0	0	5
	43244	with band ligation of esophageal and/or gastric varices	(I) 7.0	0	5
	43245	with dilation of gastric outlet for obstruction, any method	5.2	0	5
	43246	with directed placement of percutaneous gastrostomy tube	7.1	0	5
	43247	with removal of foreign body	5.2	0	5
	43248	with insertion of guide wire followed by dilation of esophagus over guide wire	(I) 5.0	0	5
	43249	with balloon dilation of esophagus (less than 30 mm diameter)	(I) 4.5	0	5
	43250	with removal of tumor(s), polyp(s), or other lesion(s) by hot biopsy forceps or bipolar cautery	(I) 5.3	0	5
	43251	with removal of tumor(s), polyp(s), or other lesion(s) by snare technique	5.4	0	5
	43255	with control of bleeding, any method	6.8	0	5
	43258	with ablation of tumor(s), polyp(s), or other lesion(s) not amenable to removal by hot biopsy forceps, bipolar cautery or snare technique	7.0	0	5
	43259	with endoscopic ultrasound examination	(I) 8.5	0	5
	43260	Endoscopic retrograde cholangiopancreatography (ERCP); diagnostic, with or without collection of specimen(s) by brushing or washing (separate procedure)	8.5	0	5
	43261	Endoscopic retrograde cholangiopancreatography (ERCP); with biopsy, single or multiple	(I) 8.5	0	5

UPD	Code	Description	Units	FUD	Anes
	43262	with sphincterotomy/papillotomy	10.5	0	5
	43263	with pressure measurement of sphincter of Oddi (pancreatic duct or common bile duct)	8.5	0	5
	43264	with endoscopic retrograde removal of stone(s) from biliary and/or pancreatic ducts	12.5	0	5
	43265	with endoscopic retrograde destruction, lithotripsy of stone(s), any method	12.5	0	5
	43267	with endoscopic retrograde insertion of nasobiliary or nasopancreatic drainage tube	10.5	0	5
	43268	with endoscopic retrograde insertion of tube or stent into bile or pancreatic duct	10.5	0	5
	43269	with endoscopic retrograde removal of foreign body and/ or change of tube or stent	8.5	0	5
	43271	with endoscopic retrograde balloon dilation of ampulla, biliary and/or pancreatic duct(s)	10.5	0	5
	43272	with ablation of tumor(s), polyp(s), or other lesion(s) not amenable to removal by hot biopsy forceps, bipolar cautery or snare technique	10.5	0	5
	43300	Esophagoplasty, (plastic repair or reconstruction), cervical approach; without repair of tracheoesophageal fistula	19.0	90	6
	43305	with repair of tracheoesophageal fistula	22.0	90	6
	43310	Esophagoplasty, (plastic repair or reconstruction), thoracic approach; without repair of tracheoesophageal fistula	25.0	90	15
	43312	Esophagoplasty, (plastic repair or reconstruction), thoracic approach; with repair of tracheoesophageal fistula	29.0	90	15
	43320	Esophagogastrostomy (cardioplasty), with or without vagotomy and pyloroplasty, transabdominal or transthoracic approach	23.0	90	7
	43324	Esophagogastric fundoplasty (eg, Nissen, Belsey IV, Hill procedures)	20.0	90	7
	43325	Esophagogastric fundoplasty; with fundic patch (Thal-Nissen procedure)	23.0	90	7
	43326	with gastroplasty (eg, Collis)	(I) 22.0	90	7
	43330	Esophagomyotomy (Heller type); abdominal approach	19.2	90	7
	43331	thoracic approach	19.2	90	15
	43340	Esophagojejunostomy (without total gastrectomy); abdominal approach	24.0	90	7
	43341	thoracic approach	25.0	90	15
	43350	Esophagostomy, fistulization of esophagus, external; abdominal approach	15.0	90	7
	43351	thoracic approach	14.0	90	15

UPD	Code	Description	Units	FUD	Anes
	43352	cervical approach	14.0	90	6
98.2	43360	Gastrointestinal reconstruction for previous esophagectomy, for obstructing esophageal lesion or fistula, or for previous esophageal exclusion; with stomach, with or without pyloroplasty	(I) 40.0	90	15
98.2	43361	with colon interposition or small bowel reconstruction, including bowel mobilization, preparation, and anastomosis(es)	(I) 45.0	90	15
	43400	Ligation, direct, esophageal varices	20.0	90	15
98.2	43401	Transection of esophagus with repair, for esophageal varices	(I) 22.0	90	15
	43405	Ligation or stapling at gastroesophageal junction for pre-existing esophageal perforation	(I) 20.0	90	7
	43410	Suture of esophageal wound or injury; cervical approach	15.0	90	6
	43415	transthoracic or transabdominal approach	19.2	90	15
	43420	Closure of esophagostomy or fistula; cervical approach	13.5	90	6
	43425	transthoracic or transabdominal approach	22.0	90	15
	43450*	Dilation of esophagus, by unguided sound or bougie, single or multiple passes	1.8	0	5
	43453	Dilation of esophagus, over guide wire	3.0	0	5
	43456	Dilation of esophagus, by balloon or dilator, retrograde	4.0	0	5
	43458	Dilation of esophagus with balloon (30 mm diameter or larger) for achalasia	3.6	0	5
98.2	43460	Esophagogastric tamponade, with balloon (Sengstaaken type)	4.0	0	15
98.2	43496	Free jejunum transfer with microvascular anastomosis	(I) 50.0	90	15
98.2	43499	Unlisted procedure, esophagus	0.0	0	15
	43500	Gastrotomy; with exploration or foreign body removal	13.5	45	7
	43501	with suture repair of bleeding ulcer	16.5	45	7
	43502	with suture repair of pre-existing esophagogastric laceration (eg, Mallory-Weiss)	(I) 19.0	45	7
	43510	with esophageal dilation and insertion of permanent intraluminal tube (eg, Celestin or Mousseaux-Barbin)	14.0	45	7
	43520	Pyloromyotomy, cutting of pyloric muscle (Fredet-Ramstedt type operation)	11.5	45	7
	43600	Biopsy of stomach; by capsule, tube, peroral (one or more specimens)	1.4	0	5
	43605	by laparotomy	13.5	45	7
	43610	Excision, local; ulcer or benign tumor of stomach	15.0	45	7
	43611	malignant tumor of stomach	(I) 21.0	90	7

UPD	Code	Description	Units	FUD	Anes
	43620	Gastrectomy, total; with esophagoenterostomy	28.0	90	7
	43621	with Roux-en-Y reconstruction	(I) 29.0	90	7
	43622	with formation of intestinal pouch, any type	(I) 31.0	90	7
	43631	Gastrectomy, partial, distal; with gastroduodenostomy	(I) 24.0	90	7
	43632	with gastrojejunostomy	(I) 24.0	90	7
	43633	with Roux-en-Y reconstruction	(I) 25.0	90	7
	43634	with formation of intestinal pouch	(I) 27.0	90	7
98.2	+ 43635	Vagotomy when performed with partial distal gastrectomy (List separately in addition to code(s) for primary procedure) Note: This code is an add-on procedure and as such is valued appropriately. Multiple procedure guidelines for reduction of value are not applicable.	3.0	0	0
	43638	Gastrectomy, partial, proximal, thoracic or abdominal approach including esophagogastrostomy, with vagotomy;	28.0	60	7
	43639	with pyloroplasty or pyloromyotomy	(I) 29.0	60	7
	43640	Vagotomy including pyloroplasty, with or without gastrostomy; truncal or selective	18.5	60	7
	43641	parietal cell (highly selective)	20.0	60	7
98.2	43750	Percutaneous placement of gastrostomy tube	4.0	0	5
	43760*	Change of gastrostomy tube	0.8	0	3
	43761	Repositioning of the gastric feeding tube through the duodenum for enteric nutrition	(I) 2.0	0	3
	43800	Pyloroplasty	14.5	45	7
	43810	Gastroduodenostomy	15.2	45	7
	43820	Gastrojejunostomy; without vagotomy	15.2	45	7
	43825	with vagotomy, any type	18.3	45	7
	43830	Gastrostomy, temporary (tube, rubber or plastic) (separate procedure);	11.5	45	7
	43831	neonatal, for feeding	8.9	30	7
	43832	Gastrostomy, permanent, with construction of gastric tube	16.0	45	7
	43840	Gastrorrhaphy, suture of perforated duodenal or gastric ulcer, wound, or injury	14.0	45	7
	43842	Gastric restrictive procedure, without gastric bypass, for morbid obesity; vertical-banded gastroplasty	(I) 17.0	45	7
	43843	other than vertical-banded gastroplasty	(I) 17.0	45	7

UPD	Code	Description	Units	FUD	Anes
	43846	Gastric restrictive procedure, with gastric bypass for morbid obesity; with short limb (less than 100 cm) Roux-en-Y gastroenterostomy	(I) 18.0	45	7
	43847	with small bowel reconstruction to limit absorption	(I) 22.0	45	7
	43848	Revision of gastric restrictive procedure for morbid obesity (separate procedure)	(I) 23.0	45	7
	43850	Revision of gastroduodenal anastomosis (gastroduodenostomy) with reconstruction; without vagotomy	20.0	60	7
	43855	with vagotomy	23.0	60	7
	43860	Revision of gastrojejunal anastomosis (gastrojejunostomy) with reconstruction, with or without partial gastrectomy or bowel resection; without vagotomy	20.0	60	7
	43865	with vagotomy	23.0	60	7
	43870	Closure of gastrostomy, surgical	10.0	45	7
	43880	Closure of gastrocolic fistula	16.0	45	7
98.2	**43999**	Unlisted procedure, stomach	BR	0	7
	44005	Enterolysis (freeing of intestinal adhesion) (separate procedure)	14.6	90	6
	44010	Duodenotomy, for exploration, biopsy(s), or foreign body removal	14.9	60	7
98.2	+ **44015**	Tube or needle catheter jejunostomy for enteral alimentation, intraoperative, any method (List separately in addition to primary procedure) Note: This code is an add-on procedure and as such is valued appropriately. Multiple procedure guidelines for reduction of value are not applicable.	8.5	60	0
	44020	Enterotomy, small bowel, other than duodenum; for exploration, biopsy(s), or foreign body removal	14.6	60	6
	44021	for decompression (eg, Baker tube)	(I) 14.0	60	6
	44025	Colotomy, for exploration, biopsy(s), or foreign body removal	15.6	60	6
	44050	Reduction of volvulus, intussusception, internal hernia, by laparotomy	14.5	90	6
98.2	**44055**	Correction of malrotation by lysis of duodenal bands and/or reduction of midgut volvulus (eg, Ladd procedure)	(I) 14.0	60	7
98.2	**44100**	Biopsy of intestine by capsule, tube, peroral (one or more specimens)	2.6	0	5
	44110	Excision of one or more lesions of small or large bowel not requiring anastomosis, exteriorization, or fistulization; single enterotomy	15.1	60	6
	44111	multiple enterotomies	17.0	60	6

UPD			Code	Description	Units	FUD	Anes
98.2			**44120**	Enterectomy, resection of small intestine; single resection and anastomosis	17.6	60	7
98.2	▲	+	**44121**	each additional resection and anastomosis (List separately in addition to code for primary procedure) Note: This code is an add-on procedure and as such is valued appropriately. Multiple procedure guidelines for reduction of value are not applicable.	(I) 6.5	0	0
			44125	with enterostomy	(I) 17.6	60	6
			44130	Enteroenterostomy, anastomosis of intestine, with or without cutaneous enterostomy (separate procedure)	15.0	60	6
98.2		+	**44139**	Mobilization (take-down) of splenic flexure performed in conjunction with partial colectomy (List separately in addition to primary procedure) Note: This code is an add-on procedure and as such is valued appropriately. Multiple procedure guidelines for reduction of value are not applicable.	(I) 3.2	0	0
			44140	Colectomy, partial; with anastomosis	18.5	90	6
			44141	with skin level cecostomy or colostomy	20.0	90	6
			44143	with end colostomy and closure of distal segment (Hartmann type procedure)	19.0	90	6
			44144	with resection, with colostomy or ileostomy and creation of mucofistula	18.8	90	6
			44145	with coloproctostomy (low pelvic anastomosis)	21.3	90	6
			44146	with coloproctostomy (low pelvic anastomosis), with colostomy	23.0	90	6
			44147	abdominal and transanal approach	25.0	90	6
			44150	Colectomy, total, abdominal, without proctectomy; with ileostomy or ileoproctostomy	25.0	90	7
			44151	with continent ileostomy	27.0	90	7
			44152	with rectal mucosectomy, ileoanal anastomosis, with or without loop ileostomy	32.0	90	7
			44153	with rectal mucosectomy, ileoanal anastomosis, creation of ileal reservoir (S or J), with or without loop ileostomy	42.5	90	7
			44155	Colectomy, total, abdominal, with proctectomy; with ileostomy	30.0	90	7
			44156	with continent ileostomy	32.0	90	7
			44160	Colectomy with removal of terminal ileum and ileocolostomy	19.0	60	7
			44300	Enterostomy or cecostomy, tube (eg, for decompression or feeding) (separate procedure)	9.0	60	6
			44310	Ileostomy or jejunostomy, non-tube (separate procedure)	14.5	60	6

UPD	Code	Description	Units	FUD	Anes
	44312	Revision of ileostomy; simple (release of superficial scar) (separate procedure)	2.8	60	6
	44314	complicated (reconstruction in-depth) (separate procedure)	16.0	60	6
	44316	Continent ileostomy (Kock procedure) (separate procedure)	22.0	60	6
	44320	Colostomy or skin level cecostomy; (separate procedure)	11.5	60	6
	44322	with multiple biopsies (eg, for Hirschsprung disease) (separate procedure)	12.0	60	6
	44340	Revision of colostomy; simple (release of superficial scar) (separate procedure)	2.5	60	6
	44345	complicated (reconstruction in-depth) (separate procedure)	12.0	60	6
	44346	with repair of paracolostomy hernia (separate procedure)	12.5	60	6
	44360	Small intestinal endoscopy, enteroscopy beyond second portion of duodenum, not including ileum; diagnostic, with or without collection of specimen(s) by brushing or washing (separate procedure)	4.5	0	5
	44361	with biopsy, single or multiple	5.2	0	5
	44363	with removal of foreign body	5.4	0	5
	44364	with removal of tumor(s), polyp(s), or other lesion(s) by snare technique	5.7	0	5
	44365	with removal of tumor(s), polyp(s), or other lesion(s) by hot biopsy forceps or bipolar cautery	5.6	0	5
	44366	with control of bleeding, any method	6.5	0	5
	44369	with ablation of tumor(s), polyp(s), or other lesion(s) not amenable to removal by hot biopsy forceps, bipolar cautery or snare technique	6.9	0	5
	44372	with placement of percutaneous jejunostomy tube	(I) 7.1	0	5
	44373	with conversion of percutaneous gastrostomy tube to percutaneous jejunostomy tube	(I) 7.1	0	5
	44376	Small intestinal endoscopy, enteroscopy beyond second portion of duodenum, including ileum; diagnostic, with or without collection of specimen(s) by brushing or washing (separate procedure)	(I) 9.5	0	5
	44377	with biopsy, single or multiple	(I) 10.0	0	5
	44378	with control of bleeding, any method	(I) 11.3	0	5
	44380	Ileoscopy, through stoma; diagnostic, with or without collection of specimen(s) by brushing or washing (separate procedure)	3.3	0	5
	44382	with biopsy, single or multiple	3.6	0	5

UPD		Code	Description	Units	FUD	Anes
		44385	Endoscopic evaluation of small intestinal (abdominal or pelvic) pouch; diagnostic, with or without collection of specimen(s) by brushing or washing (separate procedure)	3.6	0	5
		44386	with biopsy, single or multiple	3.9	0	5
		44388	Colonoscopy through stoma; diagnostic, with or without collection of specimen(s) by brushing or washing (separate procedure)	4.5	0	5
		44389	with biopsy, single or multiple	4.9	0	5
		44390	with removal of foreign body	5.8	0	5
		44391	with control of bleeding, any method	6.5	0	5
		44392	with removal of tumor(s), polyp(s), or other lesion(s) by hot biopsy forceps or bipolar cautery	5.7	0	5
		44393	with ablation of tumor(s), polyp(s), or other lesion(s) not amenable to removal by hot biopsy forceps, bipolar cautery or snare technique	7.0	0	5
		44394	with removal of tumor(s), polyp(s), or other lesion(s) by snare technique	(I) 6.5	0	5
98.2	⊘	44500	Introduction of long gastrointestinal tube (eg, Miller-Abbott) (separate procedure) Note: Procedure listed may be considered a necessary part of and/or procedure and in such cases, not billable. If the procedure is distinct by encounter or performed in conjunction with a procedure for which the listed service is not considered a necessary component, then multiple procedure guidelines for reduction of value do not apply for this code.	(I) 1.3	0	5
		44602	Suture of small intestine (enterorrhaphy) for perforated ulcer, diverticulum, wound, injury or rupture; single perforation	(I) 13.5	60	6
		44603	multiple perforations	(I) 17.5	60	6
		44604	Suture of large intestine (colorrhaphy) for perforated ulcer, diverticulum, wound, injury or rupture (single or multiple perforations); without colostomy	(I) 17.5	60	6
		44605	with colostomy	15.7	60	6
		44615	Intestinal stricturoplasty (enterotomy and enterorrhaphy) with or without dilation, for intestinal obstruction	(I) 17.7	60	6
		44620	Closure of enterostomy, large or small intestine;	10.0	60	6
97.2		44625	Closure of enterostomy, large or small intestine; with resection and anastomosis other than colorectal	14.5	60	6
97.2		44626	Closure of enterostomy, large or small intestine; with resection and colorectal anastomosis (eg, closure of Hartmann type procedure)	(I) 26.0	60	6
		44640	Closure of intestinal cutaneous fistula	13.0	60	6
		44650	Closure of enteroenteric or enterocolic fistula	14.0	60	6

UPD	Code	Description	Units	FUD	Anes
	44660	Closure of enterovesical fistula; without intestinal or bladder resection	14.0	60	6
	44661	with bowel and/or bladder resection	22.0	60	6
	44680	Intestinal plication (separate procedure)	18.0	60	6
97.2	44700	Exclusion of small bowel from pelvis by mesh or other prosthesis, or native tissue (eg, bladder or omentum)	(I) 21.0	90	6
98.2	44799	Unlisted procedure, intestine	BR	0	6
	44800	Excision of Meckel's diverticulum (diverticulectomy) or omphalomesenteric duct	12.0	45	6
	44820	Excision of lesion of mesentery (separate procedure)	10.0	45	6
	44850	Suture of mesentery (separate procedure)	10.5	45	6
98.2	44899	Unlisted procedure, Meckel's diverticulum and the mesentery	BR	0	6
97.2	44900	Incision and drainage of appendiceal abscess; open	10.0	45	6
98.2	44901	Incision and drainage of appendiceal abscess; percutaneous	(I) 5.0	10	3
	44950	Appendectomy;	10.0	45	6
98.2 ▲ +	44955	when done for indicated purpose at time of other major procedure (not as separate procedure) (List separately in addition to code for primary procedure) Note: This code is an add-on procedure and as such is valued appropriately. Multiple procedure guidelines for reduction of value are not applicable.	0.6	45	0
	44960	for ruptured appendix with abscess or generalized peritonitis	11.0	45	6
98.2	45000	Transrectal drainage of pelvic abscess	3.5	0	5
98.2	45005	Incision and drainage of submucosal abscess, rectum	2.4	15	5
98.2	45020	Incision and drainage of deep supralevator, pelvirectal, or retrorectal abscess	4.5	30	5
98.2	45100	Biopsy of anorectal wall, anal approach (eg, congenital megacolon)	4.0	15	5
98.2	45108	Anorectal myomectomy	8.0	90	5
	45110	Proctectomy; complete, combined abdominoperineal, with colostomy	28.0	90	7
	45111	partial resection of rectum, transabdominal approach	21.0	90	7
	45112	Proctectomy, combined abdominoperineal, pull-through procedure (eg, colo-anal anastomosis)	30.0	90	7
	45113	Proctectomy, partial, with rectal mucosectomy, ileoanal anastomosis, creation of ileal reservoir (S or J), with or without loop ileostomy	(I) 34.0	90	7
	45114	Proctectomy, partial, with anastomosis; abdominal and transsacral approach	26.0	90	7

UPD		Code	Description	Units	FUD	Anes
		45116	transacral approach only (Kraske type)	21.0	90	7
97.2		45119	Proctectomy, combined abdominoperineal pull-through procedure (eg, colo-anal anastomosis), with creation of colonic reservoir (eg, J-pouch), with or without proximal diverting ostomy	(I) 34.0	90	7
		45120	Proctectomy, complete (for congenital megacolon), abdominal and perineal approach; with pull-through procedure and anastomosis (eg, Swenson, Duhamel, or Soave type operation)	31.0	90	7
		45121	with subtotal or total colectomy, with multiple biopsies	27.5	90	7
		45123	Proctectomy, partial, without anastomosis, perineal approach	(I) 20.0	90	7
98.2	●	45126	Pelvic exenteration for colorectal malignancy, with proctectomy (with or without colostomy), with removal of bladder and ureteral transplantations, and/or hysterectomy, or cervicectomy, with or without removal of tube(s), with or without removal of ovary(s), or any combination thereof	(I) 36.0	90	8
98.2		45130	Excision of rectal procidentia, with anastomosis; perineal approach	15.0	90	5
		45135	abdominal and perineal approach	25.0	90	7
98.2		45150	Division of stricture of rectum	10.0	90	5
98.2		45160	Excision of rectal tumor by proctotomy, transacral or transcoccygeal approach	19.0	90	5
98.2		45170	Excision of rectal tumor, transanal approach	3.0	30	5
98.2		45190	Destruction of rectal tumor, any method (eg, electrodesiccation) transanal approach	(I) 12.0	90	5
98.2		45300	Proctosigmoidoscopy, rigid; diagnostic, with or without collection of specimen(s) by brushing or washing (separate procedure)	0.7	0	5
98.2		45303	with dilation, any method	0.7	0	5
98.2		45305	with biopsy, single or multiple	1.2	0	5
98.2		45307	with removal of foreign body	2.5	0	5
98.2		45308	with removal of single tumor, polyp, or other lesion by hot biopsy forceps or bipolar cautery	(I) 2.2	0	5
98.2		45309	with removal of single tumor, polyp, or other lesion by snare technique	(I) 2.7	0	5
98.2		45315	with removal of multiple tumors, polyps, or other lesions by hot biopsy forceps, bipolar cautery or snare technique	2.8	0	5
98.2		45317	with control of bleeding, any method	3.0	0	5
98.2		45320	with ablation of tumor(s), polyp(s), or other lesion(s) not amenable to removal by hot biopsy forceps, bipolar cautery or snare technique (eg, laser)	3.1	0	5
98.2		45321	with decompression of volvulus	3.0	0	5

UPD	Code	Description	Units	FUD	Anes
98.2	**45330**	Sigmoidoscopy, flexible; diagnostic, with or without collection of specimen(s) by brushing or washing (separate procedure)	1.3	0	5
98.2	**45331**	with biopsy, single or multiple	1.8	0	5
98.2	**45332**	with removal of foreign body	2.0	0	5
98.2	**45333**	with removal of tumor(s), polyp(s), or other lesion(s) by hot biopsy forceps or bipolar cautery	2.0	0	5
98.2	**45334**	with control of bleeding, any method	3.5	0	5
98.2	**45337**	with decompression of volvulus, any method	2.6	0	5
98.2	**45338**	with removal of tumor(s), polyp(s), or other lesion(s) by snare technique	(I) 2.7	0	5
98.2	**45339**	with ablation of tumor(s), polyp(s), or other lesion(s) not amenable to removal by hot biopsy forceps, bipolar cautery or snare technique	(I) 3.7	0	5
98.2	**45355**	Colonoscopy, rigid or flexible, transabdominal via colotomy, single or multiple	4.0	0	5
98.2	**45378**	Colonoscopy, flexible, proximal to splenic flexure; diagnostic, with or without collection of specimen(s) by brushing or washing, with or without colon decompression (separate procedure)	5.1	0	5
98.2	**45379**	with removal of foreign body	8.5	0	5
98.2	**45380**	with biopsy, single or multiple	6.6	0	5
98.2	**45382**	with control of bleeding, any method	8.0	0	5
98.2	**45383**	with ablation of tumor(s), polyp(s), or other lesion(s) not amenable to removal by hot biopsy forceps, bipolar cautery or snare technique	8.5	0	5
98.2	**45384**	with removal of tumor(s), polyp(s), or other lesion(s) by hot biopsy forceps or bipolar cautery	(I) 7.4	0	5
98.2	**45385**	with removal of tumor(s), polyp(s), or other lesion(s) by snare technique	8.0	0	5
98.2	**45500**	Proctoplasty; for stenosis	10.0	90	5
98.2	**45505**	for prolapse of mucous membrane	11.0	90	5
98.2	**45520**	Perirectal injection of sclerosing solution for prolapse	0.8	0	5
98.2	**45540**	Proctopexy for prolapse; abdominal approach	17.5	90	6
98.2	**45541**	perineal approach	17.8	90	5
98.2	**45550**	Proctopexy combined with sigmoid resection, abdominal approach	21.6	90	7
98.2	**45560**	Repair of rectocele (separate procedure)	7.0	90	5
98.2	**45562**	Exploration, repair, and presacral drainage for rectal injury;	(I) 17.0	90	5

UPD	Code	Description	Units	FUD	Anes
98.2	**45563**	with colostomy	(I) 26.0	90	6
98.2	**45800**	Closure of rectovesical fistula;	19.0	90	6
98.2	**45805**	with colostomy	21.0	90	6
98.2	**45820**	Closure of rectourethral fistula;	19.0	90	6
98.2	**45825**	with colostomy	21.0	90	6
98.2	**45900***	Reduction of procidentia (separate procedure) under anesthesia	2.2	0	5
98.2	**45905***	Dilation of anal sphincter (separate procedure) under anesthesia other than local	1.5	0	5
98.2	**45910**	Dilation of rectal stricture (separate procedure) under anesthesia other than local	1.5	0	5
98.2	**45915***	Removal of fecal impaction or foreign body (separate procedure) under anesthesia	2.5	0	5
98.2	**45999**	Unlisted procedure, rectum	BR	0	5
98.2	**46030***	Removal of anal seton, other marker	0.6	0	5
98.2	**46040**	Incision and drainage of ischiorectal and/or perirectal abscess (separate procedure)	2.3	15	5
98.2	**46045**	Incision and drainage of intramural, intramuscular or submucosal abscess, transanal, under anesthesia	2.3	15	5
98.2	**46050***	Incision and drainage, perianal abscess, superficial	0.8	0	5
98.2	**46060**	Incision and drainage of ischiorectal or intramural abscess, with fistulectomy or fistulotomy, submuscular, with or without placement of seton	8.5	90	5
98.2	**46070**	Incision, anal septum (infant)	1.6	0	5
98.2	**46080***	Sphincterotomy, anal, division of sphincter (separate procedure)	1.2	0	5
98.2	**46083**	Incision of thrombosed hemorrhoid, external	0.8	0	5
98.2	**46200**	Fissurectomy, with or without sphincterotomy	4.0	60	5
98.2	**46210**	Cryptectomy; single	1.5	30	5
98.2	**46211**	multiple (separate procedure)	5.0	90	5
98.2	**46220**	Papillectomy or excision of single tag, anus (separate procedure)	0.6	15	3
98.2	**46221**	Hemorrhoidectomy, by simple ligature (eg, rubber band)	2.0	30	5
98.2	**46230**	Excision of external hemorrhoid tags and/or multiple papillae	1.2	15	5
98.2	**46250**	Hemorrhoidectomy, external, complete	5.0	90	5
98.2	**46255**	Hemorrhoidectomy, internal and external, simple;	8.0	90	5
98.2	**46257**	with fissurectomy	8.5	90	5

UPD	Code	Description	Units	FUD	Anes
98.2	46258	with fistulectomy, with or without fissurectomy	9.0	90	5
98.2	46260	Hemorrhoidectomy, internal and external, complex or extensive;	8.5	90	5
98.2	46261	with fissurectomy	8.5	90	5
98.2	46262	with fistulectomy, with or without fissurectomy	9.0	90	5
98.2	46270	Surgical treatment of anal fistula (fistulectomy/fistulotomy); subcutaneous	6.0	90	5
98.2	46275	submuscular	8.3	90	5
98.2	46280	complex or multiple, with or without placement of seton	9.0	90	5
98.2	46285	second stage	2.0	30	5
98.2	46288	Closure of anal fistula with rectal advancement flap	(I) 10.5	30	5
98.2	46320*	Enucleation or excision of external thrombotic hemorrhoid	1.2	0	5
98.2	46500*	Injection of sclerosing solution, hemorrhoids	0.5	0	5
98.2	46600	Anoscopy; diagnostic, with or without collection of specimen(s) by brushing or washing (separate procedure)	(I) 0.7	0	5
98.2	46604	with dilation, any method	(I) 1.8	0	5
98.2	46606	with biopsy, single or multiple	(I) 1.1	0	5
98.2	46608	with removal of foreign body	(I) 2.1	0	5
98.2	46610	with removal of single tumor, polyp, or other lesion by hot biopsy forceps or bipolar cautery	(I) 1.8	0	5
98.2	46611	with removal of single tumor, polyp, or other lesion by snare technique	(I) 2.3	0	5
98.2	46612	with removal of multiple tumors, polyps, or other lesions by hot biopsy forceps, bipolar cautery or snare technique	(I) 2.5	0	5
98.2	46614	with control of bleeding, any method	(I) 2.8	0	5
98.2	46615	with ablation of tumor(s), polyp(s), or other lesion(s) not amenable to removal by hot biopsy forceps, bipolar cautery or snare technique	(I) 3.8	0	5
98.2	46700	Anoplasty, plastic operation for stricture; adult	9.0	90	5
98.2	46705	infant	10.0	90	5
98.2	46715	Repair of low imperforate anus; with anoperineal fistula ("cut-back" procedure)	12.0	90	5
98.2	46716	with transposition of anoperineal or anovestibular fistula	13.5	90	7
98.2	46730	Repair of high imperforate anus without fistula; perineal or sacroperineal approach	(I) 28.5	90	7
98.2	46735	combined transabdominal and sacroperineal approaches	(I) 32.0	90	7

UPD	Code	Description	Units	FUD	Anes
98.2	**46740**	Repair of high imperforate anus with rectourethral or rectovaginal fistula; perineal or sacroperineal approach	27.0	90	7
98.2	**46742**	combined transabdominal and sacroperineal approaches	(I) 36.0	90	7
98.2	**46744**	Repair of cloacal anomaly by anorectovaginoplasty and urethroplasty, sacroperineal approach	(I) 41.0	90	7
98.2	**46746**	Repair of cloacal anomaly by anorectovaginoplasty and urethroplasty, combined abdominal and sacroperineal approach;	(I) 45.0	90	7
98.2	**46748**	with vaginal lengthening by intestinal graft or pedicle flaps	(I) 50.0	90	7
98.2	**46750**	Sphincteroplasty, anal, for incontinence or prolapse; adult	10.5	90	5
98.2	**46751**	child	10.9	90	5
98.2	**46753**	Graft (Thiersch operation) for rectal incontinence and/or prolapse	15.0	90	7
98.2	**46754**	Removal of Thiersch wire or suture, anal canal	3.0	90	5
98.2	**46760**	Sphincteroplasty, anal, for incontinence, adult; muscle transplant	14.0	90	5
98.2	**46761**	levator muscle imbrication (Park posterior anal repair)	(I) 20.0	90	5
98.2	**46762**	implantation artificial sphincter	(I) 25.5	90	5
98.2	**46900***	Destruction of lesion(s), anus (eg, condyloma, papilloma, molluscum contagiosum, herpetic vesicle), simple; chemical	0.5	0	3
98.2	**46910***	electrodesiccation	0.8	0	3
98.2	**46916**	cryosurgery	0.7	7	3
98.2	**46917**	laser surgery	1.2	7	3
98.2	**46922**	surgical excision	1.0	7	5
98.2	**46924**	Destruction of lesion(s), anus (eg, condyloma, papilloma, molluscum contagiosum, herpetic vesicle), extensive, any method	4.5	7	5
98.2	**46934**	Destruction of hemorrhoids, any method; internal	1.7	15	5
98.2	**46935**	external	1.0	15	5
98.2	**46936**	internal and external	1.4	15	5
98.2	**46937**	Cryosurgery of rectal tumor; benign	1.4	15	5
98.2	**46938**	malignant	3.0	15	5
98.2	**46940**	Curettage or cauterization of anal fissure, including dilation of anal sphincter (separate procedure); initial	2.0	15	5
98.2	**46942**	subsequent	2.0	15	5
98.2	**46945**	Ligation of internal hemorrhoids; single procedure	1.7	15	5

UPD		Code	Description	Units	FUD	Anes
98.2		**46946**	multiple procedures	3.4	15	5
98.2		**46999**	Unlisted procedure, anus	BR	0	5
		47000*	Biopsy of liver, needle; percutaneous	2.0	0	4
98.2	▲ +	**47001**	when done for indicated purpose at time of other major procedure (List separately in addition to code for primary procedure) Note: This code is an add-on procedure and as such is valued appropriately. Multiple procedure guidelines for reduction of value are not applicable.	(I) 1.3	0	0
97.2		**47010**	Hepatotomy; for open drainage of abscess or cyst, one or two stages	16.0	60	7
98.2		**47011**	Hepatotomy; for percutaneous drainage of abscess or cyst, one or two stages	(I) 7.0	0	7
		47015	Laparotomy, with aspiration and/or injection of hepatic parasitic (eg, amoebic or echinococcal) cyst(s) or abscess(es)	(I) 14.0	60	7
		47100	Biopsy of liver, wedge	10.0	45	7
		47120	Hepatectomy, resection of liver; partial lobectomy	29.0	45	13
		47122	trisegmentectomy	39.0	45	13
		47125	total left lobectomy	39.0	45	13
		47130	total right lobectomy	39.0	45	13
98.2		**47133**	Donor hepatectomy, with preparation and maintenance of allograft; from cadaver donor	(I) 46.0	0	7
98.2		**47134**	partial, from living donor	(I) 75.0	30	13
		47135	Liver allotransplantation; orthotopic, partial or whole, from cadaver or living donor, any age	(I) 150.0	30	30
		47136	heterotopic, partial or whole, from cadaver or living donor, any age	(I) 130.0	30	30
	M	**47137**	with aorto-hepatic arterial conduit	(I) 152.0	30	30
	M	**47138**	with port-hepatic venous conduit	(I) 156.0	30	30
	M	**47139**	with choledochojejunostomy	(I) 148.0	30	30
	M	**47140**	with take down of portocaval shunt	(I) 152.0	30	30
	M	**47141**	with take down of splenorenal shunt, proximal	(I) 148.0	30	30
	M	**47142**	with take down splenorenal shunt, distal	(I) 148.0	30	30
	M	**47143**	with mesocaval shunt	(I) 148.0	30	30
	M	**47144**	with splenectomy for hyperslenism	(I) 150.0	30	30
		47300	Marsupialization of cyst or abscess of liver	17.0	90	7

UPD			Code	Description	Units	FUD	Anes
			47350	Management of liver hemorrhage; simple suture of liver wound or injury	(I) 17.0	90	7
			47360	complex suture of liver wound or injury, with or without hepatic artery ligation	(I) 22.0	90	7
			47361	exploration of hepatic wound, extensive debridement, coagulation and/or suture, with or without packing of liver	(I) 40.0	90	7
			47362	re-exploration of hepatic wound for removal of packing	(I) 14.5	90	7
98.2			47399	Unlisted procedure, liver	BR	0	7
			47400	Hepaticotomy or hepaticostomy with exploration, drainage, or removal of calculus	21.0	45	7
			47420	Choledochotomy or choledochostomy with exploration, drainage, or removal of calculus, with or without cholecystotomy; without transduodenal sphincterotomy or sphincteroplasty	19.0	45	7
			47425	with transduodenal sphincterotomy or sphincteroplasty	22.5	45	7
			47460	Transduodenal sphincterotomy or sphincteroplasty, with or without transduodenal extraction of calculus (separate procedure)	21.0	45	7
			47480	Cholecystotomy or cholecystostomy with exploration, drainage, or removal of calculus (separate procedure)	12.5	45	7
98.2			47490	Percutaneous cholecystostomy	4.5	0	4
			47500	Injection procedure for percutaneous transhepatic cholangiography	2.4	0	4
98.2			47505	Injection procedure for cholangiography through an existing catheter (eg, percutaneous transhepatic or T-tube)	(I) 2.7	0	3
			47510	Introduction of percutaneous transhepatic catheter for biliary drainage	7.0	45	4
			47511	Introduction of percutaneous transhepatic stent for internal and external biliary drainage	(I) 9.0	0	4
98.2			47525	Change of percutaneous biliary drainage catheter	2.5	0	3
98.2			47530	Revision and/or reinsertion of transhepatic tube	5.7	45	3
98.2	▲	+	47550	Biliary endoscopy, intraoperative (choledochoscopy) (List separately in addition to code for primary procedure) Note: This code is an add-on procedure and as such is valued appropriately. Multiple procedure guidelines for reduction of value are not applicable.	5.5	45	0
98.2			47552	Biliary endoscopy, percutaneous via T-tube or other tract; diagnostic, with or without collection of specimen(s) by brushing and/or washing (separate procedure)	6.8	14	3
98.2			47553	with biopsy, single or multiple	7.3	14	5
98.2			47554	with removal of stone(s)	10.8	14	5

UPD	Code	Description	Units	FUD	Anes
98.2	47555	with dilation of biliary duct stricture(s) without stent	9.0	14	5
98.2	47556	with dilation of biliary duct stricture(s) with stent	10.0	14	5
	47600	Cholecystectomy;	14.2	45	7
	47605	with cholangiography	16.0	45	7
	47610	Cholecystectomy with exploration of common duct;	20.0	45	7
	47612	with choledochoenterostomy	21.0	45	7
	47620	with transduodenal sphincterotomy or sphincteroplasty, with or without cholangiography	22.0	45	7
98.2	47630	Biliary duct stone extraction, percutaneous via T-tube tract, basket or snare (eg, Burhenne technique)	7.0	45	3
	47700	Exploration for congenital atresia of bile ducts, without repair, with or without liver biopsy, with or without cholangiography	18.0	45	7
	47701	Portoenterostomy (eg, Kasai procedure)	(I) 42.0	45	7
	47711	Excision of bile duct tumor, with or without primary repair of bile duct; extrahepatic	(I) 25.0	60	7
	47712	intrahepatic	(I) 35.0	60	7
	47715	Excision of choledochal cyst	(I) 20.0	60	7
	47716	Anastomosis, choledochal cyst, without excision	(I) 17.0	60	7
	47720	Cholecystoenterostomy; direct	15.0	60	7
	47721	with gastroenterostomy	19.0	60	7
	47740	Roux-en-Y	17.0	60	7
	47741	Roux-en-Y with gastroenterostomy	(I) 25.0	60	7
	47760	Anastomosis, of extrahepatic biliary ducts and gastrointestinal tract	21.0	60	7
	47765	Anastomosis, of intrahepatic ducts and gastrointestinal tract	20.0	60	7
	47780	Anastomosis, Roux-en-Y, of extrahepatic biliary ducts and gastrointestinal tract	24.0	60	7
	47785	Anastomosis, Roux-en-Y, of intrahepatic biliary ducts and gastrointestinal tract	(I) 36.0	60	7
	47800	Reconstruction, plastic, of extrahepatic biliary ducts with end-to-end anastomosis	(I) 22.0	60	7
	47801	Placement of choledochal stent	(I) 11.0	60	7
	47802	U-tube hepaticoenterostomy	(I) 18.0	60	7
	47900	Suture of extrahepatic biliary duct for pre-existing injury (separate procedure)	(I) 23.0	60	7
98.2	47999	Unlisted procedure, biliary tract	BR	0	7

UPD			Code	Description	Units	FUD	Anes
98.2			**48000**	Placement of drains, peripancreatic, for acute pancreatitis;	(I) 17.0	60	7
98.2			**48001**	with cholecystostomy, gastrostomy, and jejunostomy	(I) 19.0	60	7
98.2			**48005**	Resection or debridement of pancreas and peripancreatic tissue for acute necrotizing pancreatitis	(I) 17.0	60	7
98.2			**48020**	Removal of pancreatic calculus	20.0	60	7
98.2			**48100**	Biopsy of pancreas, open, any method (eg, fine needle aspiration, needle core biopsy, wedge biopsy)	15.0	60	7
			48102*	Biopsy of pancreas, percutaneous needle	3.0	0	4
98.2			**48120**	Excision of lesion of pancreas (eg, cyst, adenoma)	17.5	60	7
			48140	Pancreatectomy, distal subtotal, with or without splenectomy; without pancreaticojejunostomy	20.0	60	8
			48145	with pancreaticojejunostomy	24.0	60	8
			48146	Pancreatectomy, distal, near-total with preservation of duodenum (Child-type procedure)	(I) 30.0	60	8
98.2			**48148**	Excision of ampulla of Vater	18.0	60	7
			48150	Pancreatectomy, proximal subtotal with total duodenectomy, partial gastrectomy, choledochoenterostomy and gastrojejunostomy (Whipple-type procedure); with pancreatojejunostomy	35.0	60	8
			48152	without pancreatojejunostomy	(I) 33.0	60	8
			48153	Pancreatectomy, proximal subtotal with near-total duodenectomy, choledochoenterostomy and duodenojejunostomy (pylorus-sparing, Whipple-type procedure); with pancreatojejunostomy	(I) 35.0	60	8
			48154	without pancreatojejunostomy	(I) 33.0	60	8
			48155	Pancreatectomy, total	24.0	60	8
			48160	Pancreatectomy, total or subtotal, with autologous transplantation of pancreas or pancreatic islets	BR	0	8
98.2			**48180**	Pancreaticojejunostomy, side-to-side anastomosis (Puestow-type operation)	25.0	60	7
98.2	▲ +		**48400**	Injection procedure for intraoperative pancreatography (List separately in addition to code for primary procedure) Note: This code is an add-on procedure and as such is valued appropriately. Multiple procedure guidelines for reduction of value are not applicable.	(I) 2.4	0	0
98.2			**48500**	Marsupialization of cyst of pancreas	15.0	60	7
98.2			**48510**	External drainage, pseudocyst of pancreas; open	20.0	60	7
98.2			**48511**	External drainage, pseudocyst of pancreas; percutaneous	(I) 8.0	0	7
98.2			**48520**	Internal anastomosis of pancreatic cyst to gastrointestinal tract; direct	17.0	60	7

UPD	Code	Description	Units	FUD	Anes
98.2	**48540**	Roux-en-Y	20.0	60	7
98.2	**48545**	Pancreatorrhaphy for trauma	(I) 18.5	60	7
98.2	**48547**	Duodenal exclusion with gastrojejunostomy for pancreatic trauma	(I) 25.5	60	7
96.2	**48550**	Donor pancreatectomy, with preparation and maintenance of allograft from cadaver donor, with or without duodenal segment for transplantation	(I) 30.0	0	7
98.2	**48554**	Transplantation of pancreatic allograft	(I) 47.0	0	7
98.2	**48556**	Removal of transplanted pancreatic allograft	(I) 32.5	90	7
98.2	**48999**	Unlisted procedure, pancreas	BR	0	7
	49000	Exploratory laparotomy, exploratory celiotomy with or without biopsy(s) (separate procedure)	13.0	90	6
	49002	Reopening of recent laparotomy	13.5	90	6
	49010	Exploration, retroperitoneal area with or without biopsy(s) (separate procedure)	15.5	90	6
96.2	**49020**	Drainage of peritoneal abscess or localized peritonitis, exclusive of appendiceal abscess; open	12.0	90	6
98.2	**49021**	percutaneous	(I) 13.0	90	3
98.2	**49040**	Drainage of subdiaphragmatic or subphrenic abscess; open	14.0	90	7
98.2	**49041**	Drainage of subdiaphragmatic or subphrenic abscess; percutaneous	(I) 6.0	0	7
97.2	**49060**	Drainage of retroperitoneal abscess; open	12.0	90	6
98.2	**49061**	Drainage of retroperitoneal abscess; percutaneous	(I) 5.5	0	5
98.2	**49062**	Drainage of extraperitoneal lymphocele to peritoneal cavity, open	(I) 12.0	10	6
98.2	**49080***	Peritoneocentesis, abdominal paracentesis, or peritoneal lavage (diagnostic or therapeutic); initial	1.5	0	3
98.2	**49081***	subsequent	1.3	0	3
	49085	Removal of peritoneal foreign body from peritoneal cavity	11.5	90	6
98.2	**49180***	Biopsy, abdominal or retroperitoneal mass, percutaneous needle	3.0	0	5
98.2	**49200**	Excision or destruction by any method of intra-abdominal or retroperitoneal tumors or cysts or endometriomas;	14.0	60	6
98.2	**49201**	extensive	21.0	60	6
98.2	**49215**	Excision of presacral or sacrococcygeal tumor	(I) 16.5	60	10

UPD	Code	Description	Units	FUD	Anes
	49220	Staging celiotomy (laparotomy) for Hodgkin's disease or lymphoma (includes splenectomy, needle or open biopsies of both liver lobes, possibly also removal of abdominal nodes, abdominal node and/or bone marrow biopsies, ovarian repositioning)	22.0	60	7
98.2	**49250**	Umbilectomy, omphalectomy, excision of umbilicus (separate procedure)	8.0	60	6
	49255	Omentectomy, epiploectomy, resection of omentum (separate procedure)	10.0	60	7
98.2	**49400***	Injection of air or contrast into peritoneal cavity (separate procedure)	1.2	0	3
98.2	**49420***	Insertion of intraperitoneal cannula or catheter for drainage or dialysis; temporary	1.5	0	3
98.2	**49421**	permanent	3.0	0	3
98.2	**49422**	Removal of permanent intraperitoneal cannula or catheter	(I) 4.0	30	3
98.2	**49423**	Exchange of previously placed abscess or cyst drainage catheter under radiological guidance (separate procedure)	(I) 3.5	0	3
98.2	**49424**	Contrast injection for assessment of abscess or cyst via previously placed catheter (separate procedure)	(I) 2.0	0	3
98.2	**49425**	Insertion of peritoneal-venous shunt	12.5	30	7
98.2	**49426**	Revision of peritoneal-venous shunt	20.0	30	7
98.2	**49427**	Injection procedure (eg, contrast media) for evaluation of previously placed peritoneal-venous shunt	2.6	0	3
98.2	**49428**	Ligation of peritoneal-venous shunt	(I) 6.0	30	7
98.2	**49429**	Removal of peritoneal-venous shunt	(I) 9.5	30	7
	49495	Repair initial inguinal hernia, under age 6 months, with or without hydrocelectomy; reducible	(I) 10.5	45	4
96.2	**49496**	incarcerated or strangulated	(I) 13.3	45	4
	49500	Repair initial inguinal hernia, age 6 months to under 5 years, with or without hydrocelectomy; reducible	8.0	45	4
	49501	incarcerated or strangulated	(I) 10.8	45	4
	49505	Repair initial inguinal hernia, age 5 years or over; reducible	8.5	45	4
	49507	incarcerated or strangulated	(I) 11.3	45	4
	49520	Repair recurrent inguinal hernia, any age; reducible	(I) 11.0	45	4
	49521	incarcerated or strangulated	(I) 13.8	45	4
	49525	Repair inguinal hernia, sliding, any age	9.0	45	4
	49540	Repair lumbar hernia	10.3	45	6
	49550	Repair initial femoral hernia, any age, reducible;	8.9	45	4
	49553	incarcerated or strangulated	(I) 11.7	45	4

UPD		Code	Description	Units	FUD	Anes
		49555	Repair recurrent femoral hernia; reducible	10.5	45	4
		49557	incarcerated or strangulated	(I) 13.3	45	4
97.2		49560	Repair initial incisional or ventral hernia; reducible	11.5	45	6
96.2		49561	Repair initial incisional or ventral hernia; incarcerated or strangulated	(I) 14.3	45	6
97.2		49565	Repair recurrent incisional or ventral hernia; reducible	13.0	45	6
96.2		49566	Repair recurrent incisional or ventral hernia; incarcerated or strangulated	(I) 15.8	45	6
98.2	+	49568	Implantation of mesh or other prosthesis for incisional or ventral hernia repair (List separately in addition to code for the incisional or ventral hernia repair) Note: This code is an add-on procedure and as such is valued appropriately. Multiple procedure guidelines for reduction of value are not applicable.	(I) 2.0	45	0
		49570	Repair epigastric hernia (eg, preperitoneal fat); reducible (separate procedure)	4.0	45	4
		49572	incarcerated or strangulated	(I) 6.8	45	4
		49580	Repair umbilical hernia, under age 5 years; reducible	7.0	45	4
		49582	incarcerated or strangulated	(I) 9.8	45	4
		49585	Repair umbilical hernia, age 5 years or over; reducible	8.0	45	4
		49587	incarcerated or strangulated	(I) 10.8	45	4
		49590	Repair spigelian hernia	9.0	45	4
98.2		49600	Repair of small omphalocele, with primary closure	10.5	45	7
98.2		49605	Repair of large omphalocele or gastroschisis; with or without prosthesis	(I) 26.0	45	7
98.2		49606	with removal of prosthesis, final reduction and closure, in operating room	(I) 21.0	45	7
		49610	Repair of omphalocele (Gross type operation); first stage	12.0	60	7
		49611	second stage	12.0	60	7
98.2		49900	Suture, secondary, of abdominal wall for evisceration or dehiscence	6.2	30	6
98.2	+	49905	Omental flap (eg, for reconstruction of sternal and chest wall defects) (list separately in addition to code for primary procedure) Note: This code is an add-on procedure and as such is valued appropriately. Multiple procedure guidelines for reduction of value are not applicable.	(I) 12.6	30	0
96.2		49906	Free omental flap with microvascular anastomosis	(I) 32.0	90	7
98.2		49999	Unlisted procedure, abdomen, peritoneum and omentum	BR	0	7

UPD	Code	Description	Units	FUD	Anes
		Urinary System			
	50010	Renal exploration, not necessitating other specific procedures	15.0	90	7
97.2	**50020**	Drainage of perirenal or renal abscess; open	.13.5	90	7
98.2	**50021**	Drainage of perirenal or renal abscess; percutaneous	(I) 5.0	0	6
	50040	Nephrostomy, nephrotomy with drainage	18.0	90	7
	50045	Nephrotomy, with exploration	18.0	90	7
	50060	Nephrolithotomy; removal of calculus	20.0	90	7
	50065	secondary surgical operation for calculus	25.0	90	7
	50070	complicated by congenital kidney abnormality	25.0	90	7
	50075	removal of large staghorn calculus filling renal pelvis and calyces (including anatrophic pyelolithotomy)	26.0	90	7
	50080	Percutaneous nephrostolithotomy or pyelostolithotomy, with or without dilation, endoscopy, lithotripsy, stenting or basket extraction; up to 2 cm	20.0	90	7
	50081	over 2 cm	23.0	90	7
98.2	**50100**	Transection or repositioning of aberrant renal vessels (separate procedure)	16.3	90	15
	50120	Pyelotomy; with exploration	19.0	90	7
	50125	with drainage, pyelostomy	19.0	90	7
	50130	with removal of calculus (pyelolithotomy, pelviolithotomy, including coagulum pyelolithotomy)	20.0	90	7
	50135	complicated (eg, secondary operation, congenital kidney abnormality)	25.0	90	7
98.2	**50200***	Renal biopsy; percutaneous, by trocar or needle	2.8	0	6
	50205	by surgical exposure of kidney	8.0	30	7
	50220	Nephrectomy, including partial ureterectomy, any approach including rib resection;	21.0	90	7
	50225	complicated because of previous surgery on same kidney	23.7	90	7
	50230	radical, with regional lymphadenectomy and/or vena caval thrombectomy	32.5	90	7
	50234	Nephrectomy with total ureterectomy and bladder cuff; through same incision	24.0	90	7
	50236	through separate incision	28.0	90	7
	50240	Nephrectomy, partial	24.0	90	7
	50280	Excision or unroofing of cyst(s) of kidney	16.0	90	7

UPD	Code	Description	Units	FUD	Anes
98.2	50290	Excision of perinephric cyst	16.0	90	6
	50300	Donor nephrectomy, with preparation and maintenance of allograft; from cadaver donor, unilateral or bilateral	30.0	0	7
	50320	from living donor	32.5	90	7
	50340	Recipient nephrectomy (separate procedure)	25.0	90	7
	50360	Renal allotransplantation, implantation of graft; excluding donor and recipient nephrectomy	37.5	90	10
	50365	with recipient nephrectomy	50.0	90	10
	50370	Removal of transplanted renal allograft	20.0	90	7
	50380	Renal autotransplantation, reimplantation of kidney	37.5	90	10
98.2	50390*	Aspiration and/or injection of renal cyst or pelvis by needle, percutaneous	2.5	0	6
98.2	50392	Introduction of intracatheter or catheter into renal pelvis for drainage and/or injection, percutaneous	3.0	0	6
96.1	50393	Introduction of ureteral catheter or stent into ureter through renal pelvis for drainage and/or injection, percutaneous	4.0	0	6
98.2	50394	Injection procedure for pyelography (as nephrostogram, pyelostogram, antegrade pyeloureterograms) through nephrostomy or pyelostomy tube, or indwelling ureteral catheter	0.3	0	5
96.1	50395	Introduction of guide into renal pelvis and/or ureter with dilation to establish nephrostomy tract, percutaneous	5.0	0	6
98.2	50396	Manometric studies through nephrostomy or pyelostomy tube, or indwelling ureteral catheter	0.4	0	5
98.2	50398*	Change of nephrostomy or pyelostomy tube	0.6	0	5
	50400	Pyeloplasty (Foley Y-pyeloplasty), plastic operation on renal pelvis, with or without plastic operation on ureter, nephropexy, nephrostomy, pyelostomy, or ureteral splinting; simple	23.5	90	7
	50405	complicated (congenital kidney abnormality, secondary pyeloplasty, solitary kidney, calycoplasty)	26.0	90	7
	50500	Nephrorrhaphy, suture of kidney wound or injury	22.0	90	7
98.2	50520	Closure of nephrocutaneous or pyelocutaneous fistula	22.5	90	6
	50525	Closure of nephrovisceral fistula (eg, renocolic), including visceral repair; abdominal approach	24.0	90	7
98.2	50526	thoracic approach	24.0	90	13
	50540	Symphysiotomy for horseshoe kidney with or without pyeloplasty and/or other plastic procedure, unilateral or bilateral (one operation)	27.5	90	7
98.2	50551	Renal endoscopy through established nephrostomy or pyelostomy, with or without irrigation, instillation, or ureteropyelography, exclusive of radiologic service;	7.0	0	5

UPD	Code	Description	Units	FUD	Anes
98.2	**50553**	with ureteral catheterization, with or without dilation of ureter	7.6	0	5
98.2	**50555**	with biopsy	7.8	0	5
98.2	**50557**	with fulguration and/or incision, with or without biopsy	7.2	0	5
98.2	**50559**	with insertion of radioactive substance with or without biopsy and/or fulguration	8.1	0	5
98.2	**50561**	with removal of foreign body or calculus	9.1	0	5
	50570	Renal endoscopy through nephrotomy or pyelotomy, with or without irrigation, instillation, or ureteropyelography, exclusive of radiologic service;	11.7	0	6
	50572	with ureteral catheterization, with or without dilation of ureter	12.7	0	6
	50574	with biopsy	13.7	0	6
	50575	with endopyelotomy (includes cystoscopy, ureteroscopy, dilation of ureter and ureteral pelvic junction, incision of ureteral pelvic junction and insertion of endopyelotomy stent)	(I) 14.7	0	6
	50576	with fulguration and/or incision, with or without biopsy	13.6	0	6
	50578	with insertion of radioactive substance, with or without biopsy and/or fulguration	14.1	0	6
	50580	with removal of foreign body or calculus	14.7	0	6
98.2	**50590**	Lithotripsy, extracorporeal shock wave	37.5	90	5
98.2	**50600**	Ureterotomy with exploration or drainage (separate procedure)	18.5	90	7
98.2	**50605**	Ureterotomy for insertion of indwelling stent, all types	18.5	90	7
	50610	Ureterolithotomy; upper one-third of ureter	19.6	90	7
	50620	middle one-third of ureter	18.5	90	6
	50630	lower one-third of ureter	20.0	90	6
98.2	**50650**	Ureterectomy, with bladder cuff (separate procedure)	20.0	90	7
98.2	**50660**	Ureterectomy, total, ectopic ureter, combination abdominal, vaginal and/or perineal approach	28.0	90	7
98.2	**50684**	Injection procedure for ureterography or ureteropyelography through ureterostomy or indwelling ureteral catheter	0.4	0	5
98.2	**50686**	Manometric studies through ureterostomy or indwelling ureteral catheter	0.5	0	5
98.2	**50688***	Change of ureterostomy tube	1.0	0	6
	50690	Injection procedure for visualization of ileal conduit and/or ureteropyelography, exclusive of radiologic service	0.5	0	3
98.2	**50700**	Ureteroplasty, plastic operation on ureter (eg, stricture)	20.0	90	7

UPD	Code	Description	Units	FUD	Anes
98.2	**50715**	Ureterolysis, with or without repositioning of ureter for retroperitoneal fibrosis	18.0	90	7
	50722	Ureterolysis for ovarian vein syndrome	14.0	90	6
98.2	**50725**	Ureterolysis for retrocaval ureter, with reanastomosis of upper urinary tract or vena cava	25.0	90	7
	50727	Revision of urinary-cutaneous anastomosis (any type urostomy);	(I) 14.1	90	6
	50728	with repair of fascial defect and hernia	(I) 16.1	90	6
	50740	Ureteropyelostomy, anastomosis of ureter and renal pelvis	22.0	90	7
	50750	Ureterocalycostomy, anastomosis of ureter to renal calyx	25.0	90	7
	50760	Ureteroureterostomy	23.0	90	6
98.2	**50770**	Transureteroureterostomy, anastomosis of ureter to contralateral ureter	24.5	90	7
	50780	Ureteroneocystostomy; anastomosis of single ureter to bladder	22.3	90	6
	50782	anastomosis of duplicated ureter to bladder	(I) 26.4	90	6
	50783	with extensive ureteral tailoring	(I) 27.7	90	6
	50785	with vesico-psoas hitch or bladder flap	24.5	90	6
	50800	Ureteroenterostomy, direct anastomosis of ureter to intestine	22.3	90	6
	50810	Ureterosigmoidostomy, with creation of sigmoid bladder and establishment of abdominal or perineal colostomy, including bowel anastomosis	31.5	120	6
	50815	Ureterocolon conduit, including bowel anastomosis	28.5	120	6
	50820	Ureteroileal conduit (ileal bladder), including bowel anastomosis (Bricker operation)	29.0	120	6
	50825	Continent diversion, including bowel anastomosis using any segment of small and/or large bowel (Kock pouch or Camey enterocystoplasty)	40.0	120	6
	50830	Urinary undiversion (eg, taking down of ureteroileal conduit, ureterosigmoidostomy or ureteroenterostomy with ureteroureterostomy or ureteroneocystostomy)	50.0	120	6
98.2	**50840**	Replacement of all or part of ureter by bowel segment, including bowel anastomosis	29.0	120	7
	50845	Cutaneous appendico-vesicostomy	(I) 29.0	90	6
98.2	**50860**	Ureterostomy, transplantation of ureter to skin	18.1	90	7
98.2	**50900**	Ureterorrhaphy, suture of ureter (separate procedure)	20.0	90	7
98.2	**50920**	Closure of ureterocutaneous fistula	20.0	90	7
	50930	Closure of ureterovisceral fistula (including visceral repair)	23.0	90	6

UPD	Code	Description	Units	FUD	Anes
	50940	Deligation of ureter	10.0	0	6
98.2	**50951**	Ureteral endoscopy through established ureterostomy, with or without irrigation, instillation, or ureteropyelography, exclusive of radiologic service;	2.2	0	5
98.2	**50953**	with ureteral catheterization, with or without dilation of ureter	2.5	0	5
98.2	**50955**	with biopsy	2.5	0	5
98.2	**50957**	with fulguration and/or incision, with or without biopsy	2.6	0	5
98.2	**50959**	with insertion of radioactive substance, with or without biopsy and/or fulguration (not including provision of material)	2.7	0	5
98.2	**50961**	with removal of foreign body or calculus	2.6	0	5
98.2	**50970**	Ureteral endoscopy through ureterotomy, with or without irrigation, instillation, or ureteropyelography, exclusive of radiologic service;	2.3	0	6
98.2	**50972**	with ureteral catheterization, with or without dilation of ureter	2.6	0	6
98.2	**50974**	with biopsy	2.6	0	6
98.2	**50976**	with fulguration and/or incision, with or without biopsy	2.6	0	6
98.2	**50978**	with insertion of radioactive substance, with or without biopsy and/or fulguration (not including provision of material)	2.6	0	6
98.2	**50980**	with removal of foreign body or calculus	2.6	0	6
	51000*	Aspiration of bladder by needle	0.5	0	3
	51005*	Aspiration of bladder; by trocar or intracatheter	0.5	0	3
98.2	**51010**	with insertion of suprapubic catheter	1.7	0	3
98.2	**51020**	Cystotomy or cystostomy; with fulguration and/or insertion of radioactive material	13.0	90	5
	51030	with cryosurgical destruction of intravesical lesion	13.3	90	6
	51040	Cystostomy, cystotomy with drainage	12.0	90	6
	51045	Cystotomy, with insertion of ureteral catheter or stent (separate procedure)	10.5	90	6
98.2	**51050**	Cystolithotomy, cystotomy with removal of calculus, without vesical neck resection	12.0	90	5
	51060	Transvesical ureterolithotomy	22.0	90	6
	51065	Cystotomy, with stone basket extraction and/or ultrasonic or electrohydraulic fragmentation of ureteral calculus	22.0	90	6
	51080	Drainage of perivesical or prevesical space abscess	8.0	90	6

UPD	Code	Description	Units	FUD	Anes
	51500	Excision of urachal cyst or sinus, with or without umbilical hernia repair	14.0	90	6
	51520	Cystotomy; for simple excision of vesical neck (separate procedure)	15.0	90	6
	51525	for excision of bladder diverticulum, single or multiple (separate procedure)	20.0	90	6
	51530	for excision of bladder tumor	15.0	90	6
	51535	Cystotomy for excision, incision, or repair of ureterocele	15.0	90	6
	51550	Cystectomy, partial; simple	17.0	90	6
	51555	complicated (eg, postradiation, previous surgery, difficult location)	20.0	90	6
	51565	Cystectomy, partial, with reimplantation of ureter(s) into bladder (ureteroneocystostomy)	24.5	90	6
	51570	Cystectomy, complete; (separate procedure)	25.5	90	8
	51575	with bilateral pelvic lymphadenectomy, including external iliac, hypogastric and obturator nodes	37.5	90	8
	51580	Cystectomy, complete, with ureterosigmoidostomy or ureterocutaneous transplantations;	40.0	70	8
	51585	with bilateral pelvic lymphadenectomy, including external iliac, hypogastric and obturator nodes	45.0	90	8
	51590	Cystectomy, complete, with ureteroileal conduit or sigmoid bladder, including bowel anastomosis;	45.0	90	8
	51595	with bilateral pelvic lymphadenectomy, including external iliac, hypogastric and obturator nodes	50.0	90	8
	51596	Cystectomy, complete, with continent diversion, any technique, using any segment of small and/or large bowel to construct neobladder	(I) 55.0	90	8
	51597	Pelvic exenteration, complete, for vesical, prostatic or urethral malignancy, with removal of bladder and ureteral transplantations, with or without hysterectomy and/or abdominoperineal resection of rectum and colon and colostomy, or any combination thereof	48.0	90	8
	51600*	Injection procedure for cystography or voiding urethrocystography	0.3	0	3
	51605	Injection procedure and placement of chain for contrast and/or chain urethrocystography	0.4	0	3
	51610	Injection procedure for retrograde urethrocystography	0.3	0	3
	51700*	Bladder irrigation, simple, lavage and/or instillation	0.3	0	3
	51705*	Change of cystostomy tube; simple	0.5	0	3
	51710*	complicated	2.5	0	3
	51715	Endoscopic injection of implant material into the submucosal tissues of the urethra and/or bladder neck	(I) 5.0	0	3

UPD	Code	Description	Units	FUD	Anes
	51720	Bladder instillation of anticarcinogenic agent (including detention time)	0.8	0	3
	51725	Simple cystometrogram (CMG) (eg, spinal manometer)	1.3	0	3
	51726	Complex cystometrogram (eg, calibrated electronic equipment)	1.6	0	3
	51736	Simple uroflowmetry (UFR) (eg, stop-watch flow rate, mechanical uroflowmeter)	0.3	0	3
	51741	Complex uroflowmetry (eg, calibrated electronic equipment)	0.6	0	3
	51772	Urethral pressure profile studies (UPP) (urethral closure pressure profile), any technique	1.5	0	3
	51784	Electromyography studies (EMG) of anal or urethral sphincter, other than needle, any technique	2.1	0	3
	51785	Needle electromyography studies (EMG) of anal or urethral sphincter, any technique	2.1	0	3
	51792	Stimulus evoked response (eg, measurement of bulbocavernosus reflex latency time)	3.0	0	3
	51795	Voiding pressure studies (VP); bladder voiding pressure, any technique	1.3	0	3
	51797	intra-abdominal voiding pressure (AP) (rectal, gastric, intraperitoneal)	1.9	0	3
	51800	Cystoplasty or cystourethroplasty, plastic operation on bladder and/or vesical neck (anterior Y-plasty, vesical fundus resection), any procedure, with or without wedge resection of posterior vesical neck	20.0	90	6
	51820	Cystourethroplasty with unilateral or bilateral ureteroneocystostomy	30.0	90	6
97.2	51840	Anterior vesicourethropexy, or urethropexy (eg, Marshall-Marchetti-Krantz, Burch); simple	15.0	90	6
	51841	Anterior vesicourethropexy, or urethropexy (eg, Marshall-Marchetti-Krantz, Burch); complicated (eg, secondary repair)	18.0	90	6
	51845	Abdomino-vaginal vesical neck suspension, with or without endoscopic control (eg, Stamey, Raz, modified Pereyra)	20.0	90	6
	51860	Cystorrhaphy, suture of bladder wound, injury or rupture; simple	15.0	90	6
	51865	complicated	18.0	90	6
	51880	Closure of cystostomy (separate procedure)	6.5	90	6
	51900	Closure of vesicovaginal fistula, abdominal approach	30.0	90	6
	51920	Closure of vesicouterine fistula;	19.0	90	6
	51925	with hysterectomy	27.5	90	6
	51940	Closure of bladder exstrophy	45.0	90	6
	51960	Enterocystoplasty, including bowel anastomosis	30.0	90	6

UPD		Code	Description	Units	FUD	Anes
		51980	Cutaneous vesicostomy	18.0	90	6
		52000	Cystourethroscopy (separate procedure)	2.0	0	3
		52005	Cystourethroscopy, with ureteral catheterization, with or without irrigation, instillation, or ureteropyelography, exclusive of radiologic service;	3.0	0	3
		52007	with brush biopsy of ureter and/or renal pelvis	4.0	0	3
		52010	Cystourethroscopy, with ejaculatory duct catheterization, with or without irrigation, instillation, or duct radiography, exclusive of radiologic service	3.0	0	3
	M	52011	insertion and removal, indwelling stent	4.0	0	3
		52204	Cystourethroscopy, with biopsy	3.0	7	3
		52214	Cystourethroscopy, with fulguration (including cryosurgery or laser surgery) of trigone, bladder neck, prostatic fossa, urethra, or periurethral glands	3.0	7	3
		52224	Cystourethroscopy, with fulguration (including cryosurgery or laser surgery) or treatment of MINOR (less than 0.5 cm) lesion(s) with or without biopsy	3.0	7	3
98.2		52234	Cystourethroscopy, with fulguration (including cryosurgery or laser surgery) and/or resection of; SMALL bladder tumor(s) (0.5 to 2.0 cm)	5.8	15	5
98.2		52235	MEDIUM bladder tumor(s) (2.0 to 5.0 cm)	12.0	30	5
98.2		52240	LARGE bladder tumor(s)	18.0	30	5
		52250	Cystourethroscopy with insertion of radioactive substance, with or without biopsy or fulguration	4.0	7	3
		52260	Cystourethroscopy, with dilation of bladder for interstitial cystitis; general or conduction (spinal) anesthesia	3.0	7	3
98.2		52265	local anesthesia	3.0	30	3
		52270	Cystourethroscopy, with internal urethrotomy; female	3.0	15	3
		52275	male	3.5	15	3
		52276	Cystourethroscopy with direct vision internal urethrotomy	8.0	30	3
		52277	Cystourethroscopy, with resection of external sphincter (sphincterotomy)	8.5	30	3
97.2		52281	Cystourethroscopy, with calibration and/or dilation of urethral stricture or stenosis, with or without meatotomy, with or without injection procedure for cystography, male or female	3.0	0	3
97.2		52282	Cystourethroscopy, with insertion of urethral stent	(I) 8.5	30	3
		52283	Cystourethroscopy, with steroid injection into stricture	2.8	0	3

UPD		Code	Description	Units	FUD	Anes
		52285	Cystourethroscopy for treatment of the female urethral syndrome with any or all of the following: urethral meatotomy, urethral dilation, internal urethrotomy, lysis of urethrovaginal septal fibrosis, lateral incisions of the bladder neck, and fulguration of polyp(s) of urethra, bladder neck, and/or trigone	3.0	15	3
		52290	Cystourethroscopy; with ureteral meatotomy, unilateral or bilateral	4.0	15	3
96.2		52300	with resection or fulguration of orthotopic ureterocele(s), unilateral or bilateral	6.0	15	3
96.2		52301	with resection or fulguration of ectopic ureterocele(s), unilateral or bilateral	(I) 6.6	15	3
		52305	with incision or resection of orifice of bladder diverticulum, single or multiple	6.0	15	3
		52310	Cystourethroscopy, with removal of foreign body, calculus, or ureteral stent from urethra or bladder (separate procedure); simple	4.0	15	3
		52315	complicated	7.5	15	3
		52317	Litholapaxy: crushing or fragmentation of calculus by any means in bladder and removal of fragments; simple or small (less than 2.5 cm)	10.0	15	3
		52318	complicated or large (over 2.5 cm)	13.8	15	3
98.2		52320	Cystourethroscopy (including ureteral catheterization); with removal of ureteral calculus	7.5	15	5
98.2		52325	with fragmentation of ureteral calculus (eg, ultrasonic or electro-hydraulic technique)	8.0	15	5
98.2		52327	with subureteric injection of implant material	(I) 6.0	15	5
98.2		52330	with manipulation, without removal of ureteral calculus	5.0	15	5
		52332	Cystourethroscopy, with insertion of indwelling ureteral stent (eg, Gibbons or double-J type)	5.0	15	3
	M	52333	with balloon dilatation of ureteral stricture or UPJ obstruction	7.5	15	3
98.2		52334	Cystourethroscopy with insertion of ureteral guide wire through kidney to establish a percutaneous nephrostomy, retrograde	6.0	15	6
		52335	Cystourethroscopy, with ureteroscopy and/or pyeloscopy (includes dilation of the ureter and/or pyeloureteral junction by any method);	12.5	15	3
98.2		52336	with removal or manipulation of calculus (ureteral catheterization is included)	16.0	15	5
98.2		52337	with lithotripsy (ureteral catheterization is included)	18.0	15	5
		52338	with biopsy and/or fulguration of lesion	17.5	15	3
98.2		52339	with resection of tumor	(I) 12.8	15	5

UPD	Code	Description	Units	FUD	Anes
98.2	52340	Cystourethroscopy with incision, fulguration, or resection of congenital posterior urethral valves, or congenital obstructive hypertrophic mucosal folds	13.0	15	3
98.2	52450	Transurethral incision of prostate	(I) 11.0	90	3
	52500	Transurethral resection of bladder neck (separate procedure)	10.0	90	5
98.2	52510	Transurethral balloon dilation of the prostatic urethra, any method	(I) 12.6	90	3
	52601	Transurethral electrosurgical resection of prostate, including control of postoperative bleeding, complete (vasectomy, meatotomy, cystourethroscopy, urethral calibration, dilation, and internal urethrotomy are included)	20.0	90	5
	52606	Transurethral fulguration for postoperative bleeding occurring after the usual follow-up period	3.8	0	5
	52612	Transurethral resection of prostate; first stage of two-stage resection (partial resection)	13.0	90	5
	52614	second stage of two-stage resection (resection completed)		90	5
	52620	Transurethral resection; of residual obstructive tissue after 90 days postoperative	6.0	90	5
	52630	of regrowth of obstructive tissue longer than one year postoperative	20.0	90	5
	52640	of postoperative bladder neck contracture	10.0	90	5
	52647	Non-contact laser coagulation of prostate, including control of postoperative bleeding, complete (vasectomy, meatotomy, cystourethroscopy, urethral calibration and/or dilation, and internal urethrotomy are included)	(I) 16.0	90	5
	52648	Contact laser vaporization with or without transurethral resection of prostate, including control of postoperative bleeding, complete (vasectomy, meatotomy, cystourethroscopy, urethral calibration and/or dilation, and internal urethrotomy are included)	(I) 18.0	90	5
98.2	52700	Transurethral drainage of prostatic abscess	8.0	60	3
	53000	Urethrotomy or urethrostomy, external (separate procedure); pendulous urethra	2.4	15	3
	53010	perineal urethra, external	6.0	30	3
	53020	Meatotomy, cutting of meatus (separate procedure); except infant	2.0	15	3
	53025	infant	0.7	15	3
	53040	Drainage of deep periurethral abscess	3.0	30	3
	53060	Drainage of Skene's gland abscess or cyst	1.3	15	3
	53080	Drainage of perineal urinary extravasation; uncomplicated (separate procedure)	4.0	0	3
	53085	complicated	12.0	0	3

Handwritten note: TUR also see 53850 53852 52647 52648

UPD	Code	Description	Units	FUD	Anes
	53200	Biopsy of urethra	2.0	7	3
98.2	53210	Urethrectomy, total, including cystostomy; female	14.0	60	3
98.2	53215	male	18.3	60	3
	53220	Excision or fulguration of carcinoma of urethra	10.0	60	3
	53230	Excision of urethral diverticulum (separate procedure); female	13.0	60	3
	53235	male	13.0	60	3
	53240	Marsupialization of urethral diverticulum, male or female	4.0	15	3
	53250	Excision of bulbourethral gland (Cowper's gland)	4.0	15	3
	53260	Excision or fulguration; urethral polyp(s), distal urethra	1.0	15	3
	53265	urethral caruncle	2.0	15	3
	53270	Skene's glands	2.0	15	3
	53275	urethral prolapse	3.1	15	3
	53400	Urethroplasty; first stage, for fistula, diverticulum, or stricture (eg, Johannsen type)	10.0	60	3
	53405	second stage (formation of urethra), including urinary diversion	14.5	60	3
	53410	Urethroplasty, one-stage reconstruction of male anterior urethra	16.0	60	3
	53415	Urethroplasty, transpubic or perineal, one stage, for reconstruction or repair of prostatic or membranous urethra	24.0	60	3
	53420	Urethroplasty, two-stage reconstruction or repair of prostatic or membranous urethra; first stage	20.0	60	3
	53425	second stage	20.0	90	3
	53430	Urethroplasty, reconstruction of female urethra	14.1	90	3
	53440	Operation for correction of male urinary incontinence, with or without introduction of prosthesis	20.0	90	3
	53442	Removal of perineal prosthesis introduced for continence	5.0	60	3
	53443	Urethroplasty with tubularization of posterior urethra and/or lower bladder for incontinence (eg, Tenago, Leadbetter procedure)	22.0	60	3
	53445	Operation for correction of urinary incontinence with placement of inflatable urethral or bladder neck sphincter, including placement of pump and/or reservoir	27.0	90	4
	53447	Removal, repair or replacement of inflatable sphincter including pump and/or reservoir and/or cuff	6.0	60	3
	53449	Surgical correction of hydraulic abnormality of inflatable sphincter device	9.0	90	3

+ Add-on Code ⊘ Modifier -51 Exempt ▲ Revised code ● New code **M** RVSI code or deleted from CPT **(I)** Interim Value

Copyright © 1999 St. Anthony Publishing

UPD		Code	Description	Units	FUD	Anes
		53450	Urethromeatoplasty, with mucosal advancement	4.0	30	3
		53460	Urethromeatoplasty, with partial excision of distal urethral segment (Richardson type procedure)	5.0	30	3
		53502	Urethrorrhaphy, suture of urethral wound or injury, female	10.2	30	3
		53505	Urethrorrhaphy, suture of urethral wound or injury; penile	10.2	30	3
		53510	perineal	13.5	90	3
		53515	prostatomembranous	20.0	90	5
		53520	Closure of urethrostomy or urethrocutaneous fistula, male (separate procedure)	6.0	90	3
		53600*	Dilation of urethral stricture by passage of sound or urethral dilator, male; initial	0.5	0	3
		53601*	subsequent	0.4	0	3
		53605	Dilation of urethral stricture or vesical neck by passage of sound or urethral dilator, male, general or conduction (spinal) anesthesia	1.7	0	3
		53620*	Dilation of urethral stricture by passage of filiform and follower, male; initial	0.9	0	3
		53621*	subsequent	0.6	0	3
96.2	M	53640*	Passage to filiform and follower for acute vesical retention, male To report, use 53620	0.8	0	3
		53660*	Dilation of female urethra including suppository and/or instillation; initial	0.5	0	3
		53661*	subsequent	0.4	0	3
		53665	Dilation of female urethra, general or conduction (spinal) anesthesia	1.3	0	3
		53670*	Catheterization, urethra; simple	0.3	0	3
		53675*	complicated (may include difficult removal of balloon catheter)	0.6	0	3
98.2		53850	Transurethral destruction of prostate tissue; by microwave thermotherapy	(I) 11.0	90	5
98.2		53852	Transurethral destruction of prostate tissue; by radiofrequency thermotherapy	(I) 11.5	90	5
98.2		53899	Unlisted procedure, urinary system	BR	0	3

Male Genital System

UPD		Code	Description	Units	FUD	Anes
		54000	Slitting of prepuce, dorsal or lateral (separate procedure); newborn	0.8	0	3
		54001	except newborn	1.4	0	3
		54015	Incision and drainage of penis, deep	1.3	0	3

+ Add-on Code   ⊘ Modifier -51 Exempt   ▲ Revised code   ● New code   **M** RVSI code or deleted from CPT   **(I)** Interim Value

Copyright © 1999 St. Anthony Publishing

UPD	Code	Description	Units	FUD	Anes
	54050*	Destruction of lesion(s), penis (eg, condyloma, papilloma, molluscum contagiosum, herpetic vesicle), simple; chemical	0.4	0	3
	54055*	electrodesiccation	0.8	0	3
	54056	cryosurgery	1.0	7	3
	54057	laser surgery	2.0	7	3
	54060	surgical excision	2.0	7	3
	54065	Destruction of lesion(s), penis (eg, condyloma, papilloma, molluscum contagiosum, herpetic vesicle), extensive, any method	2.7	7	3
	54100	Biopsy of penis; cutaneous (separate procedure)	1.0	7	3
	54105	deep structures	1.4	7	3
	54110	Excision of penile plaque (Peyronie disease);	8.3	30	3
	54111	with graft to 5 cm in length	18.5	30	3
	54112	with graft greater than 5 cm in length	20.5	30	3
	54115	Removal foreign body from deep penile tissue (eg, plastic implant)	5.5	30	3
	54120	Amputation of penis; partial	10.0	30	3
	54125	complete	20.0	90	4
	54130	Amputation of penis, radical; with bilateral inguinofemoral lymphadenectomy	28.0	90	6
	54135	in continuity with bilateral pelvic lymphadenectomy, including external iliac, hypogastric and obturator nodes	34.0	90	8
	54150	Circumcision, using clamp or other device; newborn	0.8	15	3
	54152	except newborn	1.0	15	3
	54160	Circumcision, surgical excision other than clamp, device or dorsal slit; newborn	1.0	30	3
	54161	except newborn	3.0	30	3
	54200*	Injection procedure for Peyronie disease;	0.5	0	3
	54205	with surgical exposure of plaque	5.0	0	3
	54220	Irrigation of corpora cavernosa for priapism	1.8	0	3
	54230	Injection procedure for corpora cavernosography	1.4	7	3
	54231	Dynamic cavernosometry, including intracavernosal injection of vasoactive drugs (eg, papaverine, phentolamine)	(I) 4.0	7	3
	54235	Injection of corpora cavernosa with pharmacologic agent(s) (eg, papaverine, phentolamine)	1.4	7	3
	54240	Penile plethysmography	1.4	7	3

UPD	Code	Description	Units	FUD	Anes
	54250	Nocturnal penile tumescence and/or rigidity test	2.0	0	0
M	54251	Use of other device	0.7	0	0
	54300	Plastic operation of penis for straightening of chordee (eg, hypospadias), with or without mobilization of urethra	8.0	30	3
	54304	Plastic operation on penis for correction of chordee or for first stage hypospadias repair with or without transplantation of prepuce and/or skin flaps	14.0	90	3
	54308	Urethroplasty for second stage hypospadias repair (including urinary diversion); less than 3 cm	14.0	90	3
	54312	greater than 3 cm	16.0	90	3
	54316	Urethroplasty for second stage hypospadias repair (including urinary diversion) with free skin graft obtained from site other than genitalia	18.0	90	3
	54318	Urethroplasty for third stage hypospadias repair to release penis from scrotum (eg, third stage Cecil repair)	10.0	90	3
	54322	One stage distal hypospadias repair (with or without chordee or circumcision); with simple meatal advancement (eg, Magpi, V-flap)	12.0	90	3
	54324	with urethroplasty by local skin flaps (eg, flip-flap, prepucial flap)	14.0	90	3
	54326	with urethroplasty by local skin flaps and mobilization of urethra	16.0	90	3
	54328	with extensive dissection to correct chordee and urethroplasty with local skin flaps, skin graft patch, and/or island flap	20.5	90	3
	54332	One stage proximal penile or penoscrotal hypospadias repair requiring extensive dissection to correct chordee and urethroplasty by use of skin graft tube and/or island flap	23.0	90	3
	54336	One stage perineal hypospadias repair requiring extensive dissection to correct chordee and urethroplasty by use of skin graft tube and/or island flap	26.5	90	3
	54340	Repair of hypospadias complications (ie, fistula, stricture, diverticula); by closure, incision, or excision, simple	10.5	90	3
	54344	requiring mobilization of skin flaps and urethroplasty with flap or patch graft	16.0	90	3
	54348	requiring extensive dissection and urethroplasty with flap, patch or tubed graft (includes urinary diversion)	20.0	90	3
	54352	Repair of hypospadias cripple requiring extensive dissection and excision of previously constructed structures including re-release of chordee and reconstruction of urethra and penis by use of local skin as grafts and island flaps and skin brought in as flaps or grafts	33.5	90	3
	54360	Plastic operation on penis to correct angulation	6.0	90	3
	54380	Plastic operation on penis for epispadias distal to external sphincter;	8.0	30	3

UPD	Code	Description	Units	FUD	Anes
	54385	with incontinence	10.0	30	3
98.2	54390	with exstrophy of bladder	10.0	30	6
	54400	Insertion of penile prosthesis; non-inflatable (semi-rigid)	12.0	30	4
	54401	inflatable (self-contained)	(I) 14.0	30	4
	54402	Removal or replacement of non-inflatable (semi-rigid) or inflatable (self-contained) penile prosthesis	6.0	90	4
	54405	Insertion of inflatable (multi-component) penile prosthesis, including placement of pump, cylinders, and/or reservoir	25.0	90	4
	54407	Removal, repair, or replacement of inflatable (multi-component) penile prosthesis, including pump and/or reservoir and/or cylinders	6.0	90	4
	54409	Surgical correction of hydraulic abnormality of inflatable (multi-component) prosthesis including pump and/or reservoir and/or cylinders	7.5	90	4
M	54412	Dorsal vein ligation of penis	(I) 10.0	90	4
98.2	54420	Corpora cavernosa-saphenous vein shunt (priapism operation), unilateral or bilateral	12.5	30	3
98.2	54430	Corpora cavernosa-corpus spongiosum shunt (priapism operation), unilateral or bilateral	12.5	30	3
98.2	54435	Corpora cavernosa-glans penis fistulization (eg, biopsy needle, Winter procedure, rongeur, or punch) for priapism	3.0	30	3
	54440	Plastic operation of penis for injury	BR	0	3
	54450	Foreskin manipulation including lysis of preputial adhesions and stretching	0.8	0	3
	54500	Biopsy of testis, needle (separate procedure)	0.4	0	3
	54505	Biopsy of testis, incisional (separate procedure)	3.1	0	3
	54510	Excision of local lesion of testis	6.0	30	3
98.2	54520	Orchiectomy, simple (including subcapsular), with or without testicular prosthesis, scrotal or inguinal approach	6.3	30	3
	54530	Orchiectomy, radical, for tumor; inguinal approach	9.5	30	4
	54535	with abdominal exploration	12.5	45	6
	54550	Exploration for undescended testis (inguinal or scrotal area)	8.3	30	4
	54560	Exploration for undescended testis with abdominal exploration	11.5	30	6
	54600	Reduction of torsion of testis, surgical, with or without fixation of contralateral testis	10.0	30	3
	54620	Fixation of contralateral testis (separate procedure)	4.0	30	3
	54640	Orchiopexy, inguinal approach, with or without hernia repair	11.0	30	4

UPD	Code	Description	Units	FUD	Anes
98.2	54650	Orchiopexy, abdominal approach, for intra-abdominal testis (eg, Fowler-Stephens)	(I) 17.5	45	4
	54660	Insertion of testicular prosthesis (separate procedure)	4.0	45	3
	54670	Suture or repair of testicular injury	8.0	45	3
	54680	Transplantation of testis(es) to thigh (because of scrotal destruction)	10.0	45	3
	54700	Incision and drainage of epididymis, testis and/or scrotal space (eg, abscess or hematoma)	1.4	7	3
	54800	Biopsy of epididymis, needle	0.4	7	3
	54820	Exploration of epididymis, with or without biopsy	5.6	30	3
	54830	Excision of local lesion of epididymis	6.0	30	3
	54840	Excision of spermatocele, with or without epididymectomy	8.0	45	3
	54860	Epididymectomy; unilateral	8.0	45	3
	54861	bilateral	12.0	45	3
	54900	Epididymovasostomy, anastomosis of epididymis to vas deferens; unilateral	20.0	90	3
	54901	bilateral	30.0	90	3
	55000*	Puncture aspiration of hydrocele, tunica vaginalis, with or without injection of medication	0.3	0	3
	55040	Excision of hydrocele; unilateral	8.0	45	3
	55041	bilateral	12.0	45	3
	55060	Repair of tunica vaginalis hydrocele (Bottle type)	6.1	45	3
	55100*	Drainage of scrotal wall abscess	0.6	0	3
	55110	Scrotal exploration	5.0	0	3
	55120	Removal of foreign body in scrotum	2.5	0	3
	55150	Resection of scrotum	3.0	30	3
	55175	Scrotoplasty; simple	8.0	30	3
	55180	complicated	12.0	30	3
	55200	Vasotomy, cannulization with or without incision of vas, unilateral or bilateral (separate procedure)	3.6	30	3
	55250	Vasectomy, unilateral or bilateral (separate procedure), including postoperative semen examination(s)	4.5	30	3
	55300	Vasotomy for vasograms, seminal vesiculograms, or epididymograms, unilateral or bilateral	3.6	30	3
	55400	Vasovasostomy, vasovasorrhaphy	20.0	90	3

UPD		Code	Description	Units	FUD	Anes
		55450	Ligation (percutaneous) of vas deferens, unilateral or bilateral (separate procedure)	1.3	30	3
		55500	Excision of hydrocele of spermatic cord, unilateral (separate procedure)	6.0	45	3
		55520	Excision of lesion of spermatic cord (separate procedure)	6.0	30	3
		55530	Excision of varicocele or ligation of spermatic veins for varicocele; (separate procedure)	8.0	45	3
98.2		55535	abdominal approach	9.5	45	6
		55540	with hernia repair	9.5	45	4
		55600	Vesiculotomy;	7.0	60	6
		55605	complicated	BR	60	6
		55650	Vesiculectomy, any approach	20.0	45	6
		55680	Excision of Mullerian duct cyst	20.0	45	6
		55700	Biopsy, prostate; needle or punch, single or multiple, any approach	2.0	15	4
		55705	incisional, any approach	8.5	30	4
		55720	Prostatotomy, external drainage of prostatic abscess, any approach; simple	8.5	30	4
		55725	complicated	14.0	60	4
	M	55780	Ultrasound of prostate, complete;	2.4	0	4
	M	55782	with guidance for Bx of prostate (including Bx of prostate)	4.4	0	4
		55801	Prostatectomy, perineal, subtotal (including control of postoperative bleeding, vasectomy, meatotomy, urethral calibration and/or dilation, and internal urethrotomy)	22.0	90	6
98.2		55810	Prostatectomy, perineal radical;	26.0	90	7
98.2		55812	with lymph node biopsy(s) (limited pelvic lymphadenectomy)	28.5	90	7
98.2		55815	with bilateral pelvic lymphadenectomy, including external iliac, hypogastric and obturator nodes	35.0	90	7
98.2		55821	Prostatectomy (including control of postoperative bleeding, vasectomy, meatotomy, urethral calibration and/or dilation, and internal urethrotomy); suprapubic, subtotal, one or two stages	20.0	90	7
98.2		55831	retropubic, subtotal	20.0	90	7
98.2		55840	Prostatectomy, retropubic radical, with or without nerve sparing;	26.0	90	7
98.2		55842	with lymph node biopsy(s) (limited pelvic lymphadenectomy)	27.5	90	7

UPD	Code	Description	Units	FUD	Anes
98.2	**55845**	with bilateral pelvic lymphadenectomy, including external iliac, hypogastric and obturator nodes	35.0	90	7
98.2	**55859**	Transperineal placement of needles or catheters into prostate for interstitial radioelement application, with or without cystoscopy	(I) 20.0	90	3
	55860	Exposure of prostate, any approach, for insertion of radioactive substance;	14.0	90	6
	55862	with lymph node biopsy(s) (limited pelvic lymphadenectomy)	20.0	90	6
	55865	with bilateral pelvic lymphadenectomy, including external iliac, hypogastric and obturator nodes	30.0	90	6
98.2	**55870**	Electroejaculation	(I) 1.4	0	3
98.2	**55899**	Unlisted procedure, male genital system	BR	0	3

Intersex Surgery

UPD	Code	Description	Units	FUD	Anes
98.2	**55970**	Intersex surgery; male to female	BR	0	7
98.2	**55980**	female to male	BR	0	7

Laparoscopy/Hysteroscopy

UPD	Code	Description	Units	FUD	Anes
96.2	**56300**	Laparoscopy (peritoneoscopy), diagnostic; (separate procedure)	8.0	0	6
	56301	Laparoscopy, surgical; with fulguration of oviducts (with or without transection)	10.0	15	6
	56302	with occlusion of oviducts by device (eg, band, clip, or Falope ring)	10.0	15	6
	56303	with fulguration or excision of lesions of the ovary, pelvic viscera, or peritoneal surface by any method	10.0	15	6
97.2	**56304**	Laparoscopy, surgical; with lysis of adhesions (salpingolysis, ovariolysis) (separate procedure)	10.0	15	6
96.2	**56305**	with biopsy (single or multiple)	10.0	15	6
	56306	with aspiration (single or multiple)	10.0	15	6
	56307	with removal of adnexal structures (partial or total oophorectomy and/or salpingectomy)	14.7	15	6
	56308	with vaginal hysterectomy with or without removal of tube(s), with or without removal of ovary(s) (laparoscopic assisted vaginal hysterectomy)	(I) 20.0	15	6
97.2	**56309**	Laparoscopy, surgical; with removal of leiomyomata (single or multiple)	(I) 14.7	15	6
98.2	**56310**	Laparoscopy, surgical; enterolysis (freeing of intestinal adhesion) (separate procedure)	(I) 14.6	15	6
	56311	with retroperitoneal lymph node sampling (biopsy), single or multiple	(I) 12.0	15	6

UPD	Code	Description	Units	FUD	Anes
	56312	with bilateral total pelvic lymphadenectomy	18.0	15	6
	56313	with bilateral total pelvic lymphadenectomy and peri-aortic lymph node sampling (biopsy), single or multiple	(I) 21.0	15	6
98.2	56314	Laparoscopy, surgical; with drainage of lymphocele to peritoneal cavity	(I) 12.0	15	6
	56315	appendectomy	10.0	15	6
	56316	repair of initial inguinal hernia	(I) 8.5	15	6
	56317	repair of recurrent inguinal hernia	(I) 10.5	15	6
97.2	56318	Laparoscopy, surgical; orchiectomy	(I) 12.5	15	6
	56320	with ligation of spermatic veins for varicocele	(I) 8.0	15	6
98.2 ●	56321	with adrenalectomy, partial or complete, or exploration of adrenal gland with or without biopsy, transabdominal, lumbar or dorsal	(I) 19.5	15	6
	56322	transection of vagus nerves, truncal	(I) 14.0	15	7
	56323	transection of vagus nerves, selective or highly selective	(I) 23.0	15	7
	56324	cholecystoenterostomy	(I) 21.0	15	7
	56340	cholecystectomy (any method)	14.2	15	7
	56341	cholecystectomy with cholangiography	16.0	15	7
	56342	cholecystectomy with exploration of common duct	(I) 20.0	15	7
	56343	with salpingostomy (salpingoneostomy)	(I) 10.0	15	6
	56344	with fimbrioplasty	(I) 10.5	15	6
97.2	56345	Laparoscopy, surgical; splenectomy	(I) 16.0	15	7
97.2	56346	Laparoscopy, surgical; gastrostomy, temporary (tube or rubber or plastic) (separate procedure)	(I) 11.5	15	7
98.2	56347	Laparoscopy, surgical; jejunostomy (eg, for decompression or feeding)	(I) 14.0	15	6
98.2	56348	Laparoscopy, surgical; intestinal resection, with anastomosis (intra or extracorporeal)	(I) 17.6	15	6
97.2	56349	Laparoscopy, surgical; esophagogastric fundoplasty (eg, Nissen, Belsey IV, Hill, Toupet procedures)	(I) 20.0	15	7
	56350	Hysteroscopy, diagnostic (separate procedure)	4.0	15	4
	56351	Hysteroscopy, surgical; with sampling (biopsy) of endometrium and/or polypectomy, with or without D & C	6.0	15	4
	56352	with lysis of intrauterine adhesions (any method)	(I) 6.6	15	4
	56353	with division or resection of intrauterine septum (any method)	(I) 7.4	15	4
98.2	56354	with removal of leiomyomata	(I) 8.1	15	6

UPD		Code	Description	Units	FUD	Anes
		56355	with removal of impacted foreign body	(I) 6.5	15	4
98.2		56356	with endometrial ablation (any method)	20.0	15	6
96.2 **M**		56360	Peritoneoscopy; without biopsy To report, use 56300	4.5	0	6
96.2 **M**		56361	with biopsy To report, use 56305	4.8	0	6
96.2		56362	Laparoscopy with guided transhepatic cholangiography; without biopsy	5.0	0	6
96.2		56363	with biopsy	5.8	0	6
98.2		56399	Unlisted procedure, laparoscopy, hysteroscopy	BR	0	6

Female Genital System

UPD		Code	Description	Units	FUD	Anes
		56405*	Incision and drainage of vulva or perineal abscess	(I) 2.0	0	3
		56420*	Incision and drainage of Bartholin's gland abscess	1.0	0	3
		56440	Marsupialization of Bartholin's gland cyst	4.0	0	3
		56441	Lysis of labial adhesions	1.0	0	3
		56501	Destruction of lesion(s), vulva; simple, any method	1.0	0	3
		56515	extensive, any method	4.0	0	3
		56605*	Biopsy of vulva or perineum (separate procedure); one lesion	(I) 1.2	0	3
98.2	▲ +	56606*	each separate additional lesion (List separately in addition to code for primary procedure) Note: This code is an add-on procedure and as such is valued appropriately. Multiple procedure guidelines for reduction of value are not applicable.	(I) 0.6	0	0
		56620	Vulvectomy simple; partial	11.0	60	4
		56625	complete	15.5	60	4
		56630	Vulvectomy, radical, partial;	16.1	90	7
		56631	with unilateral inguinofemoral lymphadenectomy	(I) 22.0	90	7
		56632	with bilateral inguinofemoral lymphadenectomy	(I) 26.0	90	7
		56633	Vulvectomy, radical, complete;	(I) 19.2	90	7
		56634	with unilateral inguinofemoral lymphadenectomy	(I) 24.0	90	7
		56637	with bilateral inguinofemoral lymphadenectomy	(I) 25.3	90	7
98.2		56640	Vulvectomy, radical, complete, with inguinofemoral, iliac, and pelvic lymphadenectomy	29.0	90	7
		56700	Partial hymenectomy or revision of hymenal ring	3.5	30	3
		56720*	Hymenotomy, simple incision	1.1	0	3

UPD		Code	Description	Units	FUD	Anes
		56740	Excision of Bartholin's gland or cyst	4.3	30	3
		56800	Plastic repair of introitus	4.8	30	3
		56805	Clitoroplasty for intersex state	(I) 12.0	90	3
		56810	Perineoplasty, repair of perineum, non-obstetrical (separate procedure)	(I) 5.8	30	3
		57000	Colpotomy; with exploration	4.5	30	4
		57010	with drainage of pelvic abscess	5.5	30	4
98.2		57020*	Colpocentesis (separate procedure)	0.8	0	3
		57061	Destruction of vaginal lesion(s); simple, any method	1.0	15	3
		57065	extensive, any method	4.2	15	3
		57100*	Biopsy of vaginal mucosa; simple (separate procedure)	0.8	0	3
		57105	extensive, requiring suture (including cysts)	1.2	0	3
98.2	●	57106	Vaginectomy, partial removal of vaginal wall;	(I) 10.0	90	4
98.2	●	57107	with removal of paravaginal tissue (radical vaginectomy)	(I) 18.0	90	4
98.2	M	57108	Colpectomy, obliteration of vagina; partial To report, see 57106	10.0	30	4
98.2	●	57109	with removal of paravaginal tissue (radical vaginectomy) with bilateral total pelvic lymphadenectomy and para-aortic lymph node sampling (biopsy)	(I) 22.0	90	4
98.2	▲	57110	Vaginectomy, complete removal of vaginal wall;	14.0	90	4
98.2	●	57111	with removal of paravaginal tissue (radical vaginectomy)	(I) 22.0	90	4
98.2	●	57112	with removal of paravaginal tissue (radical vaginectomy) with bilateral total pelvic lymphadenectomy and para-aortic lymph node sampling (biopsy)	(I) 24.0	90	4
		57120	Colpocleisis (Le Fort type)	12.3	60	4
		57130	Excision of vaginal septum	5.0	7	3
		57135	Excision of vaginal cyst or tumor	4.0	30	3
		57150*	Irrigation of vagina and/or application of medicament for treatment of bacterial, parasitic, or fungoid disease	0.3	0	3
96.2		57160*	Fitting and insertion of pessary or other intravaginal support device	0.8	0	3
		57170	Diaphragm or cervical cap fitting with instructions	1.0	0	3
		57180	Introduction of any hemostatic agent or pack for spontaneous or traumatic nonobstetrical vaginal hemorrhage (separate procedure)	1.2	0	3
		57200	Colporrhaphy, suture of injury of vagina (nonobstetrical)	6.0	7	4

UPD	Code	Description	Units	FUD	Anes
	57210	Colpoperineorrhaphy, suture of injury of vagina and/or perineum (nonobstetrical)	6.5	7	4
98.2	57220	Plastic operation on urethral sphincter, vaginal approach (eg, Kelly urethral plication)	7.5	7	3
	57230	Plastic repair of urethrocele	7.0	7	4
	57240	Anterior colporrhaphy, repair of cystocele with or without repair of urethrocele	8.6	60	4
	57250	Posterior colporrhaphy, repair of rectocele with or without perineorrhaphy	8.0	60	4
	57260	Combined anteroposterior colporrhaphy;	13.0	60	4
	57265	with enterocele repair	14.5	60	4
	57268	Repair of enterocele, vaginal approach (separate procedure)	10.0	60	4
	57270	Repair of enterocele, abdominal approach (separate procedure)	12.5	60	6
	57280	Colpopexy, abdominal approach	14.0	60	6
	57282	Sacrospinous ligament fixation for prolapse of vagina	14.0	60	6
98.2	57284	Paravaginal defect repair (including repair of cystocele, stress urinary incontinence, and/or incomplete vaginal prolapse)	(I) 17.5	90	4
98.2	57288	Sling operation for stress incontinence (eg, fascia or synthetic)	14.0	60	4
98.2	57289	Pereyra procedure, including anterior colporrhaphy	12.5	60	4
98.2	57291	Construction of artificial vagina; without graft	27.5	90	7
98.2	57292	with graft	34.0	90	7
98.2	57300	Closure of rectovaginal fistula; vaginal or transanal approach	13.5	90	5
	57305	abdominal approach	17.5	90	6
	57307	abdominal approach, with concomitant colostomy	19.5	90	6
97.2	57308	Closure of rectovaginal fistula; transperineal approach, with perineal body reconstruction, with or without levator plication	(I) 15.0	90	6
98.2	57310	Closure of urethrovaginal fistula;	14.5	60	3
98.2	57311	with bulbocavernosus transplant	BR	0	3
98.2	57320	Closure of vesicovaginal fistula; vaginal approach	15.0	60	3
	57330	transvesical and vaginal approach	17.0	60	6
98.2	57335	Vaginoplasty for intersex state	(I) 27.5	90	3
	57400*	Dilation of vagina under anesthesia	2.0	0	3
	57410*	Pelvic examination under anesthesia	2.0	0	3

UPD	Code	Description	Units	FUD	Anes
	57415	Removal of impacted vaginal foreign body (separate procedure) under anesthesia	(I) 1.3	0	3
	57452*	Colposcopy (vaginoscopy); (separate procedure)	2.3	0	3
	57454*	with biopsy(s) of the cervix and/or endocervical curettage	2.6	0	3
98.2	**57460**	with loop electrode excision procedure of the cervix	(I) 4.1	0	4
	57500*	Biopsy, single or multiple, or local excision of lesion, with or without fulguration (separate procedure)	0.8	0	3
	57505	Endocervical curettage (not done as part of a dilation and curettage)	1.2	0	3
	57510	Cauterization of cervix; electro or thermal	0.8	7	3
	57511*	cryocautery, initial or repeat	1.5	0	3
	57513	laser ablation	3.5	45	3
	57520	Conization of cervix, with or without fulguration, with or without dilation and curettage, with or without repair; cold knife or laser	5.0	45	3
	57522	loop electrode excision	(I) 4.5	45	3
98.2	**57530**	Trachelectomy (cervicectomy), amputation of cervix (separate procedure)	5.0	45	3
98.2	**57531**	Radical trachelectomy, with bilateral total pelvic lymphadenectomy and para-aortic lymph node sampling biopsy, with or without removal of tube(s), with or without removal of ovary(s)	(I) 24.0	90	8
	57540	Excision of cervical stump, abdominal approach;	12.0	45	6
	57545	with pelvic floor repair	15.0	45	6
98.2	**57550**	Excision of cervical stump, vaginal approach;	12.0	45	6
98.2	**57555**	with anterior and/or posterior repair	15.0	45	6
98.2	**57556**	with repair of enterocele	15.0	45	6
	57700	Cerclage of uterine cervix, nonobstetrical	9.5	45	4
	57720	Trachelorrhaphy, plastic repair of uterine cervix, vaginal approach	5.0	45	4
	57800*	Dilation of cervical canal, instrumental (separate procedure)	0.6	0	3
	57820	Dilation and curettage of cervical stump	4.0	15	3
	58100*	Endometrial sampling (biopsy) with or without endocervical sampling (biopsy), without cervical dilation, any method (separate procedure)	1.0	0	3
	58120	Dilation and curettage, diagnostic and/or therapeutic (nonobstetrical)	4.0	0	3

UPD	Code	Description	Units	FUD	Anes
	58140	Myomectomy, excision of fibroid tumor of uterus, single or multiple (separate procedure); abdominal approach	12.0	45	6
98.2	**58145**	vaginal approach	9.0	45	6
	58150	Total abdominal hysterectomy (corpus and cervix), with or without removal of tube(s), with or without removal of ovary(s);	17.0	45	6
97.2	**58152**	Total abdominal hysterectomy (corpus and cervix), with or without removal of tube(s), with or without removal of ovary(s); with colpo-urethrocystopexy (eg, Marshall-Marchetti-Krantz, Burch)	23.0	45	6
	58180	Supracervical abdominal hysterectomy (subtotal hysterectomy), with or without removal of tube(s), with or without removal of ovary(s)	15.0	45	6
	58200	Total abdominal hysterectomy, including partial vaginectomy, with para-aortic and pelvic lymph node sampling, with or without removal of tube(s), with or without removal of ovary(s)	20.0	120	6
	58210	Radical abdominal hysterectomy, with bilateral total pelvic lymphadenectomy and para-aortic lymph node sampling (biopsy), with or without removal of tube(s), with or without removal of ovary(s)	35.0	120	8
	58240	Pelvic exenteration for gynecologic malignancy, with total abdominal hysterectomy or cervicectomy, with or without removal of tube(s), with or without removal of ovary(s), with removal of bladder and ureteral transplantations, and/or abdominoperineal resection of rectum and colon and colostomy, or any combination thereof	44.0	120	8
	58260	Vaginal hysterectomy;	19.0	45	6
	58262	with removal of tube(s), and/or ovary(s)	(I) 20.0	45	6
	58263	with removal of tube(s), and/or ovary(s), with repair of enterocele	(I) 22.0	45	6
	58267	with colpo-urethrocystopexy (Marshall-Marchetti-Krantz type, Pereyra type, with or without endoscopic control)	22.0	45	6
	58270	with repair of enterocele	20.0	45	6
	58275	Vaginal hysterectomy, with total or partial colpectomy;	20.0	45	6
	58280	with repair of enterocele	20.0	45	6
98.2	**58285**	Vaginal hysterectomy, radical (Schauta type operation)	24.0	90	6
	58300*	Insertion of intrauterine device (IUD)	1.5	0	3
	58301	Removal of intrauterine device (IUD)	0.5	0	3
	58321	Artificial insemination; intra-cervical	(I) 1.5	45	3
	58322	intra-uterine	(I) 2.0	45	3
98.2	**58323**	Sperm washing for artificial insemination	(I) 0.5	45	0

UPD			Code	Description	Units	FUD	Anes
98.2			**58340***	Catheterization and introduction of saline or contrast material for hysterosonography or hysterosalpingography	1.0	0	4
98.2			**58345**	Transcervical introduction of fallopian tube catheter for diagnosis and/or re-establishing patency (any method), with or without hysterosalpingography	(I) 6.7	45	4
98.2			**58350***	Chromotubation of oviduct, including materials	1.5	0	4
			58400	Uterine suspension, with or without shortening of round ligaments, with or without shortening of sacrouterine ligaments; (separate procedure)	12.1	45	6
			58410	with presacral sympathectomy	16.5	45	6
			58520	Hysterorrhaphy, repair of ruptured uterus (nonobstetrical)	11.0	45	6
			58540	Hysteroplasty, repair of uterine anomaly (Strassman type)	18.0	45	6
			58600	Ligation or transection of fallopian tube(s), abdominal or vaginal approach, unilateral or bilateral	10.0	45	6
			58605	Ligation or transection of fallopian tube(s), abdominal or vaginal approach, postpartum, unilateral or bilateral, during same hospitalization (separate procedure)	7.5	45	6
98.2	▲	+	**58611**	Ligation or transection of fallopian tube(s) when done at the time of cesarean section or intra-abdominal surgery (not a separate procedure) (List separately in addition to code for primary procedure) Note: This code is an add-on procedure and as such is valued appropriately. Multiple procedure guidelines for reduction of value are not applicable.	4.0	45	0
			58615	Occlusion of fallopian tube(s) by device (eg, band, clip, Falope ring) vaginal or suprapubic approach	10.0	45	6
			58700	Salpingectomy, complete or partial, unilateral or bilateral (separate procedure)	11.4	90	6
			58720	Salpingo-oophorectomy, complete or partial, unilateral or bilateral (separate procedure)	17.0	90	6
			58740	Lysis of adhesions (salpingolysis, ovariolysis)	16.5	45	6
			58750	Tubotubal anastomosis	21.0	45	6
			58752	Tubouterine implantation	16.5	45	6
			58760	Fimbrioplasty	17.0	45	6
			58770	Salpingostomy (salpingoneostomy)	17.0	45	6
98.2			**58800**	Drainage of ovarian cyst(s), unilateral or bilateral, (separate procedure); vaginal approach	5.0	15	6
			58805	abdominal approach	12.0	45	6
98.2			**58820**	Drainage of ovarian abscess; vaginal approach, open	5.0	15	6
			58822	abdominal approach	10.0	45	6

UPD	Code	Description	Units	FUD	Anes
98.2	58823	Drainage of pelvic abscess, transvaginal or transrectal approach, percutaneous (eg, ovarian, pericolic)	(I) 4.0	0	4
	58825	Transposition, ovary(s)	12.0	45	6
	58900	Biopsy of ovary, unilateral or bilateral (separate procedure)	10.5	45	6
	58920	Wedge resection or bisection of ovary, unilateral or bilateral	11.0	45	6
	58925	Ovarian cystectomy, unilateral or bilateral	11.0	45	6
	58940	Oophorectomy, partial or total, unilateral or bilateral;	11.0	45	6
	58943	for ovarian malignancy, with para-aortic and pelvic lymph node biopsies, peritoneal washings, peritoneal biopsies, diaphragmatic assessments, with or without salpingectomy(s), with or without omentectomy	20.0	45	6
	58950	Resection of ovarian malignancy with bilateral salpingo-oophorectomy and omentectomy;	16.0	60	6
98.2	58951	with total abdominal hysterectomy, pelvic and limited para-aortic lymphadenectomy	25.0	60	8
98.2	58952	with radical dissection for debulking	23.5	60	8
98.2	58960	Laparotomy, for staging or restaging of ovarian malignancy ("second look"), with or without omentectomy, peritoneal washing, biopsy of abdominal and pelvic peritoneum, diaphragmatic assessment with pelvic and limited para-aortic lymphadenectomy	(I) 20.5	60	7
98.2	58970	Follicle puncture for oocyte retrieval, any method	(I) 11.0	0	6
98.2	58974	Embryo transfer, intrauterine	(I) 9.0	0	3
98.2	58976	Gamete, zygote, or embryo intrafallopian transfer, any method	(I) 12.0	0	6
98.2	58999	Unlisted procedure, female genital system (nonobstetrical)	BR	0	3

Maternity Care and Delivery

UPD	Code	Description	Units	FUD	Anes
	59000*	Amniocentesis, any method	1.0	0	4
	59012	Cordocentesis (intrauterine), any method	(I) 4.0	0	4
	59015	Chorionic villus sampling, any method	3.0	0	4
	59020*	Fetal contraction stress test	1.0	0	0
	59025	Fetal non-stress test	1.0	0	0
	59030*	Fetal scalp blood sampling	1.0	0	4
97.2	59050	Fetal monitoring during labor by consulting physician (ie, non-attending physician) with written report; supervision and interpretation	1.8	0	3
	59051	Fetal monitoring during labor by consulting physician (ie, non-attending physician) with written report; interpretation only	(I) 1.4	0	0

UPD	Code	Description	Units	FUD	Anes
	59100	Hysterotomy, abdominal (eg, for hydatidiform mole, abortion)	16.0	45	6
	59120	Surgical treatment of ectopic pregnancy; tubal or ovarian, requiring salpingectomy and/or oophorectomy, abdominal or vaginal approach	14.0	45	6
	59121	tubal or ovarian, without salpingectomy and/or oophorectomy	14.0	45	6
	59130	abdominal pregnancy	14.5	45	6
	59135	interstitial, uterine pregnancy requiring total hysterectomy	17.5	45	6
	59136	interstitial, uterine pregnancy with partial resection of uterus	(I) 20.0	45	6
98.2	59140	cervical, with evacuation	14.0	45	3
	59150	Laparoscopic treatment of ectopic pregnancy; without salpingectomy and/or oophorectomy	(I) 11.0	45	6
	59151	with salpingectomy and/or oophorectomy	(I) 18.0	45	6
97.2	59160	Curettage, postpartum	4.2	15	3
	59200	Insertion of cervical dilator (eg, laminaria, prostaglandin) (separate procedure)	(I) 2.4	0	3
	59300	Episiotomy or vaginal repair, by other than attending physician	2.1	0	3
98.2	59320	Cerclage of cervix, during pregnancy; vaginal	(I) 3.6	0	4
98.2	59325	abdominal	(I) 6.0	0	6
	59350	Hysterorrhaphy of ruptured uterus	15.0	45	6
	59400	Routine obstetric care including antepartum care, vaginal delivery (with or without episiotomy, and/or forceps) and postpartum care	20.0	45	5
	59409	Vaginal delivery only (with or without episiotomy and/or forceps);	(I) 10.5	45	5
	59410	including postpartum care	12.5	45	5
98.2	59412	External cephalic version, with or without tocolysis (list in addition to code(s) for delivery)	3.5	0	5
	59414	Delivery of placenta (separate procedure)	(I) 2.5	0	5
	59425	Antepartum care only; 4-6 visits	5.0	0	0
	59426	7 or more visits	8.0	0	0
	59430	Postpartum care only (separate procedure)	2.0	45	0
	59510	Routine obstetric care including antepartum care, cesarean delivery, and postpartum care	25.0	45	7
	59514	Cesarean delivery only;	(I) 14.5	45	7
	59515	including postpartum care	17.5	45	7

UPD			Code	Description	Units	FUD	Anes
98.2	▲	+	59525	Subtotal or total hysterectomy after cesarean delivery (List separately in addition to code for primary procedure) Note: This code is an add-on procedure and as such is valued appropriately. Multiple procedure guidelines for reduction of value are not applicable.	8.5	45	0
			59610	Routine obstetric care including antepartum care, vaginal delivery (with or without episiotomy, and/or forceps) and postpartum care, after previous cesarean delivery	(I) 24.0	45	5
			59612	Vaginal delivery only, after previous cesarean delivery (with or without episiotomy and/or forceps);	(I) 14.5	45	5
98.2			59614	including postpartum care	(I) 16.5	45	5
98.2			59618	Routine obstetric care including antepartum care, cesarean delivery, and postpartum care, following attempted vaginal delivery after previous cesarean delivery	(I) 29.0	45	7
98.2			59620	Cesarean delivery only, following attempted vaginal delivery after previous cesarean delivery;	(I) 18.5	45	7
98.2			59622	including postpartum care	(I) 21.5	45	7
			59812	Treatment of incomplete abortion, any trimester, completed surgically	(I) 4.0	30	3
			59820	Treatment of missed abortion, completed surgically; first trimester	4.5	30	3
			59821	second trimester	5.0	30	3
			59830	Treatment of septic abortion, completed surgically	5.0	30	3
			59840	Induced abortion, by dilation and curettage	4.5	30	3
			59841	Induced abortion, by dilation and evacuation	4.5	30	3
			59850	Induced abortion, by one or more intra-amniotic injections (amniocentesis-injections), including hospital admission and visits, delivery of fetus and secundines;	7.1	30	3
			59851	with dilation and curettage and/or evacuation	9.0	30	3
			59852	with hysterotomy (failed intra-amniotic injection)	12.0	45	6
			59855	Induced abortion, by one or more vaginal suppositories (eg, prostaglandin) with or without cervical dilation (eg, laminaria), including hospital admission and visits, delivery of fetus and secundines;	(I) 8.4	30	3
			59856	with dilation and curettage and/or evacuation	(I) 10.3	30	3
98.2			59857	with hysterotomy (failed medical evaluation)	(I) 13.3	45	3
98.2			59866	Multifetal pregnancy redution(s) (MPR)	(I) 6.0	0	4
			59870	Uterine evacuation and curettage for hydatidiform mole	(I) 5.0	30	3
97.2			59871	Removal of cerclage suture under anesthesia (other than local)	(I) 3.0	0	3
			59899	Unlisted procedure, maternity care and delivery	BR	0	0

UPD			Code	Description	Units	FUD	Anes

Endocrine System

UPD			Code	Description	Units	FUD	Anes
98.2			60000*	Incision and drainage of thyroglossal cyst, infected	0.9	0	5
98.2			60001	Aspiration and/or injection, thyroid cyst	(I) 1.5	0	3
			60100*	Biopsy thyroid, percutaneous core needle	1.5	0	3
			60200	Excision of cyst or adenoma of thyroid, or transection of isthmus	10.0	30	6
			60210	Partial thyroid lobectomy, unilateral; with or without isthmusectomy	(I) 12.5	30	6
			60212	with contralateral subtotal lobectomy, including isthmusectomy	(I) 17.5	30	6
			60220	Total thyroid lobectomy, unilateral; with or without isthmusectomy	16.0	45	6
			60225	with contralateral subtotal lobectomy, including isthmusectomy	18.0	30	6
			60240	Thyroidectomy, total or complete	21.0	30	6
			60252	Thyroidectomy, total or subtotal for malignancy; with limited neck dissection	26.0	30	6
			60254	with radical neck dissection	29.0	30	6
			60260	Thyroidectomy, removal of all remaining thyroid tissue following previous removal of a portion of thyroid	17.0	30	6
			60270	Thyroidectomy, including substernal thyroid gland; sternal split or transthoracic approach	23.0	30	13
98.2			60271	cervical approach	(I) 20.0	90	6
			60280	Excision of thyroglossal duct cyst or sinus;	12.0	30	6
			60281	recurrent	12.0	30	6
			60500	Parathyroidectomy or exploration of parathyroid(s);	18.3	45	6
			60502	re-exploration	18.0	45	6
			60505	with mediastinal exploration, sternal split or transthoracic approach	23.0	30	13
98.2	▲	+	60512	Parathyroid autotransplantation (List separately in addition to code for primary procedure) Note: This code is an add-on procedure and as such is valued appropriately. Multiple procedure guidelines for reduction of value are not applicable.	(I) 6.5	30	0
98.2			60520	Thymectomy, partial or total; transcervical approach (separate procedure)	19.5	90	6
			60521	sternal split or transthoracic approach, without radical mediastinal dissection (separate procedure)	(I) 24.0	90	13

UPD			Code	Description	Units	FUD	Anes
			60522	sternal split or transthoracic approach, with radical mediastinal dissection (separate procedure)	(I) 29.0	90	13
			60540	Adrenalectomy, partial or complete, or exploration of adrenal gland with or without biopsy, transabdominal, lumbar or dorsal (separate procedure);	19.5	30	10
			60545	with excision of adjacent retroperitoneal tumor	22.5	30	10
			60600	Excision of carotid body tumor; without excision of carotid artery	20.0	30	6
			60605	with excision of carotid artery	24.5	30	10
			60699	Unlisted procedure, endocrine system	BR	0	0

Nervous System

UPD			Code	Description	Units	FUD	Anes
			61000*	Subdural tap through fontanelle, or suture, infant, unilateral or bilateral; initial	2.0	0	5
			61001*	subsequent taps	1.4	0	5
			61020*	Ventricular puncture through previous burr hole, fontanelle, suture, or implanted ventricular catheter/reservoir; without injection	2.0	0	5
			61026*	with injection of drug or other substance for diagnosis or treatment	3.0	0	5
			61050*	Cisternal or lateral cervical (C1-C2) puncture; without injection (separate procedure)	2.5	0	5
			61055*	with injection of drug or other substance for diagnosis or treatment (eg, C1-C2)	4.1	0	5
			61070*	Puncture of shunt tubing or reservoir for aspiration or injection procedure	1.6	0	5
98.2	▲		61105*	Twist drill hole for subdural or ventricular puncture;	10.0	0	9
98.2	M		61106	61106 has been deleted.	7.0	0	9
98.2		⊘	61107*	for implanting ventricular catheter or pressure recording device Note: Multiple procedure guidelines for reduction of value are not applicable for this code.	10.7	0	9
			61108	for evacuation and/or drainage of subdural hematoma	20.0	7	9
98.2	▲		61120	Burr hole(s) for ventricular puncture (including injection of gas, contrast media, dye, or radioactive material)	10.0	30	9
98.2	M		61130	61130 has been deleted.	7.0	0	9
			61140	Burr hole(s) or trephine; with biopsy of brain or intracranial lesion	22.0	30	9
			61150	with drainage of brain abscess or cyst	22.0	30	9
96.1			61151	with subsequent tapping (aspiration) of intracranial abscess or cyst	22.5	30	9

UPD		Code	Description	Units	FUD	Anes
		61154	Burr hole(s) with evacuation and/or drainage of hematoma, extradural or subdural	22.0	90	9
		61156	Burr hole(s); with aspiration of hematoma or cyst, intracerebral	21.5	90	9
98.2	⊘	61210*	for implanting ventricular catheter, reservoir, EEG electrode(s) or pressure recording device (separate procedure) Note: Procedure listed may be considered a necessary part of and/or procedure and in such cases, not billable. If the procedure is distinct by encounter or performed in conjunction with a procedure for which the listed service is not considered a necessary component, then multiple procedure guidelines for reduction of value do not apply for this code.	8.0	0	9
96.2		61215	Insertion of subcutaneous reservoir, pump or continuous infusion system for connection to ventricular catheter	(I) 7.0	0	9
		61250	Burr hole(s) or trephine, supratentorial, exploratory, not followed by other surgery	15.0	90	9
		61253	Burr hole(s) or trephine, infratentorial, unilateral or bilateral	25.5	90	9
		61304	Craniectomy or craniotomy, exploratory; supratentorial	35.0	90	11
98.2		61305	infratentorial (posterior fossa)	37.0	90	13
		61312	Craniectomy or craniotomy for evacuation of hematoma, supratentorial; extradural or subdural	36.0	90	11
		61313	intracerebral	38.0	90	11
98.2		61314	Craniectomy or craniotomy for evacuation of hematoma, infratentorial; extradural or subdural	45.0	90	13
98.2		61315	intracerebellar	49.0	90	13
		61320	Craniectomy or craniotomy, drainage of intracranial abscess; supratentorial	32.0	90	11
98.2		61321	infratentorial	35.0	90	13
		61330	Decompression of orbit only, transcranial approach	30.0	90	11
		61332	Exploration of orbit (transcranial approach); with biopsy	40.0	90	11
		61333	with removal of lesion	40.0	90	11
		61334	with removal of foreign body	40.0	90	11
		61340	Other cranial decompression (eg, subtemporal), supratentorial	22.0	90	11
98.2		61343	Craniectomy, suboccipital with cervical laminectomy for decompression of medulla and spinal cord, with or without dural graft (eg, Arnold-Chiari malformation)	45.0	90	13
98.2		61345	Other cranial decompression, posterior fossa	19.5	90	13
98.2		61440	Craniotomy for section of tentorium cerebelli (separate procedure)	26.0	90	13

UPD	Code	Description	Units	FUD	Anes
98.2	61450	Craniectomy, subtemporal, for section, compression, or decompression of sensory root of gasserian ganglion	35.0	90	13
98.2	61458	Craniectomy, suboccipital; for exploration or decompression of cranial nerves	39.0	90	13
	61460	for section of one or more cranial nerves	38.0	90	11
	61470	for medullary tractotomy	38.0	90	11
	61480	for mesencephalic tractotomy or pedunculotomy	38.0	90	11
	61490	Craniotomy for lobotomy, including cingulotomy	25.0	90	11
	61500	Craniectomy; with excision of tumor or other bone lesion of skull	36.0	90	11
	61501	for osteomyelitis	35.0	90	11
	61510	Craniectomy, trephination, bone flap craniotomy; for excision of brain tumor, supratentorial, except meningioma	40.0	90	11
	61512	for excision of meningioma, supratentorial	42.0	90	11
	61514	for excision of brain abscess, supratentorial	37.0	90	11
	61516	for excision or fenestration of cyst, supratentorial	37.0	90	11
98.2	61518	Craniectomy for excision of brain tumor, infratentorial or posterior fossa; except meningioma, cerebellopontine angle tumor, or midline tumor at base of skull	44.0	90	13
98.2	61519	meningioma	50.0	90	13
98.2	61520	cerebellopontine angle tumor	50.0	90	13
98.2	61521	midline tumor at base of skull	66.7	90	13
98.2	61522	Craniectomy, infratentorial or posterior fossa; for excision of brain abscess	44.0	90	13
98.2	61524	for excision or fenestration of cyst	44.0	90	13
98.2	61526	Craniectomy, bone flap craniotomy, transtemporal (mastoid) for excision of cerebellopontine angle tumor;	50.0	90	13
98.2	61530	combined with middle/posterior fossa craniotomy/ craniectomy	50.0	90	13
	61531	Subdural implantation of strip electrodes through one or more burr or trephine hole(s) for long term seizure monitoring	(I) 40.0	90	11
	61533	Craniotomy with elevation of bone flap; for subdural implantation of an electrode array, for long term seizure monitoring	38.5	90	11
	61534	for excision of epileptogenic focus without electrocorticography during surgery	38.0	90	11
	61535	for removal of epidural or subdural electrode array, without excision of cerebral tissue (separate procedure)	29.0	90	11

UPD	Code	Description	Units	FUD	Anes
	61536	for excision of cerebral epileptogenic focus, with electrocorticography during surgery (includes removal of electrode array)	41.0	90	11
	61538	for lobectomy with electrocorticography during surgery, temporal lobe	44.0	90	11
	61539	for lobectomy with electrocorticography during surgery, other than temporal lobe, partial or total	44.0	90	11
	61541	for transection of corpus callosum	58.5	90	11
	61542	for total hemispherectomy	53.0	90	11
	61543	for partial or subtotal hemispherectomy	(I) 30.0	90	11
	61544	for excision or coagulation of choroid plexus	38.0	90	11
	61545	for excision of craniopharyngioma	73.0	90	11
	61546	Craniotomy for hypophysectomy or excision of pituitary tumor, intracranial approach	42.5	90	11
	61548	Hypophysectomy or excision of pituitary tumor, transnasal or transseptal approach, nonstereotactic	39.5	90	11
	61550	Craniectomy for craniosynostosis; single cranial suture	25.0	90	11
	61552	multiple cranial sutures	28.0	90	11
	61556	Craniotomy for craniosynostosis; frontal or parietal bone flap	(I) 28.0	90	11
	61557	bifrontal bone flap	(I) 32.0	90	11
	61558	Extensive craniectomy for multiple cranial suture craniosynostosis (eg, cloverleaf skull); not requiring bone grafts	(I) 39.0	90	11
	61559	recontouring with multiple osteotomies and bone autografts (eg, barrel-stave procedure) (includes obtaining grafts)	(I) 44.0	90	11
	61563	Excision, intra and extracranial, benign tumor of cranial bone (eg, fibrous dysplasia); without optic nerve decompression	(I) 38.0	90	11
	61564	with optic nerve decompression	(I) 49.0	90	11
	61570	Craniectomy or craniotomy; with excision of foreign body from brain	49.0	90	11
	61571	with treatment of penetrating wound of brain	49.0	90	11
	61575	Transoral approach to skull base, brain stem or upper spinal cord for biopsy, decompression or excision of lesion;	28.0	90	11
	61576	requiring splitting of tongue and/or mandible (including tracheostomy)	29.0	90	11
	61580	Craniofacial approach to anterior cranial fossa; extradural, including lateral rhinotomy, ethmoidectomy, sphenoidectomy, without maxillectomy or orbital exenteration	(I) 40.0	90	11

UPD	Code	Description	Units	FUD	Anes
	61581	extradural, including lateral rhinotomy, orbital exenteration, ethmoidectomy, sphenoidectomy and/or maxillectomy	(I) 46.0	90	11
	61582	extradural, including unilateral or bifrontal craniotomy, elevation of frontal lobe(s), osteotomy of base of anterior cranial fossa	(I) 41.5	90	11
	61583	intradural, including unilateral or bifrontal craniotomy, elevation or resection of frontal lobe, osteotomy of base of anterior cranial fossa	(I) 47.0	90	11
	61584	Orbitocranial approach to anterior cranial fossa, extradural, including supraorbital ridge osteotomy and elevation of frontal and/or temporal lobe(s); without orbital exenteration	(I) 46.0	90	11
	61585	with orbital exenteration	(I) 51.0	90	11
96.2	61586	Bicoronal, transzygomatic and/or LeFort I osteotomy approach to anterior cranial fossa with or without internal fixation, without bone graft	(I) 35.0	90	11
	61590	Infratemporal pre-auricular approach to middle cranial fossa (parapharyngeal space, infratemporal and midline skull base, nasopharynx), with or without disarticulation of the mandible, including parotidectomy, craniotomy, decompression and/or mobilization of the facial nerve and/or petrous carotid artery	(I) 56.0	90	11
	61591	Infratemporal post-auricular approach to middle cranial fossa (internal auditory meatus, petrous apex, tentorium, cavernous sinus, parasellar area, infratemporal fossa) including mastoidectomy, resection of sigmoid sinus, with or without decompression and/or mobilization of contents of auditory canal or petrous carotid artery	(I) 58.5	90	11
	61592	Orbitocranial zygomatic approach to middle cranial fossa (cavernous sinus and carotid artery, clivus, basilar artery or petrous apex) including osteotomy of zygoma, craniotomy, extra- or intradural elevation of temporal lobe	(I) 53.0	90	11
	61595	Transtemporal approach to posterior cranial fossa, jugular foramen or midline skull base, including mastoidectomy, decompression of sigmoid sinus and/or facial nerve, with or without mobilization	(I) 39.0	90	11
	61596	Transcochlear approach to posterior cranial fossa, jugular foramen or midline skull base, including labyrinthectomy, decompression, with or without mobilization of facial nerve and/or petrous carotid artery	(I) 47.5	90	11
	61597	Transcondylar (far lateral) approach to posterior cranial fossa, jugular foramen or midline skull base, including occipital condylectomy, mastoidectomy, resection of C1-C3 vertebral body(s), decompression of vertebral artery, with or without mobilization	(I) 50.0	90	11
	61598	Transpetrosal approach to posterior cranial fossa, clivus or foramen magnum, including ligation of superior petrosal sinus and/or sigmoid sinus	(I) 44.5	90	11
	61600	Resection or excision of neoplastic, vascular or infectious lesion of base of anterior cranial fossa; extradural	(I) 34.0	90	11

UPD			Code	Description	Units	FUD	Anes
			61601	intradural, including dural repair, with or without graft	(I) 36.5	90	11
			61605	Resection or excision of neoplastic, vascular or infectious lesion of infratemporal fossa, parapharyngeal space, petrous apex; extradural	(I) 38.5	90	11
			61606	intradural, including dural repair, with or without graft	(I) 51.5	90	11
			61607	Resection or excision of neoplastic, vascular or infectious lesion of parasellar area, cavernous sinus, clivus or midline skull base; extradural	(I) 48.0	90	11
			61608	intradural, including dural repair, with or without graft	(I) 56.0	90	11
98.2	▲	+	**61609**	Transection or ligation, carotid artery in cavernous sinus; without repair (List separately in addition to code for primary procedure) Note: This code is an add-on procedure and as such is valued appropriately. Multiple procedure guidelines for reduction of value are not applicable.	(I) 13.5	0	0
98.2	▲	+	**61610**	with repair by anastomosis or graft (List separately in addition to code for primary procedure) Note: This code is an add-on procedure and as such is valued appropriately. Multiple procedure guidelines for reduction of value are not applicable.	(I) 47.5	0	0
98.2	▲	+	**61611**	Transection or ligation, carotid artery in petrous canal; without repair (List separately in addition to code for primary procedure) Note: This code is an add-on procedure and as such is valued appropriately. Multiple procedure guidelines for reduction of value are not applicable.	(I) 10.0	0	0
98.2	▲	+	**61612**	with repair by anastomosis or graft (List separately in addition to code for primary procedure) Note: This code is an add-on procedure and as such is valued appropriately. Multiple procedure guidelines for reduction of value are not applicable.	(I) 45.0	0	0
			61613	Obliteration of carotid aneurysm, arteriovenous malformation, or carotid-cavernous fistula by dissection within cavernous sinus	(I) 55.0	90	15
			61615	Resection or excision of neoplastic, vascular or infectious lesion of base of posterior cranial fossa, jugular foramen, foramen magnum, or C1-C3 vertebral bodies; extradural	(I) 42.5	90	11
			61616	intradural, including dural repair, with or without graft	(I) 57.5	90	11
			61618	Secondary repair of dura for CSF leak, anterior, middle or posterior cranial fossa following surgery of the skull base; by free tissue graft (eg, pericranium, fascia, tensor fascia lata, adipose tissue, homologous or synthetic grafts)	(I) 22.0	90	11
			61619	by local or regionalized vascularized pedicle flap or myocutaneous flap (including galea, temporalis, frontalis or occipitalis muscle)	(I) 27.0	90	11

UPD	Code	Description	Units	FUD	Anes
98.2	**61624**	Transcatheter occlusion or embolization (eg, for tumor destruction, to achieve hemostasis, to occlude a vascular malformation), percutaneous, any method; central nervous system (intracranial, spinal cord)	(I) 27.0	90	11
98.2	**61626**	non-central nervous system, head or neck (extracranial, brachiocephalic branch)	(I) 23.0	90	11
	61680	Surgery of intracranial arteriovenous malformation; supratentorial, simple	60.0	90	15
	61682	supratentorial, complex	70.0	90	15
98.2	**61684**	infratentorial, simple	65.0	90	13
98.2	**61686**	infratentorial, complex	75.0	90	13
	61690	dural, simple	65.0	90	15
	61692	dural, complex	75.0	90	15
	61700	Surgery of intracranial aneurysm, intracranial approach; carotid circulation	46.0	90	15
	61702	vertebral-basilar circulation	50.0	90	15
98.2	**61703**	Surgery of intracranial aneurysm, cervical approach by application of occluding clamp to cervical carotid artery (Selverstone-Crutchfield type)	13.0	90	15
	61705	Surgery of aneurysm, vascular malformation or carotid-cavernous fistula; by intracranial and cervical occlusion of carotid artery	54.0	90	15
	61708	by intracranial electrothrombosis	40.0	90	15
	61710	by intra-arterial embolization, injection procedure, or balloon catheter	40.0	90	15
	61711	Anastomosis, arterial, extracranial-intracranial (eg, middle cerebral/cortical) arteries	41.0	90	15
98.2	**61720**	Creation of lesion by stereotactic method, including burr hole(s) and localizing and recording techniques, single or multiple stages; globus pallidus or thalamus	34.5	90	11
	61735	subcortical structure(s) other than globus pallidus or thalamus	33.8	90	9
98.2	**61750**	Stereotactic biopsy, aspiration, or excision, including burr hole(s), for intracranial lesion;	28.8	90	11
98.2	**61751**	with computerized axial tomography	30.8	90	11
98.2	**61760**	Stereotactic implantation of depth electrodes into the cerebrum for long term seizure monitoring	(I) 31.4	90	11
98.2	**61770**	Stereotactic localization, any method, including burr hole(s), with insertion of catheter(s) for brachytherapy	19.0	90	13
98.2	**61790**	Creation of lesion by stereotactic method, percutaneous, by neurolytic agent (eg, alcohol, thermal, electrical, radiofrequency); gasserian ganglion	28.0	90	6

+ Add-on Code   ⊘ Modifier -51 Exempt   ▲ Revised code   ● New code   **M** RVSI code or deleted from CPT   **(I)** Interim Value

UPD		Code	Description	Units	FUD	Anes
98.2		**61791**	trigeminal medullary tract	34.5	90	6
98.2		**61793**	Stereotactic radiosurgery (particle beam, gamma ray or linear accelerator), one or more sessions	38.0	90	7
98.2	+	**61795**	Stereotactic computer assisted volumetric intracranial procedure (list separately in addition to code for primary procedure) Note: This code is an add-on procedure and as such is valued appropriately. Multiple procedure guidelines for reduction of value are not applicable.	(I) 5.5	0	0
		61850	Twist drill or burr hole(s) for implantation of neurostimulator electrodes; cortical	(I) 23.0	90	9
		61855	subcortical	(I) 20.0	90	9
98.2		**61860**	Craniectomy or craniotomy for implantation of neurostimulator electrodes, cerebral; cortical	(I) 17.0	90	11
98.2		**61865**	subcortical	(I) 34.0	90	11
98.2		**61870**	Craniectomy for implantation of neurostimulator electrodes, cerebellar; cortical	(I) 8.8	90	11
98.2		**61875**	subcortical	(I) 14.0	90	11
98.2		**61880**	Revision or removal of intracranial neurostimulator electrodes	(I) 8.8	90	11
		61885	Incision and subcutaneous placement of cranial neurostimulator pulse generator or receiver, direct or inductive coupling	(I) 3.7	90	5
		61888	Revision or removal of cranial neurostimulator pulse generator or receiver	(I) 5.0	90	5
98.2		**62000**	Elevation of depressed skull fracture; simple, extradural	18.0	90	9
98.2		**62005**	compound or comminuted, extradural	25.0	90	9
		62010	with repair of dura and/or debridement of brain	31.0	90	11
		62100	Craniotomy for repair of dural/CSF leak, including surgery for rhinorrhea/otorrhea	33.0	90	11
96.2		**62115**	Reduction of craniomegalic skull (eg, treated hydrocephalus); not requiring bone grafts or cranioplasty	(I) 33.0	90	11
96.2		**62116**	with simple cranioplasty	(I) 35.0	90	11
96.2		**62117**	requiring craniotomy and reconstruction with or without bone graft (includes obtaining grafts)	(I) 40.0	90	11
		62120	Repair of encephalocele, skull vault, including cranioplasty	25.0	90	11
		62121	Craniotomy for repair of encephalocele, skull base	(I) 34.0	90	11
98.2		**62140**	Cranioplasty for skull defect; up to 5 cm diameter	24.0	90	9
98.2		**62141**	larger than 5 cm diameter	29.0	90	9
98.2		**62142**	Removal of bone flap or prosthetic plate of skull	21.0	90	9

UPD	Code	Description	Units	FUD	Anes
98.2	62143	Replacement of bone flap or prosthetic plate of skull	28.0	90	9
98.2	62145	Cranioplasty for skull defect with reparative brain surgery	35.0	90	9
98.2	62146	Cranioplasty with autograft (includes obtaining bone grafts); up to 5 cm diameter	(I) 28.2	90	9
98.2	62147	larger than 5 cm diameter	(I) 33.2	90	9
98.2	62180	Ventriculocisternostomy (Torkildsen type operation)	27.0	7	10
98.2	62190	Creation of shunt; subarachnoid/subdural-atrial, -jugular, -auricular	20.0	7	10
98.2	62192	subarachnoid/subdural-peritoneal, -pleural, other terminus	20.0	7	10
98.2	62194	Replacement or irrigation, subarachnoid/subdural catheter	8.0	7	10
98.2	62200	Ventriculocisternostomy, third ventricle;	34.0	7	10
98.2	62201	stereotactic method	(I) 20.0	7	10
98.2	62220	Creation of shunt; ventriculo-atrial, -jugular, -auricular	23.0	7	10
98.2	62223	ventriculo-peritoneal, -pleural, other terminus	24.0	7	10
98.2	62225	Replacement or irrigation, ventricular catheter	9.0	7	10
98.2	62230	Replacement or revision of CSF shunt, obstructed valve, or distal catheter in shunt system	18.0	7	10
98.2	62256	Removal of complete CSF shunt system; without replacement	9.0	7	10
98.2	62258	with replacement by similar or other shunt at same operation	20.0	7	10
	62268*	Percutaneous aspiration, spinal cord cyst or syrinx	15.3	0	5
	62269*	Biopsy of spinal cord, percutaneous needle	16.8	0	5
	62270*	Spinal puncture, lumbar, diagnostic	2.0	0	5
	62272*	Spinal puncture, therapeutic, for drainage of spinal fluid (by needle or catheter)	2.0	0	5
	62273*	Injection, lumbar epidural, of blood or clot patch	1.0	0	5
	62274*	Injection of diagnostic or therapeutic anesthetic or antispasmodic substance (including narcotics); subarachnoid or subdural, single	1.0	0	8
	62275*	epidural, cervical or thoracic, single	(I) 1.5	0	8
	62276*	subarachnoid or subdural, differential	1.0	0	8
	62277*	subarachnoid or subdural, continuous	1.0	0	8
	62278*	epidural, lumbar or caudal, single	1.0	0	8
	62279*	epidural, lumbar or caudal, continuous	1.0	0	8

UPD		Code	Description	Units	FUD	Anes
		62280*	Injection of neurolytic substance (eg, alcohol, phenol, iced saline solutions); subarachnoid	3.0	0	20
		62281*	epidural, cervical or thoracic	(I) 3.2	0	20
		62282*	epidural, lumbar or caudal	3.0	0	20
	⊘	62284*	Injection procedure for myelography and/or computerized axial tomography, spinal (other than C1-C2 and posterior fossa) Note: Multiple procedure guidelines for reduction of value are not applicable for this code.	3.0	0	9
		62287	Aspiration procedure, percutaneous, of nucleus pulposus of intervertebral disk, any method, single or multiple levels, lumbar	2.9	0	8
		62288*	Injection of substance other than anesthetic, antispasmodic, contrast, or neurolytic solutions; subarachnoid (separate procedure)	2.6	0	8
		62289*	lumbar or caudal epidural (separate procedure)		0	8
		62290*	Injection procedure for diskography, each level; lumbar	3.0	0	5
98.2		62291*	cervical	3.0	0	5
98.2		62292	Injection procedure for chemonucleolysis, including diskography, intervertebral disk, single or multiple levels, lumbar	5.0	0	10
		62294	Injection procedure, arterial, for occlusion of arteriovenous malformation, spinal	3.0	0	5
		62298*	Injection of substance other than anesthetic, contrast, or neurolytic solutions, epidural, cervical or thoracic (separate procedure)	(I) 3.1	0	10
98.2		62350	Implantation, revision or repositioning of intrathecal or epidural catheter, for implantable reservoir or implantable infusion pump; without laminectomy	(I) 9.0	90	8
		62351	with laminectomy	(I) 13.2	90	10
98.2		62355	Removal of previously implanted intrathecal or epidural catheter	(I) 7.0	90	5
		62360	Implantation or replacement of device for intrathecal or epidural drug infusion; subcutaneous reservoir	(I) 3.0	90	5
		62361	non-programmable pump	(I) 7.0	90	5
		62362	programmable pump, including preparation of pump, with or without programming	(I) 9.0	90	5
		62365	Removal of subcutaneous reservoir or pump, previously implanted for intrathecal or epidural infusion	(I) 7.0	90	5
		62367	Electronic analysis of programmable, implanted pump for intrathecal or epidural drug infusion (includes evaluation of reservoir status, alarm status, drug prescription status); without reprogramming	(I) 0.8	0	0

UPD	Code	Description	Units	FUD	Anes
	62368	with reprogramming	(I) 1.2	0	0
	63001	Laminectomy with exploration and/or decompression of spinal cord and/or cauda equina, without facetectomy, foraminotomy or diskectomy, (eg, spinal stenosis), one or two vertebral segments; cervical	35.0	90	10
	63003	thoracic	35.0	90	10
	63005	lumbar, except for spondylolisthesis	33.0	90	8
	63011	sacral	31.0	90	8
	63012	Laminectomy with removal of abnormal facets and/or pars inter-articularis with decompression of cauda equina and nerve roots for spondylolisthesis, lumbar (Gill type procedure)	31.0	90	8
	63015	Laminectomy with exploration and/or decompression of spinal cord and/or cauda equina, without facetectomy, foraminotomy or diskectomy, (eg, spinal stenosis), more than 2 vertebral segments; cervical	40.0	90	10
	63016	thoracic	40.0	90	10
	63017	lumbar	40.0	90	8
	63020	Laminotomy (hemilaminectomy), with decompression of nerve root(s), including partial facetectomy, foraminotomy and/or excision of herniated intervertebral disk; one interspace, cervical	32.0	90	10
	63030	one interspace, lumbar	30.0	90	8
98.2 ▲ +	**63035**	each additional interspace, cervical or lumbar (List separately in addition to code for primary procedure) Note: This code is an add-on procedure and as such is valued appropriately. Multiple procedure guidelines for reduction of value are not applicable.	6.0	90	0
	63040	Laminotomy (hemilaminectomy), with decompression of nerve root(s), including partial facetectomy, foraminotomy and/or excision of herniated intervertebral disk, re-exploration; cervical	35.0	90	10
	63042	lumbar	35.0	90	8
	63045	Laminectomy, facetectomy and foraminotomy (unilateral or bilateral with decompression of spinal cord, cauda equina and/or nerve root(s), (eg, spinal or lateral recess stenosis), single vertebral segment; cervical	35.0	90	10
	63046	thoracic	35.0	90	10
	63047	lumbar	35.0	90	8
98.2 ▲ +	**63048**	each additional segment, cervical, thoracic, or lumbar (List separately in addition to code for primary procedure)	7.0	90	0

UPD			Code	Description	Units	FUD	Anes
				Note: This code is an add-on procedure and as such is valued appropriately. Multiple procedure guidelines for reduction of value are not applicable.			
			63055	Transpedicular approach with decompression of spinal cord, equina and/or nerve root(s) (eg, herniated intervertebral disk), single segment; thoracic	(I) 36.0	90	10
			63056	lumbar	(I) 34.0	90	8
98.2	▲	+	63057	each additional segment, thoracic or lumbar (List separately in addition to code for primary procedure)	5.0	90	0
				Note: This code is an add-on procedure and as such is valued appropriately. Multiple procedure guidelines for reduction of value are not applicable.			
			63064	Costovertebral approach with decompression of spinal cord or nerve root(s), (eg, herniated intervertebral disk), thoracic; single segment	38.0	90	10
98.2	▲	+	63066	each additional segment (List separately in addition to code for primary procedure)	5.5	90	0
				Note: This code is an add-on procedure and as such is valued appropriately. Multiple procedure guidelines for reduction of value are not applicable.			
			63075	Diskectomy, anterior, with decompression of spinal cord and/or nerve root(s), including osteophytectomy; cervical, single interspace	28.0	90	10
98.2	▲	+	63076	cervical, each additional interspace (List separately in addition to code for primary procedure)	7.5	90	0
				Note: This code is an add-on procedure and as such is valued appropriately. Multiple procedure guidelines for reduction of value are not applicable.			
			63077	thoracic, single interspace	30.0	90	10
98.2	▲	+	63078	thoracic, each additional interspace (List separately in addition to code for primary procedure)	7.5	90	0
				Note: This code is an add-on procedure and as such is valued appropriately. Multiple procedure guidelines for reduction of value are not applicable.			
			63081	Vertebral corpectomy (vertebral body resection), partial or complete, anterior approach with decompression of spinal cord and/or nerve root(s); cervical, single segment	42.0	90	10
98.2	▲	+	63082	cervical, each additional segment (List separately in addition to code for primary procedure)	9.0	90	0
				Note: This code is an add-on procedure and as such is valued appropriately. Multiple procedure guidelines for reduction of value are not applicable.			
98.2			63085	Vertebral corpectomy (vertebral body resection), partial or complete, transthoracic approach with decompression of spinal cord and/or nerve root(s); thoracic, single segment	45.0	90	13

UPD			Code	Description	Units	FUD	Anes
98.2	▲	+	63086	thoracic, each additional segment (List separately in addition to code for primary procedure) Note: This code is an add-on procedure and as such is valued appropriately. Multiple procedure guidelines for reduction of value are not applicable.	9.0	90	0
98.2			63087	Vertebral corpectomy (vertebral body resection), partial or complete, combined thoracolumbar approach with decompression of spinal cord, cauda equina or nerve root(s), lower thoracic or lumbar; single segment	45.0	90	13
98.2	▲	+	63088	each additional segment (List separately in addition to code for primary procedure) Note: This code is an add-on procedure and as such is valued appropriately. Multiple procedure guidelines for reduction of value are not applicable.	9.0	90	0
			63090	Vertebral corpectomy (vertebral body resection), partial or complete, transperitoneal or retroperitoneal approach with decompression of spinal cord, cauda equina or nerve root(s), lower thoracic, lumbar, or sacral; single segment	42.0	90	8
98.2	▲	+	63091	each additional segment (List separately in addition to code for primary procedure) Note: This code is an add-on procedure and as such is valued appropriately. Multiple procedure guidelines for reduction of value are not applicable.	7.0	90	0
98.2			63170	Laminectomy with myelotomy (eg, Bischof or DREZ type), cervical, thoracic or thoracolumbar	42.0	90	13
98.2			63172	Laminectomy with drainage of intramedullary cyst/syrinx; to subarachnoid space	34.0	90	13
98.2			63173	to peritoneal space	34.0	90	13
98.2			63180	Laminectomy and section of dentate ligaments, with or without dural graft, cervical; one or two segments	42.0	90	13
			63182	more than two segments	46.0	90	10
98.2			63185	Laminectomy with rhizotomy; one or two segments	34.0	90	8
98.2			63190	more than two segments	37.0	90	8
			63191	Laminectomy with section of spinal accessory nerve	37.0	90	10
98.2			63194	Laminectomy with cordotomy, with section of one spinothalamic tract, one stage; cervical	37.0	90	13
			63195	thoracic	37.0	90	10
98.2			63196	Laminectomy with cordotomy, with section of both spinothalamic tracts, one stage; cervical	38.0	90	13
			63197	thoracic	38.0	90	10
98.2			63198	Laminectomy with cordotomy with section of both spinothalamic tracts, two stages within 14 days; cervical	43.5	90	13
			63199	thoracic	43.5	90	10

UPD	Code	Description	Units	FUD	Anes
	63200	Laminectomy, with release of tethered spinal cord, lumbar	37.5	90	8
98.2	63250	Laminectomy for excision or occlusion of arteriovenous malformation of spinal cord; cervical	45.0	90	13
98.2	63251	thoracic	45.0	90	13
98.2	63252	thoracolumbar	55.0	90	13
98.2	63265	Laminectomy for excision or evacuation of intraspinal lesion other than neoplasm, extradural; cervical	40.0	90	13
	63266	thoracic	40.0	90	10
	63267	lumbar	36.0	90	8
	63268	sacral	36.0	90	8
	63270	Laminectomy for excision of intraspinal lesion other than neoplasm, intradural; cervical	42.0	90	10
	63271	thoracic	42.0	90	10
	63272	lumbar	38.0	90	8
	63273	sacral	38.0	90	8
	63275	Laminectomy for biopsy/excision of intraspinal neoplasm; extradural, cervical	40.0	90	10
	63276	extradural, thoracic	40.0	90	10
	63277	extradural, lumbar	36.0	90	8
	63278	extradural, sacral	36.0	90	8
	63280	intradural, extramedullary, cervical	42.0	90	10
	63281	intradural, extramedullary, thoracic	42.0	90	10
	63282	intradural, extramedullary, lumbar	38.0	90	8
98.2	63283	intradural, sacral	38.0	90	6
	63285	intradural, intramedullary, cervical	50.0	90	10
	63286	intradural, intramedullary, thoracic	50.0	90	10
98.2	63287	intradural, intramedullary, thoracolumbar	50.0	90	8
98.2	63290	combined extradural-intradural lesion, any level	(I) 52.0	90	13
	63300	Vertebral corpectomy (vertebral body resection), partial or complete, for excision of intraspinal lesion, single segment; extradural, cervical	45.0	90	10
	63301	extradural, thoracic by transthoracic approach	50.0	90	10
	63302	extradural, thoracic by thoracolumbar approach	50.0	90	10
	63303	extradural, lumbar or sacral by transperitoneal or retroperitoneal approach	50.0	90	8

UPD			Code	Description	Units	FUD	Anes
			63304	intradural, cervical	45.0	90	10
			63305	intradural, thoracic by transthoracic approach	50.0	90	10
			63306	intradural, thoracic by thoracolumbar approach	50.0	90	10
			63307	intradural, lumbar or sacral by transperitoneal or retroperitoneal approach	50.0	90	8
98.2	▲	+	63308	each additional segment (List separately in addition to codes for single segment) Note: This code is an add-on procedure and as such is valued appropriately. Multiple procedure guidelines for reduction of value are not applicable.	6.0	90	0
98.2			63600	Creation of lesion of spinal cord by stereotactic method, percutaneous, any modality (including stimulation and/or recording)	24.0	90	3
98.2			63610	Stereotactic stimulation of spinal cord, percutaneous, separate procedure not followed by other surgery	24.0	90	3
98.2			63615	Stereotactic biopsy, aspiration, or excision of lesion, spinal cord	29.0	90	3
98.2	▲		63650	Percutaneous implantation of neurostimulator electrode array, epidural	(I) 11.0	90	3
98.2	▲		63655	Laminectomy for implantation of neurostimulator electrodes, plate/paddle, epidural	(I) 14.0	90	8
98.2	▲		63660	Revision or removal of spinal neurostimulator electrode percutaneous array(s) or plate/paddle(s)	(I) 8.5	90	8
98.2			63685	Incision and subcutaneous placement of spinal neurostimulator pulse generator or receiver, direct or inductive coupling	(I) 9.6	90	5
98.2			63688	Revision or removal of implanted spinal neurostimulator pulse generator or receiver	(I) 7.0	90	5
98.2	M		63690	Electronic analysis of implanted neurostimulator pulse generator system (may include rate, pulse amplitude and duration, configuration of wave form, battery status, electrode selectability, output modulation, cycling, impedance and patient compliance measurements); without reprogramming of pulse generator To report, see 95970, 95971	(I) 1.0	0	8
98.2	M		63691	with reprogramming of pulse generator To report, see 95970, 95971	(I) 1.5	0	8
98.2			63700	Repair of meningocele; less than 5 cm diameter	26.0	90	8
98.2			63702	larger than 5 cm diameter	28.0	90	8
98.2			63704	Repair of myelomeningocele; less than 5 cm diameter	30.0	90	8
98.2			63706	larger than 5 cm diameter	32.0	90	8
98.2			63707	Repair of dural/CSF leak, not requiring laminectomy	32.0	90	8

UPD			Code	Description	Units	FUD	Anes
98.2			**63709**	Repair of dural/CSF leak or pseudomeningocele, with laminectomy	32.0	90	8
98.2			**63710**	Dural graft, spinal	31.0	90	8
98.2			**63740**	Creation of shunt, lumbar, subarachnoid-peritoneal, -pleural, or other; including laminectomy	26.0	7	8
			63741	percutaneous, not requiring laminectomy	(I) 18.0	7	8
98.2			**63744**	Replacement, irrigation or revision of lumbosubarachnoid shunt	13.0	7	8
98.2			**63746**	Removal of entire lumbosubarachnoid shunt system without replacement	10.0	7	8
			64400*	Injection, anesthetic agent; trigeminal nerve, any division or branch	2.5	0	10
			64402*	facial nerve	1.8	0	7
			64405*	greater occipital nerve	0.7	0	5
			64408*	vagus nerve	1.2	0	7
			64410*	phrenic nerve	1.2	0	8
			64412*	spinal accessory nerve	1.2	0	7
			64413*	cervical plexus	1.2	0	8
			64415*	brachial plexus	1.5	0	8
			64417*	axillary nerve	1.5	0	8
			64418*	suprascapular nerve	1.5	0	5
			64420*	intercostal nerve, single	1.5	0	5
			64421*	intercostal nerves, multiple, regional block	1.5	0	7
			64425*	ilioinguinal, iliohypogastric nerves	1.5	0	5
			64430*	pudendal nerve	1.5	0	5
			64435*	paracervical (uterine) nerve	1.5	0	5
			64440*	paravertebral nerve (thoracic, lumbar, sacral, coccygeal), single vertebral level	1.5	0	7
			64441*	paravertebral nerves, multiple levels (eg, regional block)	(I) 3.1	0	10
			64442*	paravertebral facet joint nerve, lumbar, single level		0	10
98.2	▲	+	**64443***	paravertebral facet joint nerve, lumbar, each additional level (List separately in addition to code for primary procedure) Note: This code is an add-on procedure and as such is valued appropriately. Multiple procedure guidelines for reduction of value are not applicable.	1.1	0	0
			64445*	sciatic nerve	1.5	0	7

UPD	Code	Description	Units	FUD	Anes
	64450*	other peripheral nerve or branch	0.6	0	5
	64505*	Injection, anesthetic agent; sphenopalatine ganglion	1.3	0	10
	64508*	carotid sinus (separate procedure)	1.3	0	7
	64510*	stellate ganglion (cervical sympathetic)	1.3	0	7
	64520*	lumbar or thoracic (paravertebral sympathetic)	1.5	0	7
	64530*	celiac plexus, with or without radiologic monitoring	1.3	0	7
	64550	Application of surface (transcutaneous) neurostimulator	1.0	0	0
98.2	64553	Percutaneous implantation of neurostimulator electrodes; cranial nerve	3.5	0	5
98.2	64555	peripheral nerve	2.8	0	4
98.2	64560	autonomic nerve	2.8	0	5
98.2	64565	neuromuscular	2.8	0	4
98.2	64573	Incision for implantation of neurostimulator electrodes; cranial nerve	6.0	0	5
98.2	64575	peripheral nerve	5.2	0	4
98.2	64577	autonomic nerve	5.2	0	5
98.2	64580	neuromuscular	5.2	0	4
98.2	64585	Revision or removal of peripheral neurostimulator electrodes	4.5	0	5
98.2	64590	Incision and subcutaneous placement of peripheral neurostimulator pulse generator or receiver, direct or inductive coupling	4.9	0	5
98.2	64595	Revision or removal of peripheral neurostimulator pulse generator or receiver	3.3	0	5
	64600	Destruction by neurolytic agent, trigeminal nerve; supraorbital, infraorbital, mental, or inferior alveolar branch	2.5	7	20
	64605	second and third division branches at foramen ovale	4.5	7	20
	64610	second and third division branches at foramen ovale under radiologic monitoring	5.5	7	20
	64612	Destruction by neurolytic agent (chemodenervation of muscle endplate); muscles enervated by facial nerve (eg, for blepharospasm, hemifacial spasm)	(I) 2.4	7	20
	64613	cervical spinal muscles (eg, for spasmodic torticollis)	(I) 2.4	7	20
	64620	Destruction by neurolytic agent; intercostal nerve	1.5	7	10
	64622	paravertebral facet joint nerve, lumbar, single level	2.5	7	10

UPD			Code	Description	Units	FUD	Anes
98.2	▲	+	64623	paravertebral facet joint nerve, lumbar, each additional level (List separately in addition to code for primary procedure) Note: This code is an add-on procedure and as such is valued appropriately. Multiple procedure guidelines for reduction of value are not applicable.	0.5	7	0
			64630	pudendal nerve	0.8	7	10
98.2			64640	other peripheral nerve or branch	0.8	7	3
			64680	Destruction by neurolytic agent, celiac plexus, with or without radiologic monitoring	0.8	7	20
			64702	Neuroplasty; digital, one or both, same digit	5.0	90	3
			64704	nerve of hand or foot	8.0	90	3
98.2			64708	Neuroplasty, major peripheral nerve, arm or leg; other than specified	10.0	90	3
98.2			64712	sciatic nerve	14.0	90	4
98.2			64713	brachial plexus	13.0	90	5
98.2			64714	lumbar plexus	13.0	90	8
			64716	Neuroplasty and/or transposition; cranial nerve (specify)	15.0	90	5
			64718	ulnar nerve at elbow	11.0	90	3
			64719	ulnar nerve at wrist	7.9	90	3
			64721	median nerve at carpal tunnel	8.4	90	3
98.2			64722	Decompression; unspecified nerve(s) (specify)	10.0	90	4
			64726	plantar digital nerve	4.8	90	3
98.2	▲	+	64727	Internal neurolysis, requiring use of operating microscope (List separately in addition to code for neuroplasty) (Neuroplasty includes external neurolysis) Note: This code is an add-on procedure and as such is valued appropriately. Multiple procedure guidelines for reduction of value are not applicable.	BR	0	0
			64732	Transection or avulsion of; supraorbital nerve	7.0	30	5
			64734	infraorbital nerve	7.0	30	5
			64736	mental nerve	10.0	30	5
			64738	inferior alveolar nerve by osteotomy	10.0	30	5
			64740	lingual nerve	5.0	30	5
			64742	facial nerve, differential or complete	10.0	30	5
			64744	greater occipital nerve	7.5	30	5
98.2			64746	phrenic nerve	5.0	30	5

UPD			Code	Description	Units	FUD	Anes
			64752	vagus nerve (vagotomy), transthoracic	14.5	45	13
			64755	vagi limited to proximal stomach (selective proximal vagotomy, proximal gastric vagotomy, parietal cell vagotomy, supra- or highly selective vagotomy)	23.0	60	7
			64760	vagus nerve (vagotomy), abdominal	14.0	45	7
			64761	pudendal nerve	5.0	45	3
98.2			64763	Transection or avulsion of obturator nerve, extrapelvic, with or without adductor tenotomy	6.0	45	3
98.2			64766	Transection or avulsion of obturator nerve, intrapelvic, with or without adductor tenotomy	10.0	45	4
98.2			64771	Transection or avulsion of other cranial nerve, extradural	11.0	30	11
98.2			64772	Transection or avulsion of other spinal nerve, extradural	6.0	30	10
98.2			64774	Excision of neuroma; cutaneous nerve, surgically identifiable	4.0	30	5
			64776	digital nerve, one or both, same digit	4.0	30	3
98.2	▲	+	64778	digital nerve, each additional digit (List separately in addition to code for primary procedure) Note: This code is an add-on procedure and as such is valued appropriately. Multiple procedure guidelines for reduction of value are not applicable.	2.0	30	0
			64782	hand or foot, except digital nerve	6.0	30	3
98.2	▲	+	64783	hand or foot, each additional nerve, except same digit (List separately in addition to code for primary procedure) Note: This code is an add-on procedure and as such is valued appropriately. Multiple procedure guidelines for reduction of value are not applicable.	BR	30	0
			64784	major peripheral nerve, except sciatic	9.0	30	4
98.2			64786	sciatic nerve	10.5	30	4
98.2	▲	+	64787	Implantation of nerve end into bone or muscle (List separately in addition to neuroma excision) Note: This code is an add-on procedure and as such is valued appropriately. Multiple procedure guidelines for reduction of value are not applicable.	6.3	30	0
98.2			64788	Excision of neurofibroma or neurolemmoma; cutaneous nerve	6.3	30	5
98.2			64790	major peripheral nerve	9.0	60	5
			64792	extensive (including malignant type)	11.0	60	5
98.2			64795	Biopsy of nerve	3.0	0	5
98.2			64802	Sympathectomy, cervical	14.5	60	10
98.2			64804	Sympathectomy, cervicothoracic	20.0	60	10

UPD			Code	Description	Units	FUD	Anes
			64809	Sympathectomy, thoracolumbar	20.0	60	13
			64818	Sympathectomy, lumbar	12.0	60	7
98.2			64820	Sympathectomy, digital arteries, with magnification, each digit	(I) 15.0	90	3
			64831	Suture of digital nerve, hand or foot; one nerve	5.8	90	3
98.2	▲	+	64832	each additional digital nerve (List separately in addition to code for primary procedure)	2.5	90	0
				Note: This code is an add-on procedure and as such is valued appropriately. Multiple procedure guidelines for reduction of value are not applicable.			
			64834	Suture of one nerve, hand or foot; common sensory nerve	8.0	90	3
			64835	median motor thenar	10.0	90	3
			64836	ulnar motor	12.0	90	3
98.2	▲	+	64837	Suture of each additional nerve, hand or foot (List separately in addition to code for primary procedure)	6.0	90	0
				Note: This code is an add-on procedure and as such is valued appropriately. Multiple procedure guidelines for reduction of value are not applicable.			
			64840	Suture of posterior tibial nerve	12.0	90	3
			64856	Suture of major peripheral nerve, arm or leg, except sciatic; including transposition	12.0	90	3
			64857	without transposition	12.0	90	3
98.2			64858	Suture of sciatic nerve	14.7	90	3
98.2	▲	+	64859	Suture of each additional major peripheral nerve (List separately in addition to code for primary procedure)	6.0	90	0
				Note: This code is an add-on procedure and as such is valued appropriately. Multiple procedure guidelines for reduction of value are not applicable.			
98.2			64861	Suture of; brachial plexus	13.5	90	5
98.2			64862	lumbar plexus	13.5	90	8
			64864	Suture of facial nerve; extracranial	12.0	90	5
98.2			64865	infratemporal, with or without grafting	12.0	90	11
			64866	Anastomosis; facial-spinal accessory	29.5	90	5
			64868	facial-hypoglossal	29.5	90	5
			64870	facial-phrenic	29.5	90	5

UPD		Code	Description	Units	FUD	Anes
98.2	+	64872	Suture of nerve; requiring secondary or delayed suture (list separately in addition to code for primary neurorrhaphy)	(I) 4.0	90	0
			Note: This code is an add on procedure and as such is valued appropriately. Multiple procedure guidelines for reduction of value are not applicable.			
98.2	+	64874	requiring extensive mobilization, or transposition of nerve (list separately in addition to code for nerve suture)	(I) 2.5	90	0
			Note: This code is an add-on procedure and as such is valued appropriately. Multiple procedure guidelines for reduction of value are not applicable.			
98.2	+	64876	requiring shortening of bone of extremity (list separately in addition to code for nerve suture)	(I) 2.5	90	0
			Note: This code is an add-on procedure and as such is valued appropriately. Multiple procedure guidelines for reduction of value are not applicable.			
98.2		64885	Nerve graft (includes obtaining graft), head or neck; up to 4 cm in length	(I) 29.5	90	5
98.2		64886	more than 4 cm in length	(I) 32.0	90	5
		64890	Nerve graft (includes obtaining graft), single strand, hand or foot; up to 4 cm length	14.0	120	3
		64891	more than 4 cm length	16.0	120	3
98.2		64892	Nerve graft (includes obtaining graft), single strand, arm or leg; up to 4 cm length	14.0	120	4
98.2		64893	more than 4 cm length	16.0	120	4
		64895	Nerve graft (includes obtaining graft), multiple strands (cable), hand or foot; up to 4 cm length	18.0	120	3
		64896	more than 4 cm length	20.0	120	3
98.2		64897	Nerve graft (includes obtaining graft), multiple strands (cable), arm or leg; up to 4 cm length	18.0	120	4
98.2		64898	more than 4 cm length	20.0	120	4
98.2	▲ +	64901	Nerve graft, each additional nerve; single strand (List separately in addition to code for primary procedure)	2.0	120	0
			Note: This code is an add-on procedure and as such is valued appropriately. Multiple procedure guidelines for reduction of value are not applicable.			
98.2	▲ +	64902	multiple strands (cable) (List separately in addition to code for primary procedure)	4.0	120	0
			Note: This code is an add-on procedure and as such is valued appropriately. Multiple procedure guidelines for reduction of value are not applicable.			
98.2		64905	Nerve pedicle transfer; first stage	8.0	120	4
98.2		64907	second stage	8.0	120	4

UPD	Code	Description	Units	FUD	Anes
	64999	Unlisted procedure, nervous system	BR	0	0

Eye and Ocular Adnexa

UPD	Code	Description	Units	FUD	Anes
	65091	Evisceration of ocular contents; without implant	10.0	30	5
	65093	with implant	12.5	30	5
	65101	Enucleation of eye; without implant	12.5	30	5
	65103	with implant, muscles not attached to implant	14.0	30	5
	65105	with implant, muscles attached to implant	17.0	30	5
	65110	Exenteration of orbit (does not include skin graft), removal of orbital contents; only	20.0	30	5
	65112	with therapeutic removal of bone	22.5	30	5
	65114	with muscle or myocutaneous flap	26.0	30	5
	65125	Modification of ocular implant with placement or replacement of pegs (eg, drilling receptacle for prosthesis appendage) (separate procedure)	(I) 6.0	30	5
	65130	Insertion of ocular implant secondary; after evisceration, in scleral shell	11.5	30	5
	65135	after enucleation, muscles not attached to implant	12.5	30	5
	65140	after enucleation, muscles attached to implant	15.0	30	5
	65150	Reinsertion of ocular implant; with or without conjunctival graft	11.0	30	5
	65155	with use of foreign material for reinforcement and/or attachment of muscles to implant	12.0	30	5
	65175	Removal of ocular implant	7.5	30	5
98.2	65205*	Removal of foreign body, external eye; conjunctival superficial	0.7	0	5
	65210*	conjunctival embedded (includes concretions), subconjunctival, or scleral nonperforating	0.8	0	5
	65220*	corneal, without slit lamp	0.8	0	5
	65222*	corneal, with slit lamp	1.2	0	5
	65235	Removal of foreign body, intraocular; from anterior chamber or lens	15.0	45	5
	65260	from posterior segment, magnetic extraction, anterior or posterior route	20.0	45	5
	65265	from posterior segment, nonmagnetic extraction	20.0	45	5
98.2	65270*	Repair of laceration; conjunctiva, with or without nonperforating laceration sclera, direct closure	2.0	0	5
98.2	65272	conjunctiva, by mobilization and rearrangement, without hospitalization	3.0	7	5

UPD	Code	Description	Units	FUD	Anes
98.2	65273	conjunctiva, by mobilization and rearrangement, with hospitalization	5.0	7	5
	65275	cornea, nonperforating, with or without removal foreign body	7.8	60	5
	65280	cornea and/or sclera, perforating, not involving uveal tissue	14.0	60	5
	65285	cornea and/or sclera, perforating, with reposition or resection of uveal tissue	15.0	60	5
	65286	application of tissue glue, wounds of cornea and/or sclera	10.0	30	5
	65290	Repair of wound, extraocular muscle, tendon and/or Tenon's capsule	10.0	30	5
	65400	Excision of lesion, cornea (keratectomy, lamellar, partial), except pterygium	8.0	30	5
	65410*	Biopsy of cornea	6.0	0	5
	65420	Excision or transposition of pterygium; without graft	5.0	30	5
	65426	with graft	7.0	30	5
	65430*	Scraping of cornea, diagnostic, for smear and/or culture	0.6	0	5
	65435*	Removal of corneal epithelium; with or without chemocauterization (abrasion, curettage)	1.0	0	5
	65436	with application of chelating agent (eg, EDTA)	2.0	0	5
	65450	Destruction of lesion of cornea by cryotherapy, photocoagulation or thermocauterization	1.3	0	5
	65600	Multiple punctures of anterior cornea (eg, for corneal erosion, tattoo)	6.0	30	5
98.2	65710	Keratoplasty (corneal transplant); lamellar	24.0	90	6
98.2	65730	penetrating (except in aphakia)	29.5	90	6
98.2	65750	penetrating (in aphakia)	35.0	90	6
98.2	65755	penetrating (in pseudophakia)	(I) 25.0	90	6
98.2	65760	Keratomileusis	32.0	90	5
98.2	65765	Keratophakia	35.0	90	6
98.2	65767	Epikeratoplasty	28.0	90	5
98.2	65770	Keratoprosthesis	30.0	90	6
98.2	65771	Radial keratotomy	14.0	90	5
98.2	65772	Corneal relaxing incision for correction of surgically induced astigmatism	17.0	90	5
98.2	65775	Corneal wedge resection for correction of surgically induced astigmatism	22.0	90	5

UPD	Code	Description	Units	FUD	Anes
	65800*	Paracentesis of anterior chamber of eye (separate procedure); with diagnostic aspiration of aqueous	3.0	0	5
	65805*	with therapeutic release of aqueous	2.5	0	5
	65810	with removal of vitreous and/or discission of anterior hyaloid membrane, with or without air injection	10.0	90	5
	65815	with removal of blood, with or without irrigation and/or air injection	15.0	90	5
98.2	65820	Goniotomy	10.5	30	4
	65850	Trabeculotomy ab externo	16.0	45	5
	65855	Trabeculoplasty by laser surgery, one or more sessions (defined treatment series)	10.0	45	5
	65860	Severing adhesions of anterior segment, laser technique (separate procedure)	(I) 4.9	30	5
	65865	Severing adhesions of anterior segment of eye, incisional technique (with or without injection of air or liquid) (separate procedure); goniosynechiae	10.5	30	5
	65870	anterior synechiae, except goniosynechiae	(I) 9.5	30	5
	65875	posterior synechiae	(I) 10.0	30	5
	65880	corneovitreal adhesions	(I) 10.5	30	5
	65900	Removal of epithelial downgrowth, anterior chamber eye	(I) 13.0	30	5
	65920	Removal of implanted material, anterior segment eye	20.0	30	5
	65930	Removal of blood clot, anterior segment eye	10.0	30	5
	66020	Injection, anterior chamber (separate procedure); air or liquid	2.5	0	5
	66030*	medication	2.7	0	5
	66130	Excision of lesion, sclera	4.0	45	5
	66150	Fistulization of sclera for glaucoma; trephination with iridectomy	14.5	45	5
	66155	thermocauterization with iridectomy	14.0	45	5
	66160	sclerectomy with punch or scissors, with iridectomy	14.0	45	5
	66165	iridencleisis or iridotasis	15.0	45	5
	66170	trabeculectomy ab externo in absence of previous surgery	15.0	45	5
	66172	trabeculectomy ab externo with scarring from previous ocular surgery or trauma (includes injection of antifibrotic agents)	(I) 18.0	45	5
	66180	Aqueous shunt to extraocular reservoir (eg, Molteno, Schocket, Denver-Krupin)	(I) 14.5	45	5
	66185	Revision of aqueous shunt to extraocular reservoir	(I) 10.5	45	5

UPD	Code	Description	Units	FUD	Anes
	66220	Repair of scleral staphyloma; without graft	20.0	90	5
	66225	with graft	24.0	90	5
	66250	Revision or repair of operative wound of anterior segment, any type, early or late, major or minor procedure	(I) 10.0	90	5
	66500	Iridotomy by stab incision (separate procedure); except transfixion	7.0	30	5
	66505	with transfixion as for iris bombe	7.0	30	5
	66600	Iridectomy, with corneoscleral or corneal section; for removal of lesion	14.0	45	6
	·66605	with cyclectomy	22.0	45	6
	66625	peripheral for glaucoma (separate procedure)	10.0	45	6
	66630	sector for glaucoma (separate proedure)	10.0	45	6
	66635	"optical" (separate procedure)	10.0	45	6
	66680	Repair of iris, ciliary body (as for iridodialysis)	12.0	45	5
	66682	Suture of iris, ciliary body (separate procedure) with retrieval of suture through small incision (eg, McCannel suture)	15.0	45	5
	66700	Ciliary body destruction; diathermy	(I) 9.0	45	5
	66710	cyclophotocoagulation	(I) 9.0	45	5
	66720	cryotherapy	(I) 9.0	45	5
	66740	cyclodialysis	(I) 9.0	45	5
98.2	66761	Iridotomy/iridectomy by laser surgery (eg, for glaucoma) (one or more sessions)	10.0	45	6
98.2	66762	Iridoplasty by photocoagulation (one or more sessions) (eg, for improvement of vision, for widening of anterior chamber angle)	6.0	30	6
	66770	Destruction of cyst or lesion iris or ciliary body (nonexcisional procedure)	7.5	30	5
	66820	Discission of secondary membranous cataract (opacified posterior lens capsule and/or anterior hyaloid); stab incision technique (Ziegler or Wheeler knife)	5.5	45	6
	66821	laser surgery (eg, YAG laser) (one or more stages)	5.5	45	6
	66825	Repositioning of intraocular lens prosthesis, requiring an incision (separate procedure)	(I) 11.2	45	6
	66830	Removal of secondary membranous cataract (opacified posterior lens capsule and/or anterior hyaloid) with corneo-scleral section, with or without iridectomy (iridocapsulotomy, iridocapsulectomy)	18.0	90	6
	66840	Removal of lens material; aspiration technique, one or more stages	18.0	90	6

UPD		Code	Description	Units	FUD	Anes
		66850	phacofragmentation technique (mechanical or ultrasonic) (eg, phacoemulsification), with aspiration	20.0	90	6
		66852	pars plana approach, with or without vitrectomy	(I) 16.0	90	6
		66920	intracapsular	20.0	90	6
		66930	intracapsular, for dislocated lens	24.0	90	6
		66940	extracapsular (other than 66840, 66850, 66852)	20.0	90	6
		66983	Intracapsular cataract extraction with insertion of intraocular lens prosthesis (one stage procedure)	28.0	90	6
		66984	Extracapsular cataract removal with insertion of intraocular lens prosthesis (one stage procedure), manual or mechanical technique (eg, irrigation and aspiration or phacoemulsification)	28.0	90	6
		66985	Insertion of intraocular lens prosthesis (secondary implant), not associated with concurrent cataract removal	20.0	120	6
		66986	Exchange of intraocular lens	(I) 22.0	90	6
98.2		66999	Unlisted procedure, anterior segment of eye	BR	0	5
98.2		67005	Removal of vitreous, anterior approach (open sky technique or limbal incision); partial removal	18.0	90	6
98.2		67010	subtotal removal with mechanical vitrectomy	25.0	90	6
98.2		67015	Aspiration or release of vitreous, subretinal or choroidal fluid, pars plana approach (posterior sclerotomy)	11.0	60	6
98.2		67025	Injection of vitreous substitute, pars plana or limbal approach, (fluid-gas exchange), with or without aspiration (separate procedure)	11.0	60	6
98.2	▲	67027	Implantation of intravitreal drug delivery system (eg, ganciclovir implant), includes concomitant removal of vitreous	(I) 5.0	60	6
98.2		67028	Intravitreal injection of a pharmacologic agent (separate procedure)	(I) 11.0	45	6
98.2		67030	Discission of vitreous strands (without removal), pars plana approach	15.0	45	6
98.2		67031	Severing of vitreous strands, vitreous face adhesions, sheets, membranes or opacities, laser surgery (one or more stages)	11.0	45	6
		67036	Vitrectomy, mechanical, pars plana approach;	35.0	60	6
		67038	with epiretinal membrane stripping	40.0	60	6
		67039	with focal endolaser photocoagulation	(I) 32.0	60	6
		67040	with endolaser panretinal photocoagulation	(I) 34.0	60	6
98.2		67101	Repair of retinal detachment, one or more sessions; cryotherapy or diathermy, with or without drainage of subretinal fluid	25.0	90	6

UPD		Code	Description	Units	FUD	Anes
98.2		**67105**	photocoagulation, with or without drainage of subretinal fluid	22.5	90	6
98.2		**67107**	Repair of retinal detachment; scleral buckling (such as lamellar scleral dissection, imbrication or encircling procedure), with or without implant, with or without cryotherapy, photocoagulation, and drainage of subretinal fluid	28.0	90	6
		67108	with vitrectomy, any method, with or without air or gas tamponade, focal endolaser photocoagulation, cryotherapy, drainage of subretinal fluid, scleral buckling, and/or removal of lens by same technique	41.0	90	6
		67110	by injection of air or other gas (eg, pneumatic retinopexy)	(I) 13.0	90	6
		67112	by scleral buckling or vitrectomy, on patient having previous ipsilateral retinal detachment repair(s) using scleral buckling or vitrectomy techniques	(I) 30.0	90	6
		67115	Release of encircling material (posterior segment)	9.0	30	5
		67120	Removal of implanted material, posterior segment; extraocular	9.0	30	5
98.2		**67121**	intraocular	12.0	30	6
98.2		**67141**	Prophylaxis of retinal detachment (eg, retinal break, lattice degeneration) without drainage, one or more sessions; cryotherapy, diathermy	9.0	30	6
98.2		**67145**	photocoagulation (laser or xenon arc)	12.0	30	6
98.2	▲	**67208**	Destruction of localized lesion of retina (eg, macular edema, tumors), one or more sessions; cryotherapy, diathermy	14.0	90	6
98.2	▲	**67210**	photocoagulation	12.0	90	6
98.2		**67218**	radiation by implantation of source (includes removal of source)	22.0	90	6
98.2	●	**67220**	Destruction of localized lesion of choroid (eg, choroidal neovascularization), one or more session, photocoagulation (laser)	(I) 15.0	90	6
98.2		**67227**	Destruction of extensive or progressive retinopathy (eg, diabetic retinopathy), one or more sessions; cryotherapy, diathermy	15.0	90	6
98.2		**67228**	photocoagulation (laser or xenon arc)	12.0	90	6
		67250	Scleral reinforcement (separate procedure); without graft	20.5	90	5
		67255	with graft	24.0	90	5
98.2		**67299**	Unlisted procedure, posterior segment	BR	0	5
98.2	▲	**67311**	Strabismus surgery, recession or resection procedure; one horizontal muscle	15.0	30	5
		67312	two horizontal muscles	18.0	30	5
		67314	one vertical muscle (excluding superior oblique)	(I) 15.0	30	5

UPD			Code	Description	Units	FUD	Anes
			67316	two or more vertical muscles (excluding superior oblique)	(I) 19.0	30	5
98.2	▲		67318	Strabismus surgery, any procedure, superior oblique muscle	(I) 16.0	30	5
98.2	▲	+	67320	Transposition procedure (eg, for paretic extraocular muscle), any extraocular muscle (specify) (List separately in addition to code for primary procedure) Note: This code is an add-on procedure and as such is valued appropriately. Multiple procedure guidelines for reduction of value are not applicable.	19.0	30	0
98.2	▲	+	67331	Strabismus surgery on patient with previous eye surgery or injury that did not involve the extraocular muscles (List separately in addition to code for primary procedure) Note: This code is an add-on procedure and as such is valued appropriately. Multiple procedure guidelines for reduction of value are not applicable.	15.0	30	0
98.2	▲	+	67332	Strabismus surgery on patient with scarring of extraocular muscles (eg, prior ocular injury, strabismus or retinal detachment surgery) or restrictive myopathy (eg, dysthyroid ophthalmopathy) (List separately in addition to code for primary procedure) Note: This code is an add-on procedure and as such is valued appropriately. Multiple procedure guidelines for reduction of value are not applicable.	20.0	30	0
98.2	▲	+	67334	Strabismus surgery by posterior fixation suture technique, with or without muscle recession (List separately in addition to code for primary procedure) Note: This code is an add-on procedure and as such is valued appropriately. Multiple procedure guidelines for reduction of value are not applicable.	(I) 15.0	30	0
98.2	▲	+	67335	Placement of adjustable suture(s) during strabismus surgery, including postoperative adjustment(s) of suture(s) (List separately in addition to code for specific strabismus surgery) Note: This code is an add-on procedure and as such is valued appropriately. Multiple procedure guidelines for reduction of value are not applicable.	(I) 4.0	0	0
98.2	▲	+	67340	Strabismus surgery involving exploration and/or repair of detached extraocular muscle(s) (List separately in addition to code for primary procedure) Note: This code is an add-on procedure and as such is valued appropriately. Multiple procedure guidelines for reduction of value are not applicable.	(I) 19.0	30	0
			67343	Release of extensive scar tissue without detaching extraocular muscle (separate procedure)	(I) 14.5	30	5
			67345	Chemodenervation of extraocular muscle	3.0	0	5
			67350	Biopsy of extraocular muscle	10.0	0	5
			67399	Unlisted procedure, ocular muscle	BR	0	5

UPD	Code	Description	Units	FUD	Anes
	67400	Orbitotomy without bone flap (frontal or transconjunctival approach); for exploration, with or without biopsy	14.0	30	5
	67405	with drainage only	14.0	30	5
	67412	with removal of lesion	20.0	60	5
	67413	with removal of foreign body	20.0	30	5
	67414	with removal of bone for decompression	(I) 21.0	30	5
	67415	Fine needle aspiration of orbital contents	3.5	0	5
	67420	Orbitotomy with bone flap or window, lateral approach (eg, Kroenlein); with removal of lesion	23.0	30	5
	67430	with removal of foreign body	21.0	30	5
	67440	with drainage	20.0	30	5
	67445	with removal of bone for decompression	(I) 22.0	30	5
	67450	for exploration, with or without biopsy	20.0	30	5
	67500*	Retrobulbar injection; medication (separate procedure, does not include supply of medication)	1.5	0	5
	67505	alcohol	1.5	7	5
	67515*	Injection of therapeutic agent into Tenon's capsule	0.8	0	5
	67550	Orbital implant (implant outside muscle cone); insertion	12.0	30	5
	67560	removal or revision	10.0	30	5
	67570	Optic nerve decompression (eg, incision or fenestration of optic nerve sheath)	(I) 9.0	30	5
	67599	Unlisted procedure, orbit	BR	0	5
	67700*	Blepharotomy, drainage of abscess, eyelid	1.5	0	5
	67710*	Severing of tarsorrhaphy	1.0	0	5
	67715*	Canthotomy (separate procedure)	1.5	0	5
	67800	Excision of chalazion; single	1.5	15	5
	67801	multiple, same lid	1.9	15	5
	67805	multiple, different lids	2.2	15	5
	67808	under general anesthesia and/or requiring hospitalization, single or multiple	3.2	15	5
	67810*	Biopsy of eyelid	1.3	0	5
	67820*	Correction of trichiasis; epilation, by forceps only	0.4	0	5
	67825*	epilation by other than forceps (eg, by electrosurgery, cryotherapy, laser surgery)	1.0	0	5
	67830	incision of lid margin	1.5	7	5

UPD	Code	Description	Units	FUD	Anes
	67835	incision of lid margin, with free mucous membrane graft	13.0	30	5
	67840*	Excision of lesion of eyelid (except chalazion) without closure or with simple direct closure	2.0	0	5
	67850*	Destruction of lesion of lid margin (up to 1 cm)	1.5	0	5
	67875	Temporary closure of eyelids by suture (eg, Frost suture)	(I) 2.5	30	5
	67880	Construction of intermarginal adhesions, median tarsorrhaphy, or canthorrhaphy;	4.5	30	5
	67882	with transposition of tarsal plate	6.5	30	5
	67900	Repair of brow ptosis (supraciliary, mid-forehead or coronal approach)	(I) 6.2	60	5
	67901	Repair of blepharoptosis; frontalis muscle technique with suture or other material	14.0	60	5
	67902	frontalis muscle technique with fascial sling (includes obtaining fascia)	16.0	60	5
	67903	(tarso)levator resection or advancement, internal approach	17.0	60	5
	67904	(tarso)levator resection or advancement, external approach	17.0	60	5
	67906	superior rectus technique with fascial sling (includes obtaining fascia)	16.0	60	5
	67908	conjunctivo-tarso-Muller's muscle-levator resection (eg, Fasanella-Servat type)	12.0	30	5
	67909	Reduction of overcorrection of ptosis	12.0	30	5
	67911	Correction of lid retraction	18.0	30	5
	67914	Repair of ectropion; suture	4.0	15	5
	67915	thermocauterization	2.0	15	5
	67916	blepharoplasty, excision tarsal wedge	9.0	30	5
	67917	blepharoplasty, extensive (eg, Kuhnt-Szymanowski or tarsal strip operations)	12.0	30	5
	67921	Repair of entropion; suture	4.0	15	5
	67922	thermocauterization	2.0	15	5
	67923	blepharoplasty, excision tarsal wedge	9.0	30	5
	67924	blepharoplasty, extensive (eg, Wheeler operation)	11.5	30	5
	67930	Suture of recent wound, eyelid, involving lid margin, tarsus, and/or palpebral conjunctiva direct closure; partial thickness	5.5	30	5
	67935	full thickness	8.0	30	5
	67938	Removal of embedded foreign body, eyelid	0.7	0	5

UPD	Code	Description	Units	FUD	Anes
	67950	Canthoplasty (reconstruction of canthus)	12.0	45	5
	67961	Excision and repair of eyelid, involving lid margin, tarsus, conjunctiva, canthus, or full thickness, may include preparation for skin graft or pedicle flap with adjacent tissue transfer or rearrangement; up to one-fourth of lid margin	14.5	60	5
	67966	over one-fourth of lid margin	16.0	60	5
	67971	Reconstruction of eyelid, full thickness by transfer of tarsoconjunctival flap from opposing eyelid; up to two-thirds of eyelid, one stage or first stage	17.0	60	5
	67973	total eyelid, lower, one stage or first stage	18.0	60	5
	67974	total eyelid, upper, one stage or first stage	20.0	60	5
	67975	second stage	8.0	60	5
	67999	Unlisted procedure, eyelids	BR	0	5
98.2	**68020**	Incision of conjunctiva, drainage of cyst	0.6	0	5
98.2	**68040**	Expression of conjunctival follicles, eg, for trachoma	0.7	0	5
98.2	**68100**	Biopsy of conjunctiva	1.5	0	5
98.2	**68110**	Excision of lesion, conjunctiva; up to 1 cm	2.0	15	5
98.2	**68115**	over 1 cm	4.0	15	5
	68130	with adjacent sclera	6.0	15	5
98.2	**68135***	Destruction of lesion, conjunctiva	2.0	0	5
98.2	**68200***	Subconjunctival injection	1.0	0	5
	68320	Conjunctivoplasty; with conjunctival graft or extensive rearrangement	13.0	30	5
	68325	with buccal mucous membrane graft (includes obtaining graft)	14.0	30	5
	68326	Conjunctivoplasty, reconstruction cul-de-sac; with conjunctival graft or extensive rearrangement	14.0	30	5
	68328	with buccal mucous membrane graft (includes obtaining graft)	16.0	30	5
	68330	Repair of symblepharon; conjunctivoplasty, without graft	10.0	30	5
	68335	with free graft conjunctiva or buccal mucous membrane (includes obtaining graft)	14.0	30	5
	68340	division of symblepharon, with or without insertion of conformer or contact lens	4.5	0	5
	68360	Conjunctival flap; bridge or partial (separate procedure)	6.0	30	5
	68362	total (such as Gunderson thin flap or purse string flap)	11.0	30	5
	68399	Unlisted procedure, conjunctiva	BR	0	5

UPD		Code	Description	Units	FUD	Anes
		68400	Incision, drainage of lacrimal gland	2.1	15	5
		68420	Incision, drainage of lacrimal sac (dacryocystotomy or dacryocystostomy)	2.0	15	5
		68440*	Snip incision of lacrimal punctum	1.0	0	5
		68500	Excision of lacrimal gland (dacryoadenectomy), except for tumor; total	12.5	45	5
		68505	partial	12.0	45	5
		68510	Biopsy of lacrimal gland	2.0	0	5
		68520	Excision of lacrimal sac (dacryocystectomy)	13.0	45	5
		68525	Biopsy of lacrimal sac	2.0	45	5
		68530	Removal of foreign body or dacryolith, lacrimal passages	10.0	30	5
		68540	Excision of lacrimal gland tumor; frontal approach	15.0	45	5
		68550	involving osteotomy	17.0	45	5
		68700	Plastic repair of canaliculi	12.0	30	5
		68705	Correction of everted punctum, cautery	1.5	15	5
		68720	Dacryocystorhinostomy (fistulization of lacrimal sac to nasal cavity)	15.0	60	5
		68745	Conjunctivorhinostomy (fistulization of conjunctiva to nasal cavity); without tube	16.0	90	5
		68750	with insertion of tube or stent	17.0	15	5
		68760	Closure of the lacrimal punctum; by thermocauterization, ligation, or laser surgery	1.5	15	5
		68761	by plug, each	(I) 1.9	15	5
		68770	Closure of lacrimal fistula (separate procedure)	7.5	30	5
96.2	M	68800*	Dilation of lacrimal punctum, with or without irrigation, unilateral or bilateral To report, use 68801	0.8	0	5
96.2		68801*	Dilation of lacrimal punctum, with or without irrigation	(I) 0.8	0	5
98.2		68810*	Probing of nasolacrimal duct, with or without irrigation;	(I) 1.5	0	5
96.2		68811	requiring general anesthesia	(I) 3.2	0	5
98.2		68815	with insertion of tube or stent	(I) 4.2	0	5
96.2	M	68820*	Probing of nasolacrimal duct, with or without irrigation, unilateral or bilateral; To report, see 68810, 68811, or 68815	1.2	0	0
96.2	M	68825	requiring general anesthesia To report, see 68810, 68811, or 68815	2.5	7	5

UPD		Code	Description	Units	FUD	Anes
96.2	M	68830	with insertion of tube or stent To report, see 68810, 68811, or 68815	3.5	15	5
		68840*	Probing of lacrimal canaliculi, with or without irrigation	0.8	0	5
		68850*	Injection of contrast medium for dacryocystography	0.7	0	5
		68899	Unlisted procedure, lacrimal system	BR	0	5

Auditory System

UPD	Code	Description	Units	FUD	Anes
	69000*	Drainage external ear, abscess or hematoma; simple	1.0	0	5
	69005	complicated	3.3	0	5
	69020*	Drainage external auditory canal, abscess	1.5	0	5
	69090	Ear piercing	0.8	0	0
98.2	69100	Biopsy external ear	0.8	0	5
98.2	69105	Biopsy external auditory canal	1.2	0	5
98.2	69110	Excision external ear; partial, simple repair	6.0	30	5
98.2	69120	complete amputation	8.0	90	5
98.2	69140	Excision exostosis(es), external auditory canal	11.5	90	5
	69145	Excision soft tissue lesion, external auditory canal	2.0	90	5
	69150	Radical excision external auditory canal lesion; without neck dissection	15.0	90	5
98.2	69155	with neck dissection	23.5	90	6
98.2	69200	Removal foreign body from external auditory canal; without general anesthesia	0.8	0	4
98.2	69205	with general anesthesia	2.0	0	4
98.2	69210	Removal impacted cerumen (separate procedure), one or both ears	0.6	0	4
98.2	69220	Debridement, mastoidectomy cavity, simple (eg, routine cleaning)	0.6	7	5
98.2	69222	Debridement, mastoidectomy cavity, complex (eg, with anesthesia or more than routine cleaning)	1.5	14	5
	69300	Otoplasty, protruding ear, with or without size reduction	12.0	180	5
	69310	Reconstruction of external auditory canal (meatoplasty) (eg, for stenosis due to trauma, infection) (separate procedure)	20.0	180	5
	69320	Reconstruction external auditory canal for congenital atresia, single stage	20.0	180	5
98.2	69399	Unlisted procedure, external ear	BR	0	5
98.2	69400	Eustachian tube inflation, transnasal; with catheterization	0.3	0	5

UPD	Code	Description	Units	FUD	Anes
98.2	69401	without catheterization	0.3	0	5
98.2	69405	Eustachian tube catheterization, transtympanic	0.3	0	5
98.2	69410	Focal application of phase control substance, middle ear (baffle technique)	(I) 0.2	0	5
	69420*	Myringotomy including aspiration and/or eustachian tube inflation	1.0	0	4
	69421*	Myringotomy including aspiration and/or eustachian tube inflation requiring general anesthesia	2.1	0	4
	69424	Ventilating tube removal when originally inserted by another physician	0.8	0	4
	69433*	Tympanostomy (requiring insertion of ventilating tube), local or topical anesthesia	2.0	0	5
	69436	Tympanostomy (requiring insertion of ventilating tube), general anesthesia	4.3	30	5
	69440	Middle ear exploration through postauricular or ear canal incision	11.0	30	5
	69450	Tympanolysis, transcanal	11.5	30	5
	69501	Transmastoid antrotomy ("simple" mastoidectomy)	12.4	90	5
	69502	Mastoidectomy; complete	15.0	90	5
	69505	modified radical	22.6	90	5
	69511	radical	25.7	90	5
	69530	Petrous apicectomy including radical mastoidectomy	30.9	180	5
	69535	Resection temporal bone, external approach	30.9	90	5
	69540	Excision aural polyp	1.1	15	5
	69550	Excision aural glomus tumor; transcanal	20.6	90	5
	69552	transmastoid	30.9	90	5
	69554	extended (extratemporal)	41.2	90	5
	69601	Revision mastoidectomy; resulting in complete mastoidectomy	15.5	90	5
	69602	resulting in modified radical mastoidectomy	18.3	90	5
	69603	resulting in radical mastoidectomy	23.5	90	5
	69604	resulting in tympanoplasty	21.7	90	5
	69605	with apicectomy	23.5	90	5
	69610	Tympanic membrane repair, with or without site preparation or perforation for closure, with or without patch	1.5	7	5
	69620	Myringoplasty (surgery confined to drumhead and donor area)	17.5	90	5

UPD	Code	Description	Units	FUD	Anes
	69631	Tympanoplasty without mastoidectomy (including canalplasty, atticotomy and/or middle ear surgery), initial or revision; without ossicular chain reconstruction	23.5	90	5
	69632	Tympanoplasty without mastoidectomy (including canalplasty, atticotomy and/or middle ear surgery), initial or revision; with ossicular chain reconstruction (eg, postfenestration)	25.5	90	5
	69633	with ossicular chain reconstruction and synthetic prosthesis (eg, partial ossicular replacement prosthesis, (PORP), total ossicular replacement prosthesis (TORP))	25.5	90	5
	69635	Tympanoplasty with antrotomy or mastoidotomy (including canalplasty, atticotomy, middle ear surgery, and/or tympanic membrane repair); without ossicular chain reconstruction	24.5	90	5
	69636	with ossicular chain reconstruction	25.5	90	5
	69637	with ossicular chain reconstruction and synthetic prosthesis (eg, partial ossicular replacement prosthesis, (PORP), total ossicular replacement prosthesis (TORP))	25.5	90	5
	69641	Tympanoplasty with mastoidectomy (including canalplasty, middle ear surgery, tympanic membrane repair); without ossicular chain reconstruction	28.0	90	5
	69642	with ossicular chain reconstruction	31.0	90	5
	69643	with intact or reconstructed wall, without ossicular chain reconstruction	30.0	90	5
	69644	with intact or reconstructed canal wall, with ossicular chain reconstruction	30.0	90	5
	69645	radical or complete, without ossicular chain reconstruction	28.0	90	5
	69646	radical or complete, with ossicular chain reconstruction	31.0	90	5
	69650	Stapes mobilization	13.5	90	5
	69660	Stapedectomy or stapedotomy with reestablishment of ossicular continuity, with or without use of foreign material;	23.5	90	5
96.2	69661	with footplate drill out	28.0	90	5
	69662	Revision of stapedectomy or stapedotomy	(I) 26.0	90	5
	69666	Repair oval window fistula	20.0	90	5
	69667	Repair round window fistula	19.5	90	5
	69670	Mastoid obliteration (separate procedure)	20.0	90	5
	69676	Tympanic neurectomy	18.0	90	5
	69700	Closure postauricular fistula, mastoid (separate procedure)	7.0	90	5
	69710	Implantation or replacement of electromagnetic bone conduction hearing device in temporal bone	(I) 10.0	90	5
	69711	Removal or repair of electromagnetic bone conduction hearing device in temporal bone	(I) 7.5	90	5

UPD	Code	Description	Units	FUD	Anes
	69720	Decompression facial nerve, intratemporal; lateral to geniculate ganglion	26.0	90	5
	69725	including medial to geniculate ganglion	40.0	90	5
	69740	Suture facial nerve, intratemporal, with or without graft or decompression; lateral to geniculate ganglion	30.0	90	5
	69745	including medial to geniculate ganglion	37.0	90	5
98.2	69799	Unlisted procedure, middle ear	BR	0	5
96.2	69801	Labyrinthotomy, with or without cryosurgery including other nonexcisional destructive procedures or perfusion of vestibuloactive drugs (single or multiple perfusions); transcanal	21.0	90	5
	69802	with mastoidectomy	28.0	90	5
	69805	Endolymphatic sac operation; without shunt	25.0	90	5
	69806	with shunt	29.0	90	5
	69820	Fenestration semicircular canal	25.0	90	5
	69840	Revision fenestration operation	17.0	90	5
	69905	Labyrinthectomy; transcanal	23.5	90	5
	69910	with mastoidectomy	28.0	90	5
	69915	Vestibular nerve section, translabyrinthine approach	39.2	90	5
	69930	Cochlear device implantation, with or without mastoidectomy	33.5	90	5
98.2	69949	Unlisted procedure, inner ear	BR	0	5
	69950	Vestibular nerve section, transcranial approach	38.0	90	11
	69955	Total facial nerve decompression and/or repair (may include graft)	39.0	90	5
	69960	Decompression internal auditory canal	36.0	90	5
98.2	69970	Removal of tumor, temporal bone	45.0	90	5
98.2	69979	Unlisted procedure, temporal bone, middle fossa approach	BR	0	11
98.2	● + 69990	Use of operating microscope (List separately in addition to code for primary procedure) Note: This code is an add-on procedure and as such is valued appropriately. Multiple procedure guidelines for reduction of value are not applicable.	RNE	—	—

Radiology

Guidelines

I. **General:** Listed values for radiology procedures apply only when these services are performed by or under the supervision of a physician.

.   **Total:** The unit value listed in the Total column represents the global value of the procedure. The five digit code is used to represent this service, including the professional services and technical value of providing that service. The following sections, professional and technical, provide additional definitions for each component.

B. **Professional:** The unit value listed in the Professional column is used to designate professional services. Modifier -26 is added to the procedure code to indicate the use of this value. The professional component includes examination of the patient, when indicated, performance and/or supervision of the procedure, interpretation and written report of the examination, and consultation with referring physicians.

C. **Technical:** The unit value listed in the Technical column is used to designate the technical value of providing the service. Modifier -27 may be used to designate this component. (Note: Modifier -27 is not CPT compatible and may not be accepted by all payers. Check with the specific payer prior to use of this modifier.) The technical component includes personnel, materials, space, equipment, and other allocated facility overhead normally included in providing the service.

II. **Supervision and Interpretation Only:** code designated as Supervision and Interpretation Only is used to indicate radiological services provided by a radiologist and staff, in conjunction with services provided by another physician (i.e., injection, insertion of catheter). In this instance, a physician other than the radiologist should list separately the appropriate procedure code, and the radiologist should bill using the appropriate Supervision and Interpretation code. If the Radiologist and Staff provide both portions of the service, current CPT requires reporting with the Supervision and Interpretation code and the appropriate procedure code. RVP contains the deleted complete procedures which include all aspects of the given procedure under one code. Some payers may accept these codes, others may not. Check with the payer for appropriate reporting.

III. **Complete Procedures:** Procedures designated as a "complete" procedure are used to denote radiological services that are performed by the radiologist and staff only. If other physicians provide some part of the procedure, see SUPERVISION AND INTERPRETATION ONLY.

IV. **Unlisted Services or Procedure:** service or procedure that is not identified by a particular code should be listed under the appropriate "Unlisted Procedure." These procedures often have 99 as the final two digits. Values should be substantiated by report (See BY REPORT).

V. **Procedures Without Values:** Procedures that have a BR or RNE in the units column require a report (See BY REPORT) to substantiate value.

VI. **Unusual Service or Procedure:** When a procedure of unusual nature is performed, modifier -22 should be added and value substantiated by report (See BY REPORT).

VII **By Report:** Value of a procedure should be established for any by report circumstance by identifying a similar service and justifying value difference. Procedures that require a report should include the following:

1. Accurate definition;

2. Clinical history;

3.   Related procedure values; and

4.   Reason for value adjustment.

VIII.   **Separate or Multiple Procedures:** Multiple procedures performed on the same date should be listed using modifier - 51. Customarily each procedure is allowed 100% of the listed value.

IX.   **Reduced Value:** If a physician elects to reduce the value of a procedure, modifier -52 should be added to the procedure code. Modifier -52 and the appropriate code may be used to indicate a limited or follow-up CT scan.

X.   **Services or Procedures Listed in Other Sections:** Services or procedures provided by a radiologist may be listed in an alternate section of the book (i.e., consultations listed in MEDICINE). The radiologist should use these procedure codes following the guidelines appropriate to that section. Note: The conversion factor for each section generally differs.

XI.   **Modifiers:** comprehensive listing of modifiers is provided in the introduction. Value adjustments significant to radiology and modifiers for those adjustments are listed above.

Magnetic Resonance Imaging

Upon review of procedural descriptions and their usage, the editors of RVP have elected to drop the L, S, and E identifiers. The MRI codes listed and their corresponding unit values correspond to the existing expanded MRI procedures. This is due to the common practice of utilizing 25 or more slices for each MRI service performed.

Radiology

UPD	Code	Description	Prof	Tech	Total
Diagnostic Radiology (Diagnostic Imaging)					
98.2	**70010**	Myelography, posterior fossa, radiological supervision and interpretation	5.1	8.5	13.6
	70015	Cisternography, positive contrast, radiological supervision and interpretation	5.1	8.5	13.6
98.2	**70030**	Radiologic examination, eye, for detection of foreign body	1.1	2.0	3.1
98.2	**70100**	Radiologic examination, mandible; partial, less than four views	1.0	2.0	3.0
98.2	**70110**	complete, minimum of four views	1.4	2.4	3.8
98.2	**70120**	Radiologic examination, mastoids; less than three views per side	1.0	1.8	2.8
98.2	**70130**	complete, minimum of three views per side	2.0	2.5	4.5
98.2	**70134**	Radiologic examination, internal auditory meati, complete	1.8	2.2	4.0
98.2	**70140**	Radiologic examination, facial bones; less than three views	1.0	1.8	2.8
98.2	**70150**	complete, minimum of three views	1.4	2.6	4.0
98.2	**70160**	Radiologic examination, nasal bones, complete, minimum of three views	1.0	2.0	3.0
98.2	**70170**	Dacryocystography, nasolacrimal duct, radiological supervision and interpretation	1.6	2.7	4.3
98.2	**70190**	Radiologic examination; optic foramina	1.0	2.0	3.0
98.2	**70200**	orbits, complete, minimum of four views	1.4	2.6	4.0
98.2	**70210**	Radiologic examination, sinuses, paranasal, less than three views	1.0	2.0	3.0
98.2	**70220**	Radiologic examination, sinuses, paranasal, complete, minimum of three views	1.4	2.3	3.7
98.2	**70240**	Radiologic examination, sella turcica	1.0	1.4	2.4
98.2	**70250**	Radiologic examination, skull; less than four views, with or without stereo	1.3	1.8	3.1
98.2	**70260**	complete, minimum of four views, with or without stereo	2.0	3.0	5.0
98.2	**70300**	Radiologic examination, teeth; single view	0.6	0.8	1.4
98.2	**70310**	partial examination, less than full mouth	0.9	1.4	2.3
98.2	**70320**	complete, full mouth	1.3	2.3	3.6

UPD	Code	Description	Prof	Tech	Total
98.2	70328	Radiologic examination, temporomandibular joint, open and closed mouth; unilateral	1.0	1.6	2.6
98.2	70330	bilateral	1.4	2.6	4.0
98.2	70332	Temporomandibular joint arthrography, radiological supervision and interpretation	3.2	6.2	9.4
98.2	70336	Magnetic resonance (eg, proton) imaging, temporomandibular joint	10.0	45.0	55.0
98.2	70350	Cephalogram, orthodontic	1.0	1.4	2.4
98.2	70355	Orthopantogram	1.2	2.3	3.5
98.2	70360	Radiologic examination; neck, soft tissue	1.0	1.4	2.4
98.2	70370	pharynx or larynx, including fluoroscopy and/ or magnification technique	1.8	4.0	5.8
98.2	70371	Complex dynamic pharyngeal and speech evaluation by cine or video recording	4.9	6.0	10.9
98.2	70373	Laryngography, contrast, radiological supervision and interpretation	3.0	5.1	8.1
98.2	70380	Radiologic examination, salivary gland for calculus	1.0	2.0	3.0
98.2	70390	Sialography, radiological supervision and interpretation	2.3	5.1	7.4
98.2	70450	Computerized axial tomography, head or brain; without contrast material	5.4	16.3	21.7
98.2	70460	with contrast material(s)	6.5	18.9	25.4
98.2	70470	without contrast material, followed by contrast material(s) and further sections	7.4	24.2	31.6
98.2	70480	Computerized axial tomography, orbit, sella, or posterior fossa or outer, middle, or inner ear; without contrast material	7.5	16.3	23.8
98.2	70481	with contrast material(s)	8.0	18.9	26.9
98.2	70482	without contrast material, followed by contrast material(s) and further sections	8.5	24.2	32.7
98.2	70486	Computerized axial tomography, maxillofacial area; without contrast material	6.5	16.3	22.8
98.2	70487	with contrast material(s)	7.5	18.9	26.4
98.2	70488	without contrast material, followed by contrast material(s) and further sections	8.0	24.2	32.2
98.2	70490	Computerized axial tomography, soft tissue neck; without contrast material	7.5	16.3	23.8
98.2	70491	with contrast material(s)	8.0	18.9	26.9
98.2	70492	without contrast material followed by contrast material(s) and further sections	8.5	24.2	32.7

UPD	Code	Description	Prof	Tech	Total
98.2	**70540**	Magnetic resonance (eg, proton) imaging, orbit, face, and neck	10.0	45.0	55.0
98.2	**70541**	Magnetic resonance angiography, head and/or neck, with or without contrast material(s)	(I) 11.0	(I) 47.5	(I) 58.5
98.2	**70551**	Magnetic resonance (eg, proton) imaging, brain (including brain stem); without contrast material	10.0	45.0	55.0
98.2	**70552**	with contrast material(s)	12.0	50.0	62.0
98.2	**70553**	without contrast material, followed by contrast material(s) and further sequences	15.0	55.0	70.0
98.2	**71010**	Radiologic examination, chest; single view, frontal	1.0	1.4	2.4
98.2	**71015**	stereo, frontal	1.2	1.8	3.0
98.2	**71020**	Radiologic examination, chest, two views, frontal and lateral;	1.3	1.9	3.2
98.2	**71021**	with apical lordotic procedure	1.5	2.5	4.0
98.2	**71022**	with oblique projections	1.8	2.5	4.3
98.2	**71023**	with fluoroscopy	2.0	2.5	4.5
98.2	**71030**	Radiologic examination, chest, complete, minimum of four views;	1.8	2.5	4.3
98.2	**71034**	with fluoroscopy	2.8	4.3	7.1
98.2	**71035**	Radiologic examination, chest, special views (eg, lateral decubitus, Bucky studies)	1.5	2.0	3.5
	71036	Needle biopsy of intrathoracic lesion, including follow-up films, fluoroscopic localization only, radiological supervision and interpretation	3.2	4.5	7.7
98.2　M	**71038**	Fluoroscopic localization for transbronchial biopsy or brushing To report, use 31628	3.1	5.0	8.1
	71040	Bronchography, unilateral, radiological supervision and interpretation	3.5	4.5	8.0
	71060	Bronchography, bilateral, radiological supervision and interpretation	4.5	6.5	11.0
	71090	Insertion pacemaker, fluoroscopy and radiography, radiological supervision and interpretation	3.3	5.0	8.3
98.2	**71100**	Radiologic examination, ribs, unilateral; two views	1.5	2.0	3.5
98.2	**71101**	including posteroanterior chest, minimum of three views	1.7	2.3	4.0
98.2	**71110**	Radiologic examination, ribs, bilateral; three views	1.7	2.6	4.3
98.2	**71111**	including posteroanterior chest, minimum of four views	1.9	2.9	4.8
98.2	**71120**	Radiologic examination; sternum, minimum of two views	1.0	2.0	3.0

UPD	Code	Description	Prof	Tech	Total
98.2	**71130**	sternoclavicular joint or joints, minimum of three views	1.2	2.0	3.2
98.2	**71250**	Computerized axial tomography, thorax; without contrast material	7.0	19.4	26.4
98.2	**71260**	with contrast material(s)	7.7	22.7	30.4
98.2	**71270**	without contrast material, followed by contrast material(s) and further sections	8.7	28.3	37.0
98.2	**71550**	Magnetic resonance (eg, proton) imaging, chest (eg, for evaluation of hilar and mediastinal lymphadenopathy)	10.0	45.0	55.0
98.2	**71555**	Magnetic resonance angiography, chest (excluding myocardium), with or without contrast material(s)	(I) 11.0	(I) 47.5	(I) 58.5
98.2	**72010**	Radiologic examination, spine, entire, survey study, anteroposterior and lateral	2.6	4.0	6.6
98.2	**72020**	Radiologic examination, spine, single view, specify level	1.0	1.2	2.2
98.2	**72040**	Radiologic examination, spine, cervical; anteroposterior and lateral	1.0	2.0	3.0
98.2	**72050**	minimum of four views	1.7	3.1	4.8
98.2	**72052**	complete, including oblique and flexion and/or extension studies	2.0	4.0	6.0
98.2	**72069**	Radiologic examination, spine, thoracolumbar, standing (scoliosis)	1.2	2.3	3.5
98.2	**72070**	Radiologic examination, spine; thoracic, anteroposterior and lateral	1.3	2.0	3.3
98.2	**72072**	thoracic, anteroposterior and lateral, including swimmer's view of the cervicothoracic junction	1.4	2.5	3.9
98.2	**72074**	thoracic, complete, including obliques, minimum of four views	1.2	3.0	4.2
98.2	**72080**	thoracolumbar, anteroposterior and lateral	1.5	2.0	3.5
98.2	**72090**	scoliosis study, including supine and erect studies	1.6	2.0	3.6
98.2	**72100**	Radiologic examination, spine, lumbosacral; anteroposterior and lateral	1.3	2.0	3.3
98.2	**72110**	complete, with oblique views	1.8	2.7	4.5
98.2	**72114**	complete, including bending views	2.0	3.4	5.4
98.2	**72120**	Radiologic examination, spine, lumbosacral, bending views only, minimum of four views	1.3	2.5	3.8
98.2	**72125**	Computerized axial tomography, cervical spine; without contrast material	6.8	19.2	26.0
98.2	**72126**	with contrast material	7.0	23.0	30.0

UPD	Code	Description	Prof	Tech	Total
98.2	**72127**	without contrast material, followed by contrast material(s) and further sections	7.2	28.8	36.0
98.2	**72128**	Computerized axial tomography, thoracic spine; without contrast material	6.8	19.2	26.0
98.2	**72129**	with contrast material	7.0	23.0	30.0
98.2	**72130**	without contrast material, followed by contrast material(s) and further sections	7.2	28.8	36.0
98.2	**72131**	Computerized axial tomography, lumbar spine; without contrast material	6.8	19.2	26.0
98.2	**72132**	with contrast material	7.0	23.0	30.0
98.2	**72133**	without contrast material, followed by contrast material(s) and further sections	7.2	28.8	36.0
98.2	**72141**	Magnetic resonance (eg, proton) imaging, spinal canal and contents, cervical; without contrast material	10.0	45.0	55.0
98.2	**72142**	with contrast material(s)	12.0	50.0	62.0
98.2	**72146**	Magnetic resonance (eg, proton) imaging, spinal canal and contents, thoracic; without contrast material	10.0	45.0	55.0
98.2	**72147**	with contrast material(s)	12.0	50.0	62.0
98.2	**72148**	Magnetic resonance (eg, proton) imaging, spinal canal and contents, lumbar; without contrast material	10.0	45.0	55.0
98.2	**72149**	with contrast material(s)	12.0	50.0	62.0
98.2	**72156**	Magnetic resonance (eg, proton) imaging, spinal canal and contents, without contrast material, followed by contrast material(s) and further sequences; cervical	15.0	55.0	70.0
98.2	**72157**	thoracic	15.0	55.0	70.0
98.2	**72158**	lumbar	15.0	55.0	70.0
98.2	**72159**	Magnetic resonance angiography, spinal canal and contents, with or without contrast material(s)	(I) 11.0	(I) 47.5	(I) 58.5
98.2	**72170**	Radiologic examination, pelvis; anteroposterior only	1.0	2.0	3.0
98.2	**72190**	complete, minimum of three views	1.3	2.3	3.6
98.2	**72192**	Computerized axial tomography, pelvis; without contrast material	6.0	19.5	25.5
98.2	**72193**	with contrast material(s)	6.5	22.0	28.5
98.2	**72194**	without contrast material, followed by contrast material(s) and further sections	7.0	27.5	34.5
98.2	**72196**	Magnetic resonance (eg, proton) imaging, pelvis	10.0	45.0	55.0

UPD	Code	Description	Prof	Tech	Total
98.2	**72198**	Magnetic resonance angiography, pelvis, with or without contrast material(s)	(I) 11.0	(I) 47.5	(I) 58.5
98.2	**72200**	Radiologic examination, sacroiliac joints; less than three views	1.3	1.7	3.0
98.2	**72202**	three or more views	1.4	1.8	3.2
98.2	**72220**	Radiologic examination, sacrum and coccyx, minimum of two views	1.3	1.7	3.0
98.2	**72240**	Myelography, cervical, radiological supervision and interpretation	4.5	6.3	10.8
98.2	**72255**	Myelography, thoracic, radiological supervision and interpretation	4.2	6.1	10.3
98.2	**72265**	Myelography, lumbosacral, radiological supervision and interpretation	4.2	6.1	10.3
98.2	**72270**	Myelography, entire spinal canal, radiological supervision and interpretation	6.0	10.0	16.0
	72285	Diskography, cervical, radiological supervision and interpretation	4.5	24.5	29.0
	72295	Diskography, lumbar, radiological supervision and interpretation	4.5	23.0	27.5
98.2	**73000**	Radiologic examination; clavicle, complete	0.9	1.5	2.4
98.2	**73010**	scapula, complete	1.0	1.7	2.7
98.2	**73020**	Radiologic examination, shoulder; one view	0.8	1.4	2.2
98.2	**73030**	complete, minimum of two views	1.1	1.6	2.7
	73040	Radiologic examination, shoulder, arthrography, radiological supervision and interpretation	3.5	6.0	9.5
98.2	**73050**	Radiologic examination; acromioclavicular joints, bilateral, with or without weighted distraction	1.0	2.0	3.0
98.2	**73060**	humerus, minimum of two views	1.0	1.8	2.8
98.2	**73070**	Radiologic examination, elbow; anteroposterior and lateral views	0.8	1.8	2.6
98.2	**73080**	complete, minimum of three views	1.0	1.7	2.7
98.2	**73085**	Radiologic examination, elbow, arthrography, radiological supervision and interpretation	3.5	6.0	9.5
98.2	**73090**	Radiologic examination; forearm, anteroposterior and lateral views	1.0	1.5	2.5
98.2	**73092**	upper extremity, infant, minimum of two views	1.0	1.5	2.5
98.2	**73100**	Radiologic examination, wrist; anteroposterior and lateral views	1.0	1.5	2.5
98.2	**73110**	complete, minimum of three views	1.1	1.6	2.7

UPD		Code	Description	Prof	Tech	Total
		73115	Radiologic examination, wrist, arthrography, radiological supervision and interpretation	3.2	4.7	7.9
98.2		**73120**	Radiologic examination, hand; two views	0.8	1.4	2.2
98.2		**73130**	minimum of three views	1.0	1.8	2.8
98.2		**73140**	Radiologic examination, finger(s), minimum of two views	0.8	1.3	2.1
98.2		**73200**	Computerized axial tomography, upper extremity; without contrast material	6.0	17.0	23.0
98.2		**73201**	with contrast material(s)	6.5	19.5	26.0
98.2		**73202**	without contrast material, followed by contrast material(s) and further sections	7.0	24.5	31.5
98.2		**73220**	Magnetic resonance (eg, proton) imaging, upper extremity, other than joint	10.0	45.0	55.0
98.2		**73221**	Magnetic resonance (eg, proton) imaging, any joint of upper extremity	10.0	45.0	55.0
98.2		**73225**	Magnetic resonance angiography, upper extremity, with or without contrast material(s)	(I) 11.0	(I) 47.5	(I) 58.5
98.2		**73500**	Radiologic examination, hip unilateral; one view	1.0	1.5	2.5
98.2		**73510**	complete, minimum of two views	1.0	2.0	3.0
98.2		**73520**	Radiologic examination, hips, bilateral, minimum of two views of each hip, including anteroposterior view of pelvis	1.4	2.1	3.5
98.2		**73525**	Radiologic examination, hip, arthrography, radiological supervision and interpretation	3.5	6.0	9.5
98.2		**73530**	Radiologic examination, hip, during operative procedure	1.8	2.0	3.8
98.2		**73540**	Radiologic examination, pelvis and hips, infant or child, minimum of two views	1.0	1.9	2.9
98.2		**73550**	Radiologic examination, femur, anteroposterior and lateral views	1.0	1.8	2.8
98.2	▲	**73560**	Radiologic examination, knee; one or two views	0.9	1.6	2.5
98.2	▲	**73562**	three views	1.0	1.8	2.8
98.2	▲	**73564**	complete, four or more views	1.2	1.8	3.0
98.2		**73565**	both knees, standing, anteroposterior	0.9	1.6	2.5
		73580	Radiologic examination, knee, arthrography, radiological supervision and interpretation	3.3	7.7	11.0
98.2		**73590**	Radiologic examination; tibia and fibula, anteroposterior and lateral views	0.8	1.7	2.5
98.2		**73592**	lower extremity, infant, minimum of two views	0.8	1.5	2.3

UPD	Code	Description	Prof	Tech	Total
98.2	**73600**	Radiologic examination, ankle; anteroposterior and lateral views	0.8	1.5	2.3
98.2	**73610**	complete, minimum of three views	1.0	1.8	2.8
98.2	**73615**	Radiologic examination, ankle, arthrography, radiological supervision and interpretation	3.5	6.0	9.5
98.2	**73620**	Radiologic examination, foot; anteroposterior and lateral views	0.9	1.4	2.3
98.2	**73630**	complete, minimum of three views	1.1	1.6	2.7
98.2	**73650**	Radiologic examination; calcaneus, minimum of two views	0.8	1.5	2.3
98.2	**73660**	toe(s), minimum of two views	0.7	1.3	2.0
98.2	**73700**	Computerized axial tomography, lower extremity; without contrast material	6.0	17.0	23.0
98.2	**73701**	with contrast material(s)	6.5	19.5	26.0
98.2	**73702**	without contrast material, followed by contrast material(s) and further sections	7.0	24.5	31.5
98.2	**73720**	Magnetic resonance (eg, proton) imaging, lower extremity, other than joint	10.0	45.0	55.0
98.2	**73721**	Magnetic resonance (eg, proton) imaging, any joint of lower extremity	10.0	45.0	55.0
98.2	**73725**	Magnetic resonance angiography, lower extremity, with or without contrast material(s)	(I) 11.0	(I) 47.5	(I) 58.5
98.2	**74000**	Radiologic examination, abdomen; single anteroposterior view	1.0	1.6	2.6
98.2	**74010**	anteroposterior and additional oblique and cone views	1.2	1.7	2.9
98.2	**74020**	complete, including decubitus and/or erect views	1.6	2.5	4.1
98.2	**74022**	complete acute abdomen series, including supine, erect, and/or decubitus views, upright PA chest	1.9	2.6	4.5
98.2	**74150**	Computerized axial tomography, abdomen; without contrast material	7.0	18.0	25.0
98.2	**74160**	with contrast material(s)	7.4	22.4	29.8
98.2	**74170**	without contrast material, followed by contrast material(s) and further sections	8.0	28.0	36.0
98.2	**74181**	Magnetic resonance (eg, proton) imaging, abdomen	10.0	45.0	55.0
98.2	**74185**	Magnetic resonance angiography, abdomen, with or without contrast material(s)	(I) 11.0	(I) 47.5	(I) 58.5
98.2	**74190**	Peritoneogram (eg, after injection of air or contrast), radiological supervision and interpretation	(I) 5.8	(I) 8.7	(I) 14.5

UPD			Code	Description	Prof	Tech	Total
98.2			**74210**	Radiologic examination; pharynx and/or cervical esophagus	2.0	3.4	5.4
98.2			**74220**	esophagus	2.6	3.4	6.0
98.2			**74230**	Swallowing function, pharynx and/or esophagus, with cineradiography and/or video	3.1	3.9	7.0
			74235	Removal of foreign body(s), esophageal, with use of balloon catheter, radiological supervision and interpretation	6.6	7.8	14.4
98.2			**74240**	Radiologic examination, gastrointestinal tract, upper; with or without delayed films, without KUB	4.0	4.2	8.2
98.2			**74241**	with or without delayed films, with KUB	4.1	4.3	8.4
98.2			**74245**	with small bowel, includes multiple serial films	5.0	7.0	12.0
98.2			**74246**	Radiological examination, gastrointestinal tract, upper, air contrast, with specific high density barium, effervescent agent, with or without glucagon; with or without delayed films, without KUB	4.0	4.8	8.8
98.2			**74247**	with or without delayed films, with KUB	4.1	4.9	9.0
98.2			**74249**	with small bowel follow-through	5.2	7.5	12.7
98.2			**74250**	Radiologic examination, small bowel, includes multiple serial films;	2.8	3.8	6.6
98.2			**74251**	via enteroclysis tube	(I) 4.2	(I) 6.8	(I) 11.0
98.2			**74260**	Duodenography, hypotonic	3.0	4.2	7.2
98.2			**74270**	Radiologic examination, colon; barium enema, with or without KUB	4.0	5.0	9.0
98.2			**74280**	air contrast with specific high density barium, with or without glucagon	5.5	6.5	12.0
98.2			**74283**	Therapeutic enema, contrast or air, for reduction of intussusception or other intraluminal obstruction (eg, meconium ileus)	(I) 6.8	(I) 4.0	(I) 10.8
98.2			**74290**	Cholecystography, oral contrast;	1.8	2.2	4.0
98.2			**74291**	additional or repeat examination or multiple day examination	1.2	1.3	2.5
			74300	Cholangiography and/or pancreatography; intraoperative, radiological supervision and interpretation	2.4	3.0	5.4
98.2	▲	+	**74301**	additional set intraoperative, radiological supervision and interpretation (List separately in addition to code for primary procedure)	1.1	1.4	2.5
			74305	postoperative, radiological supervision and interpretation	2.5	2.4	4.9
			74320	Cholangiography, percutaneous, transhepatic, radiological supervision and interpretation	3.2	9.3	12.5

UPD		Code	Description	Prof	Tech	Total
		74327	Postoperative biliary duct stone removal, percutaneous via T-tube tract, basket or snare (eg, Burhenne technique), radiological supervision and interpretation	15.0	6.0	21.0
		74328	Endoscopic catheterization of the biliary ductal system, radiological supervision and interpretation	4.0	9.3	13.3
		74329	Endoscopic catheterization of the pancreatic ductal system, radiological supervision and interpretation	4.0	9.3	13.3 .
		74330	Combined endoscopic catheterization of the biliary and pancreatic ductal systems, radiological supervision and interpretation	4.0	9.3	13.3
		74340	Introduction of long gastrointestinal tube (eg, Miller-Abbott), including multiple fluoroscopies and films, radiological supervision and interpretation	3.3	7.7	11.0
		74350	Percutaneous placement of gastrostomy tube, radiological supervision and interpretation	4.3	7.6	11.9
		74355	Percutaneous placement of enteroclysis tube, radiological supervision and interpretation	4.3	7.6	11.9
		74360	Intraluminal dilation of strictures and/or obstructions (eg, esophagus), radiological supervision and interpretation	3.1	9.2	12.3
		74363	Percutaneous transhepatic dilatation of biliary duct stricture with or without placement of stent, radiological supervision and interpretation	(I) 17.0	(I) 11.1	(I) 28.1
98.2		74400	Urography (pyelography), intravenous, with or without KUB, with or without tomography;	2.8	5.0	7.8
98.2	M	74405	with special hypertensive contrast concentration and/or clearance studies To report, see 74400, 74410, or 74415	2.8	6.0	8.8
98.2		74410	Urography, infusion, drip technique and/or bolus technique;	3.0	5.4	8.4
98.2		74415	with nephrotomography	3.0	6.0	9.0
98.2		74420	Urography, retrograde, with or without KUB	2.0	7.5	9.5
98.2		74425	Urography, antegrade, (pyelostogram, nephrostogram, loopogram), radiological supervision and interpretation	2.0	4.0	6.0
		74430	Cystography, minimum of three views, radiological supervision and interpretation	2.0	3.0	5.0
		74440	Vasography, vesiculography, or epididymography, radiological supervision and interpretation	2.0	3.5	5.5
		74445	Corpora cavernosography, radiological supervision and interpretation	6.5	3.5	10.0
		74450	Urethrocystography, retrograde, radiological supervision and interpretation	2.0	4.2	6.2

UPD	Code	Description	Prof	Tech	Total
	74455	Urethrocystography, voiding, radiological supervision and interpretation	2.2	4.6	6.8
	74470	Radiologic examination, renal cyst study, translumbar, contrast visualization, radiological supervision and interpretation	3.2	3.5	6.7
	74475	Introduction of intracatheter or catheter into renal pelvis for drainage and/or injection, percutaneous, radiological supervision and interpretation	4.5	15.0	19.5
	74480	Introduction of ureteral catheter or stent into ureter through renal pelvis for drainage and/or injection, percutaneous, radiological supervision and interpretation	8.5	15.0	23.5
	74485	Dilation of nephrostomy, ureters, or urethra, radiological supervision and interpretation	3.2	9.1	12.3
98.2	74710	Pelvimetry, with or without placental localization	2.0	3.2	5.2
	74740	Hysterosalpingography, radiological supervision and interpretation	2.0	4.0	6.0
	74742	Transcervical catheterization of fallopian tube, radiological supervision and interpretation	(I) 3.6	(I) 9.4	(I) 13.0
98.2	74775	Perineogram (eg, vaginogram, for sex determination or extent of anomalies)	3.5	4.3	7.8
98.2	75552	Cardiac magnetic resonance imaging for morphology; without contrast material	10.0	45.0	55.0
98.2	75553	with contrast material	12.0	50.0	62.0
98.2	75554	Cardiac magnetic resonance imaging for funciton, with or without morphology; complete study	10.0	45.0	55.0
98.2	75555	limited study	7.0	33.0	40.0
98.2	75556	Cardiac magnetic resonance imaging for velocity flow mapping	10.0	45.0	55.0
98.2	75600	Aortography, thoracic, without serialography, radiological supervision and interpretation	2.5	6.3	8.8
98.2	75605	Aortography, thoracic, by serialography, radiological supervision and interpretation	3.8	10.6	14.4
98.2	75625	Aortography, abdominal, by serialography, radiological supervision and interpretation	5.0	15.0	20.0
98.2	75630	Aortography, abdominal plus bilateral iliofemoral lower extremity, catheter, by serialography, radiological supervision and interpretation	12.0	13.0	25.0
98.2	75650	Angiography, cervicocerebral, catheter, including vessel origin, radiological supervision and interpretation	5.0	15.0	20.0
98.2	75658	Angiography, brachial, retrograde, radiological supervision and interpretation	5.0	15.0	20.0

UPD	Code	Description	Prof	Tech	Total
98.2	75660	Angiography, external carotid, unilateral, selective, radiological supervision and interpretation	5.0	15.0	20.0
98.2	75662	Angiography, external carotid, bilateral, selective, radiological supervision and interpretation	10.0	22.0	32.0
98.2	75665	Angiography, carotid, cerebral, unilateral, radiological supervision and interpretation	5.0	15.0	20.0
98.2	75671	Angiography, carotid, cerebral, bilateral, radiological supervision and interpretation	10.0	15.0	25.0
98.2	75676	Angiography, carotid, cervical, unilateral, radiological supervision and interpretation	5.0	15.0	20.0
98.2	75680	Angiography, carotid, cervical, bilateral, radiological supervision and interpretation	10.0	25.0	35.0
98.2	75685	Angiography, vertebral, cervical, and/or intracranial, radiological supervision and interpretation	5.0	15.0	20.0
98.2	75705	Angiography, spinal, selective, radiological supervision and interpretation	6.0	24.5	30.5
98.2	75710	Angiography, extremity, unilateral, radiological supervision and interpretation	3.0	9.0	12.0
98.2	75716	Angiography, extremity, bilateral, radiological supervision and interpretation	4.0	12.0	16.0
98.2	75722	Angiography, renal, unilateral, selective (including flush aortogram), radiological supervision and interpretation	5.0	15.0	20.0
98.2	75724	Angiography, renal, bilateral, selective (including flush aortogram), radiological supervision and interpretation	7.5	17.5	25.0
98.2	75726	Angiography, visceral, selective or supraselective, (with or without flush aortogram), radiological supervision and interpretation	7.5	14.5	22.0
98.2	75731	Angiography, adrenal, unilateral, selective, radiological supervision and interpretation	5.0	15.0	20.0
98.2	75733	Angiography, adrenal, bilateral, selective, radiological supervision and interpretation	7.5	19.5	27.0
98.2	75736	Angiography, pelvic, selective or supraselective, radiological supervision and interpretation	5.0	15.0	20.0
98.2	75741	Angiography, pulmonary, unilateral, selective, radiological supervision and interpretation	6.4	12.0	18.4
98.2	75743	Angiography, pulmonary, bilateral, selective, radiological supervision and interpretation	7.2	15.0	22.2
98.2	75746	Angiography, pulmonary, by nonselective catheter or venous injection, radiological supervision and interpretation	5.0	5.0	10.0
98.2	75756	Angiography, internal mammary, radiological supervision and interpretation	5.0	9.5	14.5

UPD			Code	Description	Prof	Tech	Total
98.2	▲	+	75774	Angiography, selective, each additional vessel studied after basic examination, radiological supervision and interpretation (List separately in addition to code for primary procedure)	2.3	9.0	11.3
98.2			75790	Angiography, arteriovenous shunt (eg, dialysis patient), radiological supervision and interpretation	10.3	15.4	25.7
			75801	Lymphangiography, extremity only, unilateral, radiological supervision and interpretation	5.0	11.8	16.8
			75803	Lymphangiography, extremity only, bilateral, radiological supervision and interpretation	5.0	15.0	20.0
			75805	Lymphangiography, pelvic/abdominal, unilateral, radiological supervision and interpretation	5.0	12.5	17.5
			75807	Lymphangiography, pelvic/abdominal, bilateral, radiological supervision and interpretation	5.4	14.6	20.0
98.2			75809	Shuntogram for investigation of previously placed indwelling nonvascular shunt (eg, LeVeen shunt, ventriculoperitoneal shunt), radiological supervision and interpretation	(I) 2.0	(I) 5.0	(I) 7.0
			75810	Splenoportography, radiological supervision and interpretation	3.2	8.8	12.0
			75820	Venography, extremity, unilateral, radiological supervision and interpretation	2.3	5.7	8.0
			75822	Venography, extremity, bilateral, radiological supervision and interpretation	3.4	8.6	12.0
			75825	Venography, caval, inferior, with serialography, radiological supervision and interpretation	4.0	11.0	15.0
			75827	Venography, caval, superior, with serialography, radiological supervision and interpretation	4.0	11.0	15.0
			75831	Venography, renal, unilateral, selective, radiological supervision and interpretation	4.0	11.0	15.0
			75833	Venography, renal, bilateral, selective, radiological supervision and interpretation	6.0	11.0	17.0
			75840	Venography, adrenal, unilateral, selective, radiological supervision and interpretation	4.0	11.0	15.0
			75842	Venography, adrenal, bilateral, selective, radiological supervision and interpretation	6.0	11.0	17.0
			75860	Venography, sinus or jugular, catheter, radiological supervision and interpretation	4.0	11.0	15.0
			75870	Venography, superior sagittal sinus, radiological supervision and interpretation	4.0	11.0	15.0
			75872	Venography, epidural, radiological supervision and interpretation	4.0	11.0	15.0
			75880	Venography, orbital, radiological supervision and interpretation	3.0	11.0	14.0

UPD	Code	Description	Prof	Tech	Total
	75885	Percutaneous transhepatic portography with hemodynamic evaluation, radiological supervision and interpretation	6.0	11.0	17.0
	75887	Percutaneous transhepatic portography without hemodynamic evaluation, radiological supervision and interpretation	6.0	11.0	17.0
	75889	Hepatic venography, wedged or free, with hemodynamic evaluation, radiological supervision and interpretation	4.0	11.0	15.0
	75891	Hepatic venography, wedged or free, without hemodynamic evaluation, radiological supervision and interpretation	4.0	11.0	15.0
	75893	Venous sampling through catheter, with or without angiography (eg, for parathyroid hormone, renin), radiological supervision and interpretation	14.0	11.0	25.0
	75894	Transcatheter therapy, embolization, any method, radiological supervision and interpretation	5.0	15.0	20.0
	75896	Transcatheter therapy, infusion, any method (eg, thrombolysis other than coronary), radiological supervision and interpretation	5.0	15.0	20.0
98.2	**75898**	Angiogram through existing catheter for follow-up study for transcatheter therapy, embolization or infusion	9.5	3.0	12.5
98.2	**75900**	Exchange of a previously placed arterial catheter during thrombolytic therapy with contrast monitoring, radiological supervision and interpretation	(I) 8.0	(I) 15.0	(I) 23.0
	75940	Percutaneous placement of IVC filter, radiological supervision and interpretation	2.5	7.5	10.0
96.2	**75945**	Intravascular ultrasound (non-coronary vessel), radiological supervision and interpretation; initial vessel	(I) 2.0	(I) 10.0	(I) 12.0
98.2 ▲ +	**75946**	each additional non-coronary vessel (List separately in addition to code for primary procedure)	(I) 2.0	(I) 5.0	(I) 7.0
	75960	Transcatheter introduction of intravascular stent(s), (non-coronary vessel), percutaneous and/or open, radiological supervision and interpretation, each vessel	(I) 7.2	(I) 15.0	(I) 22.2
	75961	Transcatheter retrieval, percutaneous, of intravascular foreign body (eg, fractured venous or arterial catheter), radiological supervision and interpretation	27.0	10.0	37.0
	75962	Transluminal balloon angioplasty, peripheral artery, radiological supervision and interpretation	(I) 10.0	(I) 15.0	(I) 25.0
98.2 ▲ +	**75964**	Transluminal balloon angioplasty, each additional peripheral artery, radiological supervision and interpretation (List separately in addition to code for primary procedure)	(I) 4.0	(I) 15.0	(I) 19.0

UPD			Code	Description	Prof	Tech	Total
			75966	Transluminal balloon angioplasty, renal or other visceral artery, radiological supervision and interpretation	(I) 10.0	(I) 15.0	(I) 25.0
98.2	▲	+	75968	Transluminal balloon angioplasty, each additional visceral artery, radiological supervision and interpretation (List separately in addition to code for primary procedure)	(I) 5.0	(I) 15.0	(I) 20.0
			75970	Transcatheter biopsy, radiological supervision and interpretation	4.0	13.0	17.0
			75978	Transluminal balloon angioplasty, venous (eg, subclavian stenosis), radiological supervision and interpretation	(I) 7.0	(I) 12.0	(I) 19.0
			75980	Percutaneous transhepatic biliary drainage with contrast monitoring, radiological supervision and interpretation	8.0	12.0	20.0
			75982	Percutaneous placement of drainage catheter for combined internal and external biliary drainage or of a drainage stent for internal biliary drainage in patients with an inoperable mechanical biliary obstruction, radiological supervision and interpretation	11.0	10.0	21.0
			75984	Change of percutaneous tube or drainage catheter with contrast monitoring (eg, gastrointestinal system, genitourinary system, abscess), radiological supervision and interpretation	4.0	5.8	9.8
97.2			75989	Radiological guidance for percutaneous drainage of abscess, or specimen collection (ie, fluoroscopy, ultrasound, or computed tomography), with placement of indwelling catheter, radiological supervision and interpretation	15.0	6.0	21.0
			75992	Transluminal atherectomy, peripheral artery, radiological supervision and interpretation	(I) 2.5	(I) 42.5	(I) 45.0
98.2	▲	+	75993	Transluminal atherectomy, each additional peripheral artery, radiological supervision and interpretation (List separately in addition to code for primary procedure)	(I) 1.5	(I) 23.0	(I) 24.5
			75994	Transluminal atherectomy, renal, radiological supervision and interpretation	(I) 5.5	(I) 43.0	(I) 48.5
			75995	Transluminal atherectomy, visceral, radiological supervision and interpretation	(I) 5.5	(I) 43.0	(I) 48.5
98.2	▲	+	75996	Transluminal atherectomy, each additional visceral artery, radiological supervision and interpretation (List separately in addition to code for primary procedure)	(I) 1.5	(I) 23.0	(I) 24.5
98.2			76000	Fluoroscopy (separate procedure), up to one hour physician time, other than 71023 or 71034 (eg, cardiac fluoroscopy)	1.0	4.0	5.0

UPD		Code	Description	Prof	Tech	Total
98.2		76001	Fluoroscopy, physician time more than one hour, assisting a non-radiologic physician (eg, nephrostolithotomy, ERCP, bronchoscopy, transbronchial biopsy)	3.8	7.6	11.4
98.2		76003	Fluoroscopic localization for needle biopsy or fine needle aspiration	3.1	3.8	6.9
98.2	●	76006	Radiologic examination, stress view(s), any joint, stress applied by a physician (includes comparison views)	(I) 1.2	(I) 0.8	(I) 2.0
98.2		76010	Radiologic examination from nose to rectum for foreign body, single film, child	1.0	1.5	2.5
98.2		76020	Bone age studies	1.0	2.2	3.2
98.2		76040	Bone length studies (orthoroentgenogram, scanogram)	1.5	2.3	3.8
98.2		76061	Radiologic examination, osseous survey; limited (eg, for metastases)	2.8	3.2	6.0
98.2		76062	complete (axial and appendicular skeleton)	3.5	4.5	8.0
98.2		76065	Radiologic examination, osseous survey, infant	1.5	2.4	3.9
98.2		76066	Joint survey, single view, one or more joints (specify)	1.7	3.2	4.9
98.2		76070	Computerized tomography bone mineral density study, one or more sites	1.4	9.5	10.9
98.2		76075	Dual energy x-ray absorptiometry (DEXA), bone density study, one or more sites; axial skeleton (eg, hips, pelvis, spine)	(I) 1.3	(I) 8.4	(I) 9.7
98.2		76076	Dual energy x-ray absorptiometry (DEXA), bone density study, one or more sites; appendicular skeleton (peripheral) (eg, radius, wrist, heel)	(I) 1.0	(I) 5.0	(I) 6.0
98.2		76078	Radiographic absorptiometry (photodensitometry), one or more sites	(I) 1.0	(I) 2.0	(I) 3.0
98.2		76080	Radiologic examination, abscess, fistula or sinus tract study, radiological supervision and interpretation	3.2	3.2	6.4
98.2		76086	Mammary ductogram or galactogram, single duct, radiological supervision and interpretation	2.0	7.8	9.8
98.2		76088	Mammary ductogram or galactogram, multiple ducts, radiological supervision and interpretation	2.5	10.8	13.3
98.2		76090	Mammography; unilateral	1.4	3.1	4.5
98.2		76091	bilateral	2.4	4.0	6.4
98.2		76092	Screening mammography, bilateral (two view film study of each breast)	(I) 1.4	(I) 3.1	(I) 4.5
98.2		76093	Magnetic resonance imaging, breast, without and/or with contrast material(s); unilateral	(I) 11.0	(I) 47.5	(I) 58.5

UPD		Code	Description	Prof	Tech	Total
98.2		**76094**	bilateral	(I) 17.5	(I) 67.5	(I) 84.0
		76095	Stereotactic localization for breast biopsy, each lesion, radiological supervision and interpretation	(I) 9.4	(I) 18.0	(I) 27.4
		76096	Preoperative placement of needle localization wire, breast, radiological supervision and interpretation	3.3	6.8	10.1
98.2		**76098**	Radiological examination, surgical specimen	0.8	1.2	2.0
98.2		**76100**	Radiologic examination, single plane body section (eg, tomography), other than with urography	3.4	3.6	7.0
98.2		**76101**	Radiologic examination, complex motion (ie, hypercycloidal) body section (eg, mastoid polytomography), other than with urography; unilateral	3.4	4.0	7.4
98.2		**76102**	bilateral	3.5	5.0	8.5
98.2		**76120**	Cineradiography, except where specifically included	2.2	3.0	5.2
98.2	▲ +	**76125**	Cineradiography to complement routine examination (List separately in addition to code for primary procedure)	1.5	2.5	4.0
98.2		**76140**	Consultation on x-ray examination made elsewhere, written report	2.5	0.0	2.5
98.2		**76150**	Xeroradiography	0.0	2.0	2.0
98.2		**76350**	Subtraction in conjunction with contrast studies	1.8	0.0	1.8
98.2		**76355**	Computerized tomography guidance for stereotactic localization	7.0	27.0	34.0
		76360	Computerized tomography guidance for needle biopsy, radiological supervision and interpretation	7.0	27.0	34.0
		76365	Computerized tomography guidance for cyst aspiration, radiological supervision and interpretation	7.0	27.0	34.0
98.2		**76370**	Computerized tomography guidance for placement of radiation therapy fields	4.8	9.6	14.4
98.2		**76375**	Coronal, sagittal, multiplanar, oblique, 3-dimensional and/or holographic reconstruction of computerized tomography, magnetic resonance imaging, or other tomographic modality	1.0	11.2	12.2
98.2		**76380**	Computerized tomography, limited or localized follow-up study	(I) 4.8	(I) 11.5	(I) 16.3
98.2		**76390**	Magnetic resonance spectroscopy	(I) 8.0	(I) 42.0	(I) 50.0
98.2		**76400**	Magnetic resonance (eg, proton) imaging, bone marrow blood supply	10.0	45.0	55.0
98.2		**76499**	Unlisted diagnostic radiologic procedure	BR	BR	BR

UPD	Code	Description	Prof	Tech	Total

Diagnostic Ultrasound

UPD	Code	Description	Prof	Tech	Total
98.2	76506	Echoencephalography, B-scan and/or real time with image documentation (gray scale) (for determination of ventricular size, delineation of cerebral contents and detection of fluid masses or other intracranial abnormalities), including -mode encephalography as secondary component where indicated	3.8	4.0	7.8
98.2	76511	Ophthalmic ultrasound, echography, diagnostic; -scan only, with amplitude quantification	3.5	3.8	7.3
98.2	76512	contact B-scan (with or without simultaneous -scan)	3.8	4.5	8.3
98.2	76513	immersion (water bath) B-scan	3.8	4.5	8.3
98.2	76516	Ophthalmic biometry by ultrasound echography, -scan;	3.2	3.6	6.8
98.2	76519	with intraocular lens power calculation	3.2	3.6	6.8
98.2	76529	Ophthalmic ultrasonic foreign body localization	3.5	4.0	7.5
98.2	76536	Echography, soft tissues of head and neck (eg, thyroid, parathyroid, parotid), B-scan and/or real time with image documentation	3.4	4.0	7.4
98.2	76604	Echography, chest, B-scan (includes mediastinum) and/or real time with image documentation	3.0	4.0	7.0
98.2	76645	Echography, breast(s) (unilateral or bilateral), B-scan and/or real time with image documentation	3.5	3.5	7.0
98.2	76700	Echography, abdominal, B-scan and/or real time with image documentation; complete	4.8	5.5	10.3
98.2	76705	limited (eg, single organ, quadrant, follow-up)	3.5	4.2	7.7
98.2	76770	Echography, retroperitoneal (eg, renal, aorta, nodes), B-scan and/or real time with image documentation; complete	4.4	5.6	10.0
98.2	76775	limited	3.5	4.2	7.7
98.2	76778	Echography of transplanted kidney, B-scan and/or real time with image documentation, with or without duplex Doppler studies	(I) 5.0	(I) 5.5	(I) 10.5
98.2	76800	Echography, spinal canal and contents	(I) 5.2	(I) 6.0	(I) 11.2
98.2	76805	Echography, pregnant uterus, B-scan and/or real time with image documentation; complete (complete fetal and maternal evaluation)	5.5	6.0	11.5
98.2	76810	complete (complete fetal and maternal evaluation), multiple gestation, after the first trimester	(I) 9.6	(I) 13.7	(I) 23.3

UPD	Code	Description	Prof	Tech	Total
98.2	**76815**	Echography, pregnant uterus, B-scan and/or real time with image documentation; limited (fetal size, heart beat, placental location, fetal position, or emergency in the delivery room)	3.5	4.3	7.8
98.2	**76816**	follow-up or repeat	3.3	3.2	6.5
98.2	**76818**	Fetal biophysical profile	4.3	4.7	9.0
98.2	**76825**	Echocardiography, fetal, cardiovascular system, real time with image documentation (2D) with or without M-mode recording;	4.3	5.7	10.0
98.2	**76826**	follow-up or repeat study	(I) 4.1	(I) 4.6	(I) 8.7
98.2	**76827**	Doppler echocardiography, fetal, cardiovascular system, pulsed wave and/or continuous wave with spectral display; complete	(I) 4.2	(I) 5.3	(I) 9.5
98.2	**76828**	follow-up or repeat study	(I) 3.5	(I) 4.0	(I) 7.5
98.2	**76830**	Echography, transvaginal	4.3	5.7	10.0
98.2	**76831**	Hysterosonography, with or without color flow Doppler	(I) 4.3	(I) 5.7	(I) 10.0
98.2	**76856**	Echography, pelvic (nonobstetric), B-scan and/or real time with image documentation; complete	4.0	5.0	9.0
98.2	**76857**	limited or follow-up (eg, for follicles)	2.1	3.0	5.1
98.2	**76870**	Echography, scrotum and contents	3.5	4.5	8.0
98.2	**76872**	Echography, transrectal	6.8	7.0	13.8
98.2	**76880**	Echography, extremity, non-vascular, B-scan and/or real time with image documentation	3.5	4.5	8.0
98.2	**76885**	Echography of infant hips, real time with imaging documentation; dynamic (eg, requiring manipulation)	(I) 4.5	(I) 5.8	(I) 10.3
98.2	**76886**	Echography of infant hips, real time with imaging documentation; limited, static (eg, not requiring manipulation)	(I) 4.0	(I) 5.0	(I) 9.0
98.2	**76930**	Ultrasonic guidance for pericardiocentesis, radiological supervision and interpretation	3.8	4.5	8.3
98.2	**76932**	Ultrasonic guidance for endomyocardial biopsy, radiological supervision and interpretation	(I) 4.2	(I) 4.5	(I) 8.7
98.2	**76934**	Ultrasonic guidance for thoracentesis or abdominal paracentesis, radiological supervision and interpretation	4.0	4.5	8.5
98.2	**76936**	Ultrasound guided compression repair of arterial pseudo-aneurysm or arteriovenous fistulae (includes diagnostic ultrasound evaluation, compression of lesion and imaging)	(I) 7.0	(I) 5.0	(I) 12.0
98.2	**76938**	Ultrasonic guidance for cyst (any location), or renal pelvis aspiration, radiological supervision and interpretation	4.0	4.5	8.5

UPD		Code	Description	Prof	Tech	Total
98.2		**76941**	Ultrasonic guidance for intrauterine fetal transfusion or cordocentesis, radiological supervision and interpretation	(I) 4.2	(I) 4.5	(I) 8.7
98.2		**76942**	Ultrasonic guidance for needle biopsy, radiological supervision and interpretation	4.0	4.5	8.5
98.2		**76945**	Ultrasonic guidance for chorionic villus sampling, radiological supervision and interpretation	(I) 3.7	(I) 4.5	(I) 8.2
98.2		**76946**	Ultrasonic guidance for amniocentesis, radiological supervision and interpretation	2.5	4.5	7.0
98.2		**76948**	Ultrasonic guidance for aspiration of ova, radiological supervision and interpretation	2.1	4.5	6.6
98.2		**76950**	Echography for placement of radiation therapy fields, B-scan	3.3	3.8	7.1
98.2		**76960**	Ultrasonic guidance for placement of radiation therapy fields, except for B-scan echography	3.3	3.8	7.1
98.2		**76965**	Ultrasonic guidance for interstitial radioelement application	(I) 7.8	(I) 8.5	(I) 16.3
98.2		**76970**	Ultrasound study follow-up (specify)	2.3	3.0	5.3
98.2		**76975**	Gastrointestinal endoscopic ultrasound, radiological supervision and interpretation	(I) 5.8	(I) 7.0	(I) 12.8
98.2	●	**76977**	Ultrasound bone density measurement and interpretation, peripheral site(s), any method	(I) 3.0	(I) 1.0	(I) 4.0
98.2		**76986**	Echography, intraoperative	6.8	8.1	14.9
98.2		**76999**	Unlisted ultrasound procedure	BR	BR	BR

Radiation Oncology

UPD	Code	Description	Prof	Tech	Total
	77261	Therapeutic radiology treatment planning; simple	10.2	0.0	10.2
	77262	intermediate	13.0	0.0	13.0
	77263	complex	18.0	0.0	18.0
	77280	Therapeutic radiology simulation-aided field setting; simple	3.9	9.0	12.9
	77285	intermediate	6.0	14.0	20.0
	77290	complex	8.8	16.5	25.3
97.2	**77295**	Therapeutic radiology simulation-aided field setting; three-dimensional	(I) 20.0	(I) 75.0	(I) 95.0
	77299	Unlisted procedure, therapeutic radiology clinical treatment planning	BR	BR	BR
	77300	Basic radiation dosimetry calculation, central axis depth dose, TDF, NSD, gap calculation, off axis factor, tissue inhomogeneity factors, as required during course of treatment, only when prescribed by the treating physician	3.5	3.5	7.0

UPD		Code	Description	Prof	Tech	Total
		77305	Teletherapy, isodose plan (whether hand or computer calculated); simple (one or two parallel opposed unmodified ports directed to a single area of interest)	4.0	4.8	8.8
		77310	intermediate (three or more treatment ports directed to a single area of interest)	6.0	6.0	12.0
		77315	complex (mantle or inverted Y, tangential ports, the use of wedges, compensators, complex blocking, rotational beam, or special beam considerations)	8.9	7.0	15.9
		77321	Special teletherapy port plan, particles, hemibody, total body	5.3	10.2	15.5
		77326	Brachytherapy isodose calculation; simple (calculation made from single plane, one to four sources/ribbon application, remote afterloading brachytherapy, 1 to 8 sources)	5.0	6.0	11.0
		77327	intermediate (multiplane dosage calculations, application involving five to ten sources/ribbons, remote afterloading brachytherapy, 9 to 12 sources)	8.0	8.0	16.0
		77328	complex (multiplane isodose plan, volume implant calculations, over 10 sources/ribbons used, special spatial reconstruction, remote afterloading brachytherapy, over 12 sources)	11.5	12.5	24.0
		77331	Special dosimetry (eg, TLD, microdosimetry) (specify), only when prescribed by the treating physician	4.9	1.3	6.2
		77332	Treatment devices, design and construction; simple (simple block, simple bolus)	3.1	3.4	·6.5
		77333	intermediate (multiple blocks, stents, bite blocks, special bolus)	4.7	4.8	9.5
		77334	complex (irregular blocks, special shields, compensators, wedges, molds or casts)	7.1	8.4	15.5
98.2	▲	77336	Continuing medical physics consultation, including assessment of treatment parameters, quality assurance of dose delivery, and review of patient treatment documentation in support of the radiation oncologist, reported per week of therapy	0.0	8.5	8.5
		77370	Special medical radiation physics consultation	0.0	9.5	9.5
98.2	●	77380	Proton beam delivery to a single treatment area, single port, custom block, with or without compensation, with treatment set-up and verification images	RNE	RNE	RNE
98.2	●	77381	Proton beam treatment to one or two treatment areas, two or more ports, two or more custom blocks, and two or more compensators, with treatment set-up and verification images	RNE	RNE	RNE

UPD		Code	Description	Prof	Tech	Total
98.2	▲	77399	Unlisted procedure, medical radiation physics, dosimetry and treatment devices, and special services	BR	BR	BR
98.2		77401	Radiation treatment delivery, superficial and/or ortho voltage	0.0	6.5	6.5
98.2		77402	Radiation treatment delivery, single treatment area, single port or parallel opposed ports, simple blocks or no blocks; up to 5 MeV	(I) 0.0	(I) 6.5	(I) 6.5
98.2		77403	6-10 MeV	(I) 0.0	(I) 7.0	(I) 7.0
98.2		77404	11-19 MeV	(I) 0.0	(I) 8.0	(I) 8.0
98.2		77406	20 MeV or greater	(I) 0.0	(I) 9.0	(I) 9.0
98.2		77407	Radiation treatment delivery, two separate treatment areas, three or more ports on a single treatment area, use of multiple blocks; up to 5 MeV	(I) 0.0	(I) 8.5	(I) 8.5
98.2		77408	6-10 MeV	(I) 0.0	(I) 9.0	(I) 9.0
98.2		77409	11-19 MeV	(I) 0.0	(I) 10.0	(I) 10.0
98.2		77411	20 MeV or greater	(I) 0.0	(I) 11.0	(I) 11.0
98.2		77412	Radiation treatment delivery, three or more separate treatment areas, custom blocking, tangential ports, wedges, rotational beam, compensators, special particle beam (eg, electron or neutrons); up to 5 MeV	(I) 0.0	(I) 10.5	(I) 10.5
98.2		77413	6-10 MeV	(I) 0.0	(I) 11.0	(I) 11.0
98.2		77414	11-19 MeV	(I) 0.0	(I) 12.0	(I) 12.0
98.2		77416	20 MeV or greater	(I) 0.0	(I) 13.0	(I) 13.0
98.2		77417	Therapeutic radiology port film(s)	(I) 0.0	(I) 1.0	(I) 1.0
		77419	Weekly radiation therapy management; conformal	(I) 22.0	0.0	(I) 22.0
		77420	simple	29.0	0.0	29.0
		77425	intermediate	34.0	0.0	34.0
		77430	complex	40.0	0.0	40.0
		77431	Radiation therapy management with complete course of therapy consisting of one or two fractions only	(I) 11.0	0.0	(I) 11.0
		77432	Stereotactic radiation treatment management of cerebral lesion(s) (complete course of treatment consisting of one session)	(I) 48.0	0.0	(I) 48.0
96.1		77470	Special treatment procedure (eg, total body irradiation, hemibody irradiation, per oral, vaginal cone irradiation)	(I) 4.2	(I) 25.0	(I) 29.2
		77499	Unlisted procedure, therapeutic radiology clinical treatment management	BR	BR	BR

UPD	Code	Description	Prof	Tech	Total
98.2	**77600**	Hyperthermia, externally generated; superficial (ie, heating to a depth of 4 cm or less)	8.8	8.8	17.6
98.2	**77605**	deep (ie, heating to depths greater than 4 cm)	11.7	11.7	23.4
98.2	**77610**	Hyperthermia generated by interstitial probe(s); 5 or fewer interstitial applicators	8.8	8.8	17.6
98.2	**77615**	more than 5 interstitial applicators	11.7	11.7	23.4
98.2	**77620**	Hyperthermia generated by intracavitary probe(s)	8.8	8.8	17.6
98.2	**77750**	Infusion or instillation of radioelement solution	25.7	4.0	29.7
98.2	**77761**	Intracavitary radioelement application; simple	21.0	6.0	27.0
98.2	**77762**	intermediate	30.0	9.0	39.0
98.2	**77763**	complex	45.0	11.0	56.0
98.2	**77776**	Interstitial radioelement application; simple	26.1	6.1	32.2
98.2	**77777**	intermediate	39.1	12.3	51.4
98.2	**77778**	complex	58.0	14.0	72.0
98.2	**77781**	Remote afterloading high intensity brachytherapy; 1-4 source positions or catheters	(I) 9.0	(I) 78.0	(I) 87.0
98.2	**77782**	5-8 source positions or catheters	(I) 13.5	(I) 78.0	(I) 91.5
98.2	**77783**	9-12 source positions or catheters	(I) 20.0	(I) 78.0	(I) 98.0
98.2	**77784**	over 12 source positions or catheters	(I) 30.0	(I) 78.0	(I) 108.0
98.2	**77789**	Surface application of radioelement	5.8	1.3	7.1
98.2	**77790**	Supervision, handling, loading of radioelement	5.8	1.3	7.1
	77799	Unlisted procedure, clinical brachytherapy	BR	BR	BR

Nuclear Medicine

UPD	Code	Description	Prof	Tech	Total
	78000	Thyroid uptake; single determination	1.0	3.0	4.0
	78001	multiple determinations	1.5	3.8	5.3
	78003	stimulation, suppression or discharge (not including initial uptake studies)	1.8	2.8	4.6
	78006	Thyroid imaging, with uptake; single determination	3.0	7.0	10.0
	78007	multiple determinations	3.0	7.8	10.8
	78010	Thyroid imaging; only	2.2	5.5	7.7
	78011	with vascular flow	2.6	7.0	9.6
	78015	Thyroid carcinoma metastases imaging; limited area (eg, neck and chest only)	3.8	7.5	11.3
	78016	with additional studies (eg, urinary recovery)	4.8	10.2	15.0

UPD			Code	Description	Prof	Tech	Total
98.2	**M**		**78017**	multiple areas To report, see 78018	4.9	10.9	15.8
			78018	whole body	5.8	15.7	21.5
98.2	●	+	**78020**	Thyroid carcinoma metastases uptake (List separately in addition to code for primary procedure)	(I) 1.8	(I) 1.2	(I) 3.0
			78070	Parathyroid imaging	(I) 4.0	(I) 4.3	(I) 8.3
			78075	Adrenal imaging, cortex and/or medulla	4.5	15.8	20.3
			78099	Unlisted endocrine procedure, diagnostic nuclear medicine	BR	BR	BR
			78102	Bone marrow imaging; limited area	3.3	5.9	9.2
			78103	multiple areas	4.3	9.2	13.5
			78104	whole body	4.8	11.5	16.3
			78110	Plasma volume, radiopharmaceutical volume-dilution technique (separate procedure); single sampling	1.0	2.9	3.9
			78111	multiple samplings	1.3	7.5	8.8
			78120	Red cell volume determination (separate procedure); single sampling	1.3	5.0	6.3
			78121	multiple samplings	1.7	8.8	10.5
			78122	Whole blood volume determination, including separate measurement of plasma volume and red cell volume (radiopharmaceutical volume-dilution technique)	2.5	13.3	15.8
			78130	Red cell survival study;	3.5	8.5	12.0
			78135	differential organ/tissue kinetics, (eg, splenic and/or hepatic sequestration)	3.8	14.2	18.0
			78140	Labeled red cell sequestration, differential organ/tissue, (eg, splenic and/or hepatic)	3.8	11.2	15.0
			78160	Plasma radioiron disappearance (turnover) rate	2.0	11.8	13.8
			78162	Radioiron oral absorption	2.5	9.2	11.7
			78170	Radioiron red cell utilization	2.5	13.5	16.0
			78172	Chelatable iron for estimation of total body iron	3.0	4.6	7.6
			78185	Spleen imaging only, with or without vascular flow	2.5	6.5	9.0
			78190	Kinetics, study of platelet survival, with or without differential organ/tissue localization	(I) 5.0	(I) 21.2	(I) 26.2
			78191	Platelet survival study	3.5	21.2	24.7
98.2			**78195**	Lymphatics and lymph glands imaging	4.0	11.8	15.8

UPD		Code	Description	Prof	Tech	Total
98.2		78199	Unlisted hematopoietic, reticuloendothelial and lymphatic procedure, diagnostic nuclear medicine	BR	BR	BR
98.2		78201	Liver imaging; static only	2.5	6.8	9.3
98.2		78202	with vascular flow	3.0	8.3	11.3
98.2		78205	Liver imaging (SPECT)	4.0	17.1	21.1
98.2	●	78206	with vascular flow	(I) 5.0	(I) 17.1	(I) 22.1
98.2		78215	Liver and spleen imaging; static only	2.9	8.5	11.4
98.2		78216	with vascular flow	3.4	10.1	13.5
98.2		78220	Liver function study with hepatobiliary agents, with serial images	3.0	10.9	13.9
98.2		78223	Hepatobiliary ductal system imaging, including gallbladder, with or without pharmacologic intervention, with or without quantitative measurement of gallbladder function	4.8	10.4	15.2
98.2		78230	Salivary gland imaging;	2.5	6.5	9.0
98.2		78231	with serial images	3.0	9.3	12.3
98.2		78232	Salivary gland function study	2.8	10.5	13.3
98.2		78258	Esophageal motility	4.2	8.3	12.5
98.2		78261	Gastric mucosa imaging	4.0	12.0	16.0
98.2		78262	Gastroesophageal reflux study	4.0	12.2	16.2
98.2		78264	Gastric emptying study	4.5	11.9	16.4
98.2		78270	Vitamin B-12 absorption study (eg, Schilling test); without intrinsic factor	1.3	4.7	6.0
98.2		78271	with intrinsic factor	1.4	4.8	6.2
98.2		78272	Vitamin B-12 absorption studies combined, with and without intrinsic factor	2.0	6.6	8.6
98.2		78278	Acute gastrointestinal blood loss imaging	5.5	14.3	19.8
98.2		78282	Gastrointestinal protein loss	3.0	4.5	7.5
98.2		78290	Bowel imaging (eg, ectopic gastric mucosa, Meckel's localization, volvulus)	4.0	8.8	12.8
98.2		78291	Peritoneal-venous shunt patency test (eg, for LeVeen, Denver shunt)	4.9	8.9	13.8
98.2		78299	Unlisted gastrointestinal procedure, diagnostic nuclear medicine	BR	BR	BR
98.2		78300	Bone and/or joint imaging; limited area	3.5	8.0	11.5
98.2		78305	multiple areas	4.5	11.0	15.5
98.2		78306	whole body	4.5	12.5	17.0

UPD	Code	Description	Prof	Tech	Total
98.2	78315	three phase study	5.0	13.8	18.8
98.2	78320	tomographic (SPECT)	5.8	17.1	22.9
98.2	78350	Bone density (bone mineral content) study, one or more sites; single photon asorptiometry	1.2	2.2	3.4
98.2	78351	Bone density (bone mineral content) study, one or more sites; dual photon absorptiometry, one or more sites	1.4	5.1	6.5
98.2	78399	Unlisted musculoskeletal procedure, diagnostic nuclear medicine	BR	BR	BR
98.2	78414	Determination of central c-v hemodynamics (non-imaging) (eg, ejection fraction with probe technique) with or without pharmacologic intervention or exercise, single or multiple determinations	5.0	20.0	25.0
98.2	78428	Cardiac shunt detection	4.5	6.5	11.0
98.2	78445	Non-cardiac vascular flow imaging (ie, angiography, venography)	3.0	5.5	8.5
98.2	78455	Venous thrombosis study (eg, radioactive fibrinogen)	4.4	11.1	15.5
98.2	78457	Venous thrombosis imaging (eg, venogram); unilateral	4.5	7.5	12.0
98.2	78458	bilateral	5.0	11.9	16.9
98.2	78459	Myocardial imaging, positron emission tomography (PET), metabolic evaluation	(I) 17.0	(I) 83.0	(I) 100.0
98.2	78460	Myocardial perfusion imaging; (planar) single study, at rest or stress (exercise and/or pharmacologic), with or without quantification	4.8	6.9	11.7
98.2	78461	multiple studies, (planar) at rest and/or stress (exercise and/or pharmacologic), and redistribution and/or rest injection, with or without quantification	6.9	13.7	20.6
98.2	78464	tomographic (SPECT), single study at rest or stress (exercise and/or pharmacologic), with or without quantification	6.1	20.5	26.6
98.2	78465	tomographic (SPECT), multiple studies, at rest and/or stress (exercise and/or pharmacologic) and redistribution and/or rest injection, with or without quantification	8.2	34.1	42.3
98.2	78466	Myocardial imaging, infarct avid, planar; qualitative or quantitative	3.9	7.6	11.5
98.2	78468	with ejection fraction by first pass technique	4.5	10.6	15.1
98.2	78469	tomographic SPECT with or without quantification	5.1	15.2	20.3

UPD		Code	Description	Prof	Tech	Total
98.2	▲	78472	Cardiac blood pool imaging, gated equilibrium; planar, single study at rest or stress (exercise and/or pharmacologic), wall motion study plus ejection fraction, with or without additional quantitative processing	5.5	15.9	21.4
98.2		78473	multiple studies, wall motion study plus ejection fraction, at rest and stress (exercise and/or pharmacologic), with or without additional quantification	(I) 7.2	(I) 27.0	(I) 34.2
98.2	▲ +	78478	Myocardial perfusion study with wall motion, qualitative or quantitative study (List separately in addition to code for primary procedure)	(I) 3.0	(I) 5.1	(I) 8.1
98.2	▲ +	78480	Myocardial perfusion study with ejection fraction (List separately in addition to code for primary procedure)	(I) 3.0	(I) 5.1	(I) 8.1
98.2		78481	Cardiac blood pool imaging, (planar), first pass technique; single study, at rest or with stress (exercise and/or pharmacologic), wall motion study plus ejection fraction, with or without quantification	5.5	15.1	20.6
98.2		78483	multiple studies, at rest and with stress (exercise and/or pharmacologic), wall motion study plus ejection fraction, with or without quantification	(I) 7.2	(I) 25.8	(I) 33.0
98.2		78491	Myocardial imaging, positron emission tomography (PET), perfusion; single study at rest or stress	(I) 20.0	(I) 97.0	(I) 117.0
98.2		78492	Myocardial imaging, positron emission tomography (PET), perfusion; multiple studies at rest and/or stress	(I) 24.0	(I) 117.0	(I) 141.0
98.2	●	78494	Cardiac blood pool imaging, gated equilibrium, SPECT, at rest, wall motion study plus ejection fraction, with or without quantitative processing	(I) 5.0	(I) 17.5	(I) 22.5
98.2	● +	78496	Cardiac blood pool imaging, gated equilibrium, single study, at rest, with right ventricular ejection fraction by first pass technique (List separately in addition to code for primary procedure)	(I) 2.5	(I) 6.0	(I) 8.5
98.2		78499	Unlisted cardiovascular procedure, diagnostic nuclear medicine	BR	BR	BR
98.2		78580	Pulmonary perfusion imaging, particulate	4.4	10.0	14.4
98.2		78584	Pulmonary perfusion imaging, particulate, with ventilation; single breath	5.5	9.5	15.0
98.2		78585	rebreathing and washout, with or without single breath	6.0	16.0	22.0
98.2		78586	Pulmonary ventilation imaging, aerosol; single projection	2.5	7.5	10.0
98.2		78587	multiple projections (eg, anterior, posterior, lateral views)	2.8	8.2	11.0

+ Add-on Code   ⊘ Modifier -51 Exempt   ▲ Revised code   ● New code   **M** RVSI code or deleted from CPT   **(I)** Interim Value
CPT codes and descriptions only copyright © 1998 American Medical Association

UPD		Code	Description	Prof	Tech	Total
98.2	●	78588	Pulmonary perfusion imaging, particulate, with ventilation imaging, aerosol, one or multiple projections	(I) 5.0	(I) 12.0	(I) 17.0
98.2		78591	Pulmonary ventilation imaging, gaseous, single breath, single projection	2.3	8.2	10.5
98.2		78593	Pulmonary ventilation imaging, gaseous, with rebreathing and washout with or without single breath; single projection	2.7	10.3	13.0
98.2		78594	multiple projections (eg, anterior, posterior, lateral views)	3.0	14.5	17.5
98.2		78596	Pulmonary quantitative differential function (ventilation/perfusion) study	(I) 7.5	(I) 11.5	(I) 19.0
98.2		78599	Unlisted respiratory procedure, diagnostic nuclear medicine	BR	BR	BR
98.2		78600	Brain imaging, limited procedure; static	2.5	8.5	11.0
98.2		78601	with vascular flow	3.0	9.8	12.8
98.2		78605	Brain imaging, complete study; static	3.0	9.8	12.8
98.2		78606	with vascular flow	3.5	11.5	15.0
98.2		78607	tomographic (SPECT)	6.9	19.0	25.9
98.2		78608	Brain imaging, positron emission tomography (PET); metabolic evaluation	(I) 17.0	(I) 83.0	(I) 100.0
98.2		78609	perfusion evaluation	(I) 20.0	(I) 97.0	(I) 117.0
98.2		78610	Brain imaging, vascular flow only	1.7	4.8	6.5
98.2		78615	Cerebral blood flow	2.4	11.1	13.5
98.2		78630	Cerebrospinal fluid flow, imaging (not including introduction of material); cisternography	4.0	14.8	18.8
98.2		78635	ventriculography	3.5	7.5	11.0
98.2		78645	shunt evaluation	3.5	9.8	13.3
98.2		78647	tomographic (SPECT)	(I) 5.7	(I) 18.0	(I) 23.7
98.2		78650	CSF leakage detection and localization	3.5	13.3	16.8
98.2		78660	Radiopharmaceutical dacryocystography	3.0	6.1	9.1
98.2		78699	Unlisted nervous system procedure, diagnostic nuclear medicine	BR	BR	BR
98.2		78700	Kidney imaging; static only	2.5	8.9	11.4
98.2		78701	with vascular flow	2.8	10.7	13.5
98.2		78704	with function study (ie, imaging renogram)	4.2	11.3	15.5
98.2		78707	Kidney imaging with vascular flow and function; single study without pharmacological intervention	5.3	13.2	18.5

UPD		Code	Description	Prof	Tech	Total
98.2		**78708**	Kidney imaging with vascular flow and function; single study, with pharmacological intervention (eg, angiotensin converting enzyme inhibitor and/or diuretic	(I) 7.0	(I) 13.2	(I) 20.2
98.2		**78709**	Kidney imaging with vascular flow and function; multiple studies, with and without pharmacological intervention (eg, angiotensin converting enzyme inhibitor and/or diuretic)	(I) 8.4	(I) 15.8	(I) 24.2
98.2		**78710**	Kidney imaging, tomographic (SPECT)	3.7	17.1	20.8
98.2		**78715**	Kidney vascular flow only	2.0	4.5	6.5
98.2	▲	**78725**	Kidney function study, non-imaging radioisotopic study	2.0	5.5	7.5
97.2	M	**78726**	Kidney function study including pharmacologic intervention To report, use 78799	4.9	8.6	13.5
97.2	M	**78727**	Kidney transplant evaluation To report, use 78700-78707	5.5	11.5	17.0
98.2		**78730**	Urinary bladder residual study	2.3	4.0	6.3
98.2		**78740**	Ureteral reflux study (radiopharmaceutical voiding cystogram)	3.5	6.5	10.0
98.2		**78760**	Testicular imaging;	4.0	7.5	11.5
98.2		**78761**	with vascular flow	4.2	9.2	13.4
98.2		**78799**	Unlisted genitourinary procedure, diagnostic nuclear medicine	BR	BR	BR
98.2		**78800**	Radiopharmaceutical localization of tumor; limited area	3.8	10.1	13.9
98.2		**78801**	multiple areas	4.5	12.5	17.0
98.2		**78802**	whole body	5.0	16.0	21.0
98.2		**78803**	tomographic (SPECT)	6.1	19.0	25.1
98.2		**78805**	Radiopharmaceutical localization of abscess; limited area	4.0	10.0	14.0
98.2		**78806**	whole body	4.7	16.2	20.9
98.2		**78807**	tomographic (SPECT)	(I) 6.9	(I) 19.0	(I) 25.9
98.2		**78810**	Tumor imaging, positron emission tomography (PET), metabolic evaluation	(I) 17.0	(I) 83.0	(I) 100.0
98.2		**78890**	Generation of automated data: interactive process involving nuclear physician and/or allied health professional personnel; simple manipulations and interpretation, not to exceed 30 minutes	0.3	3.7	4.0
98.2		**78891**	complex manipulations and interpretation, exceeding 30 minutes	0.8	7.2	8.0

UPD	Code	Description	Prof	Tech	Total
98.2	78990	Provision of diagnostic radiopharmaceutical(s)	0.0	4.0	4.0
98.2	78999	Unlisted miscellaneous procedure, diagnostic nuclear medicine	BR	BR	BR
	79000	Radiopharmaceutical therapy, hyperthyroidism; initial, including evaluation of patient	11.0	7.5	18.5
	79001	subsequent, each therapy	6.0	4.0	10.0
	79020	Radiopharmaceutical therapy, thyroid suppression (euthyroid cardiac disease), including evaluation of patient	10.5	7.5	18.0
	79030	Radiopharmaceutical ablation of gland for thyroid carcinoma	11.8	7.5	19.3
	79035	Radiopharmaceutical therapy for metastases of thyroid carcinoma	14.3	7.5	21.8
	79100	Radiopharmaceutical therapy, polycythemia vera, chronic leukemia, each treatment	7.5	7.5	15.0
98.2	79200	Intracavitary radioactive colloid therapy	11.5	7.5	19.0
98.2	79300	Interstitial radioactive colloid therapy	25.0	7.5	32.5
	79400	Radiopharmaceutical therapy, nonthyroid, nonhematologic	11.0	7.5	18.5
98.2	79420	Intravascular radiopharmaceutical therapy, particulate	11.5	7.5	19.0
98.2	79440	Intra-articular radiopharmaceutical therapy	11.5	7.5	19.0
	79900	Provision of therapeutic radiopharmaceutical(s)	BR	BR	BR
	79999	Unlisted radiopharmaceutical therapeutic procedure	BR	BR	BR

Pathology and Laboratory

Guidelines

I. **General:** Values in this section include recording of the specimen, performance of the test, and reporting of the result. They do not include specimen collection, transfer or individual patient administrative services.

    A. **Total:** The unit value listed in the Total column represents the global value of the procedure. The five digit code is used to represent this service, including the professional services and technical cost of providing that service. The following sections, professional and technical, provide additional definitions for each component.

    B. **Professional:** The unit value listed in the Professional column is used to designate professional services. Modifier -26 is added to the procedure code to indicate the use of this value. The professional component includes examination of the patient, when indicated, performance and/or supervision of the procedure, or lab test, interpretation and/or written report concerning the examination or lab test, and consultation with referring physicians.

    C. **Technical:** The unit value listed in the Technical column is used to designate the technical value of providing the service. Modifier -27 may be used to designate this component. (Note: Modifier -27 is not CPT compatible and may not be accepted by all payers. Check with the specific payer prior to use of this modifier.) The technical component includes personnel, materials, space, equipment, and other allocated facility overhead normally included in providing the service.

II. **Unlisted Service or Procedure:** A service or procedure that is not identified by a particular code should be listed under the appropriate "Unlisted Procedure." These procedures often have 99 as the final two digits. Values should be substantiated by report (See BY REPORT).

III. **Procedures Without Values:** Procedures that have a BR or RNE in the units column require a report (See BY REPORT) to substantiate value.

IV. **Unusual Service or Procedure:** When a procedure of unusual nature is performed, modifier -22 should be added and value substantiated by report (See BY REPORT).

V. **By Report:** The value of a procedure should be established for any "by report" circumstance by identifying a similar service and justifying the difference. Procedures that require a report should include the following:

    1. Accurate Definition;

    2. Clinical History;

    3. Related Procedure Values; and

    4. Reason for Value Adjustment.

VI. **Reference (Outside) Laboratory:** The laboratory tests and services listed in this section, when performed by other than the physician, shall use the applicable procedure number with the appropriate modifier (-90).

VII. **Collection and Handling:** Procedure codes for the collection and handling of samples for pathology tests are listed in MEDICINE at codes 99000 and 99001 and SURGERY at code 36415. See GUIDELINES for each appropriate section and use the appropriate conversion factor.

+ Add-on Code   Ø Modifier -51 Exempt   ▲ Revised code   ● New code   **M** RVSI code or deleted from CPT   **(I)** Interim Value
CPT codes and descriptions only copyright © 1998 American Medical Association   Copyright © 1999 St. Anthony Publishing

VIII. **Separate or Multiple Procedures:** Multiple procedures performed on the same date should be listed using modifier -51. Customarily each procedure is allowed 100% of the listed value.

IX. **Reduced Value:** If a physician elects to reduce the value of a procedure, modifier-52 should be added to the procedure code.

X. **Consultation:** Several consultation codes are listed for various types of pathology consults (See 80500-02, 88321 -52). Medicine codes may also be used if appropriate (see below).

XI. **Services or Procedures Listed in Other Sections:** Services or procedures provided by a pathologist may be listed in an alternate section of the book (i.e., consultations listed in MEDICINE). The Pathologist should use these procedure codes following the guidelines appropriate to that section.

Note: The conversion factor for each section generally differs.

XII. **Modifiers:** A comprehensive listing of modifiers is provided in the introduction. Value adjustments significant to Pathlogy and modifiers for those adjustments are listed above.

Pathology and Laboratory Section

UPD		Code	Description	Prof	Tech	Total
97.2	M	80002	Automated multichannel test: 1 or 2 clinical chemistry test(s) To report, see codes under Organ or disease Oriented Panels.	0.3	0.5	0.8
97.2	M	80003	3 clinical chemistry tests To report, see codes under Organ or disease Oriented Panels.	0.4	0.7	1.1
97.2	M	80004	4 clinical chemistry tests To report, see codes under Organ or disease Oriented Panels.	0.4	0.7	1.1
97.2	M	80005	5 clinical chemistry tests To report, see codes under Organ or disease Oriented Panels.	0.4	0.8	1.2
97.2	M	80006	6 clinical chemistry tests To report, see codes under Organ or disease Oriented Panels.	0.4	0.8	1.2
97.2	M	80007	7 clinical chemistry tests To report, see codes under Organ or disease Oriented Panels.	0.4	0.8	1.2
97.2	M	80008	8 clinical chemistry tests To report, see codes under Organ or disease Oriented Panels.	0.5	0.8	1.3
97.2	M	80009	9 clinical chemistry tests To report, see codes under Organ or disease Oriented Panels.	0.5	0.8	1.3
97.2	M	80010	10 clinical chemistry tests To report, see codes under Organ or disease Oriented Panels.	0.5	0.8	1.3
97.2	M	80011	11 clinical chemistry tests To report, see codes under Organ or disease Oriented Panels.	0.5	0.8	1.3
97.2	M	80012	12 clinical chemistry tests To report, see codes under Organ or disease Oriented Panels.	0.5	0.9	1.4
97.2	M	80016	13-16 clinical chemistry tests To report, see codes under Organ or disease Oriented Panels.	0.6	1.0	1.6
97.2	M	80018	17-18 clinical chemistry tests To report, see codes under Organ or disease Oriented Panels.	0.6	1.0	1.6
97.2	M	80019	19 clinical chemistry tests To report, see codes under Organ or disease Oriented Panels.	0.7	1.0	1.7

UPD		Code	Description	Prof	Tech	Total

Organ or Disease Oriented Panels

UPD		Code	Description	Prof	Tech	Total
98.2		**80049**	Basic metabolic panel This panel must include the following: carbon dioxide (82374), chloride (82435), creatinine (82565), glucose (82947), potassium (84132), sodium (84295), urea nitrogen (BUN) (84520)	0.4	1.8	2.2
97.2		**80050**	General health panel This panel must include the following: comprehensive metabolic panel (80054), hemogram, automated, and manual differential WBC count (CBC) (85022) OR hemogram and platelet count, automated, and automated complete differential WBC count (CBC) (85025), thyroid stimulating hormone (TSH) (84443)	2.2	3.2	5.4
98.2		**80051**	Electrolyte panel This panel must include the following: carbon dioxide (82374), chloride (82435), potassium (84132), sodium (84295)	0.6	0.9	1.5
98.2	▲	**80054**	Comprehensive metabolic panel This panel must include the following: Albumin (82040) Bilirubin, total (82247) Calcium (82310) Carbon dioxide (bicarbonate) (82374) Chloride (82435) Creatinine (82565) Glucose (82947) Phosphatase, alkaline (84075) Potassium (84132) Protein, total (84155) Sodium (84295) Transferase, aspartate amino (AST) (SGOT) (84450) Urea Nitrogen (BUN) (84520)	(I) 0.8	(I) 1.5	(I) 2.3
98.1		**80055**	Obstetric panel This panel must include the following: Hemogram, automated, and manual differential WBC count (CBC) (85022) OR Hemogram and platelet count, automated, and automated complete differential WBC count (CBC) (85025) Hepatitis B surface antigen (HBsAg) (87340) Antibody, rubella (86762) Syphilis test, qualitative (eg, VDRL, RPR, ART) (86592) Antibody screen, RBC, each serum technique (86850) Blood typing, ABO (86900) AND Blood typing, Rh (D) (86901)	2.0	4.0	6.0
98.2	▲	**80058**	Hepatic function panel This panel must include the following: Albumin (82040) Bilirubin, total (82247) Bilirubin, direct (82248) Phosphatase, alkaline (84075) Transferase, alanine amino (ALT) (SGPT) (84460) Transferase, aspartate amino (AST) (SGOT) (84450)	0.7	1.0	1.7
		80059	Hepatitis panel This panel must include the following: Hepatitis B surface antigen (HBsAg) (87340) Hepatitis B surface antibody (HBsAb) (86706) Hepatitis B core antibody (HBcAb), IgG and IgM (86704) Hepatitis A antibody (HAAb), IgG and IgM (86708) Hepatitis C antibody (86803)	4.0	5.8	9.8
		80061	Lipid panel This panel must include the following: Cholesterol, serum, total (82465) Lipoprotein, direct measurement, high density cholesterol (HDL cholesterol) (83718) Triglycerides (84478)	1.0	1.8	2.8

UPD	Code	Description	Prof	Tech	Total
	80072	Arthritis panel This panel must include the following: Uric acid, blood, chemical (84550) Sedimentation rate, erythrocyte, non-automated (85651) Fluorescent antibody, screen, each antibody (86255) Rheumatoid factor, qualitative (86430)	1.4	2.5	3.9
	80090	TORCH antibody panel This panel must include the following tests: Antibody, cytomegalovirus (CMV) (86644) Antibody, herpes simplex, non-specific type test (86694) Antibody, rubella (86762) Antibody, toxoplasma (86777)	3.6	5.0	8.6
	80091	Thyroid panel This panel must include the following tests: Thyroxine, total (84436) Thyroid hormone (T3 or T4) uptake or thyroid hormone binding ratio (THBR) (84479)	0.9	1.4	2.3
	80092	with thyroid stimulating hormone (TSH) (84443)	1.6	3.6	5.2

Drug Testing

UPD	Code	Description	Prof	Tech	Total
98.2	80100	Drug, screen; multiple drug classes, each procedure	1.0	2.5	3.5
98.2	80101	single drug class, each drug class	0.9	2.3	3.2
98.2	80102	Drug, confirmation, each procedure	0.8	2.0	2.8
98.2	80103	Tissue preparation for drug analysis	0.4	0.7	1.1

Therapeutic Drug Assays

UPD	Code	Description	Prof	Tech	Total
	80150	Amikacin	1.2	2.5	3.7
	80152	Amitriptyline	2.7	1.3	4.0
	80154	Benzodiazepines	3.1	1.4	4.5
	80156	Carbamazepine	2.2	1.0	3.2
98.2	80158	Cyclosporine	1.1	2.1	3.2
98.2	80160	Desipramine	1.1	2.1	3.2
	80162	Digoxin	2.1	0.9	3.0
98.2	80164	Dipropylacetic acid (valproic acid)	1.3	2.7	4.0
	80166	Doxepin	0.9	2.3	3.2
	80168	Ethosuximide	1.6	2.4	4.0
	80170	Gentamicin	1.4	2.7	4.1
	80172	Gold	1.2	2.9	4.1
	80174	Imipramine	1.1	2.7	3.8
	80176	Lidocaine	1.0	2.2	3.2
	80178	Lithium	0.6	1.0	1.6

UPD	Code	Description	Prof	Tech	Total
98.2	**80182**	Nortriptyline	1.3	2.7	4.0
98.2	**80184**	Phenobarbital	0.9	2.2	3.1
	80185	Phenytoin; total	0.9	2.4	3.3
98.2	**80186**	free	1.0	2.5	3.5
	80188	Primidone	1.0	2.2	3.2
	80190	Procainamide;	1.2	2.6	3.8
98.2	**80192**	with metabolites (eg, n-acetyl procainamide)	1.6	2.5	4.1
	80194	Quinidine	0.9	2.0	3.0
	80196	Salicylate	0.5	1.2	1.7
98.2	**80197**	Tacrolimus	1.0	2.1	3.1
	80198	Theophylline	0.6	1.9	2.5
	80200	Tobramycin	1.3	2.6	3.9
98.2	**80201**	Topiramate	(I) 1.0	(I) 2.0	(I) 3.0
98.2	**80202**	Vancomycin	1.3	2.6	3.9
	80299	Quantitation of drug, not elsewhere specified	BR	BR	BR

Evocative/Suppression Testing

UPD	Code	Description	Prof	Tech	Total
98.2	**80400**	ACTH stimulation panel; for adrenal insufficiency This panel must include the following: Cortisol (82533 x 2)	1.7	3.3	5.0
98.2	**80402**	for 21 hydroxylase deficiency This panel must include the following: Cortisol (82533 x 2) 17 hydroxyprogesterone (83498 x 2)	3.9	8.6	12.5
98.2	**80406**	for 3 beta-hydroxydehydrogenase deficiency This panel must include the following: Cortisol (82533 x 2) 17 hydroxypregnenolone (84143 x 2)	3.9	8.6	12.5
98.2	**80408**	Aldosterone suppression evaluation panel (eg, saline infusion) This panel must include the following: Aldosterone (82088 x 2) Renin (84244 x 2)	7.0	12.3	19.3
98.2	**80410**	Calcitonin stimulation panel (eg, calcium, pentagastrin) This panel must include the following: Calcitonin (82308 x 3)	5.0	10.0	15.0
98.2	**80412**	Corticotropic releasing hormone (CRH) stimulation panel This panel must include the following: Cortisol (82533 x 6) Adrenocorticotropic hormone (ACTH) (82024 x 6)	16.0	32.0	48.0
98.2	**80414**	Chorionic gonadotropin stimulation panel; testosterone response This panel must include the following: Testosterone (84403 x 2 on three pooled blood samples)	2.5	5.5	8.0

UPD	Code	Description	Prof	Tech	Total
98.2	**80415**	estradiol response This panel must include the following: Estradiol (82670 x 2 on three pooled blood samples)	2.6	5.8	8.4
98.2	**80416**	Renal vein renin stimulation panel (eg, captopril) This panel must include the following: Renin (84244 x 6)	8.0	15.0	23.0
98.2	**80417**	Peripheral vein renin stimulation panel (eg, captopril) This panel must include the following: Renin (84244 x 2)	8.0	15.0	23.0
98.2	**80418**	Combined rapid anterior pituitary evaluation panel This panel must include the following: Adrenocorticotropic hormone (ACTH) (82024 x 4) Luteinizing hormone (LH) (83002 x 4) Follicle stimulating hormone (FSH) (83001 x 4) Prolactin (84146 x 4) Human growth hormone (HGH) (83003 x 4) Cortisol (82533 x 4) Thyroid stimulating hormone (TSH) (84443 x 4)	24.0	60.0	84.0
98.2	**80420**	Dexamethasone suppression panel, 48 hour This panel must include the following: Free cortisol, urine (82530 x 2) Cortisol (82533 x 2) Volume measurement for timed collection (81050 x 2) (For single dose dexamethasone, use 82533)	3.0	6.7	9.7
98.2	**80422**	Glucagon tolerance panel; for insulinoma This panel must include the following: Glucose (82947 x 3) Insulin (83525 x 3)	1.7	4.0	5.7
98.2	**80424**	for pheochromocytoma This panel must include the following: Catecholamines, fractionated (82384 x 2)	2.5	6.0	8.5
98.2	**80426**	Gonadotropin releasing hormone stimulation panel This panel must include the following: Follicle stimulating hormone (FSH) (83001 x 4) Luteinizing hormone (LH) (83002 x 4)	5.0	16.0	21.0
98.2	**80428**	Growth hormone stimulation panel (eg, arginine infusion, l-dopa administration) This panel must include the following: Human growth hormone (HGH) (83003 x 4)	1.8	6.6	8.4
98.2	**80430**	Growth hormone suppression panel (glucose administration) This panel must include the following: Glucose (82947 x 3) Human growth hormone (HGH) (83003 x 4)	2.3	6.7	9.0
98.2	**80432**	Insulin-induced C-peptide suppression panel This panel must include the following: Insulin (83525) C-peptide (84681 x 5) Glucose (82947 x 5)	5.2	16.8	22.0
98.2	**80434**	Insulin tolerance panel; for ACTH insufficiency This panel must include the following: Cortisol (82533 x 5) Glucose (82947 x 5)	4.5	10.0	14.5
98.2	**80435**	for growth hormone deficiency This panel must include the following: Glucose (82947 x 5) Human growth hormone (HGH) (83003 x 5)	4.5	10.5	15.0

UPD	Code	Description	Prof	Tech	Total
98.2	**80436**	Metyrapone panel This panel must include the following: Cortisol (82533 x 2) 11 deoxycortisol (82634 x 2)	3.2	7.7	10.9
98.2	**80438**	Thyrotropin releasing hormone (TRH) stimulation panel; one hour This panel must include the following: Thyroid stimulating hormone (TSH) (84443 x 3)	2.3	5.2	7.5
98.2	**80439**	two hour This panel must include the following: Thyroid stimulating hormone (TSH) (84443 x 4)	3.0	13.0	16.0
98.2	**80440**	for hyperprolactinemia This panel must include the following: Prolactin (84146 x 3)	3.3	13.7	17.0

Consultations (Clinical Pathology)

UPD	Code	Description	Prof	Tech	Total
	80500	Clinical pathology consultation; limited, without review of patient's history and medical records	3.1	0.0	3.1
	80502	comprehensive, for a complex diagnostic problem, with review of patient's history and medical records	6.5	0.0	6.5

Urinalysis

UPD	Code	Description	Prof	Tech	Total
	81000	Urinalysis, by dip stick or tablet reagent for bilirubin, glucose, hemoglobin, ketones, leukocytes, nitrite, pH, protein, specific gravity, urobilinogen, any number of these constituents; non-automated, with microscopy	0.3	0.4	0.7
	81001	automated, with microscopy	0.3	0.4	0.7
	81002	non-automated, without microscopy	0.2	0.2	0.4
	81003	automated, without microscopy	0.1	0.2	0.3
	81005	Urinalysis; qualitative or semiquantitative, except immunoassays	0.1	0.2	0.3
	81007	bacteriuria screen, by non-culture technique, commercial kit (specify type)	0.1	0.2	0.3
	81015	microscopic only	0.2	0.3	0.5
	81020	two or three glass test	0.3	0.5	0.8
	81025	Urine pregnancy test, by visual color comparison methods	0.2	0.2	0.4
98.2	**81050**	Volume measurement for timed collection, each	1.0	2.0	3.0
	81099	Unlisted urinalysis procedure	BR	BR	BR

Chemistry

UPD	Code	Description	Prof	Tech	Total
	82000	Acetaldehyde, blood	0.7	1.6	2.3
	82003	Acetaminophen	0.9	2.4	3.3

UPD		Code	Description	Prof	Tech	Total
		82009	Acetone or other ketone bodies, serum; qualitative	0.3	0.6	0.9
		82010	quantitative	0.7	1.4	2.1
		82013	Acetylcholinesterase	0.7	1.6	2.3
98.2	●	82016	Acylcarnitines; qualitative, each specimen	RNE	RNE	RNE
98.2	●	82017	quantitative, each specimen (for carnitine, see 82379)	RNE	RNE	RNE
		82024	Adrenocorticotropic hormone (ACTH)	2.1	4.9	7.0
		82030	Adenosine, 5'-monophosphate, cyclic (cyclic AMP)	1.6	2.4	4.0
		82040	Albumin; serum	0.3	0.7	1.0
		82042	urine, quantitative	0.3	0.8	1.1
98.2		82043	urine, microalbumin, quantitative	0.4	0.9	1.3
98.2		82044	urine, microalbumin, semiquantitative (eg, reagent strip assay)	0.2	0.5	0.7
		82055	Alcohol (ethanol); any specimen except breath	0.9	2.1	3.0
		82075	breath	0.9	2.0	2.9
		82085	Aldolase	0.7	1.6	2.3
		82088	Aldosterone	2.6	5.7	8.3
		82101	Alkaloids, urine, quantitative	1.7	3.8	5.5
98.2		82103	Alpha-1-antitrypsin; total	0.7	1.3	2.0
98.2		82104	phenotype	0.7	1.4	2.1
98.2		82105	Alpha-fetoprotein; serum	0.8	1.7	2.5
98.2		82106	amniotic fluid	0.8	1.7	2.5
		82108	Aluminum	1.3	2.9	4.2
98.2	●	82127	Amino acids; single, qualitative, each specimen	(I) 1.0	(I) 2.0	(I) 3.0
98.2	▲	82128	multiple, qualitative, each specimen	(I) 1.0	(I) 2.0	(I) 3.0
98.2	M	82130	Amino acids, urine or plasma, chromatographic fractionation To report, use 82131, 82136, 82139	(I) 3.6	(I) 8.3	(I) 11.9
98.2	▲	82131	single, quantitative, each specimen	(I) 1.2	(I) 4.1	(I) 5.3
		82135	Aminolevulinic acid, delta (ALA)			
98.2	●	82136	Amino acids, 2 to 5 amino acids, quantitative, each specimen	(I) 1.3	(I) 2.2	(I) 3.5
98.2	●	82139	Amino acids, 6 or more amino acids, quantitative, each specimen	(I) 1.3	(I) 2.2	(I) 3.5
		82140	Ammonia	1.1	2.6	3.7

UPD		Code	Description	Prof	Tech	Total
		82143	Amniotic fluid scan (spectrophotometric)	0.8	1.8	2.6
		82145	Amphetamine or methamphetamine	0.9	2.3	3.2
		82150	Amylase	0.5	1.0	1.5
98.2		82154	Androstanediol glucuronide	(I) 2.0	(I) 3.5	(I) 5.5
		82157	Androstenedione	3.7	1.6	5.3
		82160	Androsterone	2.0	4.0	6.0
		82163	Angiotensin II	1.1	2.8	3.9
		82164	Angiotensin I - converting enzyme (ACE)	0.9	2.0	2.9
		82172	Apolipoprotein, each	1.0	2.2	3.2
		82175	Arsenic	1.4	3.0	4.4
		82180	Ascorbic acid (Vitamin C), blood	0.8	1.6	2.4
98.2		82190	Atomic absorption spectroscopy, each analyte	0.8	1.5	2.3
		82205	Barbiturates, not elsewhere specified	0.9	2.2	3.1
		82232	Beta-2 microglobulin	1.3	2.7	4.0
98.2		82239	Bile acids; total	0.8	1.4	2.2
		82240	cholylglycine	1.4	3.1	4.5
98.2	●	82247	Bilirubin; total	(I) 0.3	(I) 0.7	(I) 1.0
98.2	●	82248	direct	(I) 0.3	(I) 0.7	(I) 1.0
98.2	M	82250	Bilirubin; total OR direct To report, see 82247, 82248 as appropriate	0.4	0.8	1.2
		82251	total AND direct	0.4	0.9	1.3
		82252	feces, qualitative	0.3	0.7	1.0
98.2	●	82261	Biotinidase, each specimen	(I) 1.2	(I) 2.3	(I) 3.5
97.2		82270	Blood, occult; feces 1-3 simultaneous determinations	0.2	0.3	0.5
		82273	other sources, qualitative	0.2	0.6	0.8
		82286	Bradykinin	0.3	0.8	1.1
		82300	Cadmium	1.4	3.0	4.4
		82306	Calcifediol (25-OH Vitamin D-3)	2.4	4.8	7.2
		82307	Calciferol (Vitamin D)	1.8	3.5	5.3
		82308	Calcitonin	1.7	4.0	5.7
		82310	Calcium; total	0.3	0.7	1.0

UPD		Code	Description	Prof	Tech	Total
		82330	ionized	1.0	2.4	3.4
		82331	after calcium infusion test	0.4	0.9	1.3
		82340	urine quantitative, timed specimen	0.4	0.8	1.2
		82355	Calculus (stone); qualitative analysis	0.9	1.9	2.8
		82360	quantitative analysis, chemical	0.9	1.9	2.8
		82365	infrared spectroscopy	0.8	2.0	2.8
		82370	x-ray diffraction	0.7	1.4	2.1
		82374	Carbon dioxide (bicarbonate)	0.3	0.6	0.9
		82375	Carbon monoxide, (carboxyhemoglobin); quantitative	0.9	2.2	3.1
		82376	qualitative	0.3	0.7	1.0
98.2		82378	Carcinoembryonic antigen (CEA)	0.8	2.0	2.8
98.2	●	82379	Carnitine (total and free), quantitative, each specimen	(I) 1.2	(I) 2.3	(I) 3.5
		82380	Carotene	0.6	1.4	2.0
		82382	Catecholamines; total urine	1.1	2.4	3.5
		82383	blood	1.7	4.0	5.7
		82384	fractionated	1.7	4.0	5.7
98.2		82387	Cathepsin-D	0.9	2.2	3.1
		82390	Ceruloplasmin	0.7	1.6	2.3
98.2		82397	Chemiluminescent assay	0.7	1.4	2.1
		82415	Chloramphenicol	0.8	1.8	2.6
		82435	Chloride; blood	0.2	0.6	0.8
		82436	urine	0.4	0.9	1.3
98.2		82438	other source	0.4	0.8	1.2
		82441	Chlorinated hydrocarbons, screen	0.5	1.0	1.5
		82465	Cholesterol, serum, total	0.2	0.6	0.8
		82480	Cholinesterase; serum	0.6	1.6	2.2
		82482	RBC	0.8	1.8	2.6
		82485	Chondroitin B sulfate, quantitative	0.8	2.6	3.4
98.2	▲	82486	Chromatography, qualitative; column (eg, gas liquid or HPLC), analyte not elsewhere specified	1.3	2.6	3.9
		82487	paper, 1-dimensional, analyte not elsewhere specified	1.3	2.7	4.0

UPD		Code	Description	Prof	Tech	Total
		82488	paper, 2-dimensional, analyte not elsewhere specified	1.8	3.5	5.3
		82489	thin layer, analyte not elsewhere specified	1.4	2.9	4.3
98.2	▲	82491	Chromatography, quantitative, column (eg, gas liquid or HPLC); single analyte not elsewhere specified, single stationary and mobile phase	(I) 1.6	(I) 3.8	(I) 5.4
98.2	●	82492	multiple analytes, single stationary and mobile phase	(I) 1.2	(I) 2.6	(I) 3.8
		82495	Chromium	1.5	2.9	4.4
		82507	Citrate	1.5	3.6	5.1
		82520	Cocaine or metabolite	0.8	1.7	2.5
98.2		82523	Collagen cross links, any method	(I) 1.6	(I) 2.4	(I) 4.0
		82525	Copper	0.9	2.2	3.1
		82528	Corticosterone	1.2	2.5	3.7
98.2		82530	Cortisol; free	1.1	2.4	3.5
		82533	total	0.9	2.3	3.2
		82540	Creatine	0.3	0.6	0.9
98.2	●	82541	Column chromatography/mass spectometry (eg, GC/MS, or HPLC/MS), analyte not elsewhere specified; qualitative, single stationary and mobile phase	(I) 1.2	(I) 2.6	(I) 3.8
98.2	●	82542	quantitative, single stationary and mobile phase	(I) 1.2	(I) 2.6	(I) 3.8
98.2	●	82543	stable isotope dilution, single analyte, quantitative, single stationary and mobile phase	(I) 1.2	(I) 2.6	(I) 3.8
98.2	●	82544	stable isotope dilution, multiple analytes, quantitative, single stationary and mobile phase	(I) 1.2	(I) 2.6	(I) 3.8
		82550	Creatine kinase (CK), (CPK); total	0.4	1.1	1.5
		82552	isoenzymes	0.9	2.1	3.0
98.2		82553	MB fraction only	0.6	1.2	1.8
98.2		82554	isoforms	0.6	1.2	1.8
		82565	Creatinine; blood	0.2	1.0	1.2
98.2		82570	other source	0.3	0.9	1.2
		82575	clearance	0.8	1.6	2.4
		82585	Cryofibrinogen	0.3	1.1	1.4
		82595	Cryoglobulin	0.5	1.1	1.6
		82600	Cyanide	1.1	2.6	3.7

UPD		Code	Description	Prof	Tech	Total
		82607	Cyanocobalamin (Vitamin B-12);	1.1	2.7	3.8
		82608	unsaturated binding capacity	1.2	2.5	3.7
		82615	Cystine and homocystine, urine, qualitative	0.5	1.1	1.6
		82626	Dehydroepiandrosterone (DHEA)	1.8	3.7	5.5
98.2		82627	Dehydroepiandrosterone-sulfate (DHEA-S)	1.1	2.3	3.4
		82633	Desoxycorticosterone, 11-	2.2	5.2	7.4
		82634	Deoxycortisol, 11-	2.2	5.2	7.4
		82638	Dibucaine number	0.7	1.5	2.2
		82646	Dihydrocodeinone	1.0	2.4	3.4
		82649	Dihydromorphinone	1.6	2.4	4.0
		82651	Dihydrotestosterone (DHT)	1.6	2.4	4.0
		82652	Dihydroxyvitamin D, 1,25-	2.4	5.7	8.1
		82654	Dimethadione	1.0	2.4	3.4
98.2	●	82657	Enzyme activity in blood cells, cultured cells, or tissue, not elsewhere specified; nonradioactive substrate, each specimen	(I) 1.2	(I) 2.6	(I) 3.8
98.2	●	82658	radioactive substrate, each specimen	(I) 1.2	(I) 2.6	(I) 3.8
		82664	Electrophoretic technique, not elsewhere specified	1.2	2.5	3.7
		82666	Epiandrosterone	1.6	3.8	5.4
		82668	Erythropoietin	1.3	2.9	4.2
		82670	Estradiol	1.7	3.9	5.6
		82671	Estrogens; fractionated	1.6	4.0	5.6
		82672	total	1.5	3.8	5.3
		82677	Estriol	1.6	3.2	4.8
		82679	Estrone	1.9	4.4	6.3
		82690	Ethchlorvynol	2.0	2.9	4.9
98.2		82693	Ethylene glycol	0.7	1.5	2.2
		82696	Etiocholanolone	1.8	3.5	5.3
		82705	Fat or lipids, feces; qualitative	0.5	0.8	1.3
		82710	quantitative	1.2	2.7	3.9
		82715	Fat differential, feces, quantitative	1.0	2.0	3.0
		82725	Fatty acids, nonesterified	0.8	1.8	2.6

UPD		Code	Description	Prof	Tech	Total
98.2	●	82726	Very long chain fatty acids	(I) 1.2	(I) 2.6	(I) 3.8
		82728	Ferritin	0.7	1.6	2.3
98.2	●	82731	Fetal fibronectin, cervicovaginal secretions, semi-quantitative	(I) 1.0	(I) 2.0	(I) 3.0
		82735	Fluoride	1.1	2.2	3.3
		82742	Flurazepam	1.2	2.7	3.9
		82746	Folic acid; serum	1.2	2.4	3.6
98.2		82747	RBC	0.9	1.8	2.7
		82757	Fructose, semen	1.0	2.3	3.3
		82759	Galactokinase, RBC	1.1	2.4	3.5
		82760	Galactose	0.8	1.7	2.5
		82775	Galactose-1-phosphate uridyl transferase; quantitative	1.3	3.0	4.3
		82776	screen	0.3	1.0	1.3
		82784	Gammaglobulin; IgA, IgD, IgG, IgM, each	0.4	1.0	1.4
		82785	IgE	1.0	2.0	3.0
98.2		82787	immunoglobulin subclasses, (IgG1, 2, 3, and 4)	1.6	3.4	5.0
		82800	Gases, blood, pH only	0.6	1.5	2.1
		82803	Gases, blood, any combination of pH, pCO2, pO2, CO2, HCO3 (including calculated O2 saturation);	1.5	3.4	4.9
98.2		82805	with O2 saturation, by direct measurement, except pulse oximetry	(I) 1.9	(I) 2.6	(I) 5.5
98.2		82810	Gases, blood, O2 saturation only, by direct measurement, except pulse oximetry	0.8	1.8	2.6
98.2		82820	Hemoglobin-oxygen affinity (pO2 for 50% hemoglobin saturation with oxygen)	0.5	1.0	1.5
		82926	Gastric acid, free and total, each specimen	0.5	1.4	1.9
		82928	Gastric acid, free or total; each specimen	0.4	0.7	1.1
		82938	Gastrin after secretin stimulation	1.5	2.9	4.4
		82941	Gastrin	1.4	2.9	4.3
		82943	Glucagon	1.1	2.4	3.5
		82946	Glucagon tolerance test	0.7	2.0	2.7
		82947	Glucose; quantitative	0.3	0.7	1.0
		82948	blood, reagent strip	0.2	0.3	0.5
		82950	post glucose dose (includes glucose)	0.4	0.7	1.1

UPD		Code	Description	Prof	Tech	Total
		82951	tolerance test (GTT), three specimens (includes glucose)	0.7	1.4	2.1
		82952	tolerance test, each additional beyond three specimens	0.3	0.7	.0
		82953	tolbutamide tolerance test	1.3	2.5	3.8
		82955	Glucose-6-phosphate dehydrogenase (G6PD); quantitative	0.7	1.7	2.4
		82960	screen	0.4	0.9	1.3
98.2		**82962**	Glucose, blood by glucose monitoring device(s) cleared by the FDA specifically for home use	0.1	0.4	0.5
		82963	Glucosidase, beta	1.6	3.4	5.0
		82965	Glutamate dehydrogenase	0.6	1.2	1.8
		82975	Glutamine (glutamic acid amide)	0.8	1.8	2.6
		82977	Glutamyltransferase, gamma (GGT)	0.4	1.1	1.5
		82978	Glutathione	0.7	1.7	2.4
		82979	Glutathione reductase, RBC	0.5	1.2	1.7
		82980	Glutethimide	0.9	3.0	3.9
		82985	Glycated protein	1.1	2.7	3.8
		83001	Gonadotropin; follicle stimulating hormone (FSH)	1.1	2.6	3.7
		83002	luteinizing hormone (LH)	1.2	2.7	3.9
		83003	Growth hormone, human (HGH) (somatotropin)	0.9	2.4	3.3
		83008	Guanosine monophosphate (GMP), cyclic	0.9	2.2	3.1
		83010	Haptoglobin; quantitative	0.8	1.7	2.5
		83012	phenotypes	1.3	2.0	3.3
98.2	●	**83013**	Helicobacter pylori, breath test analysis;	(I) 3.5	(I) 8.5	(I) 12.0
98.2	●	**83014**	drug administration and sample collection	(I) 0.6	(I) 1.2	(I) 1.8
		83015	Heavy metal (arsenic, barium, beryllium, bismuth, antimony, mercury); screen	1.4	3.3	4.7
		83018	quantitative, each	1.5	3.7	5.2
98.2	M	**83019**	Helicobacter pylori, breath test (including drug and breath sample collection kit) To report, see 83013, 83014	RNE	RNE	RNE
98.2	▲	**83020**	Hemoglobin fractionation and quantitation; electrophoresis (eg, A2, S, C, and/or F)	0.6	1.7	2.3
98.2	●	**83021**	chromatography (eg, A2, S, C, and/or F)	(I) 1.2	(I) 2.4	(I) 3.6

UPD		Code	Description	Prof	Tech	Total
98.2		83026	Hemoglobin; by copper sulfate method, non-automated	0.5	0.3	0.8
		83030	F(fetal), chemical	0.6	1.1	1.7
		83033	F(fetal), qualitative (APT) test, fecal	0.4	1.0	1.4
		83036	glycated	0.5	0.9	1.4
		83045	methemoglobin, qualitative	0.4	0.8	1.2
		83050	methemoglobin, quantitative	0.6	1.2	1.8
		83051	plasma	0.6	1.2	1.8
		83055	sulfhemoglobin, qualitative	0.4	0.8	1.2
		83060	sulfhemoglobin, quantitative	0.6	1.5	2.1
		83065	thermolabile	0.6	1.1	1.7
		83068	unstable, screen	0.5	1.4	1.9
		83069	urine	0.3	0.7	1.0
		83070	Hemosiderin; qualitative	0.4	0.8	1.2
		83071	quantitative	0.5	1.2	1.7
98.2	●	83080	b-Hexosaminidase, each assay	(I) 1.0	(I) 2.5	(I) 3.5
		83088	Histamine	1.7	3.8	5.5
		83150	Homovanillic acid (HVA)	1.5	3.0	4.5
		83491	Hydroxycorticosteroids, 17- (17-OHCS)	1.0	2.4	3.4
		83497	Hydroxyindolacetic acid, 5-(HIAA)	1.0	2.2	3.2
		83498	Hydroxyprogesterone, 17-d	1.9	3.8	5.7
		83499	Hydroxyprogesterone, 20-	1.4	3.3	4.7
		83500	Hydroxyproline; free	2.0	4.2	6.2
		83505	total	2.0	5.0	7.0
98.2	▲	83516	Immunoassay for analyte other than infectious agent antibody or infectious agent antigen, qualitative or semiquantitative; multiple step method	(I) 0.8	(I) 1.7	(I) 2.5
98.2		83518	single step method (eg, reagent strip)	0.7	1.3	2.0
98.2		83519	Immunoassay, analyte, quantitative; by radiopharmaceutical technique (eg, RIA)	0.7	1.3	2.0
98.2		83520	not otherwise specified	0.6	1.3	1.9
98.2		83525	Insulin; total	0.8	2.0	2.8
98.2		83527	free	1.0	2.2	3.2

UPD	Code	Description	Prof	Tech	Total
	83528	Intrinsic factor	1.3	2.7	4.0
	83540	Iron	0.4	1.2	1.6
	83550	Iron binding capacity	0.5	.4	1.9
	83570	Isocitric dehydrogenase (IDH)	0.7	1.5	2.2
	83582	Ketogenic steroids, fractionation	0.8	2.3	3.1
	83586	Ketosteroids, 17- (17-KS); total	1.2	2.3	3.5
	83593	fractionation	1.7	3.8	5.5
	83605	Lactate (lactic acid)	0.6	1.2	1.8
	83615	Lactate dehydrogenase (LD), (LDH);	0.5	1.0	1.5
	83625	isoenzymes, separation and quantitation	0.6	1.6	2.2
	83632	Lactogen, human placental (HPL) human chorionic somatomammotropin	1.3	2.6	3.9
	83633	Lactose, urine; qualitative	0.4	1.0	1.4
	83634	quantitative	0.9	2.0	2.9
	83655	Lead	0.8	2.0	2.8
	83661	Lecithin-sphingomyelin ratio (L/S ratio); quantitative	0.5	1.1	1.6
98.2	**83662**	foam stability test	0.9	1.7	2.6
	83670	Leucine aminopeptidase (LAP)	0.5	1.2	1.7
	83690	Lipase	0.6	1.1	1.7
	83715	Lipoprotein, blood; electrophoretic separation and quantitation	0.5	1.5	2.0
98.2 ●	**83716**	high resolution fractionation and quantitation of lipoprotein cholesterols (eg, electrophoresis, nuclear magnetic resonance, ultracentrifugation)	(I) 1.8	(I) 3.2	(I) 5.0
98.2 M	**83717**	ultracentrifugation and quantitation To report, see 83716	1.4	3.3	4.7
	83718	Lipoprotein, direct measurement; high density cholesterol (HDL cholesterol)	0.5	1.3	1.8
96.2	**83719**	direct measurement VLDL cholesterol	1.3	2.6	3.9
98.2	**83721**	direct measurement LDL cholesterol	0.5	1.0	1.5
	83727	Luteinizing releasing factor (LRH)	1.3	2.7	4.0
	83735	Magnesium	0.5	0.9	1.4
	83775	Malate dehydrogenase	0.5	1.1	1.6
	83785	Manganese	1.6	3.8	5.4

UPD		Code	Description	Prof	Tech	Total
98.2	●	83788	Mass spectrometry and tandem mass spectrometry (MS, MS/MS), analyte not elsewhere specified; qualitative, each specimen	(I) 1.2	(I) 2.4	(I) 3.6
98.2	●	83789	quantitative, each specimen	(I) 1.2	(I) 2.4	(I) 3.6
		83805	Meprobamate	1.4	2.7	4.1
		83825	Mercury, quantitative	1.0	2.1	3.1
		83835	Metanephrines	1.1	2.7	3.8
		83840	Methadone	1.3	2.6	3.9
		83857	Methemalbumin	0.8	1.7	2.5
		83858	Methsuximide	1.1	2.3	3.4
		83864	Mucopolysaccharides, acid; quantitative	0.8	2.1	2.9
		83866	screen	0.7	1.8	2.5
		83872	Mucin, synovial fluid (Ropes test)	0.4	0.8	1.2
		83873	Myelin basic protein, CSF	1.7	3.3	5.0
		83874	Myoglobin	0.8	1.6	2.4
98.2		83883	Nephelometry, each analyte not elsewhere specified	0.3	0.7	1.0
		83885	Nickel	1.3	2.9	4.2
		83887	Nicotine	1.6	3.8	5.4
98.2		83890	Molecular diagnostics; molecular isolation or extraction	0.2	0.5	0.7
98.2	●	83891	isolation or extraction of highly purified nucleic acid	(I) 0.2	(I) 0.5	(I) 0.7
98.2		83892	enzymatic digestion	0.2	0.5	0.7
98.2	●	83893	dot/slot blot production	(I) 0.2	(I) 0.5	(I) 0.7
98.2	▲	83894	separation by gel electrophoresis (eg, agarose, polyacrylamide)	(I) 0.2	(I) 0.5	(I) 0.7
98.2		83896	nucleic acid probe, each	0.2	0.5	0.7
98.2	●	83897	nucleic acid transfer (eg, Southern, Northern)	RNE	RNE	RNE
98.2	▲	83898	amplification of patient nucleic acid (eg, PCR, LCR, RT-PCR), single primer pair, each primer pair	(I) 1.3	(I) 2.7	(I) 4.0
98.2	●	83901	amplification of patient nucleic acid, multiplex, each multiplex reaction	(I) 1.3	(I) 2.7	(I) 4.0
98.2		83902	reverse transcription	(I) 1.2	(I) 2.3	(I) 3.5

UPD		Code	Description	Prof	Tech	Total
98.2	●	83903	mutation scanning, by physical properties (eg, single strand conformational polymorphisms (SSCP), heteroduplex, denaturing gradient gel electrophoresis (DGGE), RNA'ase A), single segment, each	(I) 1.3	(I) 2.7	(I) 4.0
98.2	●	83904	mutation identification by sequencing, single segment, each segment	(I) 1.3	(I) 2.7	(I) 4.0
98.2	●	83905	mutation identification by allele specific transcription, single segment, each segment	(I) 1.3	(I) 2.7	(I) 4.0
98.2	●	83906	mutation identification by allele specific translation, single segment, each segment	(I) 1.3	(I) 2.7	(I) 4.0
		83912	interpretation and report	1.0	2.6	3.6
		83915	Nucleotidase 5'-	0.9	1.9	2.8
		83916	Oligoclonal immunoglobulin (oligoclonal bands)	1.7	3.3	5.0
98.2	▲	83918	Organic acids; quantitative, each specimen	1.1	2.7	3.8
98.2	●	83919	qualitative, each specimen	(I) 1.1	(I) 2.7	(I) 3.8
98.2		83925	Opiates, (eg, morphine, mepcridine)	(I) 1.7	(I) 2.5	(I) 4.2
		83930	Osmolality; blood	0.5	1.1	1.6
		83935	urine	0.5	1.1	1.6
98.2		83937	Osteocalcin (bone gla protein)	(I) 1.8	(I) 3.8	(I) 5.6
		83945	Oxalate	1.0	1.9	2.9
		83970	Parathormone (parathyroid hormone)	2.8	5.7	8.5
		83986	pH, body fluid, except blood	0.3	0.5	0.8
		83992	Phencyclidine (PCP)	1.1	2.6	3.7
		84022	Phenothiazine	1.2	2.6	3.8
		84030	Phenylalanine (PKU), blood	0.3	0.7	1.0
		84035	Phenylketones, qualitative	0.3	0.8	1.1
		84060	Phosphatase, acid; total	1.1	2.2	3.3
98.2		84061	forensic examination	0.4	0.9	1.3
		84066	prostatic	0.6	1.1	1.7
		84075	Phosphatase, alkaline;	0.3	0.8	1.1
		84078	heat stable (total not included)	0.5	1.3	1.8
		84080	isoenzymes	1.0	2.3	3.3
		84081	Phosphatidylglycerol	1.4	2.8	4.2
		84085	Phosphogluconate, 6-, dehydrogenase, RBC	0.5	0.9	1.4

UPD		Code	Description	Prof	Tech	Total
		84087	Phosphohexose isomerase	0.7	1.7	2.4
		84100	Phosphorus inorganic (phosphate);	0.3	0.7	1.0
		84105	urine	0.3	0.7	1.0
		84106	Porphobilinogen, urine; qualitative	0.2	0.7	0.9
		84110	quantitative	0.6	1.4	2.0
		84119	Porphyrins, urine; qualitative	0.6	1.4	2.0
		84120	quantitation and fractionation	1.0	2.5	3.5
		84126	Porphyrins, feces; quantitative	1.9	4.5	6.4
98.2		84127	qualitative	0.6	1.1	1.7
		84132	Potassium; serum	0.3	0.7	1.0
		84133	urine	0.3	0.7	1.0
98.2		84134	Prealbumin	0.7	1.6	2.3
		84135	Pregnanediol	1.8	3.5	5.3
		84138	Pregnanetriol	1.7	3.5	5.2
98.2		84140	Pregnenolone	0.8	3.0	3.8
98.2		84143	17-hydroxypregnenolone	1.9	3.8	5.7
		84144	Progesterone	0.7	2.8	3.5
		84146	Prolactin	1.6	3.3	4.9
		84150	Prostaglandin, each	1.9	4.3	6.2
98.2	▲	84153	Prostate specific antigen (PSA); total	(I) 1.0	(I) 2.0	(I) 3.0
98.2	●	84154	free	(I) 1.0	(I) 2.0	(I) 3.0
		84155	Protein; total, except refractometry	0.4	0.7	1.1
		84160	refractometric	0.4	0.7	1.1
		84165	electrophoretic fractionation and quantitation	0.8	1.5	2.3
98.2		84181	Western Blot, with interpretation and report, blood or other body fluid	0.9	1.8	2.7
98.2		84182	Western Blot, with interpretation and report, blood or other body fluid, immunological probe for band identification, each	1.0	2.0	3.0
		84202	Protoporphyrin, RBC; quantitative	1.2	2.4	3.6
		84203	screen	0.5	1.0	1.5
		84206	Proinsulin	0.9	2.0	2.9
		84207	Pyridoxal phosphate (Vitamin B-6)	1.5	3.5	5.0

UPD		Code	Description	Prof	Tech	Total
		84210	Pyruvate	0.9	1.4	2.3
		84220	Pyruvate kinase	0.8	1.6	2.4
		84228	Quinine	0.9	2.0	2.9
		84233	Receptor assay; estrogen	3.2	7.4	10.6
		84234	progesterone	3.2	7.4	10.6
		84235	endocrine, other than estrogen or progesterone (specify hormone)	3.1	7.3	10.4
		84238	non-endocrine (eg, acetylcholine)	2.9	5.9	8.8
		84244	Renin	1.6	3.1	4.7
		84252	Riboflavin (Vitamin B-2)	1.3	.0	4.3
		84255	Selenium	1.6	3.8	5.4
		84260	Serotonin	1.5	3.5	5.0
98.2		**84270**	Sex hormone binding globulin (SHBG)	1.0	2.3	3.3
		84275	Sialic acid	1.0	2.4	3.4
		84285	Silica	1.6	3.9	5.5
		84295	Sodium; serum	0.3	0.6	0.9
		84300	urine	0.3	0.6	0.9
98.2		**84305**	Somatomedin	1.0	2.1	3.1
98.2		**84307**	Somatostatin	0.8	1.7	2.5
98.2		**84311**	Spectrophotometry, analyte not elsewhere specified	0.3	0.7	1.0
		84315	Specific gravity (except urine)	0.2	0.3	0.5
		84375	Sugars, chromatographic, TLC or paper chromatography	1.0	2.4	3.4
98.2	●	**84376**	Sugars (mon-, di, and oligosaccharides); single qualitative, each specimen	(I) 0.3	(I) 0.7	(I) 1.0
98.2	●	**84377**	multiple qualitative, each specimen	(I) 0.3	(I) 0.7	(I) 1.0
98.2	●	**84378**	single quantitative, each specimen	(I) 0.8	(I) 1.6	(I) 2.4
98.2	●	**84379**	multiple quantitative, each specimen	(I) 0.8	(I) 1.6	(I) 2.4
98.2		**84392**	Sulfate, urine	0.2	0.6	0.8
98.2		**84402**	Testosterone; free	2.0	4.5	6.5
		84403	total	1.8	4.2	6.0
		84425	Thiamine (Vitamin B-1)	1.6	3.4	5.0
		84430	Thiocyanate	0.9	1.9	2.8

UPD	Code	Description	Prof	Tech	Total
98.2	**84432**	Thyroglobulin	0.8	1.8	2.6
	84436	Thyroxine; total	0.3	1.0	1.3
	84437	requiring elution (eg, neonatal)	0.4	0.8	1.2
	84439	free	0.4	1.1	1.5
	84442	Thyroxine binding globulin (TBG)	0.6	1.8	2.4
	84443	Thyroid stimulating hormone (TSH)	0.7	2.2	2.9
	84445	Thyroid stimulating immunoglobulins (TSI)	2.7	6.2	8.9
	84446	Tocopherol alpha (Vitamin E)	1.0	2.2	3.2
98.2	**84449**	Transcortin (cortisol binding globulin)	1.2	2.3	3.5
	84450	Transferase; aspartate amino (AST) (SGOT)	0.3	0.7	1.0
	84460	alanine amino (ALT) (SGPT)	0.4	0.8	1.2
98.2	**84466**	Transferrin	0.7	1.4	2.1
	84478	Triglycerides	0.3	0.8	1.1
96.2	**84479**	Thyroid hormone (T3 or T4) uptake or thyroid hormone binding ratio (THBR)	0.5	0.9	1.4
96.2	**84480**	Triiodothyronine T3; total (TT-3)	0.8	1.5	2.3
	84481	free	1.4	2.9	4.3
98.2	**84482**	Triiodothyronine (T-3); reverse	1.4	2.8	4.2
98.2	**84484**	Troponin, quantitative	(I) 0.6	(I) 1.4	(I) 2.0
	84485	Trypsin; duodenal fluid	0.4	1.0	1.4
	84488	feces, qualitative	0.4	1.0	1.4
	84490	feces, quantitative, 24-hour collection	0.4	1.0	1.4
	84510	Tyrosine	0.8	1.7	2.5
98.2	**84512**	Troponin, qualitative	(I) 0.5	(I) 1.1	(I) 1.6
	84520	Urea nitrogen; quantitative	0.3	0.8	1.1
	84525	semiquantitative (eg, reagent strip test)	0.2	0.5	0.7
	84540	Urea nitrogen, urine	0.4	0.8	1.2
	84545	Urea nitrogen, clearance	0.5	1.2	1.7
	84550	Uric acid; blood	0.4	0.7	1.1
98.2	**84560**	other source	0.3	0.8	1.1
	84577	Urobilinogen, feces, quantitative	1.0	2.1	3.1
	84578	Urobilinogen, urine; qualitative	0.2	0.5	0.7

UPD	Code	Description	Prof	Tech	Total
	84580	quantitative, timed specimen	0.5	1.1	1.6
	84583	semiquantitative	0.3	0.7	1.0
	84585	Vanillylmandelic acid (VMA), urine	1.0	2.3	3.3
98.2	84586	Vasoactive intestinal peptide (VIP)	(I) 2.2	(I) 4.4	(I) 6.6
98.2	84588	Vasopressin (antidiuretic hormone, ADH)	(I) 2.2	(I) 4.4	(I) 6.6
	84590	Vitamin A	1.0	2.0	3.0
	84597	Vitamin K	1.0	2.4	3.4
	84600	Volatiles (eg, acetic anhydride, carbon tetrachloride, dichloroethane, dichloromethane, diethylether, isopropyl alcohol, methanol)	1.2	2.8	4.0
	84620	Xylose absorption test, blood and/or urine	0.8	1.9	2.7
	84630	Zinc	0.8	1.7	2.5
	84681	C-peptide	1.6	3.2	4.8
	84702	Gonadotropin, chorionic (hCG); quantitative	1.2	2.5	3.7
	84703	qualitative	1.1	2.4	3.5
98.2	84830	Ovulation tests, by visual color comparison methods for human luteinizing hormone	0.5	1.1	1.6
	84999	Unlisted chemistry procedure	BR	BR	BR

Hematology and Coagulation

UPD	Code	Description	Prof	Tech	Total
	85002	Bleeding time	0.3	0.6	0.9
	85007	Blood count; manual differential WBC count (includes RBC morphology and platelet estimation)	0.2	0.4	0.6
98.2	85008	manual blood smear examination without differential parameters	0.2	0.3	0.5
	85009	differential WBC count, buffy coat	0.3	0.5	0.8
98.2	85013	spun microhematocrit	0.1	0.3	0.4
	85014	other than spun hematocrit	0.1	0.3	0.4
	85018	hemoglobin	0.2	0.3	0.5
	85021	hemogram, automated (RBC, WBC, Hgb, Hct and indices only)	0.3	0.7	1.0
	85022	hemogram, automated, and manual differential WBC count (CBC)	0.4	1.0	1.4
	85023	hemogram and platelet count,	0.7	1.4	2.1
	85024	hemogram and platelet count, automated, and automated partial differential WBC count (CBC)	0.6	1.4	2.0

UPD		Code	Description	Prof	Tech	Total
		85025	hemogram and platelet count, automated, and automated complete differential WBC count (CBC)	0.6	1.4	2.0
		85027	hemogram and platelet count, automated	0.6	1.2	1.8
98.2	M	85029	Additional automated hemogram indices (eg, red cell distribution width (RDW), mean platelet volume (MPV), red blood cell histogram, platelet histogram, white blood cell histogram); one to three indices To report, see 85021-85027	0.4	0.7	1.1
98.2	M	85030	four or more indices To report, see 85021-85027	0.4	0.7	1.1
		85031	Blood count; hemogram, manual, complete CBC (RBC, WBC, Hgb, Hct, differential and indices)	0.3	0.8	1.1
		85041	red blood cell (RBC) only	0.3	0.4	0.7
		85044	reticulocyte count, manual	0.3	0.6	0.9
98.2		85045	reticulocyte count, flow cytometry	0.2	0.4	0.6
98.2	●	85046	reticulocytes, hemoglobin concentration	RNE	RNE	RNE
		85048	white blood cell (WBC)	0.3	0.4	0.7
		85060	Blood smear, peripheral, interpretation by physician with written report	0.7	1.7	2.4
		85095	Bone marrow; aspiration only	2.3	5.2	7.5
		85097	smear interpretation only, with or without differential cell count	5.5	0.0	5.5
		85102	Bone marrow biopsy, needle or trocar	2.9	6.9	9.8
98.2		85130	Chromogenic substrate assay	0.6	1.2	1.8
		85170	Clot retraction	0.3	0.6	0.9
		85175	Clot lysis time, whole blood dilution	0.3	0.6	0.9
		85210	Clotting; factor II, prothrombin, specific	0.8	2.0	2.8
		85220	factor V (AcG or proaccelerin), labile factor	1.4	2.9	4.3
		85230	factor VII (proconvertin, stable factor)	1.3	3.0	4.3
		85240	factor VIII (AHG), one stage	1.4	3.0	4.4
		85244	factor VIII related antigen	1.4	3.1	4.5
98.2		85245	factor VIII, VW factor, ristocetin cofactor	1.7	3.3	5.0
98.2		85246	factor VIII, VW factor antigen	1.7	3.3	5.0
98.2		85247	factor VIII, Von Willebrand's factor, multimetric analysis	1.7	3.3	5.0

UPD	Code	Description	Prof	Tech	Total
	85250	factor IX (PTC or Christmas)	1.3	3.2	4.5
	85260	factor X (Stuart-Prower)	1.3	3.2	4.5
	85270	factor XI (PTA)	1.3	3.2	4.5
	85280	factor XII (Hageman)	1.3	3.2	4.5
	85290	factor XIII (fibrin stabilizing)	1.2	2.9	4.1
	85291	factor XIII (fibrin stabilizing), screen solubility	0.6	1.3	1.9
	85292	prekallikrein assay (Fletcher factor assay)	1.6	3.1	4.7
	85293	high molecular weight kininogen assay (Fitzgerald factor assay)	1.6	3.1	4.7
	85300	Clotting inhibitors or anticoagulants; antithrombin III, activity	0.9	1.8	2.7
	85301	antithrombin III, antigen assay	0.9	1.8	2.7
	85302	protein C, antigen	1.0	2.0	3.0
98.2	85303	protein C, activity	0.8	1.7	2.5
98.2	85305	protein S, total	0.7	1.3	2.0
98.2	85306	protein S, free	0.9	1.8	2.7
98.2	85335	Factor inhibitor test	0.7	1.3	2.0
98.2	85337	Thrombomodulin	0.6	1.2	1.8
	85345	Coagulation time; Lee and White	0.3	0.8	1.1
	85347	activated	0.2	0.6	0.8
	85348	other methods	0.3	0.6	0.9
	85360	Euglobulin lysis	0.4	1.1	1.5
	85362	Fibrin(ogen) degradation (split) products (FDP)(FSP); agglutination slide, semiquantitative	0.7	1.0	1.7
98.2	85366	paracoagulation	0.3	0.9	1.2
98.2	85370	quantitative	0.5	1.4	1.9
98.2	85378	Fibrin degradation products, D-dimer; semiquantitative	0.4	0.8	1.2
98.2	85379	quantitative	0.6	1.1	1.7
98.2	85384	Fibrinogen; activity	0.5	1.0	1.5
98.2	85385	antigen	0.5	1.0	1.5
	85390	Fibrinolysins or coagulopathy screen, interpretation and report	0.2	0.7	0.9
	85400	Fibrinolytic factors and inhibitors; plasmin	0.3	0.8	1.1

UPD	Code	Description	Prof	Tech	Total
	85410	alpha-2 antiplasmin	0.3	0.8	1.1
98.2	85415	plasminogen activator	0.9	1.7	2.6
	85420	plasminogen, except antigenic assay	0.4	1.2	1.6
	85421	plasminogen, antigenic assay	1.1	2.5	3.6
	85441	Heinz bodies; direct	0.2	0.5	0.7
	85445	induced, acetyl phenylhydrazine	0.5	1.0	1.5
	85460	Hemoglobin or RBCs, fetal, for fetomaternal hemorrhage; differential lysis (Kleihauer-Betke)	0.4	1.0	1.4
98.2	85461	rosette	0.3	0.8	1.1
98.2	85475	Hemolysin, acid	0.4	1.0	1.4
	85520	Heparin assay	0.6	1.5	2.1
98.2	85525	Heparin neutralization	0.6	1.3	1.9
	85530	Heparin-protamine tolerance test	1.1	2.5	3.6
	85535	Iron stain (RBC or bone marrow smears)	0.5	0.9	1.4
	85540	Leukocyte alkaline phosphatase with count	0.6	1.5	2.1
	85547	Mechanical fragility, RBC	0.6	1.6	2.2
	85549	Muramidase	1.4	2.8	4.2
	85555	Osmotic fragility, RBC; unincubated	0.5	1.1	1.6
	85557	incubated	0.9	2.2	3.1
	85576	Platelet; aggregation (in vitro), each agent	0.5	1.5	2.0
	85585	estimation on smear, only	0.2	0.6	0.8
	85590	manual count	0.3	0.7	1.0
	85595	automated count	0.3	0.5	0.8
98.2	85597	Platelet neutralization	0.9	2.0	2.9
	85610	Prothrombin time;	0.2	0.4	0.6
98.2	85611	substitution, plasma fractions, each	0.2	0.4	0.6
	85612	Russell viper venom time (includes venom); undiluted	0.6	1.5	2.1
98.2	85613	diluted	0.4	1.0	1.4
	85635	Reptilase test	0.8	1.7	2.5
	85651	Sedimentation rate, erythrocyte; non-automated	0.2	0.6	0.8
98.2	85652	automated	0.2	0.6	0.8
	85660	Sickling of RBC, reduction	0.3	0.6	0.9

UPD	Code	Description	Prof	Tech	Total
	85670	Thrombin time; plasma	0.3	0.9	1.2
	85675	titer	0.4	0.8	1.2
98.2	**85705**	Thromboplastin inhibition; tissue	0.4	0.8	1.2
	85730	Thromboplastin time, partial (PTT); plasma or whole blood	0.3	0.7	1.0
	85732	substitution, plasma fractions, each	0.5	1.1	1.6
	85810	Viscosity	0.4	1.4	1.8
	85999	Unlisted hematology and coagulation procedure	BR	BR	BR

Immunology

UPD	Code	Description	Prof	Tech	Total
	86000	Agglutinins, febrile (eg, Brucella, Francisella, Murine typhus, Q fever, Rocky Mountain spotted fever, scrub typhus), each antigen	0.6	1.1	1.7
98.2	**86003**	Allergen specific IgE; quantitative or semiquantitative, each allergen	0.5	1.0	1.5
98.2	**86005**	qualitative, multiallergen screen (dipstick, paddle or disk)	0.4	0.6	1.0
	86021	Antibody identification; leukocyte antibodies	1.1	2.7	3.8
	86022	platelet antibodies	1.7	3.6	5.3
	86023	platelet associated immunoglobulin assay	0.9	1.7	2.6
98.2	**86038**	Antinuclear antibodies (ANA);	0.7	1.4	2.1
98.2	**86039**	titer	0.6	1.2	1.8
	86060	Antistreptolysin 0; titer	0.3	0.9	1.2
	86063	screen	0.6	1.4	2.0
	86077	Blood bank physician services; difficult cross match and/or evaluation of irregular antibody(s), interpretation and written report	2.5	5.8	8.3
	86078	investigation of transfusion reaction including suspicion of transmissible disease, interpretation and written report	2.5	5.8	8.3
	86079	authorization for deviation from standard blood banking procedures (eg, use of outdated blood, transfusion of Rh incompatible units), with written report	2.4	4.8	7.2
	86140	C-reactive protein	0.4	0.9	1.3
98.2	**86147**	Cardiolipin (phospholipid) antibody	(I) 2.2	(I) 3.6	(I) 5.8
98.1	**86148**	Anti-phosphatidylserine (phospholipid) antibody	(I) 2.0	(I) 3.5	(I) 5.5
	86155	Chemotaxis assay, specify method	0.8	1.7	2.5

UPD		Code	Description	Prof	Tech	Total
98.2		**86156**	Cold agglutinin; screen	0.3	0.7	1.0
98.2		**86157**	titer	0.4	0.8	1.2
98.2		**86160**	Complement; antigen, each component	0.5	1.5	2.0
98.2		**86161**	functional activity, each component	0.5	1.5	2.0
		86162	total hemolytic (CH50)	1.7	3.3	5.0
		86171	Complement fixation tests, each antigen	0.7	1.7	2.4
		86185	Counterimmunoelectrophoresis, each antigen	0.6	1.2	1.8
		86215	Deoxyribonuclease, antibody	1.1	2.2	3.3
		86225	Deoxyribonucleic acid (DNA) antibody; native or double stranded	1.0	2.3	3.3
98.2		**86226**	single stranded	0.8	1.5	2.3
		86235	Extractable nuclear antigen, antibody to, any method (eg, nRNP, SS-A, SS-B, Sm, RNP, Sc170, J01), each antibody	0.9	2.1	3.0
		86243	Fc receptor	1.4	3.2	4.6
98.2	▲	**86255**	Fluorescent noninfectious agent antibody; screen, each antibody	0.8	1.6	2.4
		86256	titer, each antibody	0.8	1.6	2.4
		86277	Growth hormone, human (HGH), antibody	1.3	2.5	3.8
		86280	Hemagglutination inhibition test (HAI)	0.3	1.1	1.4
97.2	**M**	**86287**	Hepatitis B surface antigen (HBsAg) To report, use 87340	0.7	1.9	2.6
97.2	**M**	**86289**	Hepatitis B core antibody (HBcAb); IgG and IgM To report, use 86704	1.0	2.0	3.0
97.2	**M**	**86290**	IgM antibody To report, use 86705	1.0	2.2	3.2
97.2	**M**	**86291**	Hepatitis B surface antibody (HBsAb) To report, use 86706	0.8	1.5	2.3
97.2	**M**	**86293**	Hepatitis Be antigen (HBeAg) To report, use 87350	0.8	1.7	2.5
97.2	**M**	**86295**	Hepatitis Be antibody (HBeAb) To report, use 86707	0.8	1.7	2.5
97.2	**M**	**86296**	Hepatis A antibody (HAAb); IgG and IgM To report, use 86708	0.9	2.0	2.9
97.2	**M**	**86299**	IgM antibody To report, use 86709	0.9	1.8	2.7

+ Add-on Code   ⊘ Modifier -51 Exempt   ▲ Revised code   ● New code   **M** RVSI code or deleted from CPT   **(I)** Interim Value

CPT codes and descriptions only copyright © 1998 American Medical Association

Copyright © 1999 St. Anthony Publishing

UPD		Code	Description	Prof	Tech	Total
97.2	M	86302	Hepatitis C antibody; To report, use 86803	(I) 0.8	(I) 1.5	(I) 2.3
97.2	M	86303	confirmatory test (eg, immunoblot) To report, use 86804	(I) 0.8	(I) 1.7	(I) 2.5
97.2	M	86306	Hepatitis, delta agent To report, use 87380	(I) 0.8	(I) 1.8	(I) 2.6
98.2		86308	Heterophile antibodies; screening	0.3	0.5	0.8
98.2		86309	titer	0.3	0.8	1.1
		86310	titers after absorption with beef cells and guinea pig kidney	0.6	1.2	1.8
97.2	M	86311	HIV, antigen To report, see 87390, 87391	(I) 0.9	(I) 1.9	(I) 2.8
97.2	M	86313	Immunoassay for infectious agent antigen, qualitative or semiquantitative; multiple step method To report, use 87449	(I) 1.0	(I) 2.0	(I) 3.0
97.2	M	86315	single step method (eg, reagent strip) To report, use 87450	(I) 0.8	(I) 1.6	(I) 2.4
		86316	Immunoassay for tumor antigen (eg, cancer antigen 125), each	1.0	2.4	3.4
		86317	Immunoassay for infectious agent antibody, quantitative, not otherwise specified	0.9	1.9	2.8
		86318	Immunoassay for infectious agent antibody, qualitative or semiquantitative, single step method (eg, reagent strip)	0.9	1.3	2.2
		86320	Immunoelectrophoresis; serum	1.8	2.7	4.5
		86325	other fluids (eg, urine, CSF) with concentration	1.5	3.0	4.5
		86327	crossed (2-dimensional assay)	1.8	3.9	5.7
		86329	Immunodiffusion; not elsewhere specified	1.1	2.3	3.4
		86331	gel diffusion, qualitative (Ouchterlony), each antigen or antibody	0.9	2.1	3.0
98.2		86332	Immune complex assay	1.7	3.3	5.0
98.2		86334	Immunofixation electrophoresis	1.7	4.2	5.9
		86337	Insulin antibodies	1.7	3.3	5.0
		86340	Intrinsic factor antibodies	1.2	2.4	3.6
98.2		86341	Islet cell antibody	1.2	2.3	3.5
		86343	Leukocyte histamine release test (LHR)	1.0	2.0	3.0
		86344	Leukocyte phagocytosis	0.7	1.3	2.0

UPD	Code	Description	Prof	Tech	Total
	86353	Lymphocyte transformation, mitogen (phytomitogen) or antigen induced blastogenesis	2.8	6.5	9.3
98.2	86359	T cells; total count	(I) 2.3	(I) 4.7	(I) 7.0
97.2	86360	absolute CD4 and CD8 count, including ratio	(I) 6.0	(I) 3.0	(I) 9.0
98.1	86361	absolute CD4 count	(I) 2.0	(I) 4.0	(I) 6.0
	86376	Microsomal antibodies (eg, thyroid or liver-kidney), each	1.0	2.2	3.2
	86378	Migration inhibitory factor test (MIF)	1.4	2.8	4.2
	86382	Neutralization test, viral	1.3	2.9	4.2
	86384	Nitroblue tetrazolium dye test (NTD)	0.8	1.5	2.3
	86403	Particle agglutination; screen, each antibody	0.4	1.5	1.9
98.2	86406	titer, each antibody	0.5	1.5	2.0
	86430	Rheumatoid factor; qualitative	0.4	0.8	1.2
98.2	86431	quantitative	0.6	1.0	1.6
98.2	86485	Skin test; candida	0.4	0.8	1.2
	86490	coccidioidomycosis	0.5	1.1	1.6
	86510	histoplasmosis	0.4	0.8	1.2
	86580	tuberculosis, intradermal	0.4	0.8	1.2
	86585	tuberculosis, tine test	0.4	0.8	1.2
	86586	unlisted antigen, each	BR	BR	BR
98.2	86588	Streptococcus, screen, direct	0.5	1.0	1.5
	86590	Streptokinase, antibody	0.6	1.1	1.7
	86592	Syphilis test; qualitative (eg, VDRL, RPR, ART)	0.2	0.6	0.8
	86593	quantitative	0.3	0.7	1.0
98.2	86602	Antibody; actinomyces	0.5	1.1	1.6
98.2	86603	adenovirus	0.6	1.3	1.9
98.2	86606	Aspergillus	0.8	1.5	2.3
98.2	86609	bacterium, not elsewhere specified	0.6	1.3	1.9
98.2	86612	Blastomyces	0.6	1.4	2.0
98.2	86615	Bordetella	0.6	1.4	2.0
98.2	86617	Borrelia burgdorferi (Lyme disease) confirmatory test (eg, Western blot or immunoblot)	0.9	1.8	2.7
98.2	86618	Borrelia burgdorferi (Lyme disease)	0.8	1.7	2.5

UPD	Code	Description	Prof	Tech	Total
98.2	**86619**	Borrelia (relapsing fever)	0.6	1.4	2.0
98.2	**86622**	Brucella	0.5	1.0	1.5
98.2	**86625**	Campylobacter	0.6	1.4	2.0
98.2	**86628**	Candida	0.6	1.3	1.9
98.2	**86631**	Chlamydia	0.6	1.3	1.9
98.2	**86632**	Chlamydia, IgM	0.6	1.3	1.9
98.2	**86635**	Coccidioides	0.5	1.2	1.7
98.2	**86638**	Coxiella Brunetii (Q fever)	0.6	1.3	1.9
98.2	**86641**	Cryptococcus	0.7	1.3	2.0
98.2	**86644**	cytomegalovirus (CMV)	0.7	1.4	2.1
98.2	**86645**	cytomegalovirus (CMV), IgM	0.9	1.7	2.6
98.2	**86648**	Diphtheria	0.8	1.5	2.3
98.2	**86651**	encephalitis, California (La Crosse)	0.7	1.3	2.0
98.2	**86652**	encephalitis, Eastern equine	0.7	1.3	2.0
98.2	**86653**	encephalitis, St. Louis	0.7	1.3	2.0
98.2	**86654**	encephalitis, Western equine	0.7	1.3	2.0
98.2	**86658**	enterovirus (eg, coxsackie, echo, polio)	0.7	1.3	2.0
98.2	**86663**	Epstein-Barr (EB) virus, early antigen (EA)	0.7	1.3	2.0
98.2	**86664**	Epstein-Barr (EB) virus, nuclear antigen (EBNA)	0.8	1.6	2.4
98.2	**86665**	Epstein-Barr (EB) virus, viral capsid (VCA)	0.9	1.8	2.7
98.2	**86668**	Francisella Tularensis	0.5	1.1	1.6
98.2	**86671**	fungus, not elsewhere specified	0.6	1.3	1.9
98.2	**86674**	Giardia Lamblia	0.7	1.5	2.2
98.2	**86677**	Helicobacter Pylori	0.8	1.5	2.3
98.2	**86682**	helminth, not elsewhere specified	0.7	1.3	2.0
98.2	**86684**	Hemophilus influenza	0.8	1.5	2.3
98.2	**86687**	HTLV I	0.3	0.7	1.0
98.2	**86688**	HTLV-II	0.6	1.3	1.9
98.2	**86689**	HTLV or HIV antibody, confirmatory test (eg, Western Blot)	0.8	1.6	2.4
98.2	**86692**	hepatitis, delta agent	0.7	1.4	2.1
98.2	**86694**	herpes simplex, non-specific type test	0.7	1.4	2.1

UPD	Code	Description	Prof	Tech	Total
98.2	86695	herpes simplex, type I	0.7	1.3	2.0
98.2	86698	histoplasma	0.6	1.3	1.9
98.2	86701	HIV-1	0.4	0.9	1.3
98.2	86702	HIV-2	0.7	1.3	2.0
98.2	86703	HIV-1 and HIV-2, single assay	0.7	1.4	2.1
97.2	86704	Hepatitis B core antibody (HBcAb); IgG and IgM	1.0	2.0	3.0
97.2	86705	IgM antibody	1.0	2.2	3.2
97.2	86706	Hepatitis B surface antibody (HBsAb)	0.8	1.5	2.3
97.2	86707	Hepatitis Be antibody (HBeAb)	0.8	1.7	2.5
97.2	86708	Hepatitis A antibody (HAAb); IgG and IgM	0.9	2.0	2.9
97.2	86709	IgM antibody	0.9	1.8	2.7
98.2	86710	influenza virus	0.7	1.4	2.1
98.2	86713	Legionella	0.7	1.5	2.2
98.2	86717	Leishmania	0.6	1.3	1.9
98.2	86720	Leptospira	0.7	1.3	2.0
98.2	86723	Listeria monocytogenes	0.7	1.3	2.0
98.2	86727	lymphocytic choriomeningitis	0.6	1.3	1.9
98.2	86729	Lymphogranuloma Venereum	0.6	1.2	1.8
98.2	86732	mucormycosis	0.7	1.3	2.0
98.2	86735	mumps	0.7	1.3	2.0
98.2	86738	Mycoplasma	0.7	1.3	2.0
98.2	86741	Neisseria meningitidis	0.7	1.3	2.0
98.2	86744	Nocardia	0.7	1.3	2.0
98.2	86747	parvovirus	0.7	1.5	2.2
98.2	86750	Plasmodium (malaria)	0.7	1.3	2.0
98.2	86753	protozoa, not elsewhere specified	0.6	1.3	1.9
98.2	86756	respiratory syncytial virus	0.6	1.3	1.9
98.2	86759	rotavirus	0.7	1.3	2.0
98.2	86762	rubella	0.7	1.4	2.1
98.2	86765	rubeola	0.6	1.3	1.9
98.2	86768	Salmonella	0.7	1.3	2.0

UPD	Code	Description	Prof	Tech	Total
98.2	**86771**	Shigella	0.7	1.3	2.0
98.2	**86774**	tetanus	0.7	1.5	2.2
98.2	**86777**	Toxoplasma	0.7	1.4	2.1
98.2	**86778**	Toxoplasma, IgM	0.7	1.5	2.2
	86781	Treponema Pallidum, confirmatory test (eg, FTA-abs)	0.7	1.4	2.1
98.2	**86784**	trichinella	0.7	1.3	2.0
98.2	**86787**	varicella-zoster	0.6	1.3	1.9
98.2	**86790**	virus, not elsewhere specified	0.7	1.3	2.0
98.2	**86793**	Yersinia	0.7	1.3	2.0
	86800	Thyroglobulin antibody	0.8	1.7	2.5
97.2	**86803**	Hepatitis C antibody;	0.8	1.5	2.3
97.2	**86804**	confirmatory test (eg, immunoblot)	0.8	1.7	2.5
98.2	**86805**	Lymphocytotoxicity assay, visual crossmatch; with titration	3.0	5.8	8.8
98.2	**86806**	without titration	2.6	5.3	7.9
98.2	**86807**	Serum screening for cytotoxic percent reactive antibody (PRA); standard method	2.0	4.7	6.7
98.2	**86808**	quick method	1.4	3.4	4.8
	86812	HLA typing; A, B, or C (eg, A10, B7, B27), single antigen	3.6	8.4	12.0
	86813	A, B, or C, multiple antigens	2.8	6.4	9.2
	86816	DR/DQ, single antigen	1.7	4.1	5.8
	86817	DR/DQ, multiple antigens	3.6	8.5	12.1
	86821	lymphocyte culture, mixed (MLC)	3.3	7.8	11.1
	86822	lymphocyte culture, primed (PLC)	2.5	5.8	8.7
	86849	Unlisted immunology procedure	BR	BR	BR

Transfusion Medicine

UPD	Code	Description	Prof	Tech	Total
98.2	**86850**	Antibody screen, RBC, each serum technique	0.4	0.7	1.1
98.2	**86860**	Antibody elution (RBC), each elution	1.4	2.7	4.1
98.1	**86870**	Antibody identification, RBC antibodies, each panel for each serum technique			
98.2	**86880**	Antihuman globulin test (Coombs test); direct, each antiserum	0.4	0.8	1.2

UPD	Code	Description	Prof	Tech	Total
98.2	86885	indirect, qualitative, each antiserum	0.4	1.0	1.4
98.2	86886	indirect, titer, each antiserum	0.4	0.9	1.3
98.1	86890	Autologous blood or component, collection processing and storage; predeposited	1.0	5.0	6.0
98.2	86891	intra- or postoperative salvage	2.5	5.8	8.3
98.2	86900	Blood typing; ABO	0.3	0.7	1.0
98.2	86901	Rh (D)	0.4	0.7	1.1
98.2	86903	antigen screening for compatible blood unit using reagent serum, per unit screened	0.5	0.9	1.4
98.2	86904	antigen screening for compatible unit using patient serum, per unit screened	0.6	1.2	1.8
98.2	86905	RBC antigens, other than ABO or Rh (D), each	0.2	0.6	0.8
98.2	86906	Rh phenotyping, complete	0.3	0.7	1.0
98.2	86910	Blood typing, for paternity testing, per individual; ABO, Rh and MN	2.3	5.3	7.6
98.2	86911	each additional antigen system	0.6	1.2	1.8
98.1	86915	Bone marrow, modification or treatment to eliminate cell (eg, T-cells, metastatic carcinoma)	10.0	15.0	25.0
98.2	86920	Compatibility test each unit; immediate spin technique	0.4	1.5	1.9
98.2	86921	incubation technique	0.7	1.5	2.2
98.2	86922	antiglobulin technique	0.7	1.5	2.2
98.2	86927	Fresh frozen plasma, thawing, each unit	0.5	1.5	2.0
98.2	86930	Frozen blood, preparation for freezing, each unit;	4.2	9.8	14.0
98.2	86931	with thawing	4.2	9.8	14.0
98.2	86932	with freezing and thawing	4.4	10.1	14.5
98.2	86940	Hemolysins and agglutinins; auto, screen, each	0.5	1.2	1.7
98.2	86941	incubated	0.8	2.0	2.8
98.2	86945	Irradiation of blood product, each unit	1.0	2.2	3.2
98.2	86950	Leukocyte transfusion	2.7	6.3	9.0
98.2	86965	Pooling of platelets or other blood products	0.7	1.7	2.4
98.2	86970	Pretreatment of RBC's for use in RBC antibody detection, identification, and/or compatibility testing; incubation with chemical agents or drugs, each	1.1	2.7	3.8
98.2	86971	incubation with enzymes, each	0.5	1.4	1.9

UPD	Code	Description	Prof	Tech	Total
98.2	**86972**	by density gradient separation	0.6	1.3	1.9
98.2	**86975**	Pretreatment of serum for use in RBC antibody identification; incubation with drugs, each	1.5	3.4	4.9
98.2	**86976**	by dilution	1.5	3.4	4.9
98.2	**86977**	incubation with inhibitors, each	1.5	3.4	4.9
98.2	**86978**	by differential red cell absorption using patient RBC's or RBC's of known phenotype, each absorption	1.8	4.1	5.9
98.2	**86985**	Splitting of blood or blood products, each unit	1.0	2.0	3.0
	86999	Unlisted transfusion medicine procedure	BR	BR	BR

Microbiology

UPD	Code	Description	Prof	Tech	Total
	87001	Animal inoculation, small animal; with observation	1.0	2.2	3.2
	87003	with observation and dissection	1.2	2.5	3.7
	87015	Concentration (any type), for parasites, ova, or tubercle bacillus (TB, AFB)	0.5	1.0	1.5
	87040	Culture, bacterial, definitive; blood (includes anaerobic screen)	0.6	1.1	1.7
	87045	stool	0.7	1.4	2.1
	87060	throat or nose	0.3	0.9	1.2
	87070	any other source	0.4	0.9	1.3
	87072	Culture or direct bacterial identification method, each organism, by commercial kit, any source except urine	0.3	0.9	1.2
	87075	Culture, bacterial, any source; anaerobic (isolation)	0.6	1.1	1.7
	87076	definitive identification, each anaerobic organism, including gas chromatography	0.8	1.5	2.3
	87081	Culture, bacterial, screening only, for single organisms	0.3	0.8	1.1
	87082	Culture, presumptive, pathogenic organisms, screening only, by commercial kit (specify type); for single organisms	0.3	0.8	1.1
	87083	multiple organisms	0.6	1.1	1.7
	87084	with colony estimation from density chart	0.7	1.5	2.2
	87085	with colony count	0.7	1.5	2.2
	87086	Culture, bacterial, urine; quantitative, colony count	0.3	1.0	1.3
	87087	commercial kit	0.5	1.1	1.6
	87088	identification, in addition to quantitative or commercial kit	0.6	1.1	1.7

UPD		Code	Description	Prof	Tech	Total
		87101	Culture, fungi, isolation (with or without presumptive identification); skin	0.6	1.3	1.9
		87102	other source (except blood)	0.6	1.3	1.9
		87103	blood	1.0	1.9	2.9
		87106	Culture, fungi, definitive identification of each fungus (use in addition to codes 87101, 87102, or 87103 when appropriate)	0.7	1.7	2.4
		87109	Culture, mycoplasma, any source	0.8	1.7	2.5
		87110	Culture, chlamydia	0.9	2.1	3.0
		87116	Culture, tubercle or other acid-fast bacilli (eg, TB, AFB, mycobacteria); any source, isolation only	0.7	1.7	2.4
		87117	concentration plus isolation	0.8	1.6	2.4
		87118	Culture, mycobacteria, definitive identification of each organism	0.7	1.7	2.4
		87140	Culture, typing; fluorescent method, each antiserum	0.7	1.6	2.3
		87143	gas liquid chromatography (GLC) method	1.0	2.1	3.1
		87145	phage method	0.5	1.2	1.7
		87147	serologic method, agglutination grouping, per antiserum	0.8	1.7	2.5
		87151	serologic method, speciation	0.5	0.9	1.4
		87155	precipitin method, grouping, per antiserum	0.2	0.7	0.9
		87158	other methods	0.2	0.7	0.9
		87163	Culture, any source, additional identification methods required (use in addition to primary culture code)	0.9	1.9	2.8
		87164	Dark field examination, any source (eg, penile, vaginal, oral, skin); includes specimen collection	0.8	1.5	2.3
		87166	without collection	0.7	1.6	2.3
		87174	Endotoxin, bacterial (pyrogens); chemical	0.8	1.5	2.2
98.2		**87175**	biological assay (eg, Limulus lysate)	0.8	1.7	2.5
		87176	homogenization, tissue, for culture	0.5	1.0	1.5
		87177	Ova and parasites, direct smears, concentration and identification	0.6	1.1	1.7
97.2	**M**	**87178**	Microbial identification, nucleic acid probes, each probe used; To report, use 87797	1.2	2.2	3.4
97.2	**M**	**87179**	with amplication, eg, polymerase chain reaction (PCR) To report, use 87798	(I) 0.8	(I) 1.7	(I) 2.5

UPD	Code	Description	Prof	Tech	Total
	87181	Sensitivity studies, antibiotic; agar diffusion method, per antibiotic	0.4	0.8	1.2
96.2	87184	disk method, per plate (12 or fewer disks)	0.3	0.9	1.2
	87186	microtiter, minimum inhibitory concentration (MIC), any number of antibiotics	0.4	1.1	1.5
	87187	minimum bactericidal concentration (MBC) (use in addition to 87186 or 87188)	0.3	1.6	1.9
	87188	macrotube dilution method, each antibiotic	0.5	1.2	1.7
	87190	tubercle bacillus (TB, AFB), each drug	0.2	0.5	0.7
	87192	fungi, each drug	0.5	1.2	1.7
98.2	87197	Serum bactericidal titer (Schlicter test)	0.9	1.8	2.7
	87205	Smear, primary source, with interpretation; routine stain for bacteria, fungi, or cell types	0.3	0.7	1.0
	87206	fluorescent and/or acid fast stain for bacteria, fungi, or cell types	0.3	1.1	1.4
	87207	special stain for inclusion bodies or intracellular parasites (eg, malaria, kala azar, herpes)	0.3	0.6	0.9
	87208	direct or concentrated, dry, for ova and parasites	0.5	0.9	1.4
	87210	wet mount with simple stain, for bacteria, fungi, ova, and/or parasites	0.2	0.6	0.8
	87211	wet and dry mount, for ova and parasites	0.3	0.6	0.9
	87220	Tissue examination for fungi (eg, KOH slide)	0.4	0.7	1.1
	87230	Toxin or antitoxin assay, tissue culture (eg, Clostridium difficile toxin)	1.0	2.2	3.2
	87250	Virus identification; inoculation of embryonated eggs, or small animal, includes observation and dissection	1.2	1.8	3.0
	87252	tissue culture inoculation and observation	1.3	2.8	4.1
	87253	tissue culture, additional studies (eg, hemabsorption, neutralization) each isolate	0.9	2.1	3.0
98.2	87260	Infectious agent antigen detection by direct fluorescent antibody technique; adenovirus	(I) 0.8	(I) 1.7	(I) 2.5
98.2	87265	Bordetella pertussis/parapertussis	(I) 0.8	(I) 1.7	(I) 2.5
98.2	87270	Chlamydia trachomatis	(I) 0.8	(I) 1.7	(I) 2.5
98.2	87272	cryptosporidum/giardia	(I) 0.8	(I) 1.7	(I) 2.5
98.2	87274	Herpes simplex virus	(I) 0.8	(I) 1.7	(I) 2.5
98.2	87276	influenza A virus	(I) 0.8	(I) 1.7	(I) 2.5

UPD	Code	Description	Prof	Tech	Total
98.2	**87278**	Legionella pneumophila	(I) 0.8	(I) 1.7	(I) 2.5
98.2	**87280**	respiratory syncytial virus	(I) 0.8	(I) 1.7	(I) 2.5
98.2	**87285**	Treponema pallidum	(I) 0.8	(I) 1.7	(I) 2.5
98.2	**87290**	Varicella zoster virus	(I) 0.8	(I) 1.7	(I) 2.5
98.2	**87299**	Infectious agent antigen detection by direct fluorescent antibody technique, not otherwise specified	(I) 0.8	(I) 1.7	(I) 2.5
98.2	**87301**	Infectious agent antigen detection by enzyme immunoassay technique, qualitative or semiquantitative, multiple step method; adenovirus enteric types 40/41	(I) 0.8	(I) 1.7	(I) 2.5
98.2	**87320**	Chlamydia trachomatis	(I) 0.8	(I) 1.7	(I) 2.5
98.2	**87324**	Clostridium difficile toxin A	(I) 0.8	(I) 1.7	(I) 2.5
98.2	**87328**	cryptosporidum/giardia	(I) 0.8	(I) 1.7	(I) 2.5
98.2	**87332**	cytomegalovirus	(I) 0.8	(I) 1.7	(I) 2.5
98.2	**87335**	Escherichia coli 0157	(I) 0.8	(I) 1.7	(I) 2.5
98.1	**87340**	hepatitis B surface antigen (HBsAg)			
98.1	**87350**	hepatitis Be antigen (HBeAg)			
98.2	**87380**	hepatitis, delta agent	(I) 1.0	(I) 2.2	(I) 3.2
98.2	**87385**	Histoplasma capsulatum	(I) 0.8	(I) 1.7	(I) 2.5
98.2	**87390**	HIV-1	(I) 1.2	(I) 2.3	(I) 3.5
98.2	**87391**	HIV-2	(I) 1.2	(I) 2.3	(I) 3.5
98.2	**87420**	respiratory syncytial virus	(I) 0.8	(I) 1.7	(I) 2.5
98.2	**87425**	rotavirus	(I) 0.8	(I) 1.7	(I) 2.5
98.2	**87430**	Streptococcus, group A	(I) 0.8	(I) 1.7	(I) 2.5
98.2	**87449**	Infectious agent antigen detection by enzyme immunoassay technique, qualitative or semiquantitative; multiple step method, not otherwise specified	(I) 0.8	(I) 1.7	(I) 2.5
98.2	**87450**	single step method, not otherwise specified	(I) 0.6	(I) 1.4	(I) 2.0
98.2	**87470**	Infectious agent detection by nucleic acid (DNA or RNA); Bartonella henselae and Bartonella quintana, direct probe technique	(I) 1.2	(I) 2.6	(I) 3.8
98.2	**87471**	Bartonella henselae and Bartonella quintana, amplified probe technique	(I) 2.2	(I) 4.4	(I) 6.6
98.2	**87472**	Bartonella henselae and Bartonella quintana, quantification	(I) 2.6	(I) 5.4	(I) 8.0
98.2	**87475**	Borrelia burgdorferi, direct probe technique	(I) 1.2	(I) 2.5	(I) 3.7

UPD	Code	Description	Prof	Tech	Total
98.2	**87476**	Borrelia burgdorferi, amplified probe technique	(I) 2.2	(I) 4.4	(I) 6.6
98.2	**87477**	Borrelia burgdorferi, quantification	(I) 2.6	(I) 5.4	(I) 8.0
98.2	**87480**	Candida species, direct probe technique	(I) 1.2	(I) 2.6	(I) 3.8
98.2	**87481**	Candida species, amplified probe technique	(I) 2.2	(I) 4.4	(I) 6.6
98.2	**87482**	Candida species, quantification	(I) 2.6	(I) 5.2	(I) 7.8
98.2	**87485**	Chlamydia pneumoniae, direct probe technique	(I) 1.2	(I) 2.6	(I) 3.8
98.2	**87486**	Chlamydia pneumoniae, amplified probe technique	(I) 2.2	(I) 4.4	(I) 6.6
98.2	**87487**	Chlamydia pneumoniae, quantification	(I) 2.6	(I) 5.4	(I) 8.0
98.2	**87490**	Chlamydia trachomatis, direct probe technique	(I) 1.2	(I) 2.6	(I) 3.8
98.2	**87491**	Chlamydia trachomatis, amplified probe technique	(I) 2.2	(I) 4.4	(I) 6.6
98.2	**87492**	Chlamydia trachomatis, quantification	(I) 2.2	(I) 4.4	(I) 6.6
98.2	**87495**	cytomegalovirus, direct probe technique	(I) 1.2	(I) 2.6	(I) 3.8
98.2	**87496**	cytomegalovirus, amplified probe technique	(I) 2.2	(I) 4.4	(I) 6.6
98.2	**87497**	cytomegalovirus, quantification	(I) 2.6	(I) 5.4	(I) 8.0
98.2	**87510**	Gardnerella vaginalis, direct probe technique	(I) 1.2	(I) 2.6	(I) 3.8
98.2	**87511**	Gardnerella vaginalis, amplified probe technique	(I) 2.2	(I) 4.4	(I) 6.6
98.2	**87512**	Gardnerella vaginalis, quantification	(I) 2.6	(I) 5.2	(I) 7.8
98.2	**87515**	hepatitis B virus, direct probe technique	(I) 1.2	(I) 2.6	(I) 3.8
98.2	**87516**	hepatitis B virus, amplified probe technique	(I) 2.2	(I) 4.4	(I) 6.6
98.2	**87517**	hepatitis B virus, quantification	(I) 2.6	(I) 5.4	(I) 8.0
98.2	**87520**	hepatitis C, direct probe technique	(I) 1.2	(I) 2.6	(I) 3.8
98.2	**87521**	hepatitis C, amplified probe technique	(I) 2.2	(I) 4.4	(I) 6.6
98.2	**87522**	hepatitis C, quantification	(I) 2.6	(I) 5.4	(I) 8.0
98.2	**87525**	hepatitis G, direct probe technique	(I) 1.2	(I) 2.6	(I) 3.8
98.2	**87526**	hepatitis G, amplified probe technique	(I) 2.2	(I) 4.4	(I) 6.6
98.2	**87527**	hepatitis G, quantification	(I) 2.6	(I) 5.2	(I) 7.8
98.2	**87528**	Herpes simplex virus, direct probe technique	(I) 1.2	(I) 2.6	(I) 3.8
98.2	**87529**	Herpes simplex virus, amplified probe technique	(I) 2.2	(I) 4.4	(I) 6.6
98.2	**87530**	Herpes simplex virus, quantification	(I) 2.6	(I) 5.4	(I) 8.0

UPD	Code	Description	Prof	Tech	Total
98.2	87531	Herpes virus-6, direct probe technique	(I) 1.2	(I) 2.6	(I) 3.8
98.2	87532	Herpes virus-6, amplified probe technique	(I) 2.2	(I) 4.4	(I) 6.6
98.2	87533	Herpes virus-6, quantification	(I) 2.6	(I) 5.2	(I) 7.8
98.2	87534	HIV-1, direct probe technique	(I) 1.2	(I) 2.6	(I) 3.8
98.2	87535	HIV-1, amplified probe technique	(I) 2.2	(I) 4.4	(I) 6.6
98.2	87536	HIV-1, quantification	(I) 2.6	(I) 5.2	(I) 7.8
98.2	87537	HIV-2, direct probe technique	(I) 1.2	(I) 2.6	(I) 3.8
98.2	87538	HIV-2, amplified probe technique	(I) 2.2	(I) 4.4	(I) 6.6
98.2	87539	HIV-2, quantification	(I) 2.6	(I) 5.4	(I) 8.0
98.2	87540	Legionella pneumophila, direct probe technique	(I) 1.2	(I) 2.6	(I) 3.8
98.2	87541	Legionella pneumophila, amplified probe technique	(I) 2.2	(I) 4.4	(I) 6.6
98.2	87542	Legionella pneumophila, quantification	(I) 2.6	(I) 5.2	(I) 7.8
98.2	87550	Mycobacteria species, direct probe technique	(I) 1.2	(I) 2.6	(I) 3.8
98.2	87551	Mycobacteria species, amplified probe technique	(I) 2.2	(I) 4.4	(I) 6.6
98.2	87552	Mycobacteria species, quantification	(I) 2.6	(I) 5.4	(I) 8.0
98.2	87555	Mycobacteria tuberculosis, direct probe technique	(I) 1.2	(I) 2.6	(I) 3.8
98.2	87556	Mycobacteria tuberculosis, amplified probe technique	(I) 2.2	(I) 4.4	(I) 6.6
98.2	87557	Mycobacteria tuberculosis, quantification	(I) 2.6	(I) 5.4	(I) 8.0
98.2	87560	Mycobacteria avium-intracellulare, direct probe technique	(I) 1.2	(I) 2.6	(I) 3.8
98.2	87561	Mycobacteria avium-intracellulare, amplified probe technique	(I) 2.2	(I) 4.4	(I) 6.6
98.2	87562	Mycobacteria avium-intracellulare, quantification	(I) 2.6	(I) 5.4	(I) 8.0
98.2	87580	Mycoplasma pneumoniae, direct probe technique	(I) 1.2	(I) 2.6	(I) 3.8
98.2	87581	Mycoplasma pneumoniae, amplified probe technique	(I) 2.2	(I) 4.4	(I) 6.6
98.2	87582	Mycoplasma pneumoniae, quantification	(I) 2.6	(I) 5.2	(I) 7.8
98.2	87590	Neisseria gonorrhoeae, direct probe technique	(I) 1.2	(I) 2.6	(I) 3.8
98.2	87591	Neisseria gonorrhoeae, amplified probe technique	(I) 2.2	(I) 4.4	(I) 6.6

UPD	Code	Description	Prof	Tech	Total
98.2	**87592**	Neisseria gonorrhoeae, quantification	(I) 2.6	(I) 5.4	(I) 8.0
98.2	**87620**	papillomavirus, human, direct probe technique	(I) 1.2	(I) 2.6	(I) 3.8
98.2	**87621**	papillomavirus, human, amplified probe technique	(I) 2.2	(I) 4.4	(I) 6.6
98.2	**87622**	papillomavirus, human, quantification	(I) 2.6	(I) 5.2	(I) 7.8
98.2	**87650**	Streptococcus, group A, direct probe technique	(I) 1.2	(I) 2.6	(I) 3.8
98.2	**87651**	Streptococcus, group A, amplified probe technique	(I) 2.2	(I) 4.4	(I) 6.6
98.2	**87652**	Streptococcus, group A, quantification	(I) 2.6	(I) 5.2	(I) 7.8
98.2	**87797**	not otherwise specified, direct probe technique	(I) 1.2	(I) 2.6	(I) 3.8
98.2	**87798**	not otherwise specified, amplified probe technique	(I) 2.2	(I) 4.4	(I) 6.6
98.2	**87799**	not otherwise specified, quantification	(I) 2.6	(I) 5.4	(I) 8.0
98.2	**87810**	Infectious agent detection by immunoassay with direct optical observation; Chlamydia trachomatis	(I) 0.8	(I) 1.7	(I) 2.5
98.2	**87850**	Neisseria gonorrhoeae	(I) 0.8	(I) 1.7	(I) 2.5
98.2	**87880**	Streptococcus, group A	(I) 0.8	(I) 1.7	(I) 2.5
98.2	**87899**	not otherwise specified	(I) 0.8	(I) 1.7	(I) 2.5
	87999	Unlisted microbiology procedure	BR	BR	BR

Anatomic Pathology

UPD	Code	Description	Prof	Tech	Total
98.2	**88000**	Necropsy (autopsy), gross examination only; without CNS	40.0	0.0	40.0
98.2	**88005**	with brain	45.0	0.0	45.0
98.2	**88007**	with brain and spinal cord	50.0	0.0	50.0
98.2	**88012**	infant with brain	42.0	0.0	42.0
98.2	**88014**	stillborn or newborn with brain	42.0	0.0	42.0
98.2	**88016**	macerated stillborn	40.0	0.0	40.0
98.2	**88020**	Necropsy (autopsy), gross and microscopic; without CNS	50.0	0.0	50.0
98.2	**88025**	with brain	55.0	0.0	55.0
98.2	**88027**	with brain and spinal cord	60.0	0.0	60.0
98.2	**88028**	infant with brain	52.0	0.0	52.0
98.2	**88029**	stillborn or newborn with brain	52.0	0.0	52.0
98.2	**88036**	Necropsy (autopsy), limited, gross and/or microscopic; regional	43.0	0.0	43.0

UPD		Code	Description	Prof	Tech	Total
98.2		**88037**	single organ	35.0	0.0	35.0
98.2		**88040**	Necropsy (autopsy); forensic examination	130.0	0.0	130.0
		88045	coroner's call	BR	BR	BR
		88099	Unlisted necropsy (autopsy) procedure	BR	BR	BR
98.1		**88104**	Cytopathology, fluids, washings or brushings, except cervical or vaginal; smears with interpretation	3.4	1.6	5.0
		88106	filter method only with interpretation	1.5	3.5	5.0
		88107	smears and filter preparation with interpretation	5.3	1.4	6.7
98.1		**88108**	Cytopathology, concentration technique, smears and interpretation (eg, Saccomanno technique)	(I) 6.0	(I) 1.5	(I) 7.5
		88125	Cytopathology, forensic (eg, sperm)	1.9	4.4	6.3
		88130	Sex chromatin identification; Barr bodies	0.7	1.7	2.4
		88140	peripheral blood smear, polymorphonuclear "drumsticks"	0.5	1.2	1.7
98.2	+	**88141**	Cytopathology, cervical or vaginal (any reporting system); requiring interpretation by physician (List separately in addition to code for technical service)	(I) 3.0	0.0	(I) 3.0
98.2	▲	**88142**	Cytopathology, cervical or vaginal (any reporting system), collected in preservative fluid, automated thin layer preparation; manual screening under physician supervision	2.0	5.5	7.5
98.2	●	**88143**	with manual screening and rescreening under physician supervision	(I) 3.0	(I) 5.5	(I) 8.5
98.2	●	**88144**	with manual screening and computer-assisted rescreening under physician supervision	(I) 2.0	(I) 7.5	(I) 9.5
98.2	●	**88145**	with manual screening and computer-assisted rescreening using cell selection and review under physician supervision	(I) 2.5	(I) 7.5	(I) 10.0
98.2	●	**88147**	Cytopathology smears, cervical or vaginal; screening by automated system under physician supervision	(I) 0.0	(I) 7.5	(I) 7.5
98.2	●	**88148**	screening by automated system with manual rescreening	(I) 2.0	(I) 7.5	(I) 9.5
98.2	▲	**88150**	Cytopathology, slides, cervical or vaginal; manual screening under physician supervision	0.6	1.6	2.2
97.2 M		**88151**	requiring interpretation by physician To report, see 88141	0.4	0.6	1.0
98.2	▲	**88152**	with manual screening and computer-assisted rescreening under physician supervision	0.8	3.5	4.3
98.2	●	**88153**	with manual screening and rescreening under physician supervision	(I) 2.0	(I) 5.5	(I) 7.5

UPD			Code	Description	Prof	Tech	Total
98.2	●		88154	with manual screening and computer-assisted rescreening using cell selection and review under physician supervision	(I) 2.0	(I) 7.5	(I) 9.5
98.2	▲	+	88155	Cytopathology, slides, cervical or vaginal, definitive hormonal evaluation (eg, maturation index, karyopyknotic index, estrogenic index) (List separately in addition to code(s) for other technical and interpretation services)	0.6	1.6	2.2
98.2	M		88156	Cytopathology, smears, cervical or vaginal, (the Bethesda System (TBS)), up to three smears; screening by technician under physician supervision To report, use 88164	1.2	2.8	4.0
97.2	M		88157	requring interpretation by physician To report, use 88141	(I) 2.5	(I) 3.5	(I) 6.0
98.2	M		88158	with manual cytotecnologist screening and automated rescreening under physician supervision To report, use 88166	0.7	6.8	7.5
98.1			88160	Cytopathology, smears, any other source; screening and interpretation	2.1	2.3	4.4
98.1			88161	preparation, screening and interpretation	2.4	3.4	5.8
			88162	extended study involving over 5 slides and/or multiple stains	2.1	4.9	7.0
98.2	●		88164	Cytopathology, slides, cervical or vaginal (the Bethesda System); manual screening under physician supervision	(I) 2.0	(I) 3.0	(I) 5.0
98.2	●		88165	with manual screening and rescreening under physician supervision	(I) 3.0	(I) 3.5	(I) 6.5
98.2	●		88166	with manual screening and computer-assisted rescreening under physician supervision	(I) 2.0	(I) 5.5	(I) 7.5
98.2	●		88167	with manual screening and computer-assisted rescreening using cell selection and review under physician supervision	(I) 2.5	(I) 5.5	(I) 8.0
			88170	Fine needle aspiration with or without preparation of smears; superficial tissue (eg, thyroid, breast, prostate)	7.2	1.8	9.0
			88171	deep tissue under radiologic guidance	2.1	6.3	8.4
98.1			88172	Evaluation of fine needle aspirate with or without preparation of smears; immediate cytohistologic study to determine adequacy of specimen(s)	(I) 5.0	(I) 1.3	(I) 6.3
98.1			88173	interpretation and report	(I) 10.0	(I) 2.5	(I) 12.5
98.2			88180	Flow cytometry; each cell surface marker	3.0	5.0	8.0
98.2			88182	cell cycle or DNA analysis	3.0	5.0	8.0
			88199	Unlisted cytopathology procedure	BR	BR	BR

UPD		Code	Description	Prof	Tech	Total
98.2	▲	88230	Tissue culture for non-neoplastic disorders; lymphocyte	(I) 5.5	(I) 13.0	(I) 18.5
98.2		88233	skin or other solid tissue biopsy	6.6	15.4	22.0
98.2		88235	amniotic fluid or chorionic villus cells	6.9	16.1	23.0
98.2	▲	88237	Tissue culture for neoplastic disorders; bone marrow, blood cells	(I) 6.0	(I) 14.0	(I) 20.0
98.2	▲	88239	solid tumor	(I) 6.9	(I) 16.1	(I) 23.0
98.2	●	88240	Cryopreservation, freezing and storage of cells, each cell line	(I) 0.6	(I) 1.4	(I) 2.0
98.2	●	88241	Thawing and expansion of frozen cells, each aliquot	(I) 0.6	(I) 1.4	(I) 2.0
98.2	▲	88245	Chromosome analysis for breakage syndromes; baseline Sister Chromatid Exchange (SCE), 20-25 cells	(I) 7.0	(I) 16.5	(I) 23.5
98.2	▲	88248	baseline breakage, score 50-100 cells, count 20 cells, 2 karyotypes (eg, for ataxia telangiectasia, Fanconi anemia, fragile X)	(I) 10.8	(I) 21.7	(I) 32.5
98.2	●	88249	score 100 cells, clastogen stress (eg, diepoxybutane, mitomycin C, ionizing radiation, UV radiation)	(I) 10.8	(I) 21.7	(I) 32.5
98.2	M	88250	Chromosome analysis for fragile X associated with fragile X-linked mental retardation, score 100 cells, count 20 cells, 2 karyotypes, with banding To report, use 88428	(I) 7.5	(I) 17.5	(I) 25.0
98.2	M	88260	Chromosome analysis; count 5 cells, screening, with banding To report, use 88261	5.3	12.5	17.8
98.2	▲	88261	Chromosome analysis; count 5 cells, 1 karyotype, with banding	8.9	20.7	29.6
		88262	count 15-20 cells, 2 karyotypes, with banding			
98.2		88263	count 45 cells for mosaicism, 2 karyotypes, with banding	7.2	16.8	24.0
98.2	●	88264	analyze 20-25 cells	(I) 8.6	(I) 9.9	(I) 18.5
		88267	Chromosome analysis, amniotic fluid or chorionic villus, count 15 cells, 1 karyotype, with banding			
98.2		88269	Chromosome analysis, in situ for amniotic fluid cells, count cells from 6-12 colonies, 1 karyotype, with banding	8.0	16.0	24.0
98.2	●	88271	Molecular cytogenetics; DNA probe, each (eg, FISH)	RNE	RNE	RNE
98.2	●	88272	chromosomal in situ hybridization, analyze 3-5 cells (eg, for derivatives and markers)	RNE	RNE	RNE
98.2	●	88273	chromosomal in situ hybridization, analyze 10-30 cells (eg, for microdeletions)	RNE	RNE	RNE

UPD		Code	Description	Prof	Tech	Total
98.2	●	88274	interphase in situ hybridization, analyze 25-99 cells	RNE	RNE	RNE
98.2	●	88275	interphase in situ hybridization, analyze 100-300 cells	RNE	RNE	RNE
		88280	Chromosome analysis; additional karyotypes, each study	1.7	3.9	5.6
98.2		88283	additional specialized banding technique (eg, NOR, C-banding)	3.3	7.7	11.0
		88285	additional cells counted, each study	0.9	2.1	3.0
98.2		88289	additional high resolution study	1.7	3.9	5.6
98.2	●	88291	Cytogenetics and molecular cytogenetics, interpretation and report	(I) 0.3	(I) 0.7	(I) 1.0
		88299	Unlisted cytogenetic study	BR	BR	BR

Surgical Pathology

UPD		Code	Description	Prof	Tech	Total
		88300	LEVEL I - Surgical pathology, gross examination only	1.8	0.5	2.3
		88302	LEVEL II - Surgical pathology, gross and microscopic examination: Appendix, Incidental; Fallopian Tube, Sterilization; Fingers/Toes, Amputation,Traumatic; Foreskin, Newborn; Hernia Sac, Any Location; Hydrocele Sac; Nerve; Skin, Plastic Repair; Sympathetic Ganglion; Testis, Castration; Vaginal Mucosa, Incidental; Vas Deferens, Sterilization	3.9	1.0	4.9
		88304	LEVEL III - Surgical pathology, gross and microscopic examination: Abortion, Induced; Abscess; Aneurysm - Arterial/Ventricular; Anus, Tag; Appendix, Other than Incidental; Artery, Atheromatous Plaque; Bartholin's Gland Cyst; Bone Fragment(s), Other than Pathologic Fracture; Bursa/Synovial Cyst; Carpal Tunnel Tissue; Cartilage, Shavings; Cholesteatoma; Colon, Colostomy Stoma; Conjunctiva - Biopsy/Pterygium; Cornea; Diverticulum - Esophagus/Small Bowel; Dupuytren's Contracture Tissue; Femoral Head, Other than Fracture; Fissure/Fistula; Foreskin, Other than Newborn; Gallbladder; Ganglion Cyst; Hematoma; Hemorrhoids; Hydatid of Morgagni; Intervertebral Disc; Joint, Loose Body; Meniscus; Mucocele, Salivary; Neuroma - Morton's/Traumatic; Pilonidal Cyst/Sinus; Polyps, Inflammatory - Nasal/Sinusoidal; Skin - Cyst/Tag/Debridement; Soft Tissue, Debridement; Soft Tissue, Lipoma; Spermatocele; Tendon/Tendon Sheath; Testicular Appendage; Thrombus or Embolus; Tonsil and/or Adenoids; Varicocele; Vas Deferens, Other than Sterilization; Vein, Varicosity	5.0	1.3	6.3

UPD		Code	Description	Prof	Tech	Total
98.2	▲	88305	Level IV - Surgical pathology, gross and microscopic examination: Abortion - Spontaneous/Missed; Artery, Biopsy; Bone Marrow, Biopsy; Bone Exostosis; Brain/meninges, Other than for Tumor Resection; Breast, Biopsy, Not Requiring Microscopic Evaluation of Surgical Margins; Breast, Reduction Mammoplasty; Bronchus, Biopsy; Cell Block Any Source; Cervix, Biopsy; Colon, Biopsy; Duodenum, Biopsy; Endocervix, Curettings/Biopsy; Endometrium, Curettings/Biopsy; Eosphagus, Biopsy; Extremity, Amputation, Traumatic; Fallopian Tube, Biopsy; Fallopian Tube, Ectopic pregnancy; Femoral Head, Fracture; Fingers/Toes, Amputation, Non-traumatic; Gingiva/Oral Mucosa, Biopsy; Heart Valve; Joint, Resection; Kidney, Biopsy; Larynx, Biopsy; Leiomyoma(s), Uterine Myomectomy - without Uterus; Lip, Biopsy/Wedge Resection; Lung, Transbronchial Biopsy; Lymph Node, biopsy; Muscle, Biopsy; Nasal Mucosa, Biopsy; Nasopharynx/Oropharynx, Biopsy; Nerve, Biopsy; Odotogenic/Dental Cyst; Omentum, Biopsy; Ovary with or without Tube, Non-neoplastic; Ovary, Biopsy/Wedge Resection; Parathyroid Gland; Peritoneum, Biopsy; Pituitary Tumor; Placenta, Other than Third Trimester; Pleura/Pericardium - Biopsy/Tissue; Polyp, Cervical/Endometrial; Polyp, Colorectal; Poly, Stomach/Small Bowel; Prostate, Needle Biopsy; Prostate, TUR; Salivary Gland, Biopsy; Sinus, Paranasal Biopsy; Skin, Other than Cyst/Tag/Debridement/Plastic Repair; Small Intestine, Biopsy; Soft Tissue, Other than Tumor/Mass/Lipoma/Debridement; Spleen; Stomach, Biopsy; Synovium; Testis, Other than Tumor/Biopsy/Castration; Thyroglossal duct/Brachial Cleft Cyst; Tongue, Biopsy; Tonsil, Biopsy; Trachea, Biopsy; Ureter, Biopsy; Urethra, Biopsy; Urinary Bladder, Biopsy; Uterus, wth or without Tubes and Ovaries, for Prolapse; Vagina, Biopsy; Vulva/Labia, Biopsy	7.8	2.0	9.8

UPD		Code	Description	Prof	Tech	Total
98.2	▲	88307	Level V - Surgical pathology, gross and microscopic examination: Adrenal, Resection; Bone - Biopsy/Curettings; Bone Gragment(s), Pathologic Fracture; Brain, Biopsy; Brain/Meninges, Tumor Resection; Breast, Excision of Lesion, Requiring Microscopic Evaluation of Surgical Margins; Breast, Mastectomy - Partial/Simple; Cervix, Conization; Colon, Segmental Resection, Other than for Tumor; Extremity, Amputation, Non-Traumatic; Eye, Enucleation; Kidney, Partial/Total Nephrectomy; Larynx, Partial/Total Resection; Liver, Biopsy - Needle/Wedge; Liver, Partial Resection; Lung, Wedge Biopsy; Lymph Nodes, Regional Resection; Mediastinum, Mass; Myocardium, Biopsy; Odontogenic Tumor; Ovary with or without Tube, Neoplastic; Pancreas, Biopsy; Placenta, Third Trimester; Prostate, Except Radical Resection; Salivary Gland; Small Intesting; Resection, Other than for Tumor; Soft Tissue Mass (except Lipoma) - Biopsy/Simple Excision; Stomach - Subtotal/Total Resection, Other than for Tumor; Testis, Biopsy; Thymus, Tumor; Thyroid, Total/Lobe; Ureter, Resection; Urinary Bladder, TUR; Uterus, with or without Tubes & Ovaries, Other than Neoplastic/Prolapse	16.0	4.0	20.0
		88309	LEVEL VI - Surgical pathology, gross and microscopic examination: Bone Resection; Breast, Mastectomy - with Regional Lymph Nodes; Colon, Segmental Resection for Tumor; Colon, Total Resection; Esophagus, Partial/Total Resection; Extremity, Disarticulation; Fetus, with Dissection; Larynx, Partial/Total Resection - with Regional Lymph Nodes; Lung - Total/Lobe/Segment Resection; Pancreas, Total/Subtotal Resection; Prostate, Radical Resection; Small Intestine, Resection for Tumor; Soft Tissue Tumor, Extensive Resection; Stomach - Subtotal/Total Resection for Tumor; Testis, Tumor; Tongue/Tonsil - Resection for Tumor; Urinary Bladder, Partial/Total Resection; Uterus, with or without Tubes & Ovaries, Neoplastic; Vulva, Total/Subtotal Resection	23.2	5.8	29.0
		88311	Decalcification procedure (List separately in addition to code for surgical pathology examination)	1.8	0.4	2.2
		88312	Special stains (List separately in addition to code for surgical pathology examination); Group I for microorganisms (eg, Gridley, acid fast, methenamine silver), each	0.7	1.5	2.2
		88313	Group II, all other, (eg, iron, trichrome), except immunocytochemistry and immunoperoxidase stains, each	0.7	1.5	2.2
		88314	histochemical staining with frozen section(s)	0.6	1.4	2.0
98.2		88318	Determinative histochemistry to identify chemical components (eg, copper, zinc)	1.3	1.7	3.0
98.2		88319	Determinative histochemistry or cytochemistry to identify enzyme constituents, each	1.2	1.3	2.5

UPD	Code	Description	Prof	Tech	Total
	88321	Consultation and report on referred slides prepared elsewhere	4.0	0.0	4.0
98.2	88323	Consultation and report on referred material requiring preparation of slides	7.0	0.0	7.0
	88325	Consultation, comprehensive, with review of records and specimens, with report on referred material	5.0	0.0	5.0
	88329	Pathology consultation during surgery;	4.7	0.0	4.7
	88331	with frozen section(s), single specimen	6.3	3.0	9.3
	88332	each additional tissue block with frozen section(s)	3.3	1.6	4.9
98.2	88342	Immunocytochemistry (including tissue immunoperoxidase), each antibody	3.3	1.6	4.9
	88346	Immunofluorescent study, each antibody; direct method	7.0	3.0	10.0
98.2	88347	indirect method	9.0	3.0	12.0
98.2	88348	Electron microscopy; diagnostic	13.1	4.1	17.2
98.2	88349	scanning	13.1	4.1	17.2
98.2	88355	Morphometric analysis; skeletal muscle	7.3	2.5	9.8
98.2	88356	nerve	7.3	2.5	9.8
98.2	88358	tumor	7.3	2.5	9.8
	88362	Nerve teasing preparations	RNE	RNE	RNE
	88365	Tissue in situ hybridization, interpretation and report	2.3	0.0	2.3
98.2	88371	Protein analysis of tissue by Western Blot, with interpretation and report;	(I) 1.5	(I) 3.0	(I) 4.5
98.2	88372	immunological probe for band identification, each	(I) 1.5	(I) 3.0	(I) 4.5
	88399	Unlisted surgical pathology procedure	BR	BR	BR

Other Procedures

UPD	Code	Description	Prof	Tech	Total
	89050	Cell count, miscellaneous body fluids (eg, CSF, joint fluid), except blood;	0.3	0.6	0.9
	89051	with differential count	0.4	0.8	1.2
	89060	Crystal identification by light microscopy with or without polarizing lens analysis, any body fluid (except urine)	0.4	0.8	1.2
	89100	Duodenal intubation and aspiration; single specimen (eg, simple bile study or afferent loop culture) plus appropriate test procedure	1.4	3.3	4.7

UPD		Code	Description	Prof	Tech	Total
		89105	collection of multiple fractional specimens with pancreatic or gallbladder stimulation, single or double lumen tube	1.8	4.1	5.9
		89125	Fat stain, feces, urine, or sputum	0.4	0.9	1.3
		89130	Gastric intubation and aspiration, diagnostic, each specimen, for chemical analyses or cytopathology;	1.2	2.9	4.1
		89132	after stimulation	0.6	1.3	1.9
		89135	Gastric intubation, aspiration, and fractional collections (eg, gastric secretory study); one hour	1.0	2.4	3.4
		89136	two hours	1.3	2.7	4.0
		89140	two hours including gastric stimulation (eg, histalog, pentagastrin)	1.5	3.1	4.6
		89141	three hours, including gastric stimulation	1.8	3.4	5.2
		89160	Meat fibers, feces	0.2	0.4	0.6
		89190	Nasal smear for eosinophils	0.3	0.6	0.9
98.2		89250	Culture and fertilization of oocyte(s)	65.0	10.0	75.0
97.2		89251	with co-culture of embryos	RNE	RNE	RNE
97.2		89252	Assisted oocyte fertilization, microtechnique (any method)	RNE	RNE	RNE
97.2		89253	Assisted embryo hatching, microtechniques (any method)	RNE	RNE	RNE
97.2		89254	Oocyte identification from follicular fluid	RNE	RNE	RNE
97.2		89255	Preparation of embryo for transfer (any method)	RNE	RNE	RNE
97.2		89256	Preparation of cryopreserved embryos for transfer (includes thaw)	RNE	RNE	RNE
97.2		89257	Sperm identification from aspiration (other than seminal fluid)	RNE	RNE	RNE
97.2		89258	Cryopreservation; embryo	RNE	RNE	RNE
97.2		89259	sperm	RNE	RNE	RNE
97.2		89260	Sperm isolation; simple prep (eg, sperm wash and swim-up) for insemination or diagnosis with semen analysis	RNE	RNE	RNE
97.2		89261	complex prep (eg, per col gradient, albumin gradient) for insemination or diagnosis with semen analysis	RNE	RNE	RNE
98.2	●	89264	Sperm identification from testis tissue, fresh or cryopreserved	RNE	RNE	RNE
		89300	Semen analysis; presence and/or motility of sperm including Huhner test (post coital)	0.7	1.4	2.1
		89310	motility and count	0.5	1.3	1.8

UPD	Code	Description	Prof	Tech	Total
	89320	complete (volume, count, motility and differential)	0.6	1.5	2.1
	89325	Sperm antibodies	0.5	1.3	1.8
	89329	Sperm evaluation; hamster penetration test	2.3	4.0	6.3
	89330	cervical mucus penetration test, with or without spinnbarkeit test	0.5	1.3	1.8
	89350	Sputum, obtaining specimen, aerosol induced technique (separate procedure)	0.6	1.1	1.7
	89355	Starch granules, feces	0.3	0.6	0.9
	89360	Sweat collection by iontophoresis	0.4	1.0	1.4
	89365	Water load test	0.7	1.6	2.3
	89399	Unlisted miscellaneous pathology test	BR	BR	BR

Medicine

Guidelines

I. **Separate Procedures:** Procedures identified as "(separate procedures)" are frequently included in the global value of other procedures. Listing of a "(separate procedure)" code and full value is appropriate if the procedure is not included in the global value of another. Listing of "(separate procedure)" codes is not appropriate when procedure is included in the global value of another.

II. **Unusual Service Or Procedure:** A service may necessitate skills and time of the physician over and above listed services and values. If substantiated "by report" (BR), additional values may be warranted. Use modifier -22 to indicate these procedures.

III. **Unlisted Service Or Procedure:** When a service or procedure provided is not adequately identified, use of the unlisted procedure code for the related anatomical area is appropriate. Most codes of this nature have 99 for the last two digits. Value should be substantiated "by report" (BR).

IV. **Procedures Without Specified Unit Values:** Procedures that have RNE or BR in the units column, should be substantiated "by report".

V. **By Report:** Value of a procedure should be established for any "by report" circumstance by identifying a similar service and justifying value difference. When a report is indicated, the report should include the following:

1. Accurate procedure definition or description;

2. Operative report;

3. Justification for procedural variance, when appropriate;

4. Similar procedure and value; and

5. Justification for value difference.

VI. **Reduced Values:** Under some circumstances, a value for a procedure may be reduced or eliminated. Use modifier -52 to identify reduced value services.

VII. **Concurrent Care:** When separate procedures or services are provided by two or more physicians on the same date, the use of modifier -75 is appropriate. Each physician would indicate his or her service(s) by adding -75 to the appropriate procedure(s). This modifier does not warrant any increase or reduction in value. This is no longer CPT compatible.

VIII. **Multiple Modifiers:** If circumstances require the use of more than one modifier with any one procedure code, modifier -99 should be added to the procedure code. Other modifiers are then attached to the procedure code and listed separately with appropriate values for each.

IX. **Materials Supplied By Physician:** Identify as 99070 or the appropriate HCPCS Level II code. The list of appropriately billable supplies for each CPT code is variable by contract. RVU's are not based on supply costs. However, traditional fees or conversion factors may be constructed to account for supplies required for a given code.

X. **Professional Component:** Values listed under the column heading "PROF" indicate the Professional Component to be billed with Modifier -26. If a Professional Component is justified, a value is listed under the heading "PROF." Values shown under the column heading "UNITS" are the appropriate value for billing that code without a modifier. Where a value appears in both the "PROF" column and the "UNITS" column, the difference between the two values ("UNITS" minus "PROF") is the Technical component, which should be billed using the code number plus Modifier -27 or -TC.

Medicine Section

UPD		Code	Description	Prof	Units	Anes

Immune Globulins

UPD		Code	Description	Prof	Units	Anes
98.2	●	90281	Immune globulin (IG), human, for intramuscular use		RNE	
98.2	●	90283	Immune globulin (IGIV), human, for intravenous use		RNE	
98.2	●	90287	Botulinum antitoxin, equine, any route		RNE	
98.2	●	90288	Botulism immune globulin, human, for intravenous use		RNE	
98.2	●	90291	Cytomegalovirus immune globulin (CMV-IGIV), human, for intravenous use		RNE	
98.2	●	90296	Diphtheria antitoxin, equine, any route		RNE	
98.2	●	90371	Hepatitis B immune globulin (HBIG), human, for intramuscular use		RNE	
98.2	●	90375	Rabies immune globulin (RIG), human, for intramuscular use and/or subcutaneous use		RNE	
98.2	●	90376	Rabies immune globulin, heat-treated (RIG-HT), human, for intramuscular and/or subcutaneous use		RNE	
98.2	●	90379	Respiratory syncytial virus immune globulin (RSV-IGIV), human, for intravenous use		RNE	
98.2	●	90384	Rho(D) immune globulin (RhIG), human, full-dose, for intramuscular use		RNE	
98.2	●	90385	Rho(D) immune globulin (RhIG), human, mini-dose, for intramuscular use		RNE	
98.2	●	90386	Rho(D) immune globulin (RhIGIV), human, for intravenous use		RNE	
98.2	●	90389	Tetanus immune globulin (TIG), human, for intramuscular use		RNE	
98.2	●	90393	Vaccinia immune globulin, human, for intramuscular use		RNE	
98.2	●	90396	Varicella-zoster immune globulin, human, for intramuscular use		RNE	
98.2	●	90399	Unlisted immune globulin		RNE	

Immunization Administration for Vaccines/Toxoids

UPD		Code	Description	Prof	Units	Anes
98.2	●	90471	Immunization administration (includes percutaneous, intradermal, subcutaneous, intramuscular and jet injections and/or intranasal or oral administration); single or combination vaccine/toxoid		(I) 2.0	
98.2	●	90472	two or more single or combination vaccines/toxoids		(I) 3.0	

UPD		Code	Description	Prof	Units	Anes

Vaccines, Toxoids

UPD		Code	Description	Prof	Units	Anes
98.2	●	90476	Adenovirus vaccine, type 4, live, for oral use		RNE	
98.2	●	90477	Adenovirus vaccine, type 7, live, for oral use		RNE	
98.2	●	90581	Anthrax vaccine, for subcutaneous use		RNE	
98.2	●	90585	Bacillus Calmette-Guerin vaccine (BCG) for tuberculosis, live, for percutaneous use		RNE	
98.2	●	90586	Bacillus Calmette-Guerin vaccine (BCG) for bladder cancer, live, for intravesical use		RNE	
98.2	●	90592	Cholera vaccine, live, for oral use		RNE	
98.2	●	90632	Hepatitis A vaccine, adult dosage, for intramuscular use		RNE	
98.2	●	90633	Hepatitis A vaccine, pediatric/adolescent dosage-2 dose schedule, for intramuscular use		RNE	
98.2	●	90634	Hepatitis A vaccine, pediatric/adolescent dosage-3 dose schedule, for intramuscular use		RNE	
98.2	●	90636	Hepatitis A and hepatitis B vaccine (HepA-HepB), adult dosage, for intramuscular use		RNE	
98.2	●	90645	Hemophilus influenza b vaccine (Hib), HbOC conjugate (4 dose schedule), for intramuscular use		RNE	
98.2	●	90646	Hemophilus influenza b vaccine (Hib), PRP-D conjugate, for booster use only, intramuscular use		RNE	
98.2	●	90647	Hemophilus influenza b vaccine (Hib), PRP-OMP conjugate (3 dose schedule), for intramuscular use		RNE	
98.2	●	90648	Hemophilus influenza b vaccine (Hib),PRP-T conjugate (4 dose schedule), for intramuscular use		RNE	
98.2	●	90657	Influenza virus vaccine, split virus, 6-35 months dosage, for intramuscular or jet injection use		RNE	
98.2	●	90658	Influenza virus vaccine, split virus, 3 years and above dosage, for intramuscular or jet injection use		RNE	
98.2	●	90659	Influenza virus vaccine, whole virus, for intramuscular or jet injection use		RNE	
98.2	●	90660	Influenza virus vaccine, live, for intranasal use		RNE	
98.2	●	90665	Lyme disease vaccine, adult dosage, for intramuscular use		RNE	
98.2	●	90669	Pneumococcal conjugate vaccine, polyvalent, for intramuscular use		RNE	
98.2	●	90675	Rabies vaccine, for intramuscular use		RNE	
98.2	●	90676	Rabies vaccine, for intradermal use		RNE	
98.2	●	90680	Rotavirus vaccine, tetravalent, live, for oral use		RNE	

UPD		Code	Description	Prof	Units	Anes
98.2	●	90690	Typhoid vaccine, live, oral		RNE	
98.2	●	90691	Typhoid vaccine, Vi capsular polysaccharide (ViCPs), for intramuscular use		RNE	
98.2	●	90692	Typhoid vaccine, heat- and phenol-inactivated (H-P), for subcutaneous or intradermal use		RNE	
98.2	●	90693	Typhoid vaccine, acetone-killed, dried (AKD), for subcutaneous or jet injection use (U.S. military)		RNE	
98.2	▲	90700	Diphtheria, tetanus toxoids, and acellular pertussis vaccine (DTaP), for intramuscular use		(I) 4.5	
98.2	▲	90701	Diphtheria, tetanus toxoids, and whole cell pertussis vaccine (DTP), for intramuscular use		(I) 4.0	
98.2	▲	90702	Diphtheria and tetanus toxoids (DT) adsorbed for pediatric use, for intramuscular use		(I) 2.5	
98.2	▲	90703	Tetanus toxoid adsorbed, for intramuscular or jet injection use		(I) 2.0	
98.2	▲	90704	Mumps virus vaccine, live, for subcutaneous or jet injection use		(I) 2.5	
98.2	▲	90705	Measles virus vaccine, live, for subcutaneous or jet injection use		(I) 2.5	
98.2	▲	90706	Rubella virus vaccine, live, for subcutaneous or jet injection use		(I) 2.5	
98.2	▲	90707	Measles, mumps and rubella virus vaccine (MMR), live, for subcutaneous or jet injection use		(I) 5.5	
98.2	▲	90708	Measles and rubella virus vaccine, live, for subcutaneous or jet injection use		(I) 3.5	
98.2	▲	90709	Rubella and mumps virus vaccine, live, for subcutaneous use		(I) 3.5	
98.2	▲	90710	Measles, mumps, rubella, and varicella vaccine (MMRV), live, for subcutaneous use		(I) 6.0	
98.2	▲	90712	Poliovirus vaccine, (any type(s)) (OPV), live, for oral use		(I) 3.0	
98.2	▲	90713	Poliovirus vaccine, inactivated, (IPV), for subcutaneous use		(I) 2.0	
98.2	▲	90716	Varicella virus vaccine, live, for subcutaneous use		(I) 7.5	
98.2	▲	90717	Yellow fever vaccine, live, for subcutaneous use		(I) 3.0	
98.2	▲	90718	Tetanus and diphtheria toxoids (Td) adsorbed for adult use, for intramuscular or jet injection		(I) 1.5	
98.2	▲	90719	Diphtheria toxoid, for intramuscular use		(I) 1.0	
98.2	▲	90720	Diphtheria, tetanus toxoids, and whole cell pertussis vaccine and Hemophilus influenza B vaccine (DTP-Hib), for intramuscular use		(I) 5.0	

UPD			Code	Description	Prof	Units	Anes
98.2		▲	**90721**	Diphtheria, tetanus toxoids, and acellular pertussis vaccine and Hemophilus influenza B vaccine (DtaP-Hib), for intramsucular use		(I) 6.0	
98.2	M		**90724**	90724 has been deleted. To report, see 90585, 90586		(I) 4.0	
98.2	M	▲	**90725**	Cholera vaccine for injectable use		(I) 3.0	
98.2	M		**90726**	90726 has been deleted. To report, see 90675, 90676		(I) 4.0	
98.2		▲	**90727**	Plague vaccine, for intramuscular or jet injection use		(I) 1.5	
98.2	M		**90728**	90728 has been deleted. To report, see 90585, 90586		(I) 3.0	
98.2	M		**90730**	90730 has been deleted. To report, see 90632-90634		(I) 8.7	
98.2		▲	**90732**	Pneumococcal polysaccharide vaccine, 23-valent, adult dosage, for subcutaneous or intramuscular use		(I) 4.0	
98.2		▲	**90733**	Meningocococcal polysaccharide vaccine (any group(s)), for subcutaneous or jet injection use		(I) 4.5	
98.2		▲	**90735**	Japanese encephalitis virus vaccine, for subcutaneous use		(I) 3.0	
98.2	M		**90737**	90737 has been deleted. To report, see 90645-90648		(I) 5.0	
98.2	M		**90741**	90741 has been deleted. To report, see 90281-90283		(I) 4.0	
98.2	M		**90742**	90742 has been deleted. To report, see90287-90399		(I) 6.5	
98.2		▲	**90744**	Hepatitis B vaccine, pediatric or pediatric/adolescent dosage, for intramuscular use		(I) 6.7	
98.2		▲	**90745**	Hepatitis B vaccine, adolescent/high risk infant dosage, for intramuscular use		(I) 7.7	
98.2		▲	**90746**	Hepatitis B vaccine, adult dosage, for intramuscular use		(I) 8.7	
98.2		▲	**90747**	Hepatitis B vaccine, dialysis or immunosuppressed patient dosage, for intramuscular use		(I) 9.7	
98.2		▲	**90748**	Hepatitis B and Hemophilus influenza b vaccine (HepB-Hib), for intramuscular use		RNE	
98.2		▲	**90749**	Unlisted vaccine/toxoid		BR	

Therapeutic or Diagnostic Infusions (Excludes Chemotherapy)

UPD			Code	Description	Prof	Units	Anes
			90780	IV infusion for therapy/diagnosis, administered by physician or under direct supervision of physician; up to one hour		11.0	
98.2		▲ +	**90781**	each additional hour, up to eight (8) hours (List separately in addition to code for primary procedure)		5.0	

Therapeutic or Diagnostic Injections

UPD	Code	Description	Prof	Units	Anes
	90782	Therapeutic or diagnostic injection (specify material injected); subcutaneous or intramuscular		2.5	
98.2	**90783**	intra-arterial		3.0	3
98.2	**90784**	intravenous		4.0	3
	90788	Intramuscular injection of antibiotic (specify)		2.5	
98.2	**90799**	Unlisted therapeutic or diagnostic injection		BR	3

Psychiatry

UPD	Code	Description	Prof	Units	Anes
97.2	**90801**	Psychiatric diagnostic interview examination		0.4 (per minute)	
97.2	**90802**	Interactive psychiatric diagnostic interview examination using play equipment, physical devices, language interpreter, or other mechanisms of communication		0.4 (per minute)	
97.2	**90804**	Individual psychotherapy, insight oriented, behavior modifying and/or supportive, in an office or outpatient facility, approximately 20 to 30 minutes face-to-face with the patient;		(I) 10.5	
97.2	**90805**	with medical evaluation and management services		(I) 13.5	
97.2	**90806**	Individual psychotherapy, insight oriented, behavior modifying and/or supportive, in an office or outpatient facility, approximately 45 to 50 minutes face-to-face with the patient;		(I) 19.0	
97.2	**90807**	with medical evaluation and management services		(I) 22.0	
97.2	**90808**	Individual psychotherapy, insight oriented, behavior modifying and/or supportive, in an office or outpatient facility, approximately 75 to 80 minutes face-to-face with the patient;		(I) 31.0	
97.2	**90809**	with medical evaluation and management services		(I) 34.0	
97.2	**90810**	Individual psychotherapy, interactive, using play equipment, physical devices, language interpreter, or other mechanisms of nonverbal communication, in an office or outpatient facility, approximately 20 to 30 minutes face-to-face with the patient;		(I) 13.5	
97.2	**90811**	with medical evaluation and management services		(I) 16.5	
97.2	**90812**	Individual psychotherapy, interactive, using play equipment, physical devices, language interpreter, or other mechanisms of nonverbal communication, in an office or outpatient facility, approximately 45 to 50 minutes face-to-face with the patient;		(I) 21.0	
97.2	**90813**	with medical evaluation and management services		(I) 24.0	

UPD		Code	Description	Prof	Units	Anes
97.2		**90814**	Individual psychotherapy, interactive, using play equipment, physical devices, language interpreter, or other mechanisms of nonverbal communication, in an office or outpatient facility, approximately 75 to 80 minutes face-to-face with the patient;		(I) 33.0	
97.2		**90815**	with medical evaluation and management services		(I) 36.0	
97.2		**90816**	Individual psychotherapy, insight oriented, behavior modifying and/or supportive, in an inpatient hospital, partial hospital or residential care setting, approximately 20 to 30 minutes face-to-face with the patient;		(I) 11.5	
97.2		**90817**	with medical evaluation and management services		(I) 14.5	
97.2		**90818**	Individual psychotherapy, insight oriented, behavior modifying and/or supportive, in an inpatient hospital, partial hospital or residential care setting, approximately 45 to 50 minutes face-to-face with the patient;		(I) 20.0	
97.2		**90819**	with medical evaluation and management services		(I) 23.0	
97.2	**M**	**90820**	Interactive medical psychiatric diagnostic interview examination To report, use 90802		0.4 (per minute)	
97.2		**90821**	Individual psychotherapy, insight oriented, behavior modifying and/or supportive, in an inpatient hospital, partial hospital or residential care setting, approximately 75 to 80 minutes face-to-face with the patient;		(I) 32.0	
97.2		**90822**	with medical evaluation and management services		(I) 35.0	
97.2		**90823**	Individual psychotherapy, interactive, using play equipment, physical devices, language interpreter, or other mechanisms of nonverbal communication, in an inpatient hospital, partial hospital or residential care setting, approximately 20 to 30 minutes face-to-face with the patient;		(I) 14.0	
97.2		**90824**	with medical evaluation and management services		(I) 17.0	
97.2	**M**	**90825**	Psychiatric evaluation of hospital records, other psychiatric reports, psychometric and/or projective tests, and other accumulated data for medical diagnostic purposes To report, use 90885		0.3 (per minute)	
97.2		**90826**	Individual psychotherapy, interactive, using play equipment, physical devices, language interpreter, or other mechanisms of nonverbal communication, in an inpatient hospital, partial hospital or residential care setting, approximately 45 to 50 minutes face-to-face with the patient;		(I) 22.0	

UPD		Code	Description	Prof	Units	Anes
97.2		**90827**	with medical evaluation and management services		(I) 25.0	
97.2		**90828**	Individual psychotherapy, interactive, using play equipment, physical devices, language interpreter, or other mechanisms of nonverbal communication, in an inpatient hospital, partial hospital or residential care setting, approximately 75 to 80 minutes face-to-face with the patient;		(I) 34.0	
97.2		**90829**	with medical evaluation and management services		(I) 37.0	
97.2	**M**	**90835**	Nacrosynthesis for psychiatric diagnostic and therapeutic purposes (eg, sodium amobarbital (Amytal) interview) To report, see 90865		0.3 (per minute)	
97.2	**M**	**90841**	Individual medical psychotherapy by a physician, with continuing medical diagnostic evaluation, and drug management when indicated, including insight oriented, behavior modifying or supportive psychotherapy (face to face with the patient); time unspecified		24.0	
97.2	**M**	**90842**	approximately 75 to 80 minutes To report, see 90808, 90809, 90821, 90822		(I) 31.0	
97.2	**M**	**90843**	approximately 20 to 30 minutes To report, see 90804, 90805, 90816, 90817		10.5	
97.2	**M**	**90844**	approximately 45 to 50 minutes To report, see 90806, 90807, 90818, 90819		19.0	
97.2		**90845**	Psychoanalysis		BR	
97.2		**90846**	Family psychotherapy (without the patient present)		0.4 (per minute)	
97.2		**90847**	Family psychotherapy (conjoint psychotherapy) (with patient present)		0.4 (per minute)	
97.2		**90849**	Multiple-family group psychotherapy		0.4 (per minute)	
97.2		**90853**	Group psychotherapy (other than of a multiple-family group)		6.2	
97.2	**M**	**90855**	Interactive individual medical psychotherapy To report, see 90810-90815, and 90823-90829		0.4 (per minute)	
97.2		**90857**	Interactive group psychotherapy		(I) 5.5	
		90862	Pharmacologic management, including prescription, use, and review of medication with no more than minimal medical psychotherapy		0.4 (per minute)	
97.2		**90865**	Narcosynthesis for psychiatric diagnostic and therapeutic purposes (eg, sodium amobarbital (Amytal) interview)		(I) 30.0	
		90870	Electroconvulsive therapy (includes necessary monitoring); single seizure		10.0	4

UPD		Code	Description	Prof	Units	Anes
		90871	multiple seizures, per day		BR	4
97.2		90875	Individual psychophysiological therapy incorporating biofeedback training by any modality (face-to-face with the patient), with psychotherapy (eg, insight oriented, behavior modifying or supportive psychotherapy); approximately 20-30 minutes		(I) 8.5	
96.2		90876	approximately 45-50 minutes		(I) 17.0	
97.2		90880	Hypnotherapy		0.4 (per minute)	
		90882	Environmental intervention for medical management purposes on a psychiatric patient's behalf with agencies, employers, or institutions		0.3 (per minute)	
97.2		90885	Psychiatric evaluation of hospital records, other psychiatric reports, psychometric and/or projective tests, and other accumulated data for medical diagnostic purposes		(I) 7.0	
		90887	Interpretation or explanation of results of psychiatric, other medical examinations and procedures, or other accumulated data to family or other responsible persons, or advising them how to assist patient		0.4 (per minute)	
		90889	Preparation of report of patient's psychiatric status, history, treatment, or progress (other than for legal or consultative purposes) for other physicians, agencies, or insurance carriers		0.3 (per minute)	
		90899	Unlisted psychiatric service or procedure		BR	

Biofeedback

UPD		Code	Description	Prof	Units	Anes
96.2	M	90900	Biofeedback training; by electromyogram application (eg, in tension headache, muscle spasm) To report, see 90901		0.3 (per minute)	
96.2		90901	Biofeedback training by any modality		0.3 (per minute)	
96.2	M	90902	in conduction disorder (eg, arrhythmia) To report, see 90901		0.3 (per minute)	
96.2	M	90904	regulation of blood pressure (eg, in essential hypertension) To report, see 90901		0.3 (per minute)	
96.2	M	90906	regulation of skin temperature or peripheral blood flow To report, see 90901		0.3 (per minute)	
96.2	M	90908	by electroencephalogram application (eg, in anxiety, insomnia) To report, see 90901		0.3 (per minute)	

UPD		Code	Description	Prof	Units	Anes
96.2	M	90910	by electro-oculogram application (eg, in blepharospasm) To report, see 90901		0.3 (per minute)	
97.2		90911	Biofeedback training, perineal muscles, anorectal or urethral sphincter, including EMG and/or manometry		0.3 (per minute)	
96.2	M	90915	Biofeedback training; other To report, see 90901		BR	

Dialysis

UPD	Code	Description	Prof	Units	Anes
	90918	End stage renal disease (ESRD) related services per full month; for patients under 2 years of age to include monitoring for the adequacy of nutrition, assessment of growth and development, and counseling of parents		(I) 160.0	
	90919	for patients between two and eleven years of age to include monitoring for the adequacy of nutrition, assessment of growth and development, and counseling of parents		(I) 120.0	
	90920	for patients between twelve and nineteen years of age to include monitoring for the adequacy of nutrition, assessment of growth and development, and counseling of parents		(I) 100.0	
	90921	for patients twenty years of age and over		(I) 55.0	
	90922	End stage renal disease (ESRD) related services (less than full month), per day; for patients under two years of age		(I) 7.5	
	90923	for patients between two and eleven years of age		(I) 5.0	
	90924	for patients between twelve and nineteen years of age		(I) 4.0	
	90925	for patients twenty years of age and over		(I) 3.0	
	90935	Hemodialysis procedure with single physician evaluation		(I) 20.0	
	90937	Hemodialysis procedure requiring repeated evaluation(s) with or without substantial revision of dialysis prescription		(I) 45.0	
	90945	Dialysis procedure other than hemodialysis (eg, peritoneal, hemofiltration), with single physician evaluation		(I) 16.0	
	90947	Dialysis procedure other than hemodialysis (eg, peritoneal, hemofiltration) requiring repeated evaluations, with or without substantial revision of dialysis prescription		(I) 38.0	
	90989	Dialysis training, patient, including helper where applicable, any mode, completed course		(I) 50.0	

UPD	Code	Description	Prof	Units	Anes
	90993	Dialysis training, patient, including helper where applicable, any mode, course not completed, per training session	(I) 12.0		
	90997	Hemoperfusion (eg, with activated charcoal or resin)		90.0	
	90999	Unlisted dialysis procedure, inpatient or outpatient		BR	

Gastroenterology

UPD	Code	Description	Prof	Units	Anes
98.2	91000	Esophageal intubation and collection of washings for cytology, including preparation of specimens (separate procedure)	(I) 10.5	13.0	5
98.2	91010	Esophageal motility (manometric study of the esophagus and/or gastroesophageal junction) study;	(I) 16.5	26.0	5
98.2	91011	with mecholyl or similar stimulant	(I) 17.5	28.0	5
98.2	91012	with acid perfusion studies	(I) 19.0	30.0	5
98.2	91020	Gastric motility (manometric) studies	(I) 8.5	30.0	5
98.2	91030	Esophagus, acid perfusion (Bernstein) test for esophagitis	(I) 8.0	12.5	5
98.2	91032	Esophagus, acid reflux test, with intraluminal pH electrode for detection of gastroesophageal reflux;	(I) 8.3	13.0	5
98.2	91033	prolonged recording	(I) 10.5	19.0	5
98.2	91052	Gastric analysis test with injection of stimulant of gastric secretion (eg, histamine, insulin, pentagastrin, calcium and secretin)	(I) 9.0	15.5	5
98.2	91055	Gastric intubation, washings, and preparing slides for cytology (separate procedure)	(I) 10.0	15.0	5
98.2	91060	Gastric saline load test	(I) 5.0	8.5	5
	91065	Breath hydrogen test (eg, for detection of lactase deficiency)	(I) 11.5	19.0	
98.2	91100	Intestinal bleeding tube, passage, positioning and monitoring		14.0	5
98.2	91105	Gastric intubation, and aspiration or lavage for treatment (eg, for ingested poisons)		8.2	5
	91122	Anorectal manometry	(I) 9.5	16.0	
98.2	91299	Unlisted diagnostic gastroenterology procedure		BR	5

Ophthalmology

UPD	Code	Description	Prof	Units	Anes
	92002	Ophthalmological services: medical examination and evaluation with initiation of diagnostic and treatment program; intermediate, new patient		11.0	
	92004	comprehensive, new patient, one or more visits		17.5	

UPD		Code	Description	Prof	Units	Anes
		92012	Ophthalmological services: medical examination and evaluation, with initiation or continuation of diagnostic and treatment program; intermediate, established patient		8.0	
		92014	comprehensive, established patient, one or more visits		14.5	
98.2		**92015**	Determination of refractive state		(I) 4.0	4
		92018	Ophthalmological examination and evaluation, under general anesthesia, with or without manipulation of globe for passive range of motion or other manipulation to facilitate diagnostic examination; complete		19.0	4
98.2		**92019**	limited		15.0	4
		92020	Gonioscopy (separate procedure)		10.0	
96.2		**92060**	Sensorimotor examination with multiple measurements of ocular deviation (eg, restrictive or paretic muscle with diplopia) with interpretation and report (separate procedure)	(I) 6.0	8.0	
96.2		**92065**	Orthoptic and/or pleoptic training, with continuing medical direction and evaluation	(I) 4.0	6.0	
98.2		**92070**	Fitting of contact lens for treatment of disease, including supply of lens		28.0	4
96.2		**92081**	Visual field examination, unilateral or bilateral, with interpretation and report; limited examination (eg, tangent screen, Autoplot, arc perimeter, or single stimulus level automated test, such as Octopus 3 or 7 equivalent)	(I) 5.5	7.5	
96.2		**92082**	intermediate examination (eg, at least 2 isopters on Goldmann perimeter, or semiquantitative, automated suprathreshold screening program, Humphrey suprathreshold automatic diagnostic test, Octopus program 33)	(I) 7.5	9.5	
96.2		**92083**	extended examination (eg, Goldmann visual fields with at least 3 isopters plotted and static determination within	(I) 10.0	12.5	
		92100	Serial tonometry (separate procedure) with multiple measurements of intraocular pressure over an extended time period with interpretation and report, same day (eg, diurnal curve or medical treatment of acute elevation of intraocular pressure)		4.0	
		92120	Tonography with interpretation and report, recording indentation tonometer method or perilimbal suction method		4.8	
		92130	Tonography with water provocation		5.0	
98.2	●	**92135**	Scanning computerized ophthalmic diagnostic imaging (eg, scanning laser) with interpretation and report, unilateral	(I) 3.0	5.0	5

UPD	Code	Description	Prof	Units	Anes
	92140	Provocative tests for glaucoma, with interpretation and report, without tonography		5.3	
	92225	Ophthalmoscopy, extended, with retinal drawing (eg, for retinal detachment, melanoma), with interpretation and report; initial		8.0	4
	92226	subsequent		7.0	4
98.2	92230	Fluorescein angioscopy with interpretation and report		20.0	5
98.2	92235	Fluorescein angiography (includes multiframe imaging) with interpretation and report	(I) 12.0	20.5	5
98.2	92240	Indocyanine-green angiography (includes multiframe imaging) with interpretation and report)	(I) 14.0	(I) 23.0	5
96.2	92250	Fundus photography with interpretation and report	(I) 13.0	16.5	4
98.2	92260	Ophthalmodynamometry		11.0	5
98.2	92265	Needle oculoelectromyography, one or more extraocular muscles, one or both eyes, with interpretation and report	(I) 15.0	17.5	5
98.2	92270	Electro-oculography with interpretation and report	(I) 15.0	17.5	5
98.2	92275	Electroretinography with interpretation and report	(I) 15.0	17.5	5
98.2	92283	Color vision examination, extended, eg, anomaloscope or equivalent	(I) 7.0	10.0	5
98.2	92284	Dark adaptation examination, with interpretation and report	(I) 6.0	8.5	5
98.2	92285	External ocular photography with interpretation and report for documentation of medical progress (eg, close-up photography, slit lamp photography, goniophotography, stereophotography)	(I) 2.5	3.5	5
98.2	92286	Special anterior segment photography with interpretation and report; with specular endothelial microscopy and cell count	(I) 13.0	15.0	5
98.2	92287	with fluorescein angiography		12.0	5
	92310	Prescription of optical and physical characteristics of and fitting of contact lens, with medical supervision of adaptation; corneal lens, both eyes, except for aphakia		24.0	
	92311	corneal lens for aphakia, one eye		26.0	
	92312	corneal lens for aphakia, both eyes		28.0	
	92313	corneoscleral lens		28.0	
	92314	Prescription of optical and physical characteristics of contact lens, with medical supervision of adaptation and direction of fitting by independent technician; corneal lens, both eyes, except for aphakia		17.0	

UPD	Code	Description	Prof	Units	Anes
	92315	corneal lens for aphakia, one eye		19.0	
	92316	corneal lens for aphakia, both eyes		21.0	
	92317	corneoscleral lens		23.0	
	92325	Modification of contact lens (separate procedure), with medical supervision of adaptation		7.0	
	92326	Replacement of contact lens		8.0	
98.2	92330	Prescription, fitting, and supply of ocular prosthesis (artificial eye), with medical supervision of adaptation		28.0	5
98.2	92335	Prescription of ocular prosthesis (artificial eye) and direction of fitting and supply by independent technician, with medical supervision of adaptation		21.0	5
	92340	Fitting of spectacles, except for aphakia; monofocal		5.0	
	92341	bifocal		6.0	
	92342	multifocal, other than bifocal		6.2	
	92352	Fitting of spectacle prosthesis for aphakia; monofocal		6.0	
	92353	multifocal		6.2	
	92354	Fitting of spectacle mounted low vision aid; single element system		6.0	
	92355	telescopic or other compound lens system		6.5	
	92358	Prosthesis service for aphakia, temporary (disposable or loan, including materials)		14.0	
	92370	Repair and refitting spectacles; except for aphakia		5.0	
	92371	spectacle prosthesis for aphakia		5.2	
	92390	Supply of spectacles, except prosthesis for aphakia and low vision aids		BR	
	92391	Supply of contact lenses, except prosthesis for aphakia		BR	
	92392	Supply of low vision aids (A low vision aid is any lens or device used to aid or improve visual function in a person whose vision cannot be normalized by conventional spectacle correction. Includes reading additions up to 4D.)		BR	
	92393	Supply of ocular prosthesis (artificial eye)		BR	
	92395	Supply of permanent prosthesis for aphakia; spectacles		BR	
	92396	contact lenses		BR	
98.2	92499	Unlisted ophthalmological service or procedure		BR	5

UPD	Code	Description	Prof	Units	Anes

Special Otorhinolaryngologic Services

UPD	Code	Description	Prof	Units	Anes
98.2	92502	Otolaryngologic examination under general anesthesia		8.0	5
	92504	Binocular microscopy (separate diagnostic procedure)		5.0	
	92506	Evaluation of speech, language, voice, communication, auditory processing, and/or aural rehabilitation status		(I) 14.7	
	92507	Treatment of speech, language, voice, communication, and/or auditory processing disorder (includes aural rehabilitation); individual		(I) 9.0	
	92508	group, two or more individuals		(I) 4.5	
	92510	Aural rehabilitation following cochlear implant (includes evaluation of aural rehabilitation status and hearing, therapeutic services) with or without speech processor programming		(I) 25.5	
98.2	92511	Nasopharyngoscopy with endoscope (separate procedure)		12.0	5
98.2	92512	Nasal function studies (eg, rhinomanometry)		BR	5
98.2	92516	Facial nerve function studies (eg, electroneuronography)		(I) 7.5	5
98.2	92520	Laryngeal function studies		BR	6
	92525	Evaluation of swallowing and oral function for feeding		(I) 27.4	
	92526	Treatment of swallowing dysfunction and/or oral function for feeding		(I) 11.0	
	92531	Spontaneous nystagmus, including gaze		2.5	
	92532	Positional nystagmus		3.4	
	92533	Caloric vestibular test, each irrigation (binaural, bithermal stimulation constitutes four tests)		2.0	
	92534	Optokinetic nystagmus		1.0	
	92541	Spontaneous nystagmus test, including gaze and fixation nystagmus, with recording	(I) 3.5	10.0	
	92542	Positional nystagmus test, minimum of 4 positions, with recording	(I) 4.0	12.0	
	92543	Caloric vestibular test, each irrigation (binaural, bithermal stimulation constitutes four tests), with recording	(I) 2.5	8.3	
	92544	Optokinetic nystagmus test, bidirectional, foveal or peripheral stimulation, with recording	(I) 1.0	(I) 5.5	
	92545	Oscillating tracking test, with recording	(I) 2.0	7.0	

UPD			Code	Description	Prof	Units	Anes
			92546	Sinusoidal vertical axis rotational testing	(I) 5.0	(I) 8.5	
98.2	▲	+	92547	Use of vertical electrodes (List separately in addition to code for primary procedure)		2.2	
96.2			92548	Computerized dynamic posturography	(I) 9.0	(I) 22.0	
			92551	Screening test, pure tone, air only		3.5	
			92552	Pure tone audiometry (threshold); air only		3.5	
			92553	air and bone		5.0	
			92555	Speech audiometry threshold;		2.5	
			92556	with speech recognition		5.0	
			92557	Comprehensive audiometry threshold evaluation and speech recognition (92553 and 92556 combined)		11.0	
			92559	Audiometric testing of groups		3.5	
			92560	Bekesy audiometry; screening		2.0	
			92561	diagnostic		4.0	
			92562	Loudness balance test, alternate binaural or monaural		1.5	
			92563	Tone decay test		1.5	
			92564	Short increment sensitivity index (SISI)		1.5	
			92565	Stenger test, pure tone		1.5	
			92567	Tympanometry (impedance testing)		2.5	
			92568	Acoustic reflex testing		2.0	
			92569	Acoustic reflex decay test		2.0	
			92571	Filtered speech test		1.5	
			92572	Staggered spondaic word test		1.6	
			92573	Lombard test		1.6	
			92575	Sensorineural acuity level test		1.6	
			92576	Synthetic sentence identification test		1.6	
			92577	Stenger test, speech		1.6	
96.2			92579	Visual reinforcement audiometry (VRA)		(I) 7.0	
			92582	Conditioning play audiometry		3.0	
			92583	Select picture audiometry		3.0	
98.2			92584	Electrocochleography		13.5	5

UPD	Code	Description	Prof	Units	Anes
	92585	Auditory evoked potentials for evoked response audiometry and/or testing of the central nervous system	6.0	30.0	
	92587	Evoked otoacoustic emissions; limited (single stimulus level, either transient or distortion products)	(I) 3.0	(I) 12.0	
	92588	comprehensive or diagnostic evaluation (comparison of transient and/or distortion product otoacoustic emissions at multiple levels and frequencies)	(I) 5.0	(I) 17.5	
	92589	Central auditory function test(s) (specify)		BR	
	92590	Hearing aid examination and selection; monaural		11.0	
	92591	binaural		16.5	
	92592	Hearing aid check; monaural		4.0	
	92593	binaural		6.0	
	92594	Electroacoustic evaluation for hearing aid; monaural		4.0	
	92595	binaural		6.0	
	92596	Ear protector attenuation measurements		6.0	
96.2	92597	Evaluation for use and/or fitting of voice prosthetic or augmentative/alternative communication device to supplement oral speech		(I) 21.0	
96.2	92598	Modification of voice prosthetic or augmentative/alternative communication device to supplement oral speech		(I) 15.0	
	92599	Unlisted otorhinolaryngological service or procedure		BR	

Cardiovascular

UPD	Code	Description	Prof	Units	Anes
	92950	Cardiopulmonary resuscitation (eg, in cardiac arrest)		37.0	
	92953	Temporary transcutaneous pacing		(I) 55.0	
98.2	92960	Cardioversion, elective, electrical conversion of arrhythmia, external		50.0	4
	92970	Cardioassist-method of circulatory assist; internal		36.5	
	92971	external		14.0	
98.2	92975	Thrombolysis, coronary; by intracoronary infusion, including selective coronary angiography		93.0	7
98.2	92977	by intravenous infusion		83.0	7

UPD			Code	Description	Prof	Units	Anes
98.2	▲	+	92978	Intravascular ultrasound (coronary vessel or graft) during therapeutic intervention including imaging supervision, interpretation and report; initial vessel (List separately in addition to code for primary procedure)	60.0	85.0	
98.2		+	92979	each additional vessel (List separately in addition to code for primary procedure)	30.0	45.0	
98.2			92980	Transcatheter placement of an intracoronary stent(s), percutaneous, with or without other therapeutic intervention, any method; single vessel		(I) 315.0	7
98.2	▲	+	92981	each additional vessel (List separately in addition to code for primary procedure)		157.5	
98.2			92982	Percutaneous transluminal coronary balloon angioplasty; single vessel		(I) 250.0	8
98.2	▲	+	92984	each additional vessel (List separately in addition to code for primary procedure)		125.0	
98.2			92986	Percutaneous balloon valvuloplasty; aortic valve		(I) 430.0	11
98.2			92987	mitral valve		(I) 350.0	11
98.2			92990	pulmonary valve		(I) 360.0	11
98.2			92992	Atrial septectomy or septostomy; transvenous method, balloon, (eg, Rashkind type) (includes cardiac catheterization)		(I) 485.0	11
98.2			92993	blade method (Park septostomy) (includes cardiac catheterization)		(I) 515.0	11
98.2			92995	Percutaneous transluminal coronary atherectomy, by mechanical or other method, with or without balloon angioplasty; single vessel		(I) 211.8	8
98.2	▲	+	92996	each additional vessel (List separately in addition to code for primary procedure)		78.2	
98.2			92997	Percutaneous transluminal pulmonary artery balloon angioplasty; single vessel		(I) 209.0	8
98.2	▲	+	92998	each additional vessel (List separately in addition to code for primary procedure)		80.0	
			93000	Electrocardiogram, routine ECG with at least 12 leads; with interpretation and report		7.8	
			93005	tracing only, without interpretation and report		4.0	
			93010	interpretation and report only		4.5	
			93012	Telephonic transmission of post-symptom electrocardiogram rhythm strip(s), per 30 day period of time; tracing only		4.0	
			93014	physician review with interpretation and report only		4.5	

UPD		Code	Description	Prof	Units	Anes
		93015	Cardiovascular stress test using maximal or submaximal treadmill or bicycle exercise, continous electrocardiographic monitoring, and/or pharmacological stress; with physician supervision, with interpretation and report		37.0	
96.1		**93016**	physician supervision only, without interpretation and report		10.0	
		93017	tracing only, without interpretation and report		19.0	
96.1		**93018**	interpretation and report only		8.0	
		93024	Ergonovine provocation test	(I) 14.0	30.0	
		93040	Rhythm ECG, one to three leads; with interpretation and report		5.0	
		93041	tracing only without interpretation and report		3.0	
		93042	interpretation and report only		4.0	
96.2	M	**93201**	Phonocardiogram with or without ECG lead; with supervision during recording with interpretation and report (when equipment is supplied by the physician) To report, use 93799		12.5	
96.2	M	**93202**	tracing only, without interpretation and report (eg, when equipment is supplied by the hospital, clinic) To report, use 93799		6.5	
96.2	M	**93204**	interpretation and report To report, use 93799		7.5	
96.2	M	**93205**	Phonocardiogram with ECG lead, with indirect carotid artery and/or jugular vein tracing, and/or apex cardiogram; with interpretation and report To report, use 93799		13.0	
96.2	M	**93208**	tracing only, without interpretation and report To report, use 93799		7.0	
96.2	M	**93209**	interpretation and report only To report, use 93799		8.0	
	M	**93210**	Phonocardiogram, intracardiac To report, use 93799	(I) 8.0	(I) 9.0	
96.2	M	**93220**	Vectorcardiogram (VCG), with or without ECG; with interpretation and report To report, use 93799		15.0	
96.2	M	**93221**	tracing only, without interpretation and report To report, use 93799		8.0	
96.2	M	**93222**	interpretation and report only To report, use 93799		9.0	

UPD	Code	Description	Prof	Units	Anes
	93224	Electrocardiographic monitoring for 24 hours by continuous original ECG waveform recording and storage, with visual superimposition scanning; includes recording, scanning analysis with report, physician review and interpretation		40.0	
	93225	recording (includes hook-up, recording, and disconnection)		15.5	
	93226	scanning analysis with report		12.5	
	93227	physician review and interpretation		17.0	
	93230	Electrocardiographic monitoring for 24 hours by continuous original ECG waveform recording and storage without superimposition scanning utilizing a device capable of producing a full miniaturized printout; includes recording, microprocessor-based analysis with report, physician review and interpretation		40.0	
	93231	recording (includes hook-up, recording, and disconnection)		15.5	
	93232	microprocessor-based analysis with report		12.5	
	93233	physician review and interpretation		17.0	
	93235	Electrocardiographic monitoring for 24 hours by continuous computerized monitoring and non-continuous recording, and real-time data analysis utilizing a device capable of producing intermittent full-sized waveform tracings, possibly patient activated; includes monitoring and real time data analysis with report, physician review and interpretation		20.0	
	93236	monitoring and real-time data analysis with report		17.5	
	93237	physician review and interpretation		18.0	
	93268	Patient demand single or multiple event recording with presymptom memory loop, per 30 day period of time; includes transmission, physician review and interpretation	(I) 5.0	(I) 25.0	
	93270	recording (includes hook-up, recording and disconnection)		(I) 8.0	
	93271	monitoring, receipt of transmissions, and analysis		(I) 15.0	
	93272	physician review and interpretation only		(I) 5.0	
	93278	Signal-averaged electrocardiography (SAECG), with or without ECG	(I) 6.1	(I) 19.0	
96.2	93303	Transthoracic echocardiography for congenital cardiac anomalies; complete	(I) 20.0	(I) 55.0	
96.2	93304	follow-up or limited study	(I) 13.0	(I) 30.0	

UPD			Code	Description	Prof	Units	Anes
98.2			93307	Echocardiography, transthoracic, real-time with image documentation (2D) with or without M-mode recording; complete	(I) 20.0	(I) 59.0	7
98.2			93308	follow-up or limited study	(I) 13.0	(I) 33.0	7
98.2			93312	Echocardiography, transesophageal, real time with image documentation (2D) (with or without M-mode recording); including probe placement, image acquisition, interpretation and report	(I) 31.0	(I) 71.0	7
98.2			93313	placement of transesophageal probe only		(I) 17.0	7
98.2			93314	image acquisition, interpretation and report only	(I) 17.0	(I) 57.0	7
96.2			93315	Transesophageal echocardiography for congential cardiac anomalies; including probe placement, image acquisiston, interpretation and report	(I) 36.0	(I) 75.0	
98.2			93316	placement of transesophageal probe only		(I) 15.0	7
96.2			93317	image acquisition, interpretation and report only	(I) 24.0	(I) 60.0	
98.2	▲	+	93320	Doppler echocardiography, pulsed wave and/or continuous wave with spectral display (List separately in addition to codes for echocardiographic imaging); complete	10.5	28.0	
98.2	▲	+	93321	follow-up or limited study (List separately in addition to codes for echocardiographic imaging)	4.0	16.0	
98.2	▲	+	93325	Doppler echocardiography color flow velocity mapping (List separately in addition to codes for echocardiography)	16.2	31.5	
98.2			93350	Echocardiography, transthoracic, real-time with image documentation (2D, with or without M-mode recording) during rest and cardiovascular stress test using treadmill, bicycle exercise and/or pharmacologically induced stress, with interpretation and report	(I) 37.0	(I) 72.5	7
98.2	⊘		93501	Right heart catheterization	60.0	210.0	4
98.2	⊘		93503	Insertion and placement of flow directed catheter (eg, Swan-Ganz) for monitoring purposes		52.0	4
98.2	⊘		93505	Endomyocardial biopsy	65.0	90.0	7
98.2	⊘		93508	Catheter placement in coronary artery(s), arterial coronary conduit(s), and/or venous coronary bypass graft(s) for coronary angiography without concomitant left heart catheterization	55.0	155.0	7
98.2	⊘		93510	Left heart catheterization, retrograde, from the brachial artery, axillary artery or femoral artery; percutaneous	60.0	410.0	7
98.2	⊘		93511	by cutdown	60.0	410.0	7

UPD	Code	Description	Prof	Units	Anes
98.2	⊘ **93514**	Left heart catheterization by left ventricular puncture	110.0	440.0	7
98.2	⊘ **93524**	Combined transseptal and retrograde left heart catheterization	110.0	550.0	7
98.2	⊘ **93526**	Combined right heart catheterization and retrograde left heart catheterization	105.0	560.0	7
98.2	⊘ **93527**	Combined right heart catheterization and transseptal left heart catheterization through intact septum (with or without retrograde left heart catheterization)	130.0	580.0	7
98.2	⊘ **93528**	Combined right heart catheterization with left ventricular puncture (with or without retrograde left heart catheterization)	120.0	570.0	7
98.2	⊘ **93529**	Combined right heart catheterization and left heart catheterization through existing septal opening (with or without retrograde left heart catheterization)	70.0	510.0	7
98.2	⊘ **93530**	Right heart catheterization, for congenital cardiac anomalies	64.0	200.0	7
98.2	⊘ **93531**	Combined right heart catheterization and retrograde left heart catheterization, for congenital cardiac anomalies	112.0	500.0	7
98.2	⊘ **93532**	Combined right heart catheterization and transseptal left heart catheterization through intact septum with or without retrograde left heart catheterization, for congenital cardiac anomalies	140.0	520.0	7
98.2	⊘ **93533**	Combined right heart catheterization and transseptal left heart catheterization through existing septal opening, with or without retrograde left heart catheterization, for congenital cardiac anomalies	78.0	455.0	7
98.2	⊘ **93536**	Percutaneous insertion of intra-aortic balloon catheter		105.0	7
98.2	⊘ **93539**	Injection procedure during cardiac catheterization; for selective opacification of arterial conduits (eg, internal mammary), whether native or used for bypass		22.0	7
98.2	⊘ **93540**	for selective opacification of aortocoronary venous bypass grafts, one or more coronary arteries		22.0	7
98.2	⊘ **93541**	for pulmonary angiography		22.0	7
98.2	⊘ **93542**	for selective right ventricular or right atrial angiography		22.0	7
98.2	⊘ **93543**	for selective left ventricular or left atrial angiography		22.0	7
98.2	⊘ **93544**	for aortography		22.0	7

UPD		Code	Description	Prof	Units	Anes
98.2	⊘	93545	for selective coronary angiography (injection of radiopaque material may be by hand)		22.0	7
98.2	⊘	93555	Imaging supervision, interpretation and report for injection procedure(s) during cardiac catheterization; ventricular and/or atrial angiography	10.5	65.0	7
98.2	⊘	93556	pulmonary angiography, aortography, and/or selective coronary angiography including venous bypass grafts and arterial conduits (whether native or used in bypass)	11.5	100.0	7
98.2		93561	Indicator dilution studies such as dye or thermal dilution, including arterial and/or venous catheterization; with cardiac output measurement (separate procedure)	(I) 23.0	(I) 30.0	7
98.2		93562	subsequent measurement of cardiac output	(I) 10.0	(I) 15.0	7
98.2	● +	93571	Intravascular doppler velocity and/or pressure derived coronary flow reserve measurement (coronary vessel or graft) during coronary angiography including pharmacologically induced stress; initial vessel (List separately in addition to code for primary procedure)	(I) 20.0	(I) 54.0	
98.2	● +	93572	each additional vessel (List separately in addition to code for primary procedure)	(I) 16.0	(I) 50.0	
98.2		93600	Bundle of His recording	28.0	(I) 65.0	10
98.2		93602	Intra-atrial recording	28.0	(I) 45.0	10
98.2		93603	Right ventricular recording	28.0	(I) 55.0	10
98.2		93607	Left ventricular recording	28.0	(I) 65.0	10
98.2		93609	Intraventricular and/or intra-atrial mapping of tachycardia site(s) with catheter manipulation to record from multiple sites to identify origin of tachycardia	(I) 43.0	(I) 145.0	10
98.2		93610	Intra-atrial pacing	28.0	(I) 60.0	10
98.2		93612	Intraventricular pacing	28.0	(I) 65.0	10
98.2		93615	Esophageal recording of atrial electrogram with or without ventricular electrogram(s);	(I) 7.0	(I) 14.5	10
98.2		93616	with pacing	(I) 13.0	(I) 28.5	10
98.2		93618	Induction of arrhythmia by electrical pacing	(I) 50.0	(I) 125.0	10
98.2		93619	Comprehensive electrophysiologic evaluation with right atrial pacing and recording, right ventricular pacing and recording, His bundle recording, including insertion and repositioning of multiple electrode catheters; without induction or attempted induction of arhythmia (This code is to be used when 93600 is combined with 93602, 93603, 93610, 93612)	(I) 150.0	(I) 225.0	10

UPD			Code	Description	Prof	Units	Anes
98.2			**93620**	with induction or attempted induction of arrhythmia (This code is to be used when 93618 is combined with 936190)	(I) 200.0	(I) 300.0	10
98.2	▲		**93621**	with left atrial recordings from coronary sinus or left atrium, with or without pacing, with induction or attempted induction of arrhythmia	230.0	330.0	10
98.2	▲		**93622**	with left ventricular recordings, with or without pacing, with induction or attempted induction of arrhythmia	230.0	330.0	10
98.2	▲	+	**93623**	Programmed stimulation and pacing after intravenous drug infusion (List separately in addition to code for primary procedure)	80.0	85.0	
98.2			**93624**	Electrophysiologic follow-up study with pacing and recording to test effectiveness of therapy, including induction or attempted induction of arrhythmia	(I) 80.0	(I) 90.0	10
98.2			**93631**	Intra-operative epicardial and endocardial pacing and mapping to localize the site of tachycardia or zone of slow conduction for surgical correction	(I) 110.0	(I) 170.0	10
98.2			**93640**	Electrophysiologic evaluation of cardioverter-defibrillator leads (includes defibrillation threshold testing and sensing function) at time of initial implantation or replacement;	(I) 70.0	(I) 140.0	10
98.2			**93641**	with testing of cardioverter-defibrillator pulse generator	(I) 125.0	(I) 180.0	10
98.2			**93642**	Electrophysiologic evaluation of cardioverter-defibrillator (includes defibrillation threshold evaluation, induction of arrhythmia, evaluation of sensing and pacing for arrhythmia termination, and programming or reprogramming of sensing or therapeutic parameters)	(I) 85.0	(I) 155.0	10
98.2			**93650**	Intracardiac catheter ablation of atrioventricular node function, atrioventricular conduction for creation of complete heart block, with or without temporary pacemaker placement	(I) 180.0	(I) 240.0	10
98.2			**93651**	Intracardiac catheter ablation of arrhythmogenic focus; for treatment of supraventricular tachycardia by ablation of fast or slow atrioventricular pathways, accessory atrioventricular connections or other atrial foci, singly or in combination	(I) 270.0	(I) 315.0	10
98.2			**93652**	for treatment of ventricular tachycardia	(I) 290.0	(I) 330.0	10
			93660	Evaluation of cardiovascular function with tilt table evaluation, with continuous ECG monitoring and intermittent blood pressure monitoring, with or without pharmacological intervention	(I) 30.0	(I) 65.0	
			93720	Plethysmography, total body; with interpretation and report		10.0	
			93721	tracing only, without interpretation and report		7.0	
			93722	interpretation and report only		3.0	

UPD	Code	Description	Prof	Units	Anes
	93724	Electronic analysis of antitachycardia pacemaker system (includes electrocardiographic recording, programming of device, induction and termination of tachycardia via implanted pacemaker, and interpretation of recordings)	(I) 70.0	(I) 105.0	
	93731	Electronic analysis of dual-chamber pacemaker system (includes evaluation of programmable parameters at rest and during activity where applicable, using electrocardiographic recording and interpretation of recordings at rest and during exercise, analysis of event markers and device response); without reprogramming	7.0	12.0	
	93732	with reprogramming	9.0	14.0	
	93733	Electronic analysis of dual chamber internal pacemaker system (may include rate, pulse amplitude and duration, configuration of wave form, and/or testing of sensory function of pacemaker), telephonic analysis	3.2	(I) 10.5	
	93734	Electronic analysis of single chamber pacemaker system (includes evaluation of programmable parameters at rest and during activity where applicable, using electrocardiographic recording and interpretation of recordings at rest and during exercise, analysis of event markers and device response); without reprogramming	5.0	(I) 8.0	
	93735	with reprogramming	7.0	12.0	
	93736	Electronic analysis of single chamber internal pacemaker system (may include rate, pulse amplitude and duration, configuration of wave form, and/or testing of sensory function of pacemaker), telephonic analysis	2.2	(I) 8.5	
	93737	Electronic analysis of cardioverter/defibrillator only (interrogation, evaluation of pulse generator status); without reprogramming	(I) 6.0	(I) 11.5	
	93738	with reprogramming	(I) 9.0	(I) 15.0	
	93740	Temperature gradient studies	(I) 9.0	13.0	
	93760	Thermogram; cephalic	(I) 20.0	24.0	
	93762	peripheral	(I) 25.0	30.0	
	93770	Determination of venous pressure	2.5	(I) 4.0	
	93784	Ambulatory blood pressure monitoring, utilizing a system such as magnetic tape and/or computer disk, for 24 hours or longer; including recording, scanning analysis, interpretation and report		(I) 32.0	
	93786	recording only		(I) 11.0	
	93788	scanning analysis with report		(I) 10.0	
	93790	physician review with interpretation and report		(I) 12.0	

UPD	Code	Description	Prof	Units	Anes
	93797	Physician services for outpatient cardiac rehabilitation; without continuous ECG monitoring (per session)		(I) 8.0	
	93798	with continuous ECG monitoring (per session)		(I) 8.0	
	93799	Unlisted cardiovascular service or procedure		BR	

Non-Invasive Vascular Diagnostic Studies

UPD	Code	Description	Prof	Units	Anes
	93875	Noninvasive physiologic studies of extracranial arteries, complete bilateral study (eg, periorbital flow direction with arterial compression, ocular pneumoplethysmography, Doppler ultrasound spectral analysis)	(I) 8.0	(I) 20.0	
	93880	Duplex scan of extracranial arteries; complete bilateral study	(I) 10.0	(I) 42.0	
	93882	unilateral or limited study	(I) 9.0	(I) 24.0	
	93886	Transcranial Doppler study of the intracranial arteries; complete study	(I) 12.0	(I) 48.0	
	93888	limited study	(I) 8.0	(I) 38.0	
	93922	Noninvasive physiologic studies of upper or lower extremity arteries, single level, bilateral (eg, ankle/brachial indices, Doppler waveform analysis, volume plethysmography, transcutaneous oxygen tension measurement)	(I) 11.5	(I) 20.0	
	93923	Non-invasive physiologic studies of upper or lower extremity arteries, multiple levels or with provocative functional maneuvers, complete bilateral study (eg, segmental blood pressure measurements, segmental Doppler waveform analysis, segmental volume plethysmography, segmental transcutaneous oxygen tension measurements, measurements with postural provocative tests, measurements with reactive hyperemia)	(I) 17.0	(I) 28.0	
	93924	Non-invasive physiologic studies of lower extremity arteries, at rest and following treadmill stress testing, complete bilateral study	(I) 18.0	(I) 29.0	
	93925	Duplex scan of lower extremity arteries or arterial bypass grafts; complete bilateral study	(I) 10.0	(I) 40.0	
	93926	unilateral or limited study	(I) 5.0	(I) 30.0	
	93930	Duplex scan of upper extremity arteries or arterial bypass grafts; complete bilateral study	(I) 8.0	(I) 44.0	
	93931	unilateral or limited study	(I) 4.0	(I) 31.0	
	93965	Non-invasive physiologic studies of extremity veins, complete bilateral study (eg, Doppler waveform analysis with responses to compression and other maneuvers, phleborheography, impedance plethysmography)	(I) 8.0	(I) 18.0	

UPD		Code	Description	Prof	Units	Anes
		93970	Duplex scan of extremity veins including responses to compression and other maneuvers; complete bilateral study	(I) 10.0	(I) 36.0	
		93971	unilateral or limited study	(I) 5.0	(I) 26.0	
96.2		93975	Duplex scan of arterial inflow and venous outflow of abdominal, pelvic, scrotal contents and/or retroperitoneal organs; complete study	(I) 21.0	(I) 52.0	
		93976	limited study	(I) 10.5	(I) 37.0	
		93978	Duplex scan of aorta, inferior vena cava, iliac vasculature, or bypass grafts; complete study	(I) 10.0	(I) 44.0	
		93979	unilateral or limited study	(I) 5.0	(I) 31.0	
		93980	Duplex scan of arterial inflow and venous outflow of penile vessels; complete study	(I) 22.0	(I) 52.0	
		93981	follow-up or limited study	(I) 11.0	(I) 37.0	
		93990	Duplex scan of hemodialysis access (including arterial inflow, body of access and venous outflow)	(I) 4.0	(I) 28.0	

Pulmonary

UPD		Code	Description	Prof	Units	Anes
97.2		94010	Spirometry, including graphic record, total and timed vital capacity, expiratory flow rate measurement(s), with or without maximal voluntary ventilation	6.0	10.5	8
98.2	●	94014	Patient initiated spirometric recording per 30 day period of time; includes reinforced education, transmission of spirometric tracing, data capture, analysis of transmitted data, periodic recalibration and physician review and interpretation	(I) 5.0	(I) 8.5	
98.2	●	94015	recording (includes hook-up, reinforced education, data transmission, data capture, trend analysis, and periodic recalibration)	(I) 5.0	(I) 10.0	
98.2	●	94016	physician review and interpretation only		(I) 5.3	
98.2	▲	94060	Bronchospasm evaluation: spirometry as in 94010, before and after bronchodilator (aerosol or parenteral)	6.0	20.0	10
98.2	▲	94070	Prolonged postexposure evaluation of bronchospasm with multiple spirometric determinations after antigen, cold air, methacholine or other chemical agent, with subsequent spirometrics	4.0	35.0	10
		94150	Vital capacity, total (separate procedure)	0.9	2.2	1
97.1	M	94160	Vital capacity screening tests: total capacity, with timed forced expiratory volume (state duration), and peak flow rate For vital capacity measurement only, see 94150. For spirometry with timed expiratory volumes, see 94010	2.5	10.0	3

UPD		Code	Description	Prof	Units	Anes
		94200	Maximum breathing capacity, maximal voluntary ventilation	3.0	5.0	2
		94240	Functional residual capacity or residual volume: helium method, nitrogen open circuit method, or other method	4.0	15.0	3
		94250	Expired gas collection, quantitative, single procedure (separate procedure)	1.2	3.5	3
		94260	Thoracic gas volume	5.0	15.0	2
		94350	Determination of maldistribution of inspired gas: multiple breath nitrogen washout curve including alveolar nitrogen or helium equilibration time	5.0	15.0	3
		94360	Determination of resistance to airflow, oscillatory or plethysmographic methods	4.0	11.0	2
		94370	Determination of airway closing volume, single breath tests	1.5	7.0	2
		94375	Respiratory flow volume loop	5.0	15.0	8
		94400	Breathing response to CO2 (CO2 response curve)	27.5	30.0	8
		94450	Breathing response to hypoxia (hypoxia response curve)	27.5	30.0	8
98.2	▲	94620	Pulmonary stress testing; simple (eg, prolonged exercise test for bronchospasm with pre- and post-spirometry)	11.0	40.0	15
98.2	●	94621	complex (including measurements of CO2 production, O2 uptake, and electrocardiographic recordings)	(I)8.0	(I) 20.0	
		94640	Nonpressurized inhalation treatment for acute airway obstruction	1.5	4.5	2
		94642	Aerosol inhalation of pentamidine for pneumocystis carinii pneumonia treatment or prophylaxis		(I) 10.0	
		94650	Intermittent positive pressure breathing (IPPB) treatment, air or oxygen, with or without nebulized medication; initial demonstration and/or evaluation	1.5	4.5	2
		94651	subsequent		4.0	1
		94652	newborn infants		8.0	4
		94656	Ventilation assist and management, initiation of pressure or volume preset ventilators for assisted or controlled breathing; first day		28.0	10
		94657	subsequent days		10.0	5
		94660	Continuous positive airway pressure ventilation (CPAP), initiation and management		28.0	10
		94662	Continuous negative pressure ventilation (CNP), initiation and management		28.0	5

UPD	Code	Description	Prof	Units	Anes
	94664	Aerosol or vapor inhalations for sputum mobilization, bronchodilation, or sputum induction for diagnostic purposes; initial demonstration and/or evaluation		8.5	3
	94665	subsequent		7.0	1
	94667	Manipulation chest wall, such as cupping, percussing, and vibration to facilitate lung function; initial demonstration and/or evaluation		5.5	4
	94668	subsequent		4.0	2
	94680	Oxygen uptake, expired gas analysis; rest and exercise, direct, simple	27.5	55.5	3
	94681	including CO2 output, percentage oxygen extracted	27.5	55.5	3
	94690	rest, indirect (separate procedure)	4.5	30.5	3
	94720	Carbon monoxide diffusing capacity, any method	4.5	12.0	3
	94725	Membrane diffusion capacity	(I) 6.0	(I) 16.0	3
	94750	Pulmonary compliance study, any method	(I) 6.0	(I) 14.0	3
	94760	Noninvasive ear or pulse oximetry for oxygen saturation; single determination		(I) 8.0	
	94761	multiple determinations (eg, during exercise)		(I) 12.0	
	94762	by continuous overnight monitoring (separate procedure)		(I) 10.0	
	94770	Carbon dioxide, expired gas determination by infrared analyzer	(I) 5.0	(I) 9.0	1
	94772	Circadian respiratory pattern recording (pediatric pneumogram), 12 to 24 hour continuous recording, infant		BR	
	94799	Unlisted pulmonary service or procedure		BR	

Allergy and Clinical Immunology

UPD	Code	Description	Prof	Units	Anes
	95004	Percutaneous tests (scratch, puncture, prick) with allergenic extracts, immediate type reaction, specify number of tests		0.7/Test	
	95010	Percutaneous tests (scratch, puncture, prick) sequential and incremental, with drugs, biologicals or venoms, immediate type reaction, specify number of tests		1.4/Test	
	95015	Intracutaneous (intradermal) tests, sequential and incremental, with drugs, biologicals, or venoms, immediate type reaction, specify number of tests		1.6/Test	
	95024	Intracutaneous (intradermal) tests with allergenic extracts, immediate type reaction, specify number of tests		1.0/Test	

UPD	Code	Description	Prof	Units	Anes
	95027	Skin end point titration		8.3	
	95028	Intracutaneous (intradermal) tests with allergenic extracts, delayed type reaction, including reading, specify number of tests		2.0/Test	
96.2	95044	Patch or application test(s) (specify number of tests)		1.5/Test	
	95052	Photo patch test(s) (specify number of tests)		0.7/Test	
	95056	Photo tests		0.7	
	95060	Ophthalmic mucous membrane tests		1.5	
	95065	Direct nasal mucous membrane test		1.5	
	95070	Inhalation bronchial challenge testing (not including necessary pulmonary function tests); with histamine, methacholine, or similar compounds		(I) 22.0	
	95071	with antigens or gases, specify		(I) 25.0	
	95075	Ingestion challenge test (sequential and incremental ingestion of test items, eg, food, drug or other substance such as metabisulfite)		(I) 18.0	
	95078	Provocative testing (eg, Rinkel test)		5.0	
	95115	Professional services for allergen immunotherapy not including provision of allergenic extracts; single injection		2.5	
	95117	two or more injections		3.5	
	95120	Professional services for allergen immunotherapy in prescribing physician's office or institution, including provision of allergenic extract; single injection		3.0	
	95125	two or more injections		4.5/ Injection	
	95130	single stinging insect venom		5.0	
	95131	two stinging insect venoms		7.0	
	95132	three stinging insect venoms		8.0	
	95133	four stinging insect venoms		9.0	
	95134	five stinging insect venoms		10.0	
	95144	Professional services for the supervision and provision of antigens for allergen immunotherapy, single or multiple antigens, single dose vials (specify number of vials)		(I) 1.4/Vial	
	95145	Professional services for the supervision and provision of antigens for allergen immunotherapy (specify number of doses); single stinging insect venom		4.0/Per dose	

UPD	Code	Description	Prof	Units	Anes
	95146	two single stinging insect venoms		4.5/Per dose	
	95147	three single stinging insect venoms		5.6/Per dose	
	95148	four single stinging insect venoms		6.7/Per dose	
	95149	five single stinging insect venoms		7.8/Per dose	
	95165	Professional services for the supervision and provision of antigens for allergen immunotherapy; single or multiple antigens (specify number of doses)		(I) 1.8/Per dose	
	95170	whole body extract of biting insect or other arthropod (specify number of doses)		BR	
	95180	Rapid desensitization procedure, each hour (eg, insulin, penicillin, horse serum)		30.0	
	95199	Unlisted allergy/clinical immunologic service or procedure		BR	

Neurology and Neuromuscular Procedures

UPD	Code	Description	Prof	Units	Anes
97.2	95805	Multiple sleep latency or maintenance of wakefulness testing, recording, analysis and interpretation of physiological measurements of sleep during multiple trials to assess sleepiness	(I) 10.0	(I) 31.0	
97.2	95806	Sleep study, simultaneous recording of ventilation, respiratory effort, ECG or heart rate, and oxygen saturation, unattended by a technologist	(I) 30.0	(I) 70.0	
97.2	95807	Sleep study, simultaneous recording of ventilation, respiratory effort, ECG or heart rate, and oxygen saturation, attended by a technologist	(I) 8.0	(I) 35.0	
	95808	Polysomnography; sleep staging with 1-3 additional parameters of sleep, attended by a technologist	(I) 16.0	(I) 62.0	
	95810	sleep staging with 4 or more additional parameters of sleep, attended by a technologist	(I) 23.0	(I) 103.0	
97.2	95811	Polysomnography; sleep staging with 4 or more additional parameters of sleep, with initiation of continuous positive airway pressure therapy or bilevel ventilation, attended by a technologist	(I) 50.0	(I) 100.0	
	95812	Electroencephalogram (EEG) extended monitoring; up to one hour	(I) 17.0	(I) 35.0	
	95813	greater than one hour	(I) 19.0	(I) 40.0	
	95816	Electroencephalogram (EEG) including recording awake and drowsy, with hyperventilation and/or photic stimulation	(I) 5.0	(I) 21.0	

UPD	Code	Description	Prof	Units	Anes
	95819	Electroencephalogram (EEG) including recording awake and asleep, with hyperventilation and/or photic stimulation	(I) 5.0	(I) 23.0	
	95822	Electroencephalogram (EEG); sleep only	(I) 4.0	(I) 19.0	
	95824	cerebral death evaluation only	(I) 7.0	(I) 25.0	
	95827	all night sleep only	BR	BR	
	95829	Electrocorticogram at surgery (separate procedure)	(I) 55.0	(I) 60.0	
	95830	Insertion by physician of sphenoidal electrodes for electroencephalographic (EEG) recording		(I) 20.0	
	95831	Muscle testing, manual (separate procedure); extremity (excluding hand) or trunk, with report		4.5	
	95832	hand (with or without comparison with normal side)		7.0	
	95833	total evaluation of body, excluding hands		15.0	
	95834	total evaluation of body, including hands		18.0	
	95851	Range of motion measurements and report (separate procedure); each extremity (excluding hand) or each trunk section (spine)		4.2	
	95852	hand, with or without comparison with normal side		6.3	
	95857	Tensilon test for myasthenia gravis;		7.5	
	95858	with electromyographic recording	12.0	(I) 20.0	
97.2	95860	Needle electromyography, one extremity with or without related paraspinal areas	(I) 13.0	(I) 17.5	
97.2	95861	Needle electromyography, two extremities with or without related paraspinal areas	(I) 18.0	(I) 24.8	
97.2	95863	Needle electromyography, three extremities with or without related paraspinal areas	(I) 23.0	(I) 32.1	
97.2	95864	Needle electromyography, four extremities with or without related paraspinal areas	(I) 28.0	(I) 39.4	
	95867	Needle electromyography, cranial nerve supplied muscles, unilateral	(I) 12.0	(I) 16.5	
	95868	Needle electromyography, cranial nerve supplied muscles, bilateral	(I) 17.0	(I) 21.5	
97.2	95869	Needle electromyography; thoracic paraspinal muscles	(I) 7.0	(I) 11.5	
97.2	95870	other than paraspinal (eg, abdomen, thorax)	(I) 5.5	(I) 7.5	
	95872	Needle electromyography using single fiber electrode, with quantitative measurement of jitter, blocking and/or fiber density, any/all sites of each muscle studied	(I) 22.0	(I) 30.0	

UPD			Code	Description	Prof	Units	Anes
96.2			95875	Ischemic limb exercise with needle electromyography, with lactic acid determination	(I) 15.0	(I) 20.0	
98.2		⊘	95900	Nerve conduction, amplitude and latency/velocity study, each nerve, any/all site(s) along the nerve; motor, without F-wave study	6.5	10.5	
98.2		⊘	95903	motor, with F-wave study	9.5	13.5	
98.2		⊘	95904	sensory	6.0	10.0	
98.2	▲	+	95920	Intraoperative neurophysiology testing, per hour (List separately in addition to code for primary procedure)	30.0	41.0	
96.2			95921	Testing of autonomic nervous system function; cardiovagal innervation (parasympathetic function), including two or more of the following; heart rate response to deep breathing with recorded R-R interval, Valsalva ratio, and 30:15 ratio	(I) 7.5	(I) 11.0	
96.2			95922	vasomotor adrenergic innervation (sympathetic adrenergic function), including beat-to-beat blood pressure and R-R interval changes during Valsalva maneuver and at least five minutes of passsive tilt	(I) 8.0	(I) 12.0	
96.2			95923	sudomotor, including one or more of the following; quantitative sudomotor axon reflex test (QSART), silastic sweat imprint, thermoregulatory sweat test, and changes in sympathetic skin potential	(I) 7.5	(I) 11.0	
			95925	Short-latency somatosensory evoked potential study, stimulation of any/all peripheral nerves or skin sites, recording from the central nervous system; in upper limbs	(I) 9.0	(I) 34.0	
			95926	in lower limbs	(I) 9.0	(I) 34.0	
			95927	in the trunk or head	(I) 9.0	(I) 34.0	
			95930	Visual evoked potential (VEP) testing central nervous system, checkerboard or flash	(I) 6.0	(I) 14.0	
			95933	Orbicularis oculi (blink) reflex, by electrodiagnostic testing	6.5	(I) 10.5	
			95934	H-reflex, amplitude and latency study; record gastrocnemius/soleus muscle	(I) 8.5	(I) 12.5	
96.1			95936	record muscle other than gastrocnemius/soleus muscle	(I) 9.5	(I) 13.5	
			95937	Neuromuscular junction testing (repetitive stimulation, paired stimuli), each nerve, any one method	6.5	(I) 10.5	
96.2			95950	Monitoring for identification and lateralization of cerebral seizure focus, electroencephalographic (eg, 8 channel EEG) recording and interpretation, each 24 hours	(I) 15.0	(I) 45.0	

UPD			Code	Description	Prof	Units	Anes
96.2			**95951**	Monitoring for localization of cerebral seizure focus by cable or radio, 16 or more channel telemetry, combined electroencephalographic (EEG) and video recording and interpretation (eg, for presurgical localization), each 24 hours	(I) 50.0	(I) 135.0	
			95953	Monitoring for localization of cerebral seizure focus by computerized portable 16 or more channel EEG; electroencephalographic (EEG) recording and interpretation, each 24 hours	(I) 30.0	(I) 80.0	
			95954	Pharmacological or physical activation requiring physician attendance during EEG recording of activation phase (eg, thiopental activation test)	(I) 30.0	(I) 35.0	
			95955	Electroencephalogram (EEG) during nonintracranial surgery (eg, carotid surgery)	(I) 15.0	(I) 30.0	
			95956	Monitoring for localization of cerebral seizure focus by cable or radio, 16 or more channel telemetry, electroencephalographic (EEG) recording and interpretation, each 24 hours	(I) 19.0	(I) 70.0	
98.2	▲		**95957**	Digital analysis of electroencephalogram (EEG) (eg, for epileptic spike analysis)	14.0	32.0	
			95958	Wada activation test for hemispheric function, including electroencephalographic (EEG) monitoring	(I) 65.0	(I) 95.0	
			95961	Functional cortical mapping by stimulation of electrodes on brain surface, or of depth electrodes, to provoke seizures or identify vital cortex; initial hour of physician attendance	(I) 30.0	(I) 40.0	
98.2	▲	+	**95962**	each additional hour of physician attendance (List separately in addition to code for primary procedure)	30.0	40.0	
98.2	●		**95970**	Electronic analysis of implanted neurostimulator pulse generator system (eg, rate, pulse amplitude and duration, configuration of wave form, battery status, electrode selectability, output modulation, cycling, impedance and patient compliance measurements); simple or complex neurostimulator pulse generator, without reprogramming		(I) 5.0	
98.2	●		**95971**	simple neurostimulator pulse generator, with intraoperative or subsequent programming		(I) 7.5	
98.2	●		**95972**	complex brain or spinal cord neurostimulator pulse generator/transmitter, with intraoperative subsequent programming, first hour		(I) 14.0	
98.2	●	+	**95973**	complex brain or spinal cord neurostimulator pulse generator/transmitter, with intraoperative subsequent programming, each additional 30 minutes after first hour (List separately in addition to code for primary procedure)		(I) 9.0	
98.2	●		**95974**	complex cranial nerve neurostimulator pulse generator/transmitter, with intraoperative or subsequent programming, with or without nerve interface testing, first hour		(I) 27.5	

UPD			Code	Description	Prof	Units	Anes
98.2	●	+	95975	complex cranial nerve neurostimulator pulse generator/transmitter, with intraoperative or subsequent programming, each additional 30 minutes after first hour (List separately in addition to code for primary procedure)		(I) 16.5	
			95999	Unlisted neurological or neuromuscular diagnostic procedure		BR	

Central Nervous System Assessments/Tests (eg, Neuro-Cognitive Mental Status, Speech Testing)

UPD		Code	Description	Prof	Units	Anes
98.2		96100	Psychological testing (includes psychodiagnostic assessment of personality, psychopathology, emotionality, intellectual abilities, eg, WAIS-R, Rorschach, MMPI) with interpretation and report, per hour		(I) 26.6	
98.2		96105	Assessment of aphasia (includes assessment of expressive and receptive speech and language function, language comprehension, speech production ability, reading, spelling, writing, eg, by Boston Diagnostic Aphasia Examination) with interpretation and report, per hour		(I) 29.2	
98.2		96110	Developmental testing; limited (eg, Developmental Screening Test II, Early Language Milestone Screen), with interpretation and report		(I) 23.5	
98.2		96111	extended (includes assessment of motor, language, social, adaptive and/or cognitive functioning by standardized developmental instruments, eg, Bayley Scales of Infant Development) with interpretation and report, per hour		(I) 26.3	
98.2		96115	Neurobehavorial status exam (clinical assessment of thinking, reasoning and judgment, eg, acquired knowledge, attention, memory, visual spatial abilities, language functions, planning) with interpretation and report, per hour		(I) 30.8	
98.2		96117	Neuropsychological testing battery (eg, Halstead-Reitan, Luria, WAIS-R) with interpretation and report, per hour		(I) 32.4	
98.1	M	96200	Biplaner Video		(I) 9.2	
98.1	M	96201	Computerized 3D kinematics — unilateral		(I) 45.8	
98.1	M	96202	Computerized 3D kinematics — bilateral		(I) 77.0	
98.1	M	96203	Force plate collection with joint kinetics — unilateral		(I) 27.5	
98.1	M	96204	Force plate collection with joint kinetics — bilateral		(I) 42.6	
98.1	M	96205	Dynamic Pedobarography		(I) 24.1	
98.1	M	96206	Stride characteristics — Measurements & Analysis		(I) 14.4	

UPD			Code	Description	Prof	Units	Anes
98.1	M		96207	Physician review and interpretation of gait analysis data		(I) 24.2	
98.1	M		96208	Surface Electromyography 1–5 muscles		(I) 26.3	
98.1	M		96209	Surface Electromyography 6–10 muscles		(I) 32.5	
98.1	M		96210	Surface Electromyography more than 10 muscles		(I) 35.1	
98.1	M		96211	Fine Wire Electromyography — one muscle		(I) 20.7	

Chemotherapy Administration

UPD			Code	Description	Prof	Units	Anes
			96400	Chemotherapy administration, subcutaneous or intramuscular, with or without local anesthesia		3.7	
			96405	Chemotherapy administration, intralesional; up to and including 7 lesions		(I) 8.0	
			96406	more than 7 lesions		(I) 12.0	
			96408	Chemotherapy administration, intravenous; push technique		(I) 9.0	
			96410	infusion technique, up to one hour		(I) 17.0	
98.2	▲	+	96412	infusion technique, one to 8 hours, each additional hour (List separately in addition to code for primary procedure)		(I) 14.0	
			96414	infusion technique, initiation of prolonged infusion (more than 8 hours), requiring the use of a portable or implantable pump		(I) 17.0	
			96420	Chemotherapy administration, intra-arterial; push technique		(I) 7.3	
			96422	infusion technique, up to one hour		(I) 15.0	
98.2	▲	+	96423	infusion technique, one to 8 hours, each additional hour (List separately in addition to code for primary procedure)		7.5/Per hour	
			96425	infusion technique, initiation of prolonged infusion (more than 8 hours), requiring the use of a portable or implantable pump		5.7/Per hour	
98.2			96440	Chemotherapy administration into pleural cavity, requiring and including thoracentesis		(I) 22.0	4
98.2			96445	Chemotherapy administration into peritoneal cavity, requiring and including peritoneocentesis		(I) 26.0	3
98.2			96450	Chemotherapy administration, into CNS (eg, intrathecal), requiring and including lumbar puncture		(I) 9.8	5
			96520	Refilling and maintenance of portable pump		(I) 9.0	
			96530	Refilling and maintenance of implantable pump or reservoir		(I) 10.0	

UPD	Code	Description	Prof	Units	Anes
	96542	Chemotherapy injection, subarachnoid or intraventricular via subcutaneous reservoir, single or multiple agents		(I) 19.5	
	96545	Provision of chemotherapy agent		(I) 7.0	
	96549	Unlisted chemotherapy procedure		BR	

Special Dermatological Procedures

UPD	Code	Description	Prof	Units	Anes
	96900	Actinotherapy (ultraviolet light)		3.0	
	96902	Microscopic examination of hairs plucked or clipped by the examiner (excluding hair collected by the patient) to determine telogen and anagen counts, or structural hair shaft abnormality		(I) 5.0	
	96910	Photochemotherapy; tar and ultraviolet B (Goeckerman treatment) or petrolatum and ultraviolet B		3.0	
	96912	psoralens and ultraviolet A (PUVA)		4.3	
	96913	Photochemotherapy (Goeckerman and/or PUVA) for severe photoresponsive dermatoses requiring at least four to eight hours of care under direct supervision of the physician (includes application of medication and dressings)		BR	
	96999	Unlisted special dermatological service or procedure		BR	

Physical Medicine and Rehabilitation

UPD	Code	Description	Prof	Units	Anes
97.2	97001	Physical therapy evaluation		(I) 16.0	
97.2	97002	Physical therapy re-evaluation		(I) 10.8	
97.2	97003	Occupational therapy evaluation		(I) 16.0	
97.2	97004	Occupational therapy re-evaluation		(I) 10.8	
	97010	Application of a modality to one or more areas; hot or cold packs		(I) 2.0	
	97012	traction, mechanical		(I) 4.5	
	97014	electrical stimulation (unattended)		(I) 3.5	
	97016	vasopneumatic devices		(I) 4.5	
	97018	paraffin bath		(I) 3.0	
	97020	microwave		(I) 3.0	
	97022	whirlpool		(I) 4.5	
	97024	diathermy		(I) 3.0	
	97026	infrared		(I) 2.0	
	97028	ultraviolet		4.0	

UPD		Code	Description	Prof	Units	Anes
		97032	Application of a modality to one or more areas; electrical stimulation (manual), each 15 minutes		(I) 4.5	
		97033	iontophoresis, each 15 minutes		(I) 5.0	
		97034	contrast baths, each 15 minutes		(I) 4.0	
		97035	ultrasound, each 15 minutes		(I) 4.0	
		97036	Hubbard tank, each 15 minutes		(I) 5.5	
		97039	Unlisted modality (specify type and time if constant attendance)		BR	
97.1	**M**	**97040**	Visit for the evaluation and management of a patient presenting with a problem which has not been evaluated or treated by the therapist which requires: an expanded problem focused history; an expanded problem focused examination, and; decision making of low complexity. The presenting problem is usually of low complexity. The average time spent with the patient is 25 minutes.		(I) 11.2	
97.1	**M**	**97041**	Visit for the evaluation and management of a patient presenting with a problem which has not been evaluated or treated by the therapist which requires: a detailed history; a detailed examination, and; decision making of moderate complexity. The presenting problem is usually of moderate complexity. The average time spent with the patient is 45 minutes.		(I) 16.0	
97.1	**M**	**97042**	Visit for the evaluation and management of a patient presenting with a problem which has not been evaluated or treated by the therapist which requires: a comprehensive history; a comprehensive examination, and; decision making of high complexity. The presenting problem is usually of high complexity. The average time spent with the patient is 70 minutes.		(I) 20.8	
97.1	**M**	**97043**	Visit for the evaluation and management of a patient presenting with a problem which has been evaluated or is being treated by the therapist which requires: a problem focused history; a problem focused examination, and; decision making of low complexity. The presenting problem is usually of low complexity. The average time spent with the patient is 15 minutes.		(I) 7.2	
97.1	**M**	**97044**	Visit for the evaluation and management of a patient presenting with a problem which has been evaluated or is being treated by the therapist which requires: an expanded problem focused history; a detailed examination, and; decision making of moderate complexity. The presenting problem is usually of moderate complexity. The average time spent with the patient is 30 minutes.		(I) 10.8	

UPD			Code	Description	Prof	Units	Anes
97.1	M		97045	Visit for the evaluation and management of a patient presenting with a problem which has been evaluated or is being treated by the therapist which requires: a detailed history; a comprehensive examination, and; decision making of high complexity. The presenting problem is usually of high complexity. The average time spent with the patient is 50 minutes.		(I) 15.6	
			97110	Therapeutic procedure, one or more areas, each 15 minutes; therapeutic exercises to develop strength and endurance, range of motion and flexibility		(I) 8.0	
			97112	neuromuscular reeducation of movement, balance, coordination, kinesthetic sense, posture, and proprioception		(I) 8.0	
			97113	aquatic therapy with therapeutic exercises		(I) 7.5	
			97116	gait training (includes stair climbing)		(I) 7.0	
98.2	M		97122	97122 has been deleted. To report, see 97140		(I) 8.0	
			97124	massage, including effleurage, petrissage and/or tapotement (stroking, compression, percussion)		(I) 6.5	
			97139	unlisted therapeutic procedure (specify)		BR	
98.2		●	97140	Manual therapy techniques (eg, mobilization/ manipulation, manual lymphatic drainage, manual traction), one or more regions, each 15 minutes		RNE	
			97150	Therapeutic procedure(s), group (2 or more individuals)		5.0	
98.2	M		97250	97250 has been deleted. To report, see 97140		8.0	
98.2	M		97260	97260, 97261 have been deleted. To report, see 97140		4.0	
98.2	M		97261	97260, 97261 have been deleted. To report, see 97140		1.2	
98.2	M		97265	97265 has been deleted. To report, see 97140		8.0	
96.2	M		97500	97500, 97501 have been deleted. To report, see 97504		4.5	
96.2	M		97501	97500, 97501 have been deleted. To report, see 97504		1.5	
96.2			97504	Orthotics fitting and training, upper and/or lower extermities, each 15 minutes		(I) 4.8	
96.2			97520	Prosthetic training, upper and/or lower extremities, each 15 minutes		4.8	
96.2	M		97521	97521 has been deleted. To report, see 97520		1.6	
			97530	Therapeutic activities, direct (one on one) patient contact by the provider (use of dynamic activities to improve functional performance), each 15 minutes		5.0	

UPD			Code	Description	Prof	Units	Anes
98.2	**M**	●	**97532**	Dynamic vertebral axial decompression, progressive; through variable timed tension destraction – relaxation cycles with continuous monitoring, recording and interpretation, per session		(I) 28.0	
			97535	Self care/home management training (eg, activities of daily living (ADL) and compensatory training, meal preparation, safety procedures, and instructions in use of adaptive equipment) direct one on one contact by provider, each 15 minutes		(I) 7.5	
			97537	Community/work reintegration training (eg, shopping, transportation, money management, avocational activities and/or work environment/ modification analysis, work task analysis), direct one on one contact by provider, each 15 minutes		(I) 7.5	
			97542	Wheelchair management/propulsion training, each 15 minutes		(I) 7.5	
			97545	Work hardening/conditioning; initial 2 hours		(I) 24.0	
98.2		▲ +	**97546**	each additional hour (List separately in addition to code for primary procedure)		(I) 12.0	
			97703	Checkout for orthotic/prosthetic use, established patient, each 15 minutes		(I) 7.5	
98.1			**97750**	Physical performance test or measurement (eg, musculoskeletal, functional capacity), with written report, each 15 minutes		(I) 9.5	
98.2			**97770**	Development of cognitive skills to improve attention, memory, problem solving, includes compensatory training and/or sensory integrative activities, direct (one on one) patient contact by the provider, each 15 minutes		(I) 9.4	
97.2			**97780**	Acupuncture, one or more needles; without electrical stimulation		(I) 1.3	
97.2			**97781**	with electrical stimulation		(I) 2.5	
			97799	Unlisted physical medicine/rehabilitation service or procedure		BR	

Osteopathic Manipulative Treatment

UPD			Code	Description	Prof	Units	Anes
96.2			**98925**	Osteopathic manipulative treatment (OMT); one to two body regions involved		(I) 7.5	
96.2			**98926**	three to four body regions involved		(I) 10.0	
96.2			**98927**	five to six body regions involved		(I) 12.0	
96.2			**98928**	seven to eight body regions involved		(I) 14.0	
96.2			**98929**	nine to ten body regions involved		(I) 15.0	

UPD	Code	Description	Prof	Units	Anes

Chiropractic Manipulative Treatment

UPD	Code	Description	Prof	Units	Anes
96.2	**98940**	Chiropractic manipulative treatment (CMT); spinal, one to two regions		(I) 8.0	
96.2	**98941**	spinal, three to four regions		(I) 9.2	
96.2	**98942**	spinal, five regions		(I) 10.4	
96.2	**98943**	extraspinal, one or more regions		(I) 7.5	

Special Services and Reports

UPD	Code	Description	Prof	Units	Anes
	99000	Handling and/or conveyance of specimen for transfer from the physician's office to a laboratory		3.0	
	99001	Handling and/or conveyance of specimen for transfer from the patient in other than a physician's office to a laboratory (distance may be indicated)		1.5	
	99002	Handling, conveyance, and/or any other service in connection with the implementation of an order involving devices (eg, designing, fitting, packaging, handling, delivery or mailing) when devices such as orthotics, protectives, prosthetics are fabricated by an outside laboratory or shop but which items have been designed, and are to be fitted and adjusted by the attending physician		1.5	
	99024	Postoperative follow-up visit, included in global service		BR	
	99025	Initial (new patient) visit when starred (*) surgical procedure constitutes major service at that visit		4.0	
	99050	Services requested after office hours in addition to basic service		4.0	
	99052	Services requested between 10:00 PM and 8:00 AM in addition to basic service		8.0	
	99054	Services requested on Sundays and holidays in addition to basic service		8.0	
	99056	Services provided at request of patient in a location other than physician's office which are normally provided in the office		4.0	
	99058	Office services provided on an emergency basis		4.0	
	99070	Supplies and materials (except spectacles), provided by the physician over and above those usually included with the office visit or other services rendered (list drugs, trays, supplies, or materials provided)		BR	
	99071	Educational supplies, such as books, tapes, and pamphlets, provided by the physician for the patient's education at cost to physician		BR	
M	**99072**	Supplies for an office based procedure room		BR	

UPD	Code	Description	Prof	Units	Anes
	99075	Medical testimony		35.0	
	99078	Physician educational services rendered to patients in a group setting (eg, prenatal, obesity, or diabetic instructions)		BR	
	99080	Special reports such as insurance forms, more than the information conveyed in the usual medical communications or standard reporting form		BR	
	99082	Unusual travel (eg, transportation and escort of patient)		BR	
	99090	Analysis of information data stored in computers (eg, ECGs, blood pressures, hematologic data)		22.0	

Sedation With or Without Analgesia (Conscious Sedation)

UPD	Code	Description	Prof	Units	Anes
98.2	⊘ **99141**	Sedation with or without analgesia (conscious sedation); intravenous, intramuscular or inhalation		(I) 13.0	
98.2	⊘ **99142**	oral, rectal and/or intranasal		(I) 10.0	

Other Services

UPD	Code	Description	Prof	Units	Anes
	99175	Ipecac or similar administration for individual emesis and continued observation until stomach adequately emptied of poison		7.0	
98.2	**99183**	Physician attendance and supervision of hyperbaric oxygen therapy, per session		(I) 14.0	0
	99185	Hypothermia; regional		(I) 5.0	
	99186	total body		(I) 17.0	
	99190	Assembly and operation of pump with oxygenator or heat exchanger (with or without ECG and/or pressure monitoring); each hour		86.0	
	99191	3/4 hour		64.0	
	99192	1/2 hour		42.5	
	99195	Phlebotomy, therapeutic (separate procedure)		5.0	
	99199	Unlisted special service or report		BR	

Evaluation and Management

Guidelines

I. **General:** Visits, examinations, consultations, and similar services as listed in this section reflect the wide variations required in time and skill. The following alphabetical list of definitions is included to aid in the determination of the correct code for the service provided. Documentation for each aspect of the service performed should be included in the patient record to substantiate the level of service. The listed relativities for each code group apply only when these services are performed by or under the responsible supervision of a physician.

Chief Complaint: A concise statement describing the symptom, problem, condition, diagnosis, or other factor that is the reason for the encounter.

Classification of Service: Each code in this section is grouped into a category. The groupings are defined by place (e.g. office, hospital, nursing home, etc.) and type of service (e.g. consultation, preventive, etc.). Some of the codes are grouped into subcategories (e.g. new patient, established patient, initial, etc.). Each code in the group represents a different level of service defined by the clinical components of a patient encounter for E/M (See Levels of Service).

Components: Each level of service recognizes seven components. The components include history, physical examination, medical decision making, counseling, coordination of care, nature of presenting problem, and time. (See Levels of Service, Key Components, History, Physical Examination, Medical Decision Making, Counseling, Problem, and Time).

Concurrent Care: The provision of similar services (e.g. hospital visits) to the same patient by more than one physician on the same day. CPT has deleted modifier -75 and does not require any special reporting for concurrent care.

Consultation: There are three categories for consultation: outpatient, inpatient, and confirmatory. Any physician may use an appropriate consultation code on any patient for any problem including one which has been previously evaluated by the consulting physician provided the following criteria are met:

1. The attending physician or appropriate source requests that the physician render advice or opinion regarding the evaluation and/or management of a specific problem.

2. The need for the consultation, the consultant's opinion, and any services ordered or performed must be well documented in the patient's record.

3. The information is communicated to the requesting physician or appropriate source.

Counseling: A discussion with the patient and/or family concerning one or more of the following:

Diagnostic results, impressions, and/or recommended diagnostic studies;
Prognosis;
Risks and benefits of management options;
Instructions for management and/or follow-up;
Importance of compliance with chosen management;
Risk factor reduction; and
Patient and family education.
(See Key components and Time)

Established Patient: A patient who has received professional services from a physician or another physician in the same specialty within the same group within the last three years. In the instance a physician is covering for or on call for another physician, the patient is classified as an established patient if the other physician or a member of the providing physician specialty group has provided services for the patient within the last three years.

Family History: A review of medical events in the patient's family that includes significant information about:

- the health status or cause of death of parents, siblings, and children;

- specific diseases related to problems identified in the Chief Complaint or History of the Present Illness, and/or System Review;

- diseases of family members that may be hereditary or place the patient at risk.

History: This key component relates to the type of history obtained during a patient encounter. The four types of history are defined as follows:

Problem focused-brief history of present illness or problem as related to the chief complaint.

Expanded problem focused-brief history of present illness relating to chief complaint and pertinent system review.

Detailed-extended history of present illness related to chief complaint, an extended system review, and pertinent past, family, and/or social history.

Comprehensive-extended history of present illness related to chief complaint, complete system review, and complete past, family, and social history.

History of Present Illness: A chronological description of the development of the patient's present illness from the first sign and/or symptom to the present. This includes a description of location, quality, severity, timing, context, modifying factors, and associated signs and symptoms significantly related to the presenting problem(s).

Key Components: Those components that are used primarily to determine the appropriate code level. These components include Medical Decision Making, Physical Examination, and History (See; History, Physical Examination, Medical Decision Making). Time is not considered a key component unless counseling constitutes more than 50% of the face to face patient/physician encounter (See Time, Counseling).

Levels of Service: Each category and subcategory contains three to five levels of service indicated by code. The services include examinations, evaluations, treatments, conferences with or concerning patients, preventative pediatric and adult health supervision, and similar services. Each level of service recognizes seven clinical components. Three of these components are considered key components (See Components of Service, History, Physical Examination, and Medical Decision Making). Each level of service may be used by all physicians.

Medical Decision Making: The complexity of establishing a diagnosis or selecting a management option. Medical decision making is divided into four categories. The level of medical decision making is determined using documentation in the patient record for three subcategories including: number of possible diagnoses and or the number of management options considered; the amount and/or complexity of medical records, diagnostic tests, and/or other information that must be obtained, reviewed, and analyzed; and the risk of significant complications, morbidity and/or mortality, as well as comorbidities, associated with the patient's presenting problem(s), the diagnostic procedure(s), and/or the possible management options. The following four classifications for level of medical decision making are used in determining the proper code.

Straight Forward: minimal number of possible diagnoses or management options, minimal or no amount and/or complexity of data to be reviewed, and minimal risk of complications and/or morbidity or mortality.

Low Complexity: limited number of possible diagnoses or management options, limited amount and/or complexity of data to be reviewed, and low risk of complications and/or morbidity or mortality.

Moderate Complexity: multiple number of possible diagnoses or management options, moderate amount and/or complexity of data to be reviewed, and moderate risk of complications and/or morbidity or mortality.

High Complexity: extensive number of possible diagnoses or management options, extensive amount and/or complexity of data to be reviewed, and high risk of complications and/or morbidity or mortality.

Nature of Presenting Problem: A presenting problem is a disease, condition, illness, injury, symptom, sign, finding, complaint, or other reason for encounter, with or without a diagnosis being established at the time of the encounter. The E/M codes recognize five types of presenting problems that are defined as follows:

Minimal: A problem that may not require the presence of the physician, but service is provided under the physician's supervision.

Self-limited or minor: A problem that runs a definite and prescribed course, is transient in nature, and is not likely to permanently alter health status, or has a good prognosis with management/compliance.

Low severity: A problem where the risk of morbidity without treatment is low; there is little to no risk of mortality without treatment; full recovery without functional impairment is expected.

Moderate severity: A problem where the risk of morbidity without treatment is moderate; there is moderate risk of mortality without treatment; uncertain prognosis, or increased probability of prolonged functioinal impairment.

High severity: A problem where the risk of morbidity without treatment is high to extreme; there is a moderate to high risk of mortality without treatment, or high probability of severe, prolonged functional impairment.

New Patient: A patient who has not received any professional services from a physician or another physician in the same specialty within the same group within the past three years. In the instance where a physician is on call for or covering for another physician, the patient is classified as a new patient if the other physician or a member of the providing physicians specialty group has not provided any professional service for the patient within three years (See Established Patient).

Past History: A review of the patient's past experiences with illnesses, injuries, and treatments that include significant information about:

- Prior major illnesses and injuries;
- Prior operations;
- Prior hospitalizations;
- Current medications;
- Allergies (eg, drug, food);
- Age appropriate immunization status;
- Age appropriate feeding/dietary status.

Physical Examination: This key component relates to the type of physical examination performed during a patient encounter. The four defined types of physical examination are:

Problem focused — an examination limited to the affected body area or organ system.

Expanded problem focused — an examination of the affected body area or organ system and other symptomatic or related organ systems.

Detailed — an extended examination of the affected body area(s) and other symptomatic or related organ system(s).

Comprehensive — a complete single system specialty examination or a complete multi-system examination.

Problem: Problem describes the nature of the problem presented as the reason for the encounter. Problem is considered to be a contributing factor and therefore is not used as a primary factor in determining level of service. Problem is classified in the following five categories:

Minimal: A problem that may not require the presence of the physician, but service is provided under the supervision of the physician.

Self-limited or minor: A problem that runs a definite and prescribed course, is transient in nature and is not likely to permanently alter health status, or has a good prognosis with management compliance.

Low severity: A problem where the risk of morbidity without treatment is low; there is little to no risk of mortality without treatment; full recovery without functional impairment is expected.

Moderate severity: A problem where the risk of morbidity without treatment is moderate; there is moderate risk of mortality without treatment; uncertain prognosis, or increased probability of prolonged functional impairment.

High severity: A problem where the risk of morbidity without treatment is high to extreme; there is moderate to high risk of mortality without treatment or high probability of severe, prolonged functional impairment.

Review of Systems: An inventory of body systems obtained through a series of questions seeking to identify signs and/or symptoms that the patient may be experiencing or has experienced. For the purposes of CPT the following elements of a system review have been identified:

- Constitutional symptoms (fever, weight loss, etc.)
- Eyes
- Ears, Nose, Mouth, Throat
- Cardiovascular
- Respiratory
- Gastrointestinal
- Genitourinary
- Musculoskeletal
- Integumentary (skin and/or breast)
- Neurological
- Psychiatric
- Endocrine
- Hematologic/Lymphatic
- Allergic/Immunologic

Social History: An age appropriate review of past and current activities that includes significant information about:

- Marital status and/or living arrangements;
- Current employment;
- Occupational history;
- Use of drugs, alcohol, and tobacco;
- Level of education;
- Sexual history;
- Other relevant social factors.

Time: Time for an outpatient is considered to be face-to-face time spent with the patient and does not include time spent in such things as record review or dictating. The time for an inpatient is considered to be the time spent "on the floor" and does include record review, dictating, and other services rendered while in the hospital unit of the patient. Times given are considered to be an average and should not be used to determine the length of time spent in the encounter. Time is considered to be a contributory factor and as such is not used to define the level of service unless 50% or more of the service performed is spent in counseling or coordinating care. In cases where 50% of the service is counseling or coordinating care, time is considered the overriding component and is used as the primary component for defining the level of service. Careful documentation of time is essential in cases where time is the defining component.

II. **Unusual Service or Procedure:** A service may necessitate skills and time of the physician over and above listed services and values. If substantiated "by report" (BR), additional values may be warranted. Use modifier -22 to indicate these procedures.

III. **Unlisted Service or Procedure:** When a service or procedure provided is not adequately identified, use of the unlisted procedure code for the related anatomical area is appropriate. Most codes of this nature have 99 for the last two digits. Value should be substantiated "by report" (BR) (See By Report).

IV. **Prolonged Evaluation and Management Service:** When a service provided is prolonged or otherwise greater than that usually required for the highest level of E/M service within a category (eg. 99205), it must be substantiated by report. Use modifier -21 to indicate this service.

V. **Unrelated E/M Service by the same physician during a Postoperative Period:** If a service that is not related to the original procedure is performed during the follow-up period, it may be billed at 100% of the listed value. Use modifier -24 to indicate this service is unrelated.

VI. **Significant, Separately Identifiable E/M service by the same physician on the day of a Procedure:** In cases where an E/M service is performed on the same day of a procedure above and beyond normal pre- and postoperative care associated with the procedure performed, it may be billed at 100% of the listed value. Services of this nature must be substantiated by report. Use modifier -25 to indicate this type of service.

VII. **E/M Service resulting in initial decision for surgery:** If an evaluation and management encounter results in the initial decision to perform surgery, modifier -57 may be attached to the E/M service code. At such time as the decision for surgery is made, meaning recommended to the patient and agreed to by the patient, the preoperative time begins and other E/M services related to the procedure are included in the global value of the procedure. The modifier does not reduce or increase the value of the service and should be billed at 100% of the listed value.

VIII. **Unrelated E/M Service during a designated preoperative period:** An evaluation and management service that is unrelated to a planned procedure provided during a designated preoperative period may be repeated using modifier -49. Modifier -49 should be billed at 100%. (Note: This modifier is not CPT compatible.)

IX. **Procedures without Specified Units Values:** Procedures that have RNE or BR in the units column, should be substantiated "by report".

X. **By Report:** The value of a procedure should be established for any "by report" circumstance by identifying a similar service and justifying value difference. When a report is indicated, the report should include the following:

1. Accurate procedure definition or description;

2. Operative report;

3. Justification for procedural variance, when appropriate;

4. Similar procedure and value; and

5. Justification for value difference.

XI. **Reduced Values:** Under some circumstances, the value for a procedure may be reduced or eliminated. Use modifier -52 to identify reduced value services.

XII. **Multiple Modifiers:** If circumstances require the use of more than one modifier with any one procedure code, modifier -99 should be added to the procedure code. Other modifiers are then attached to the procedure code and listed separately with appropriate values for each.

XIII. **Materials Supplied by Physician:** Identify as 99070 supplies and materials provided by the physician (e.g., sterile trays, drugs, etc.) over and above those usually indicated with the office visit or other services rendered.

Evaluation and Management Section

UPD	Code	Description	Units	Anes

Office or Other Outpatient Services

| | 99201 | Office or other outpatient visit for the evaluation and management of a new patient, which requires these three key components: a problem focused history; a problem focused examination; and straightforward medical decision making. Counseling and/or coordination of care with other providers or agencies are provided consistent with the nature of the problem(s) and the patient's and/or family's needs. Usually, the presenting problems are self limited or minor. Physicians typically spend 10 minutes face-to-face with the patient and/or family. | 6.5 | |

Examples

Initial office visit with 65-year-old male for reassurance about an isolated seborrheic keratosis on the upper back. (Dermatology/Plastic Surgery)

Initial office visit with an out-of-town visitor who needs a prescription refilled because she forgot her hay fever medication. (Allergy & Immunology/Internal Medicine)

Initial office visit with 9-month-old female with diaper rash. (Pediatrics)

Initial office visit with 10-year-old male with severe rash and itching for the past 24 hours, positive history for contact with poison oak 48 hours prior to the visit. (Family Medicine)

Initial office visit with 5-year-old female to remove sutures from simple wound, placed by another physician. (Plastic Surgery)

Initial office visit for a 22-year-old male with a small area of sunburn requiring first aid. (Dermatology/Family Medicine/Internal Medicine)

Initial office visit for the evaluation and management of a contusion of a finger. (Orthopaedic Surgery)

| | 99202 | Office or other outpatient visit for the evaluation and management of a new patient, which requires these three key components: an expanded problem focused history; an expanded problem focused examination; and straightforward medical decision making. Counseling and/or coordination of care with other providers or agencies are provided consistent with the nature of the problem(s) and the patient's and/or family's needs. Usually, the presenting problem(s) are of low to moderate severity. Physicians typically spend 20 minutes face-to-face with the patient and/or family. | 9.5 | |

Examples

Initial office visit, 16-year-old male with severe cystic acne, new patient. (Dermatology)

Initial office evaluation for gradual hearing loss, 58-year-old male, history and physical examination, with interpretation of complete audiogram, air bone, etc. (Otolaryngology)

Initial office visit for evaluation and management of recurrent urinary infection in female. (Internal Medicine)

Initial office visit with 10-year-old girl with history of chronic otitis media and a draining ear. (Pediatrics)

Initial office visit to advise for or against the removal of wisdom teeth, 18-year-old male referred by an orthodontist. (Oral & Maxillofacial Surgery)

Initial office visit for a 10-year-old female with acute maxillary sinusitis. (Family Medicine)

Initial office visit for a patient with recurring episodes of herpes simplex who has developed a clustering of vesicles on the upper lip. (Internal Medicine)

Initial office visit for a 25-year-old patient with single season allergic rhinitis. (Allergy & Immunology)

Initial office visit to plan transient dialysis for a 56-year-old stable dialysis patient who has accompanying records. (Nephrology)

UPD	Code	Description	Units	Anes
	99203	Office or other outpatient visit for the evaluation and management of a new patient, which requires these three key components: a detailed history; a detailed examination; and medical decision making of low complexity. Counseling and/or coordination of care with other providers or agencies are provided consistent with the nature of the problem(s) and the patient's and/or family's needs. Usually, the presenting problem(s) are of moderate severity. Physicians typically spend 30 minutes face-to-face with the patient and/or family.	14.0	

Examples

Initial office visit for evaluation of a 48-year-old man with recurrent low back pain radiating to the leg. (General Surgery)

Initial office evaluation, diagnosis and management of painless gross hematuria in new patient, without cystoscopy. (Internal Medicine)

Initial office visit with couple for counseling concerning voluntary vasectomy for sterility. Spent 30 minutes discussing procedure, risks and benefits, and answering questions. (Urology)

Initial office evaluation of 49-year-old male with nasal obstruction. Detailed exam with topical anesthesia. (Plastic Surgery)

Initial office visit for evaluation of 13-year-old female with progressive scoliosis. (Physical Medicine & Rehabilitation)

Initial office visit for 21-year-old female desiring counseling and evaluation of initiation of contraception. (Family Medicine/Internal Medicine/Obstetrics & Gynecology)

Initial office visit for 49-year-old male presenting with painless blood per rectum associated with bowel movement. (Colon & Rectal Surgery)

Initial office visit for 19-year-old football player with 3 day old acute knee injury; now with swelling and pain. (Orthopaedic Surgery)

UPD	Code	Description	Units	Anes
	99204	Office or other outpatient visit for the evaluation and management of a new patient, which requires these three key components: a comprehensive history; a comprehensive examination; and medical decision making of moderate complexity. Counseling and/or coordination of care with other providers or agencies are provided consistent with the nature of the problem(s) and the patient's and/or family's needs. Usually, the presenting problem(s) are of moderate to high severity. Physicians typically spend 45 minutes face-to-face with the patient and/or family.	20.0	

Examples

Initial office visit for evaluation of a 63-year-old male with chest pain on exertion. (Cardiology/Internal Medicine)

Initial office evaluation of a 70-year-old patient with recent onset of episodic confusion. (Internal Medicine)

Initial office visit for 7-year-old female with juvenile diabetes mellitus, new to area, past history of hospitalization times three. (Pediatrics)

Initial office visit of a 50-year-old female with progressive solid food dysphagia. (Gastroenterology)

Initial office visit for 34-year-old patient with primary infertility, including counseling. (Obstetrics & Gynecology)

Initial office evaluation of 70-year-old female with polyarthralgia. (Rheumatology)

Initial office visit for a patient with papulosquamous eruption involving 60% of the cutaneous surface with joint pain. Combinations of topical and systemic treatments discussed. (Dermatology)

Copyright © 1999 St. Anthony Publishing

UPD	Code	Description	Units	Anes
	99205	Office or other outpatient visit for the evaluation and management of a new patient, which requires these three key components: a comprehensive history; a comprehensive examination; and medical decision making of high complexity. Counseling and/or coordination of care with other providers or agencies are provided consistent with the nature of the problem(s) and the patient's and/or family's needs. Usually, the presenting problem(s) are of moderate to high severity. Physicians typically spend 60 minutes face-to-face with the patient and/or family.	26.0	

Examples

Initial office evaluation of a 65-year-old female with exertional chest pain, intermittent claudication, syncope and a murmur of aortic stenosis. (Cardiology)

Initial office visit for a 73-year-old male with an unexplained 20-pound weight loss. (Hematology/Oncology)

Initial office evaluation, patient with systemic lupus erythematosus, fever, seizures and profound thrombocytopenia. (Allergy & Immunology/Internal Medicine/Rheumatology)

Initial office evaluation and management of patient with systemic vasculitis and compromised circulation to the limbs. (Rheumatology)

Initial office visit for a 24-year-old homosexual male who has a fever, a cough, and shortness of breath. (Infectious Disease)

Initial outpatient evaluation of a 69-year-old male with severe chronic obstructive pulmonary disease, congestive heart failure, and hypertension. (Family Medicine)

Initial office visit for a 17-year-old female, who is having school problems and has told a friend she is considering suicide. The patient and her family are consulted in regards to treatment options. (Psychiatry)

Initial office visit for a female with sever hirsutism, amenorrhea, weight loss and a desire to have children. (Endocrinology/Obstetrics & Gynecology)

Initial office visit for a 42-year-old male on hypertensive medication, newly arrived to the area, with diastolic blood pressure of 110, history of recurrent renal calculi, episodic headaches, intermittent chest pain and orthopnea. (Internal Medicine)

UPD	Code	Description	Units	Anes
	99211	Office or other outpatient visit for the evaluation and management of an established patient, that may not require the presence of a physician. Usually, the presenting problem(s) are minimal. Typically, 5 minutes are spent performing or supervising these services.	3.5	

Examples

Outpatient visit with 19-year-old male, established patient, for supervised drug screen. (Addiction Medicine)

Office visit with 12-year-old male, established patient, for cursory check of hematoma one day after venipuncture. (Internal Medicine)

Office visit with 31-year-old female, established patient, for return to work certificate. (Anesthesiology)

Office visit for 42-year-old established patient to read tuberculin test results. (Allergy & Immunology)

Office visit for 14-year-old established patient to re-dress an abrasion. (Orthopedic Surgery)

Office visit for a 45-year-old female, established patient, for a blood pressure check. (Obstetrics & Gynecology)

Office visit for a 23-year-old established patient for instruction in use of peak flow meter. (Allergy & Immunology)

Office visit for prescription refill for a 35-year-old female, established patient, with schizophrenia who is stable but has run out of neuroleptic and is scheduled to be seen in a week. (Psychiatry)

UPD	Code	Description	Units	Anes
	99212	Office or other outpatient visit for the evaluation and management of an established patient, which requires at least two of these three key components: a problem focused history; a problem focused examination; straightforward medical decision making. Counseling and/or coordination of care with other providers or agencies are provided consistent with the nature of the problem(s) and the patient's and/or family's needs. Usually, the presenting problem(s) are self limited or minor. Physicians typically spend 10 minutes face-to-face with the patient and/or family.	6.0	

Examples

Outpatient visit with 19-year-old male, established patient, for supervised drug screen. (Addiction Medicine)

Office visit with 12-year-old male, established patient, for cursory check of hematoma one day after venipuncture. (Internal Medicine)

Office visit with 31-year-old female, established patient, for return to work certificate. (Anesthesiology)

Office visit for 42-year-old established patient to read tuberculin test results. (Allergy & Immunology)

Office visit for 14-year-old established patient to re-dress an abrasion. (Orthopedic Surgery)

Office visit for a 45-year-old female, established patient, for a blood pressure check. (Obstetrics & Gynecology)

Office visit for a 23-year-old established patient for instruction in use of peak flow meter. (Allergy & Immunology)

Office visit for prescription refill for a 35-year-old female, established patient, with schizophrenia who is stable but has run out of neuroleptic and is scheduled to be seen in a week. (Psychiatry)

UPD	Code	Description	Units	Anes
	99213	Office or other outpatient visit for the evaluation and management of an established patient, which requires at least two of these three key components: an expanded problem focused history; an expanded problem focused examination; medical decision making of low complexity. Counseling and coordination of care with other providers or agencies are provided consistent with the nature of the problem(s) and the patient's and/or family's needs. Usually, the presenting problem(s) are of low to moderate severity. Physicians typically spend 15 minutes face-to-face with the patient and/or family.	9.0	

Examples

Office visit with 55-year-old male, established patient for management of hypertension, mild fatique, on beta blocker/thiazide regimen. (Family Medicine/Internal Medicine)

Outpatient visit with 37-year-old male, established patient, who is 3 years post total colectomy for chronic ulcerative colitis, presents for increased irritation at his stoma. (General Surgery)

Office visit for a 70-year-old diabetic hypertensive established patient with recent change in insulin requirement. (Internal Medicine/Nephrology)

Office visit with 80-year-old female established patient, for follow-up osteoporosis, status-post compression fractures. (Rheumatology)

Office visit for an established patient with stable cirrhosis of the liver. (Gastroenterology)

Routine, follow-up office evaluation at a three-month interval for a 77-year-old female with nodular small cleaved-cell lymphoma. (Hematology/Oncology)

Quarterly follow-up office visit for a 45-year-old male, with stable chronic asthma, on steroid and bronchodilator therapy. (Pulmonary Medicine)

Office visit for a 50-year-old female, established patient, with insulin- dependent diabetes mellitus and stable coronary artery disease, for monitoring. (Family Medicine/Internal Medicine)

UPD	Code	Description	Units	Anes
	99214	Office or other outpatient visit for the evaluation and management of an established patient, which requires at least two of these three key components: a detailed history; a detailed examination; medical decision making of moderate complexity. Counseling and/or coordination of care with other providers or agencies are provided consistent with the nature of the problem(s) and the patient's and/or family's needs. Usually, the presenting problem(s) are of moderate to high severity. Physicians typically spend 25 minutes face-to-face with the patient and/or family.	13.5	

Examples

Office visit for a 68-year-old male, established patient, with stable angina, two months post myocardial infarction, who is not tolerating one of his medications. (Cardiology)

Weekly office visit for 5FU therapy for an ambulatory established patient with metastatic colon cancer and increasing shortness of breath. (Hematology/Oncology)

Follow-up office visit for a 60-year-old male, established patient, whose post-traumatic seizures have disappeared on medication, and who now raises the question of stopping the medication. (Neurology)

Office evaluation on new onset RLQ pain in 32-year-old woman, established patient. (Urology/General Surgery/Internal Medicine/Family Medicine)

Office evaluation of 28-year-old established patient with regional enteritis, diarrhea and low grade fever. (Family Medicine/Internal Medicine)

Office visit with 50-year-old female, established patient, diabetic, blood sugar controlled by diet. She now complains of frequency of urination and weight loss, blood sugar of 320 and negative ketones on dipstick. (Internal Medicine)

Follow-up office visit for a 45-year-old established patient with rheumatoid arthritis on gold, methotrexate, or immunosuppressive therapy. (Rheumatology)

Office visit with 63-year-old female, established patient, with familial polyposis, after a previous colectomy and sphincter sparing procedure, now with tenesmus, mucus, and increased stool frequency. (Colon & Rectal Surgery)

Office visit for 60-year-old male, established patient, 2-years post removal of intracranial meningioma, now with new headaches and visual disturbance. (Neurosurgery)

Office visit for a 68-year-old female, established patient, for routine review and follow-up of non-insulin dependent diabetes, obesity, hypertension and congestive heart failure. Complains of vision difficulties and admits dietary noncompliance. Patient is counseled concerning diet and current medications adjusted. (Family Medicine)

UPD	Code	Description	Units	Anes
	99215	Office or other outpatient visit for the evaluation and management of an established patient, which requires at least two of these three key components: a comprehensive history; a comprehensive examination; medical decision making of high complexity. Counseling and/or coordination of care with other providers or agencies are provided consistent with the nature of the problem(s) and the patient's and/or family's needs. Usually, the presenting problem(s) are of moderate to high severity. Physicians typically spend 40 minutes face-to-face with the patient and/or family.	19.5	

Examples

Office visit with 30-year-old male, established patient for 3 month history of fatigue, weight loss, intermittent fever, and presenting with diffuse adenopathy and splenomegaly. (Family Medicine)

Office visit for restaging of an established patient with new lymphadenopathy one year post-therapy for lymphoma. (Hematology/Oncology)

Office visit for evaluation of recent onset syncopal attacks in a 70-year-old woman, established patient. (Internal Medicine)

Follow-up visit, 40-year-old mother of 3, established patient, with acute rheumatoid arthritis, anatomical Stage 3, ARA function Class 3 rheumatoid arthritis, and deteriorating function. (Rheumatology)

Office evaluation and discussion of treatment options for a 68-year-old male, established patient, with a biopsy-proven rectal carcinoma. (General Surgery)

Follow-up visit for 65-year-old male, established patient, with a fever of recent onset while on outpatient antibiotic therapy for endocarditis. (Infectious Disease)

Office visit for a 75-year-old established patient with ALS (amyotrophic lateral sclerosis), who is no longer able to swallow. (Neurology)

Office visit for a 70-year-old female, established patient, with diabetes mellitus and hypertension, presenting with a 2 month history of increasing confusion, agitation and short-term memory loss. (Family Medicine/Internal Medicine)

Hospital Observation Services

UPD	Code	Description	Units	Anes
97.2	99217	Observation care discharge day management (This code is to be utilized by the physician to report all services provided to a patient on discharge from "observation status" if the discharge is on other than the initial date of "observation status." To report services to a patient designated as "observation status" or "inpatient status" and discharged on the same date, use the codes for Observation or Inpatient Care Services (including Admission and Discharge Services, 99234–99236 as appropriate.))	9.0	
	99218	Initial observation care, per day, for the evaluation and management of a patient which requires these three key components: a detailed or comprehensive history; a detailed or comprehensive examination; and medical decision making that is straightforward or of low complexity. Counseling and/or coordination of care with other providers or agencies are provided consistent with the nature of the problem(s) and the patient's and/or family's needs. Usually, the problem(s) requiring admission to "observation status" are of low severity.	12.0	
	99219	Initial observation care, per day, for the evaluation and management of a patient, which requires these three key components: a comprehensive history; a comprehensive examination; and medical decision making of moderate complexity. Counseling and/or coordination of care with other providers or agencies are provided consistent with the nature of the problem(s) and the patient's and/or family's needs. Usually, the problem(s) requiring admission to "observation status" are of moderate severity.	21.5	

UPD	Code	Description	Units	Anes
	99220	Initial observation care, per day, for the evaluation and management of a patient, which requires these three key components: a comprehensive history; a comprehensive examination; and medical decision making of high complexity. Counseling and/or coordination of care with other providers or agencies are provided consistent with the nature of the problem(s) and the patient's and/or family's needs. Usually, the problem(s) requiring admission to "observation status" are of high severity.	27.0	

Hospital Inpatient Services

UPD	Code	Description	Units	Anes
	99221	Initial hospital care, per day, for the evaluation and management of a patient which requires these three key components: a detailed or comprehensive history; a detailed or comprehensive examination; and medical decision making that is straightforward or of low complexity. Counseling and/or coordination of care with other providers or agencies are provided consistent with the nature of the problem(s) and the patient's and/or family's needs. Usually, the problem(s) requiring admission are of low severity. Physicians typically spend 30 minutes at the bedside and on the patient's hospital floor or unit.	12.5	

Examples

Hospital admission, examination, and initiation of treatment program for a 67-year-old male with uncomplicated pneumonia who requires IV antibiotic therapy. (Internal Medicine)

Hospital admission for an 18-month-old child with 10 percent dehydration. (Pediatrics)

Hospital admission for a 12-year-old with a laceration of the upper eyelid involving the lid margin and superior canaliculus, admitted prior to surgery for IV antibiotic therapy. (Cphthalmology)

Hospital admission of a 32-year-old female with severe flank pain, hematuria and presumed diagnosis of ureteral calculus as determined by Emergency Department physician. (Urology)

Initial hospital visit for a patient with several large venous stasis ulcers not responding to outpatient therapy. (Dermatology)

Initial hospital visit for 21-year-old pregnant patient (9 weeks gestation) with hyperemesis gravidarum. (Obstetrics & Gynecology)

Initial hospital visit for a 73-year-old female with acute pyelonephritis who is otherwise generally healthy. (Geriatrics)

Initial hospital visit for 62-year-old patient with cellulitis of the foot requiring bedrest and intravenous antibiotics. (Orthopaedic Surgery)

UPD	Code	Description	Units	Anes
	99222	Initial hospital care, per day, for the evaluation and management of a patient, which requires these three key components: a comprehensive history; a comprehensive examination; and medical decision making of moderate complexity. Counseling and/or coordination of care with other providers or agencies are provided consistent with the nature of the problem(s) and the patient's and/or family's needs. Usually, the problem(s) requiring admission are of moderate severity. Physicians typically spend 50 minutes at the bedside and on the patient's hospital floor or unit.	22.0	

Examples

Hospital admission, young adult patient, failed previous therapy and now presents in acute asthmatic attack. (Family Medicine/Allergy & Immunology)

Hospital admission of a 62-year-old smoker, established patient, with bronchitis in acute respiratory distress. (Internal Medicine/Pulmonary Medicine)

Hospital admission, examination, and initiation of a treatment program for a 65-year-old female with new onset of right-sided paralysis and aphasia. (Neurology)

Hospital admission for a 50-year-old with left lower quadrant abdominal pain and increased temperature, but without septic picture. (General Surgery)

Hospital admission, examination, and initiation of treatment program for a 66-year old chronic hemodialysis patient with fever and a new pulmonary infiltrate. (Nephrology)

Hospital admission for a 3-year-old with high temperature, limp and painful hip motion of 18 hours duration. (Orthopedic Surgery)

Initial hospital visit for an 8-year-old febrile patient with chronic sinusitis and sever headache, unresponsive to oral antibiotics. (Allergy & Immunology)

Initial hospital visit for a 40-year-old male with submaxillary cellulitis and trismus from infected lower molar. (Oral & Maxillofacial Surgery)

UPD	Code	Description	Units	Anes
	99223	Initial hospital care, per day, for the evaluation and management of a patient, which requires these three key components: a comprehensive history; a comprehensive examination; and medical decision making of high complexity. Counseling and/or coordination of care with other providers or agencies are provided consistent with the nature of the problem(s) and the patient's and/or family's needs. Usually, the problem(s) requiring admission are of high severity. Physicians typically spend 70 minutes at the bedside and on the patient's hospital floor or unit.	28.5	

Examples

Hospital admission, examination, and initiation of treatment program for a previously unknown 58-year-old male who presents with acute chest pain. (Cardiology)

Hospital admission, examination, and initiation of induction chemotherapy for a 42-year-old patient with newly diagnosed acute myelogenous leukemia. (Hematology/Oncology)

Hospital admission following a motor vehicle accident of a 24-year-old male with fracture dislocation of C5-6; neurologically intact. (Neurosurgery)

Hospital admission for a 78-year-old female with left lower lobe pneumonia and a history of coronary artery disease, congestive heart failure, osteoarthritis and gout. (Family Medicine)

Hospital admission, examination, and initiation of treatment program for a 65-year-old immunosuppressed male with confusion, fever, and a headache. (Infectious Disease)

Hospital admission for a 9-year-old with vomiting, dehydration,fever, tachypnea and an admitting diagnosis of diabetic ketoacidosis. (Pediatrics)

Initial hospital visit for a 65-year-old male who presents with acute myocardial infarction, oliguria, hypotension, and altered state of consciousness. (Cardiology)

Initial hospital visit for a hostile/resistant adolescent patient who is severely depressed and involved in poly-substance abuse. Patient is experiencing significant conflict in his chaotic family situation and was suspended from school following an attack on a teacher with a baseball bat. (Psychiatry)

Initial hospital visit for 89-year-old female with fulminant hepatic failure and encephalopathy. (Gastroenterology)

Initial hospital visit for a 42-year-old female with rapidly progressing scleroderma, malignant hypertension, digital infarcts, and oligourea. (Rheumatology)

UPD	Code	Description	Units	Anes
	99231	Subsequent hospital care, per day, for the evaluation and management of a patient, which requires at least two of these three key components: a problem focused interval history; a problem focused examination; medical decision making that is straightforward or of low complexity. Counseling and/or coordination of care with other providers or agencies are provided consistent with the nature of the problem(s) and the patient's and/or family's needs. Usually, the patient is stable, recovering or improving. Physicians typically spend 15 minutes at the bedside and on the patient's hospital floor or unit.	7.5	

Examples

Subsequent hospital visit for a 50-year-old male with uncomplicated myocardial infarction who is clinically stable and without chest pain. (Family Medicine/Cardiology/Internal Medicine)

Subsequent hospital visit for a stable 72-year-old lung cancer patient undergoing a five day course of infusion chemotherapy. (Hematology/Oncology)

Subsequent hospital visit, two days post admission for a 65-year-old male with a CVA (cerebral vascular accident) and left hemiparesis, who is clinically stable. (Neurology/Physical Medicine & Rehabilitation)

Subsequent hospital visit for now stable, 33-year-old male, status post lower gastrointestinal bleeding. (General Surgery)

Subsequent visit on third day of hospitalization for a 60-year-old female recovering from an uncomplicated pneumonia. (Infectious Disease/Internal Medicine/Pulmonary Medicine)

Subsequent hospital visit for a 3-year-old patient in traction for a congenital dislocation of the hip. (Orthopedic Surgery)

Subsequent hospital visit for a 4-year-old female, admitted for acute gastroenteritis and dehydration, requiring IV hydration; now stable. (Family Medicine/Internal Medicine)

Subsequent hospital visit for 50-year-old female with resolving uncomplicated acute pancreatitis. (Gastroenterology)

UPD	Code	Description	Units	Anes
	99232	Subsequent hospital care, per day, for the evaluation and management of a patient, which requires at least two of these three key components: an expanded problem focused interval history; an expanded problem focused examination; medical decision making of moderate complexity. Counseling and/or coordination of care with other providers or agencies are provided consistent with the nature of the problem(s) and the patient's and/or family's needs. Usually, the patient is responding inadequately to therapy or has developed a minor complication. Physicians typically spend 25 minutes at the bedside and on the patient's hospital floor or unit.	12.0	

Examples

Subsequent hospital visit for a 54-year-old patient, Post MI (myocardial infarction), who is out of the CCU (coronary care unit) but is now having frequent premature ventricular contractions on telemetry. (Cardiology/Internal Medicine)

Subsequent hospital visit for a patient with neutropenia, a fever responding to antibiotics, and continued slow gastrointestinal bleeding on platelet support. (Hematology/Oncology)

Subsequent hospital visit for a 50-year-old male admitted two days ago for sub-acute renal allograft rejection. (Nephrology)

Subsequent hospital visit for a 35-year-old drug addict, not responding to initial antibiotic therapy for pyelonephritis. (Urology)

Subsequent hospital visit of a 81-year-old male with abdominal distention, nausea, and vomiting. (General Surgery)

Subsequent hospital care for a 62-year-old female with congestive heart failure, who remains dyspneic and febrile. (Internal Medicine)

Subsequent hospital visit for a 73-year-old female with recently diagnosed lung cancer, who complains of unsteady gait. (Pulmonary Medicine)

Subsequent hospital visit for a 20-month-old male with bacterial meningitis treated 1 week with antibiotic therapy; has now developed temperature of 101.0° (Pediatrics)

Subsequent hospital visit for 13-year-old male admitted with left lower quadrant abdominal pain and fever, not responding to therapy. (General Surgery)

Subsequent hospital visit for a 65-year-old male with hemiplegia and painful paretic shoulder. (Physical Medicine & Rehabilitation)

UPD	Code	Description	Units	Anes
	99233	Subsequent hospital care, per day, for the evaluation and management of a patient, which requires at least two of these three key components: a detailed interval history; a detailed examination; medical decision making of high complexity. Counseling and/or coordination of care with other providers or agencies are provided consistent with the nature of the problem(s) and the patient's and/or family's needs. Usually, the patient is unstable or has developed a significant complication or a significant new problem. Physicians typically spend 35 minutes at the bedside and on the patient's hospital floor or unit.	20.0	

Examples

Subsequent hospital visit for a 60-year-old female, 4 days post uncomplicated inferior myocardial infarction who has developed sever chest pain, dyspnea, diaphoresis and nausea. (Family Medicine)

Subsequent hospital visit for a patient with AML (acute myelogenous leukemia), fever, elevated white count and uric acid undergoing induction chemotherapy. (Hematology/Oncology)

Subsequent hospital visit for a 38-year-old quadriplegic male with acute autonomic hyperreflexia, who is not responsive to initial care. (Physical Medicine & Rehabilitation)

Subsequent hospital visit for a 65-year-old female post-op resection of abdominal aortic aneurysm, with suspected ischemic bowel. (General Surgery)

Subsequent hospital visit for a 60-year-old female with persistent leukocytosis and a fever seven days after a sigmoid colon resection for carcinoma. (Infectious Disease)

Subsequent hospital visit for a chronic renal failure patient on dialysis, who develops chest pain, shortness of breath and new onset of pericardial friction rub. (Nephrology)

Subsequent hospital visit for a 65-year-old male with acute myocardial infarction who now demonstrates complete heart block and congestive heart failure. (Cardiology)

Subsequent hospital visit for a 25-year-old female with hypertension and systemic lupus erythmatosus, admitted for fever and respiratory distress. On the third hospital day, the patient presented with purpuric skin lesions and acute renal failure. (Rheumatology)

Subsequent hospital visit for a 55-year-old male with severe chronic obstructive pulmonary disease and bronchospasm; initially admitted for acute respiratory distress requiring ventilatory support in the ICU. The patient was stabilized, extubated and transferred to the floor, but now has developed acute fever, dyspnea, left lower lobe rhonchi and laboratory evidence of carbon dioxide retention and hypoxemia. (Family Medicine/Internal Medicine)

Subsequent hospital visit for 46-year-old female, known liver cirrhosis patient, with recent upper gastrointestinal hemorrhage from varices; now with worsening ascites and encephalopathy. (Gastroenterology)

Subsequent hospital visit for 62-year-old female admitted with acute subarachnoid hemorrhage, negative cerebral arteriogram, increased lethargy and hemiparesis with fever. (Neurosurgery)

UPD	Code	Description	Units	Anes
97.2	99234	Observation or inpatient hospital care, for the evaluation and management of a patient including admission and discharge on the same date which requires these three key components: a detailed or comprehensive history; a detailed or comprehensive examination; and medical decision making that is straightforward or of low complexity. Counseling and/or coordination of care with other providers or agencies are provided consistent with the nature of the problem(s) and the patient's and/or family's needs. Usually the presenting problem(s) requiring admission are of low severity.	(I) 23.0	
97.2	99235	Observation or inpatient hospital care, for the evaluation and management of a patient including admission and discharge on the same date which requires these three key components: a comprehensive history; a comprehensive examination; and medical decision making of moderate complexity. Counseling and/or coordination of care with other providers or agencies are provided consistent with the nature of the problem(s) and the patient's and/or family's needs. Usually the presenting problem(s) requiring admission are of moderate severity.	(I) 32.5	

UPD	Code	Description	Units	Anes
97.2	**99236**	Observation or inpatient hospital care, for the evaluation and management of a patient including admission and discharge on the same date which requires these three key components: a comprehensive history; a comprehensive examination; and medical decision making of high complexity. Counseling and/or coordination of care with other providers or agencies are provided consistent with the nature of the problem(s) and the patient's and/or family's needs. Usually the presenting problem(s) requiring admission are of high severity.	(I) 39.0	
	99238	Hospital discharge day management; 30 minutes or less	(I) 18.0	
	99239	more than 30 minutes	(I) 30.0	

Consultations

	Code	Description	Units	Anes
	99241	Office consultation for a new or established patient, which requires these three key components: a problem focused history; a problem focused examination; and straightforward medical decision making. Counseling and/or coordination of care with other providers or agencies are provided consistent with the nature of the problem(s) and the patient's and/or family's needs. Usually, the presenting problem(s) are self limited or minor. Physicians typically spend 15 minutes face-to-face with the patient and/or family.	12.0	

Examples

Office consultation with 25-year-old postpartum female with severe symptomatic hemorrhoids. (Colon & Rectal Surgery)

Office consultation with 58-year-old male, referred for follow-up of creatinine level and evaluation of obstructive uropathy, relieved two months ago. (Nephrology)

Office consultation for 30-year-old female tennis player with sprain or contusion of the forearm. (Orthopedic Surgery)

Office consultation for a 45-year-old male, requested by his internist, with asymptomatic torus palatinus requiring no further treatment. (Oral & Maxillofacial Surgery)

	Code	Description	Units	Anes
	99242	Office consultation for a new or established patient, which requires these three key components: an expanded problem focused history; an expanded problem focused examination; and straightforward medical decision making. Counseling and/or coordination of care with other providers or agencies are provided consistent with the nature of the problem(s) and the patient(s) and/or family's needs. Usually, the presenting problem(s) are of low severity. Physicians typically spend 30 minutes face-to-face with the patient and/or family.	17.0	

Examples

Office consultation for management of systolic hypertension in a 70-year-old male scheduled for elective prostate resection. (Geriatrics)

Office consultation with 27-year-old female, with old amputation, for evaluation of existing above-knee prosthesis. (Physical Medicine & Rehabilitation)

Office consultation with 66-year-old female with wrist and hand pain, and finger numbness, secondary to suspected carpal tunnel syndrome. (Orthopedic Surgery)

Office consultation for 61-year-old female, recently on antibiotic therapy, now with diarrhea and leukocytosis. (Abdominal Surgery)

Office consultation for a patient with papulosquamous eruption of elbow with pitting of nails and itchy scalp. (Dermatology)

Office consultation for a 30-year-old female with single season allergic rhinitis. (Allergy & Immunology)

Copyright © 1999 St. Anthony Publishing

UPD	Code	Description	Units	Anes
	99243	Office consultation for a new or established patient, which requires these three key components: a detailed history; a detailed examination; and medical decision making of low complexity. Counseling and/or coordination of care with other providers or agencies are provided consistent with the nature of the problem(s) and the patient's and/or family's needs. Usually, the presenting problem(s) are of moderate severity. Physicians typically spend 40 minutes face-to-face with the patient and/or family.	22.0	

Examples

Office consultation for a 65-year-old female with persistent bronchitis. (Infectious Disease)

Office consultation for a 65-year-old man with chronic low-back pain radiating to the leg. (Neurosurgery)

Office consultation for 23-year-old female with Crohn's disease not responding to therapy. (Abdominal Surgery/Colon & Rectal Surgery)

Office consultation for 25-year-old patient with symptomatic knee pain and swelling, with torn anterior cruciate ligament and/or torn meniscus. (Orthopedic Surgery)

Office consultation for a 67-year-old patient with osteoporosis and mandibular atrophy with regard to reconstructive alternatives. (Oral & Maxillofacial Surgery)

Office consultation for 39-year-old patient referred at a perimenopausal age for irregular menses and menopausal symptoms. (Obstetrics & Gynecology)

UPD	Code	Description	Units	Anes
	99244	Office consultation for a new or established patient, which requires these three key components: a comprehensive history; a comprehensive examination; and medical decision making of moderate complexity. Counseling and/or coordination of care with other providers or agencies are provided consistent with the nature of the problem(s) and the patient's and/or family's needs. Usually, the presenting problem(s) are of moderate to high severity. Physicians typically spend 60 minutes face-to-face with the patient and/or family.	28.0	

Examples

Office consultation with 38-year-old female, with inflammatory bowel disease, who now presents with right lower quadrant pain and suspected intra-abdominal abscess. (General Surgery/Colon & Rectal Surgery)

Office consultation with 72-year-old male with esophageal carcinoma, symptoms of dysphagia and reflux. (Thoracic Surgery)

Office consultation for discussion of treatment options for a 40-year-old female with a two-centimeter adenocarcinoma of the breast. (Radiation Oncology)

Office consultation for young patient referred by pediatrician because of patient's short attention span, easy distractibility and hyperactivity. (Psychiatry)

Office consultation for 66-year-old female, history of colon resection for adenocarcinoma 6 years earlier, now with severe mid-back pain; x-rays showing osteoporosis and multiple vertebral compression fractures. (Neurosurgery)

Office consultation for a patient with chronic pelvic inflammatory disease who now has left lower quadrant pain with a palpable pelvic mass. (Obstetrics & Gynecology)

Office consultation for a patient with long-standing psoriasis with acute onset of erythroderma, pustular lesions, chills, and fever. Combinations of topical and systemic treatments discussed and instituted. (Dermatology)

UPD	Code	Description	Units	Anes
	99245	Office consultation for a new or established patient, which requires these three key components: a comprehensive history; a comprehensive examination; and medical decision making of high complexity. Counseling and/or coordination of care with other providers or agencies are provided consistent with the nature of the problem(s) and the patient's and/or family's needs. Usually, the presenting problem(s) are of moderate to high severity. Physicians typically spend 80 minutes face-to-face with the patient and/or family.	38.0	

Examples

Office consultation in the emergency room for a 25-year-old male with severe, acute, closed head injury. (Neurosurgery)

Office consultation for a 23-year-old female with Stage II A Hodgkins disease with positive supraclavicular and mediastinal nodes. (Radiation Oncology)

Office consultation for a 27-year-old juvenile diabetic patient with severe diabetic retinopathy, gastric atony, nephrotic syndrome and progressive renal failure, now with serum creatinine of 2.7, and a blood pressure of 170/114. (Nephrology)

Office consultation for independent medical evaluation of a patient with a history of complicated low back and neck problems with previous multiple failed back surgeries. (Othopedic Surgery)

Office consultation for adolescent referred by pediatrician for recent onset of violent and self-injurious behavior. (Psychiatry)

Office consultation for a 6-year-old male for evaluation of severe muscle and joint pain and a diffuse rash. Well until 4-6 weeks earlier when he developed arthralgia, myalgias, and a fever of 102° for 1 week. (Rheumatology)

UPD	Code	Description	Units	Anes
	99251	Initial inpatient consultation for a new or established patient, which requires these three key components: a problem focused history; a problem focused examination; and straightforward medical decision making. Counseling and/or coordination of care with other providers or agencies are provided consistent with the nature of the problem(s) and the patient's and/or family's needs. Usually, the presenting problem(s) are self limited or minor. Physicians typically spend 20 minutes at the bedside and on the patient's hospital floor or unit.	13.0	

Examples

Initial inpatient consultation for a 30-year-old female complaining of vaginal itching, post orthopedic surgery. (Obstetrics & Gynecology)

Initial inpatient consultation for a 36-year-old male on orthopedic service with complaint of localized dental pain. (Oral & Maxillofacial Surgery)

UPD	Code	Description	Units	Anes
	99252	Initial inpatient consultation for a new or established patient, which requires these three key components: an expanded problem focused history; an expanded problem focused examination; and straightforward medical decision making. Counseling and/or coordination of care with other providers or agencies are provided consistent with the nature of the problem(s) and the patient's and/or family's needs. Usually, the presenting problem(s) are of low severity. Physicians typically spend 40 minutes at the bedside and on the patient's hospital floor or unit.	18.0	

Examples

Initial inpatient consultation for recommendation of antibiotic prophylaxis for a patient with a synthetic heart valve who will undergo urologic surgery. (Internal Medicine)

Initial inpatient consultation for possible drug eruption in 50-year-old male. (Dermatology)

Preoperative inpatient consultation for evaluation of hypertension in a 60 year-old man who will undergo a cholecystectomy. Patient had a normal annual check-up in your office four months ago. (Internal Medicine)

Initial inpatient consultation for 66-year-old patient with wrist and hand pain and finger numbness, secondary to carpal tunnel syndrome. (Orthopedic Surgery/Plastic Surgery)

Initial inpatient consultation of a 66-year-old male smoker referred for pain management immediately status post-biliary track surgery done via sub-costal incision. (Anesthesiology/Pain Medicine)

Initial inpatient consultation for a 45-year-old male previously abstinent alcoholic, who relapsed and was admitted for management of gastritis. The patient readily accepts the need for further treatment. (Addiction Medicine)

UPD	Code	Description	Units	Anes
	99253	Initial inpatient consultation for a new or established patient, which requires these three key components: a detailed history; a detailed examination; and medical decision making of low complexity. Counseling and/or coordination of care with other providers or agencies are provided consistent with the nature of the problem(s) and the patient's and/or family's needs. Usually, the presenting problem(s) are of moderate severity. Physicians typically spend 55 minutes at the bedside and on the patient's hospital floor or unit.	23.0	

Examples

Initial inpatient consultation for a 57-year-old male, post lower endoscopy, for evaluation of abdominal pain and fever. (General Surgery)

Initial inpatient consultation for rehabilitation of a 73-year-old female one week after surgical management of a hip fracture. (Physical Medicine & Rehabilitation)

Initial inpatient consultation for diagnosis/management of fever following abdominal surgery. (Internal Medicine)

Initial inpatient consultation for a 35-year-old female with a fever and pulmonary infiltrate following caesarean section. (Pulmonary Medicine)

Initial inpatient consultation for a 42-year-old non-diabetic patient post-op cholecystectomy, now with an acute urinary tract infection. (Nephrology)

Initial inpatient consultation for 53-year-old female with moderate uncomplicated pancreatitis. (Gastroenterology)

Initial inpatient consultation for 45-year-old patient with chronic neck pain with radicular pain of the left arm. (Orthopedic Surgery)

Initial inpatient consultation for 8-year-old patient with new onset of seizures who has a normal examination and previous history. (Neurology)

UPD	Code	Description	Units	Anes
	99254	Initial inpatient consultation for a new or established patient, which requires three key components: a comprehensive history; a comprehensive examination; and medical decision making of moderate complexity. Counseling and/or coordination of care with other providers or agencies are provided consistent with the nature of the problem(s) and the patient's and/or family's needs. Usually, the presenting problem(s) are of moderate to high severity. Physicians typically spend 80 minutes at the bedside and on the patient's hospital floor or unit.	30.0	

Examples

Initial inpatient consultation of a 63-year-old in the ICU with diabetes and chronic renal failure who develops acute respiratory distress syndrome 36 hours after a mitral valve replacement. (Anesthesiology)

Initial inpatient consultation for a 66-year-old female with enlarged supraclavicular lymph nodes, found on biopsy to be malignant. (Hematology/Oncology)

Initial inpatient consultation for a 43-year-old female for evaluation of sudden painful visual loss, optic neuritis and episodic paresthesia. (Ophthalmology)

Initial inpatient consultation for evaluation of a 71-year-old male with hyponatremia (serum sodium 114) who was admitted to the hospital with pneumonia. (Nephrology)

Initial hospital consultation for a 72-year-old male with emergency admission for possible bowel obstruction. (Internal Medicine/General Surgery)

Initial inpatient consultation for a 35-year-old female with fever, swollen joints, and rash 1 week duration. (Rheumatology)

UPD	Code	Description	Units	Anes
	99255	Initial inpatient consultation for a new or established patient, which requires these three key components: a comprehensive history; a comprehensive examination; and medical decision making of high complexity. Counseling and/or coordination of care with other providers or agencies are provided consistent with the nature of the problem(s) and the patient's and/or family's needs. Usually, the presenting problem(s) are of moderate to high severity. Physicians typically spend 110 minutes at the bedside and on the patient's hospital floor or unit.	40.0	

Examples

Initial inpatient consultation in the ICU for a 70-year-old male who experienced a cardiac arrest during surgery and was resuscitated. (Cardiology)

Initial inpatient consultation for a patient with sever pancreatitis complicated by respiratory insufficiency, acute renal failure and abscess formation. (Gastroenterology)

Initial inpatient consultation for a 70-year-old cirrhotic male admitted with ascites, jaundice, encephalopathy, and massive hematemesis. (Gastroenterology)

Initial inpatient consultation in the ICU for a 51-year-old patient who is on a ventilator and has a fever two weeks after renal transplantation. (Infectious Disease)

Initial inpatient consultation for evaluation and formulation of plan for management of multiple trauma patient with complex pelvic fracture, 35-year-old male. (General Surgery/Orthopedics)

Initial inpatient consultation for a 50-year-old male with a history of previous myocardial infarction, now with acute pulmonary edema and hypotension. (Cardiology)

Initial inpatient consultation for 45-year-old male with recent, acute subarachnoid hemorrhage, hesitant speech, mildly confused, drowsy. High risk group for HIV+ status. (Neurosurgery)

Initial inpatient consultation for 36-year-old female referred by her internist to evaluate a patient being followed for abdominal pain and fever. The patient has developed diffuse abdominal pain, guarding rigidity and increased fever. (Obstetrics & Gynecology)

UPD	Code	Description	Units	Anes
	99261	Follow-up inpatient consultation for an established patient, which requires at least two of these three key components: a problem focused interval history; a problem focused examination; medical decision making that is straightforward or of low complexity. Counseling and/or coordination of care with other providers or agencies are provided consistent with nature of the problem(s) and the patient's and/or family's needs. Usually, the patient is stable, recovering or improving. Physicians typically spend 10 minutes at the bedside and on the patient's hospital floor or unit.	6.0	

Examples

Follow-up inpatient consultation with 35-year-old female with pulmonary embolism post-op cesarean section, now stable, for assessment of response to anticoagulation and recommended adjustment of heparin dose. (Pulmonary Medicine)

Follow-up inpatient consultation for a 74-year-old male whose postoperative facial paralysis after a cholecystectomy is now resolving. (Neurology)

Follow-up inpatient consultation with 67-year-old female, established patient for review of diagnostic studies ordered at time of first contact. (Internal Medicine)

Follow-up inpatient consultation for 78-year-old female nursing home resident for evaluation of medical management of pruritis ani. (General Surgery/ Colon & Rectal Surgery)

Follow-up inpatient consultation for a 36-year-old female 2 days after spontaneous passage of 3mm stone. (Urology)

Follow-up inpatient consultation for a 94-year-old male nursing home resident for re-evaluation of hemorrhoids following conservative therapy. (Colon & Rectal Surgery/General Surgery/Geriatrics)

Follow-up inpatient consultation for a 50-year-old male, asymptomatic with borderline ECG abnormality, needs preoperative opinion after a thallium exercise perfusion scan. (Cardiology)

UPD	Code	Description	Units	Anes
	99262	Follow-up inpatient consultation for an established patient which requires at least two of these three key components: an expanded problem focused interval history; an expanded problem focused examination; medical decision making of moderate complexity. Counseling and/or coordination of care with other providers or agencies are provided consistent with the nature of the problem(s) and the patient's and/or family's needs. Usually, the patient is responding inadequately to therapy or has developed a minor complication. Physicians typically spend 20 minutes at the bedside and on the patient's hospital floor or unit.	9.0	

Examples

Follow-up inpatient consultation with 72-year-old female, established patient with bullous pemphigoid on combined oral therapy steroids and immunosuppressive to evaluate progress of cutaneous care orders and adjustment of oral/parenteral therapy dosages. (Dermatology)

Follow-up inpatient consultation for a 71-year-old male who has developed a maculopapular skin rash while on antibiotics that you recommended for an uncomplicated pneumonia. (Infectious Disease)

Follow-up inpatient consultation with 68-year-old, incapacitated male, with spinal stenosis and failure to respond to bedrest, analgesics, and PT. (Neurosurgery)

Follow-up inpatient consultation with 51-year-old male, for evaluation and determination of etiology of postoperative hyponatremia following TURP. (Family Medicine)

Follow-up inpatient consultation for reevaluation of a stroke patient, and development of plan for initial rehabilitation services. (Neurology)

Follow-up inpatient consultation with 45-year-old male, established patient for discussion of CT scan which demonstrates a cavernous hemangioma. (Ophthalmology)

Follow-up inpatient consultation for an asymptomatic 35-year-old Type I diabetic patient with hyperkalemic, hyperchloremia acidosis, to review lab results. (Nephrology)

Follow-up inpatient consultation for an elderly male with perioperative myocardial infarction requiring adjustment of vasoactive medications. (Anesthesiology)

UPD	Code	Description	Units	Anes
	99263	Follow-up inpatient consultation for an established patient which requires at least two of these three key components: a detailed interval history; a detailed examination; medical decision making of high complexity. Counseling and/or coordination of care with other providers or agencies are provided consistent with the nature of the problem(s) and the patient's and/or family's needs. Usually, the patient is unstable or has developed a significant complication or a significant new problem. Physicians typically spend 30 minutes at the bedside and on the patient's hospital floor or unit.	11.5	

Examples

Follow-up inpatient consultation with 72-year-old male established patient admitted for management of alcohol withdrawal, now confused and febrile. (Addiction Medicine)

Follow-up inpatient consultation for an HIV-positive patient with an increasing fever following ten days of antibiotic therapy for pneumocystis carinii pneumonia. (Infectious Disease)

Follow-up inpatient consultation with 58-year-old diabetic female, with bacterial endocarditis, continued fever after 2 weeks of intravenous antibiotic therapy, and new onset ventricular ectopia. (Cardiology)

Follow-up inpatient consultation for a 90-year-old female with urinary incontinence who has a complicated medical history requiring reassessment of multiple medical problems, recommendations for placement, further recommendation for management of incontinence and reevaluation of cognitive status because of competency issues. (Geriatrics/Psychiatry)

Follow-up inpatient consultation for 42-year-old male with persistent gastrointestinal bleeding, etiology undetermined, not responding to conservative therapy of transfusions. (General Surgery/Colon & Rectal Surgery)

Follow-up inpatient consultation for a 62-year-old female with steroid-dependent asthma, diabetes mellitus, thyrotoxicosis, abdominal pain and possible vasculitis. (Rhematology)

Follow-up inpatient consultation for a 62-year-old male, status post-op acute small bowel obstruction; now with acute renal failure. (Family Medicine)

UPD	Code	Description	Units	Anes
	99271	Confirmatory consultation for a new or established patient, which requires these three key components: a problem focused history; a problem focused examination; and straightforward medical decision making. Counseling and/or coordination of care with other providers or agencies are provided consistent with the nature of the problem(s) and the patient's and/or family's needs. Usually, the presenting problem(s) are self limited or minor.	8.0	
	99272	Confirmatory consultation for a new or established patient, which requires these three key components: an expanded problem focused history; an expanded problem focused examination; and straightforward medical decision making. Counseling and/or coordination of care with other providers or agencies are provided consistent with the nature of the problem(s) and the patient's and/or family's needs. Usually, the presenting problem(s) are of low severity.	12.0	
	99273	Confirmatory consultation for a new or established patient, which requires these three key components: a detailed history; a detailed examination; and medical decision making of low complexity. Counseling and/or coordination of care with other providers or agencies are provided consistent with the nature of the problem(s) and the patient's and/or family's needs. Usually, the presenting problem(s) are of moderate severity.	16.0	
	99274	Confirmatory consultation for a patient, which requires these three key components: a comprehensive history; a comprehensive examination; and medical decision making of moderate complexity. Counseling and/or coordination of care with other providers or agencies are provided consistent with the nature of the problem(s) and the patient's and/or family's needs. Usually, the presenting problem(s) are of moderate to high severity.	22.0	

UPD	Code	Description	Units	Anes
	99275	Confirmatory consultation for a patient, which requires these three key components: a comprehensive history; a comprehensive examination; and medical decision making of high complexity. Counseling and/or coordination of care with other providers or agencies are provided consistent with the nature of the problem(s) and the patient's and/or family's needs. Usually, the presenting problem(s) are of moderate to high severity.	29.0	

Emergency Department Services

UPD	Code	Description	Units	Anes
	99281	Emergency department visit for the evaluation and management of a patient, which requires these three key components: a problem focused history; a problem focused examination; and straightforward medical decision making. Counseling and/or coordination of care with other providers or agencies are provided consistent with the nature of the problem(s) and the patient's and/or family's needs. Usually, the presenting problem(s) are self limited or minor.	6.2	

Examples

Emergency department visit for a patient for removal of sutures from a well-healed, uncomplicated laceration. (Emergency Medicine)

Emergency department visit for a patient for tetanus toxid immunization. (Emergency Medicine)

Emergency department visit for a patient with several uncomplicated insect bites. (Emergency Medicine)

UPD	Code	Description	Units	Anes
	99282	Emergency department visit for the evaluation and management of a patient, which requires these three key components: an expanded problem focused history; an expanded problem focused examination; and medical decision making of low complexity. Counseling and/or coordination of care with other providers or agencies are provided consistent with the nature of the problem(s) and the patient's and/or family's needs. Usually, the presenting problem(s) are of low to moderate severity.	10.0	

Examples

Emergency department visit for a 20-year-old student who presents with a painful sunburn with blister formation on the back. (Emergency Medicine)

Emergency department visit for a child presenting with impetigo localized to the face. (Emergency Medicine)

Emergency department visit for a patient with a minor traumatic injury of an extremity with localized pain, swelling, and bruising. (Emergency Medicine)

Emergency department visit for an otherwise healthy patient whose chief complaint is a red, swollen cystic lesion on his/her back. (Emergency Medicine)

Emergency department visit for a patient presenting with a rash on both legs after exposure to poison ivy. (Emergency Medicine)

Emergency department visit for a young adult patient with infected sclera and purulent discharge from both eyes without pain, visual disturbance or history of foreign body in either eye. (Emergency Medicine)

UPD	Code	Description	Units	Anes
	99283	Emergency department visit for the evaluation and management of a patient, which requires these three key components: an expanded problem focused history; an expanded problem focused examination; and medical decision making of moderate complexity. Counseling and/or coordination of care with other providers or agencies are provided consistent with the nature of the problem(s) and the patient's and/or family's needs. Usually, the presenting problem(s) are of moderate severity.	16.5	

Examples

Emergency department visit for a sexually active female complaining of vaginal discharge who is afebrile and denies experiencing abdominal or back pain. (Emergency Medicine)

Emergency department visit for a well-appearing 8-year-old child who has a fever, diarrhea and abdominal cramps, is tolerating oral fluids and is not vomiting. (Emergency Medicine)

Emergency department visit for a patient with an inversion ankle injury, who is unable to bear weight on the injured foot and ankle. (Emergency Medicine)

Emergency department visit for a patient who has a complaint of acute pain associated with a suspected foreign body in the painful eye. (Emergency Medicine)

Emergency department visit for a healthy, young adult patient who sustained a blunt head injury with local swelling and bruising without subsequent confusion, loss of consciousness or memory deficit. (Emergency Medicine)

UPD	Code	Description	Units	Anes
	99284	Emergency department visit for the evaluation and management of a patient, which requires these three key components: a detailed history; a detailed examination; and medical decision making of moderate complexity. Counseling and/or coordination of care with other providers or agencies are provided consistent with the nature of the problem(s) and the patient's and/or family's needs. Usually, the presenting problem(s) are of high severity, and require urgent evaluation by the physician but do not pose an immediate significant threat to life or physiologic function.	25.0	

Examples

Emergency department visit for a 4-year-old child who fell off a bike sustaining a head injury with brief loss of consciousness. (Emergency Medicine)

Emergency department visit for an elderly female who has fallen and is now complaining of pain in her right hip and is unable to walk. (Emergency Medicine)

Emergency department visit for a patient with flank pain and hematuria. (Emergency Medicine)

Emergency department visit for a female presenting with lower abdominal pain and vaginal discharge. (Emergency Medicine)

UPD	Code	Description	Units	Anes
	99285	Emergency department visit for the evaluation and management of a patient, which requires these three key components within the constraints imposed by the urgency of the patient's clinical condition and mental status: a comprehensive history; a comprehensive examination; and medical decision making of high complexity. Counseling and/or coordination of care with other providers or agencies are provided consistent with the nature of the problem(s) and the patient's and/or family's needs. Usually, the presenting problem(s) are of high severity and pose an immediate significant threat to life or physiologic function.	37.0	

Examples

Emergency department visit for a patient with a complicated overdose requiring aggressive management to prevent side effects from the ingested materials. (Emergency Medicine)

Emergency department visit for a patient with a new onset of rapid heart rate requiring IV drugs. (Emergency Medicine)

Emergency department visit for patient exhibiting active, upper gastrointestinal bleeding. (Emergency Medicine)

Emergency department visit for a previously healthy young adult patient who is injured in an automobile accident and is brought to the emergency department immobilized and has symptoms compatible with intra-abdominal injuries or multiple extremity injuries. (Emergency Department)

Emergency department visit for a patient with an acute onset of chest pain compatible with symptoms of cardiac ischemia and/or pulmonary embolus. (Emergency Medicine)

Emergency department visit for a patient who presents with a sudden onset of "the worst headache of her life," and complains of a stiff neck, nausea, and inability to concentrate. (Emergency Medicine)

Emergency department visit for a patient with a new onset of a cerebral vascular accident. (Emergency Medicine)

Emergency department visit for acute febrile illness in an adult associated with shortness of breath and an altered level of alertness. (Emergency Medicine)

UPD	Code	Description	Units	Anes
	99288	Physician direction of emergency medical systems (EMS) emergency care, advanced life support	40.0	

Critical Care Services

UPD	Code	Description	Units	Anes
	99291	Critical care, evaluation and management of the unstable critically ill or unstable critically injured patient, requiring the constant attendance of the physician; first hour	42.0	
98.2 ▲ +	99292	each additional 30 minutes (List separately in addition to code for primary service)	21.0	

Neonatal Intensive Care

UPD	Code	Description	Units	Anes
	99295	Initial neonatal intensive care, per day, for the evaluation and management of a critically ill neonate or infant: This code is reserved for the date of admission for neonates who are critically ill. Critically ill neonates require cardiac and/or respiratory supporting (including ventilator or nasal CpaP), continuous or frequent vital sign moniotiring, laboratory and blood gas interpretations, follow-up physician reevaluations, and constant observation by the health ar team under direct physician suervision. Immediate preoperative evaluation and stabilization of neonates with life threatening surgical or cardiac conditions are included under this code.	(I) 150.0	

UPD	Code	Description	Units	Anes
	99296	Subsequent neonatal intensive care, per day, for the evaluation and management of a critically ill and unstable neonate or infant: A critically ill and unstable neonate will require cardiac an/or respiratory support (including enitlator or nasal CPAP), continuous or frequent vital sign monitoring, laboratory and blood gas interpretations, follow-up physician re-evaluations throughout a 24-hour period, and constant observation by the health care team nder direct physician supervision. In additio, most will require frequent ventilator changes, intravenous fluid alterations, and/or early initiation of pareneteral nutrition. Neonates in the immediate post-operative period or those who become critically ill and unstable during the hospital stay will commonly qualify for this level of care. This code encompasses intensive care provided on dates subsequent to the admission date.	(I) 80.0	
	99297	Subsequent neonatal intensive care, per day, for the evaluation and management of a critically ill though stable neonate or infant: Critically ill though stable neonates require cardiac and/or respiratory support (including ventilator and nasal CPAP), continuous or frequent vital sign monioring, laboratory and blood gas interpretations, follow-up physician re-evaluations throughout a 24-hour period, and constant observation by the health care team under direct physician supervision. neonates at this livel of care would be expected to require less frequent changes in respiratory, cardiovascular and fluid and electrolyte therapy as those included under code 99296. This code encompasses intensive care provided on dates subsequent to the admission date.	(I) 40.0	
98.2 ●	99298	Subsequent neonatal intensive care, per day, for the evaluation and management of the recovering very low birth weight infant (less than 1500 grams) Very low birth weight neonates who are no longer critically ill continue to require intensive cardiac and respiratory monitoring, continuous and/or frequent vital sign monitoring, heat maintenance, enteral and/or parenteral nutritional adjustments, laboratory and oxygen monitoring and constant observation by the health care team under direct physician supervision. Neonates of this level of care would be expected to require infrequent changes in respiratory, cardiovascular and/or fluid and electrolyte therapy as those induced under 99296 or 99297. This code encompasses intensive care provided on days subsequent to the admission date.	RNE	

Nursing Facility Services

UPD	Code	Description	Units	Anes
	99301	Evaluation and management of a new or established patient involving an annual nursing facility assessment which requires these three key components: a detailed interval history; a comprehensive examination; and medical decision making that is straightforward or of low complexity. Counseling and/or coordination of care with other providers or agencies are provided consistent with the nature of the problem(s) and the patient's and/or family's needs. Usually, the patient is stable, recovering or improving. The review and affirmation of the medical plan of care is required. Physicians typically spend 30 minutes at the bedside and on the patient's facility floor or unit.	13.0	

Examples

Annual nursing facility history and physical and MDS/RAI evaluation for a 2-year nursing facility resident who is an 84-year-old female with multiple chronic health problems, including: stable controlled hypertension, chronic constipation, osteoarthritis, and moderated stable dementia.

Nursing facility visit for an assessment of a resident with non-insulin dependent diabetes, stable angina, and chronic obstructive pulmonary disease (COPD) one year after previous MDS/RAI

UPD	Code	Description	Units	Anes
	99302	Evaluation and management of a new or established patient involving a nursing facility assessment which requires these three key components: a detailed interval history; a comprehensive examination; and medical decision making of moderate to high complexity. Counseling and/or coordination of care with other providers or agencies are provided consistent with the nature of the problem(s) and the patient's and/or family's needs. Usually, the patient has developed a significant complication or a significant new problem and has had a major permanent change in status. The creation of a new medical plan of care is required. Physicians typically spend 40 minutes at the bedside and on the patient's facility floor or unit.	17.5	

Examples

Nursing facility visit one year after previous MDS/RAI to assess an 80-year-old woman with Parkinson's disease, chronic hypertension and degenerative arthritis. Visit reveals stage II decubitus.

Nursing facility assessment of a 28-year-old diabetic, male resident with a new stage IV pressure ulcer on his left lateral malleolus that is unresponsive to treatment, thus triggering the need for a new MDS/RAI and new medical plan of care.

Nursing facility assessment of an 88-year-old male resident with a permanent change in status following a new cerebral vascular accident (CVA) that has triggered the need for a new MDS/RAI and medical plan of care.

Nursing facility visit and assessment to take over the primary care of 75-year-old diabetic, previously stable, who was on oral hypoglycemic agents, but who now requires initiation of insulin therapy, a new MDS/RAI, and medical plan of care.

Nursing facility visit and assessment for an 81-year-old female resident with dementia who under structured guidance and intensive nutritional support has regained significant levels of function in three activities of daily living—and is now able to feed and dress herself and ambulate with appliance and who now thus requires a new MDS/RAI and medical plan of care.

UPD	Code	Description	Units	Anes
	99303	Evaluation and management of a new or established patient involving a nursing facility assessment at the time of initial admission or readmission to the facility, which requires these three key components: a comprehensive history; a comprehensive examination; and medical decision making of moderate to high complexity. Counseling and/or coordination of care with other providers or agencies are provided consistent with the nature of the problem(s) and the patient's and/or family's needs. The creation of a medical plan of care is required. Physicians typically spend 50 minutes at the bedside and on the patient's facility floor or unit.	23.5	

Examples

Initial nursing facility assessment (MDS/RAI and medical plan of care) of a 72-year-old insulin dependent diabetic amputee with hearing and visual impairments and possible dementia seen in the office the day before and judged to require nursing facility care.

Sub-acute nursing facility assessment of a previously independent living 90-year-old male who suffered a recent cerebral vascular accident (CVA) and is transferred to the hospital sub-acute rehabilitiation unit for further rehabilitation supportive services.

Initial nursing facility visit to evaluate a 72-year-old woman found confused and wandering, admitted by Adult Protective Services without a qualifying hospital stay or inpatient work. The patient lives alone and has no relatives or significant others in the community.

Nursing facility assessment and creation of medical plan of care upon readmission to the nursing facility of an 82-year-old male who was previously discharged. The patient has just been discharged from the hospital where he had been treated for an acute gastric ulcer bleed associated with transient delirium. The patient returns to the nursing facility debilitated, protein depleted, and with a stage III coccygeal decubitus.

UPD	Code	Description	Units	Anes
	99311	Subsequent nursing facility care, per day, for the evaluation and management of a new or established patient, which requires at least two of these three key components: a problem focused interval history; a problem focused examination; medical decision making that is straightforward or of low complexity. Counseling and/or coordination of care with other providers or agencies are provided consistent with the nature of the problem(s) and the patient's and/or family's needs. Usually, the patient is stable, recovering or improving. Physicians typically spend 15 minutes at the bedside and on the patient's facility floor or unit.	7.5	

Examples

Scheduled follow-up visit for a known 70-year-old stable paraplegic with no status change noted during visit.

Scheduled monthly nursing home visit with a patient who has mild senile dementia, Alzheimer's type, with no change in status, stable hypertension, and who is ambulating with a walker one year past stroke.

Follow-up in skilled nursing facility with a 70-year-old patient following a ten day treatment of a cellulitis of the foot.

UPD	Code	Description	Units	Anes
	99312	Subsequent nursing facility care, per day, for the evaluation and management of a new or established patient, which requires at least two of these three key components: an expanded problem focused interval history; an expanded problem focused examination; medical decision making of moderate complexity. Counseling and/or coordination of care with other providers or agencies are provided consistent with the nature of the problem(s) and the patient's and/or family's needs. Usually, the patient is responding inadequately to therapy or has developed a minor complication. Physicians typically spend 25 minutes at the bedside and on the patient's facility floor or unit.	12.0	

Examples

Scheduled follow-up visit to a resident with controlled dementia, hypertension and diabetes. During visit, patient seems to exhibit flu symptoms.

Scheduled nursing facility visit with an afebrile demented resident who also has a mild cough, requiring no change in the medical plan of care.

Subsequent visit in a skilled nursing facility with a patient who is six months post stroke and now has a fever and mild cough.

Scheduled nursing facility visit for an 84-year-old male with chronic renal insufficiency, on digitalis and diuretics, requiring adjustment of medications and revision of medical plan of care.

Nursing facility visit of a resident with multiple chronic health problems who is six months past stroke and now has a fever and mild cough, to evaluate for possible pneumonia. Requires the development of a new medical plan of care, but not a revised MDS/RAI.

UPD	Code	Description	Units	Anes
	99313	Subsequent nursing facility care, per day, for the evaluation and management of a new or established patient, which requires at least two of these three key components: a detailed interval history; a detailed examination; medical decision making of moderate to high complexity. Counseling and/or coordination of care with other providers or agencies are provided consistent with the nature of the problem(s) and the patient's and/or family's needs. Usually, the patient has developed a significant complication or a significant new problem. Physicians typically spend 35 minutes at the bedside and on the patient's facility floor or unit.	19.5	

Examples

Follow-up nursing facility visit to evaluate the reason for frequent falls by a 90-year-old ataxic resident, and to determine possible need for change in medications and medical care plan.

Re-admission of a 75-year-old man with stroke who was hospitalized with pneumonia for his illness and who returns to the nursing facility with no permanent change in status from his condition prior to hospitalization; no new MDS/RAI is required.

Nursing facility visit with a diabetic resident who has developed Stage II decubitus ulcers with cellulitis, requiring a revision in the medical plan of care.

Nursing facility visit to develop a new plan of care for an amputee with atherosclerosis obliterans who has refused to eat for three days and has developed decreased urinary output.

Nursing facility visit for a 78-year-old resident with chronic atrial fibrillation and a history of heart failure to evaluate an acute confusional state and to revise the medical plan of care.

Unscheduled nursing facility visit for evaluation of a patient with fever and obtundation who is determined not to require hospital admission or new MDS, but who does require workup and revision of medical plan of care.

UPD	Code	Description	Units	Anes
97.2	99315	Nursing facility discharge day management; 30 minutes or less	(I) 14.0	
97.2	99316	more than 30 minutes	(I) 16.0	

Domiciliary, Rest Home (eg, Boarding Home), or Custodial Care Services

UPD	Code	Description	Units	Anes
	99321	Domiciliary or rest home visit for the evaluation and management of a new patient which requires these three key components: a problem focused history; a problem focused examination; and medical decision making that is straightforward or of low complexity. Counseling and/or coordination of care with other providers or agencies are provided consistent with the nature of the problem(s) and the patient's and/or family's needs. Usually, the presenting problem(s) are of low severity.	8.3	
	99322	Domiciliary or rest home visit for the evaluation and management of a new patient, which requires these three key components: an expanded problem focused history; an expanded problem focused examination; and medical decision making of moderate complexity. Counseling and/or coordination of care with other providers or agencies are provided consistent with the nature of the problem(s) and the patient's and/or family's needs. Usually, the presenting problem(s) are of moderate severity.	12.5	
	99323	Domiciliary or rest home visit for the evaluation and management of a new patient, which requires these three key components: a detailed history; a detailed examination; and medical decision making of high complexity. Counseling and/or coordination of care with other providers or agencies are provided consistent with the nature of the problem(s) and the patient's and/or family's needs. Usually, the presenting problem(s) are of high complexity.	19.0	

UPD	Code	Description	Units	Anes
	99331	Domiciliary or rest home visit for the evaluation and management of an established patient, which requires at least two of these three key components: a problem focused interval history; a problem focused examination; medical decision making that is straightforward or of low complexity. Counseling and/or coordination of care with other providers or agencies are provided consistent with the nature of the problem(s) and the patient's and/or family's needs. Usually, the patient is stable, recovering or improving.	7.3	
	99332	Domiciliary or rest home visit for the evaluation and management of an established patient, which requires at least two of these three key components: an expanded problem focused interval history; an expanded problem focused examination; medical decision making of moderate complexity. Counseling and/or coordination of care with other providers or agencies are provided consistent with the nature of the problem(s) and the patient's and/or family's needs. Usually, the patient is responding inadequately to therapy or has developed a minor complication.	10.0	
	99333	Domiciliary or rest home visit for the evaluation and management of an established patient, which requires at least two of these three key components: a detailed interval history; a detailed examination; medical decision making of high complexity. Counseling and/or coordination of care with other providers or agencies are provided consistent with the nature of the problem(s) and the patient's and/or family's needs. Usually, the patient is unstable or has developed a significant complication or a significant new problem.	13.0	

Home Services

UPD	Code	Description	Units	Anes
97.2	99341	Home visit for the evaluation and management of a new patient, which requires these three key components: a problem focused history; a problem focused examination; and straightforward medical decision making. Counseling and/or coordination of care with other providers or agencies are provided consistent with the nature of the problem(s) and the patient's and/or family's needs. Usually, the presenting problem(s) are of low severity. Physicians typically spend 20 minutes face-to-face with the patient and/or family.	10.0	
97.2	99342	Home visit for the evaluation and management of a new patient, which requires these three key components: an expanded problem focused history; an expanded problem focused examination; and medical decision making of low complexity. Counseling and/or coordination of care with other providers or agencies are provided consistent with the nature of the problem(s) and the patient's and/or family's needs. Usually, the presenting problem(s) are of moderate severity. Physicians typically spend 30 minutes face-to-face with the patient and/or family.	12.5	
97.2	99343	Home visit for the evaluation and management of a new patient, which requires these three key components: a detailed history; a detailed examination; and medical decision making of moderate complexity. Counseling and/or coordination of care with other providers or agencies are provided consistent with the nature of the problem(s) and the patient's and/or family's needs. Usually, the presenting problem(s) are of moderate to high severity. Physicians typically spend 45 minutes face-to-face with the patient and/or family.	16.8	
97.2	99344	Home visit for the evaluation and management of a new patient, which requires these three key components: a comprehensive history; a comprehensive examination; and medical decision making of moderate complexity. Counseling and/or coordination of care with other providers or agencies are provided consistent with the nature of the problem(s) and the patient's and/or family's needs. Usually, the presenting problem(s) are of high severity. Physicians typically spend 60 minutes face-to-face with the patient and/or family.	(I) 22.0	

UPD	Code	Description	Units	Anes
97.2	**99345**	Home visit for the evaluation and management of a new patient, which requires these three key components: a comprehensive history; a comprehensive examination; and medical decision making of high complexity. Counseling and/or coordination of care with other providers or agencies are provided consistent with the nature of the problem(s) and the patient's and/or family's needs. Usually, the patient is unstable or has developed a significant new problem requiring immediate physician attention. Physicians typically spend 75 minutes face-to-face with the patient and/or family.	(I) 29.0	
97.2	**99347**	Home visit for the evaluation and management of an established patient, which requires at least two of these three key components: a problem focused interval history; a problem focused examination; straightforward medical decision making. Counseling and/or coordination of care with other providers or agencies are provided consistent with the nature of the problem(s) and the patient's and/or family's needs. Usually, the presenting problem(s) are self-limited or minor. Physicians typically spend 15 minutes face-to-face with the patient and/or family.	(I) 8.0	
97.2	**99348**	Home visit for the evaluation and management of an established patient, which requires at least two of these three components: an expanded problem focused interval history; an expanded problem focused examination; medical decision making of low complexity. Counseling and/or coordination of care with other providers or agencies are provided consistent with the nature of the problem(s) and the patient's and/or family's needs. Usually, the presenting problem(s) are of low to moderate severity. Physicians typically spend 25 minutes face-to-face with the patient and/or family.	(I) 11.0	
97.2	**99349**	Home visit for the evaluation and management of an established patient, which requires at least two of these three key components: a detailed interval history; a detailed examination; medical decision making of moderate complexity. Counseling and/or coordination of care with other providers or agencies are provided consistent with the nature of the problem(s) and the patient's and/or family's needs. Usually, the presenting problem(s) are moderate to high severity. Physicians typically spend 40 minutes face-to-face with the patient and/or family.	(I) 15.3	
97.2	**99350**	Home visit for the evaluation and management of an established patient, which requires at least two of these three key components: a comprehensive interval history; a comprehensive examination; medical decision making of moderate to high complexity. Counseling and/or coordination of care with other providers or agencies are provided consistent with the nature of the problem(s) and the patient's and/or family's needs. Usually, the presenting problem(s) are of moderate to high severity. The patient may be unstable or may have developed a significant new problem requiring immediate physician attention. Physicians typically spend 60 minutes face-to-face with the patient and/or family.	(I) 25.0	

Prolonged Services

UPD	Code	Description	Units	Anes
97.2	**99351**	99351 has been deleted. To report, see 99347	9.0	
97.2	**99352**	99352 has been deleted. To report, see 99348	12.0	
97.2	**99353**	99353 has been deleted. To report, see 99349	16.3	
98.2 ▲ +	**99354**	Prolonged physician service in the office or other outpatient setting requiring direct (face-to-face) patient contact beyond the usual service (eg, prolonged care and treatment of an acute asthmatic patient in an outpatient setting); first hour (List separately in addition to code for office or other outpatient Evaluation and Management service)	(I) 20.0	

UPD		Code	Description	Units	Anes
98.2	▲ +	99355	each additional 30 minutes (List separately in addition to code for prolonged physician service)	(I) 10.0	
98.2	▲ +	99356	Prolonged physician service in the inpatient setting, requiring direct (face-to-face) patient contact beyond the usual service (eg, maternal fetal monitoring for high risk delivery or other physiological monitoring, prolonged care of an acutely ill inpatient); first hour (List separately in addition to code for inpatient Evaluation and Management service)	(I) 22.0	
98.2	▲ +	99357	each additional 30 minutes (List separately in addition to code for prolonged physician service)	(I) 11.0	
98.2	▲ +	99358	Prolonged evaluation and management service before and/or after direct (face-to-face) patient care (eg, review of extensive records and tests, communication with other professionals and/or the patient/family); first hour (List separately in addition to code(s) for other physician service(s) and/or inpatient or outpatient Evaluation and Management service)	(I) 16.0	
98.2	▲ +	99359	each additional 30 minutes (List separately in addition to code for prolonged physician service)	(I) 8.0	
97.2		99360	Physician standby service, requiring prolonged physician attendance, each 30 minutes (eg, operative standby, standby for frozen section, for cesarean/high risk delivery, for monitoring EEG)	(I) 15.0	

Case Management Services

		Code	Description	Units	Anes
		99361	Medical conference by a physician with interdisciplinary team of health professionals or representatives of community agencies to coordinate activities of patient care (patient not present); approximately 30 minutes	10.0	
		99362	approximately 60 minutes	18.0	
		99371	Telephone call by a physician to patient or for consultation or medical management or for coordinating medical management with other health care professionals (eg, nurses, therapists, social workers, nutritionists, physicians, pharmacists); simple or brief (eg, to report on tests and/or laboratory results, to clarify or alter previous instructions, to integrate new information from other health professionals into the medical treatment plan, or to adjust therapy)	2.0	
		99372	intermediate (eg, to provide advice to an established patient on a new problem, to initiate therapy that can be handled by telephone, to discuss test results in detail, to coordinate medical management of a new problem in an established patient, to discuss and evaluate new information and details, or to initiate new plan of care)	4.0	
		99373	complex or lengthy (eg, lengthy counseling session with anxious or distraught patient, detailed or prolonged discussion with family members regarding seriously ill patient, lengthy communication necessary to coordinate complex services of several different health professionals working on different aspects of the total patient care plan)	6.0	

Care Plan Oversight Services

		Code	Description	Units	Anes
97.2		99374	Physician supervision of a patient under care of home health agency (patient not present) requiring complex and multidisciplinary care modalities involving regular physician development and/or revision of care plans, review of subsequent reports of patient status, review of laboratory and other studies, communication (including telephone calls) with other health care professionals involved in patient's care, integration of new information into the medical treatment plan and/or adjustment of medical therapy, within a calendar month; 15–29 minutes	(I) 9.0	

UPD	Code	Description	Units	Anes
97.2	**99375**	30 minutes or more	(I) 17.0	
97.2	**99376**	This code has been deleted.	(I) 20.0	
97.2	**99377**	Physician supervision of a hospice patient (patient not present) requiring complex and multidisciplinary care modalities involving regular physician development and/or revision of care plans, review of subsequent reports of patient status, review of related laboratory and other studies, communication (including telephone calls) with other health care professionals involved in patient's care, integration of new information into the medical treatment plan and/or adjustment of medical therapy, within a calendar month; 15–29 minutes	(I) 9.0	
97.2	**99378**	30 minutes or more	(I) 17.0	
97.2	**99379**	Physician supervision of a nursing facility patient (patient not present) requiring complex and multidisciplinary care modalities involving regular physician development and/or revision of care plans, review of subsequent reports of patient status, review of related laboratory and other studies, communication (including telephone calls) with other health care professionals involved in patient's care, integration of new information into the medical treatment plan and/or adjustment of medical therapy, within a calendar month; 15–29 minutes	(I) 9.0	
97.2	**99380**	30 minutes or more	(I) 17.0	

Preventive Medicine Services

UPD	Code	Description	Units	Anes
97.1	**99381**	Initial preventive medicine evaluation and management of an individual including a comprehensive history, a comprehensive examination, counseling/anticipatory guidance/risk factor reduction interventions, and the ordering of appropriate laboratory/diagnostic procedures, new patient; infant (age under 1 year)	19.0	
97.1	**99382**	early childhood (age 1 through 4 years)	20.0	
97.1	**99383**	late childhood (age 5 through 11 years)	22.0	
97.1	**99384**	adolescent (age 12 through 17 years)	24.0	
97.1	**99385**	18-39 years	26.0	
97.1	**99386**	40-64 years	27.0	
97.1	**99387**	65 years and over	29.0	
97.1	**99391**	Periodic preventive medicine reevaluation and management of an individual including a comprehensive history, comprehensive examination, counseling/anticipatory guidance/risk factor reduction interventions, and the ordering of appropriate laboratory/diagnostic procedures, established patient; infant (age under 1 year)	16.0	
97.1	**99392**	early childhood (age 1 through 4 years)	17.0	
97.1	**99393**	late childhood (age 5 through 11 years)	18.0	
97.1	**99394**	adolescent (age 12 through 17 years)	19.0	
97.1	**99395**	18-39 years	20.0	
97.1	**99396**	40-64 years	21.0	
97.1	**99397**	65 years and over	22.0	

UPD	Code	Description	Units	Anes
	99401	Preventive medicine counseling and/or risk factor reduction intervention(s) provided to an individual (separate procedure); approximately 15 minutes	4.0	
	99402	approximately 30 minutes	8.0	
	99403	approximately 45 minutes	12.0	
	99404	approximately 60 minutes	16.0	
	99411	Preventive medicine counseling and/or risk factor reduction intervention(s) provided to individuals in a group setting (separate procedure); approximately 30 minutes	9.0	
	99412	approximately 60 minutes	18.0	
96.2	99420	Administration and interpretation of health risk assessment instrument (eg, health hazard appraisal)	(I) 16.0	
	99429	Unlisted preventive medicine service	0.0	

Newborn Care

UPD	Code	Description	Units	Anes
	99431	History and examination of the normal newborn infant, initiation of diagnostic and treatment programs and preparation of hospital records. (This code should also be used for birthing room deliveries.)	22.0	
	99432	Normal newborn care in other than hospital or birthing room setting, including physical examination of baby and conference(s) with parent(s)	18.0	
	99433	Subsequent hospital care, for the evaluation and management of a normal newborn, per day	10.0	
	99435	History and examination of the normal newborn infant, including the preparation of medical records (this code should only be used for newborns assessed and discharged from the hospital or birthing room on the same date)	(I) 25.5	
97.2	99436	Attendance at delivery (when requested by delivering physician) and initial stabilization of newborn	(I) 25.5	
	99440	Newborn resuscitation: provision of positive pressure ventilation and/or chest compressions in the presence of acute inadequate ventilation and/or cardiac output	28.0	

Special Evaluation and Management Services

UPD	Code	Description	Units	Anes
96.2	99450	Basic life and/or disability examination that includes: •measurement of height, weight and blood pressure; •completion of a medical history following a life insurance pro forma; •collection of blood sample and/or urinalysis complying with "chain of custody" protocols; and •completion of necessary documentation/certificates	(I) 19.0	
96.2	99455	Work related or medical disability examination by the treating physician that includes: •completion of a medical history commensurate with the patient's condition; •performance of an examination commensurate with the patient's condition; •formulation of a diagnosis, assessment of capabilities and stability, and calculation of impairment; •development of future medical treatment plan; and •completion of necessary documentation/certificates and report.	(I) 26.0	

UPD	Code	Description	Units	Anes
96.2	**99456**	Work related or medical disability examination by other than the treating physician that includes: •completion of a medical history commensurate with the patient's condition; •performance of an examination commensurate with the patient's condition; •formulation of a diagnosis, assessment of capabilities and stability, and calculation of impairment; •development of future medical treatment plan; and •completion of necessary documentation/certificates and report.	(I) 30.0	

Other Evaluation and Management Services

	Code	Description	Units	Anes
	99499	Unlisted evaluation and management service	BR	

HCPCS

HCPCS Introduction

RVP now includes a listing of HCPCS Level II codes as they relate to physician services. The following is a list of these codes as developed by the Health Care Financing Administration (HCFA) for the current year. The editors are researching a methodology for assigning values to all HCPCS codes. Many of these procedures have relative values or value guidelines for use with the conversion factor used for Medicine. Other codes list or include the cost of medical equipment and supplies. These codes are supplied in the comprehensive listing for your convenience. Values cannot be determined under the current relative value structure. The editors are researching fees for these procedures with the intention of publishing a fee range for each medical equipment or supply code in the future. The editors have elected to indicate that a relative value is not available for procedures with a "—" in the Units column. These codes should be treated as a "by report" code, and substantiating documentation should accompany the code submission.

"Physician's Current Procedural Terminology," fourth edition, copyrighted by the American Medical Association (CPT-4) is a listing of descriptive terms and numeric identifying codes and modifiers for reporting medical services and procedures performed by physicians. This Health Care Financing Administration common procedure coding system (HCPCS) includes CPT-4 descriptive terms and numeric identifying codes and modifiers for reporting medical services and procedures and other materials contained in CPT-4 that are copyrighted by the American Medical Association. Participants will be authorized to use copies of CPT-4 material in HCPCS only for the purposes directly related to participating in HCFA programs. Permission for any other use must be obtained from the AMA.

Note: The "D" codes for HCPCS are not included in this publication. These codes are related to dental procedures and have no unit values assigned.

HCPCS Disclaimer

HCPCS is designed to promote uniform medical services reporting and statistical data collection. Inclusion of a service, product, or supply does not constitute endorsement by the HCPCS editorial panel that it is noninvestigational or is commonly and customarily recognized as appropriate for medical care and treatment. Inclusion or exclusion of a procedure, product, or supply does not imply any health insurance coverage or reimbursement policy.

Note concerning the detailed portion of the HCPCS record:

The following fields are updated annually as necessary: Maintenance Date (M/D), Action Code (A/C), Coverage (COV), Control Statement (CNST), Cross Reference (X/R), The Independent Laboratory Certification (ILC), Coverage Issues Manual (CIM), and Medicare Carriers Manual (MCM). All Medicare carriers update their individual systems and records with current coverage information throughout the year. That information is not reflected in the aggregate HCPCS listing that follows. Absence of a code in FD-08 (COV) does not mean the item is automatically covered but that the carrier has the authority to determine coverage and payment policy.

-AA   Anesthesia services performed personally by anesthesiologist
-AB   Medical direction of own employee(s) by anesthesiologist (not more than four employees)
-AC   Medical direction of other than own employees by anesthesiologist (not more than four individuals)
-AD   Medical supervision by a physician: more than four concurrent anesthesia procedures
-AE   Direction of residents in furnishing not more than two concurrent anesthesia services - attending physician relationship met
-AF   Anesthesia complicated by total body hypothermia
-AG   Anesthesia for emergency surgery on a patient who is moribund or who has an incapacitating systemic disease that is a constant threat to life (may warrant additional charge)
-AH   Clinical psychologist

-AJ   Clinical social worker

-AK   (-AK. This modifier was deleted in 1999)

-AL   (-AL. This modifier was deleted in 1999)

-AM   Physician, team member service

-AN   (-AN. This modifier was deleted in 1999)

-AP   Determination of refractive state was not performed in the course of diagnostic ophthalmological examination

-AS   Physician assistant, nurse practitioner, or clinical nurse specialist services for assistant at surgery

-AT   Acute treatment (this modifier should be used when reporting service 98940, 98941, 98942)

-AU   (-AU. This modifier was deleted in 1999)

-AV   (-AV. This modifier was deleted in 1999)

-AW   (-AW. This modifier was deleted in 1999)

-AY   (-AY. This modifier was deleted in 1999)

-BP   The beneficiary has been informed of the purchase and rental options and has elected to purchase the item

-BR   The beneficiary has been informed of the purchase and rental options and has elected to rent the item

-BU   The beneficiary has been informed of the purchase and rental options and after 30 days has not informed the supplier of his/her decision

-CC   Procedure code change (use 'CC' when the procedure code submitted was changed either for administrative reasons or because an incorrect code was filed)

-DD   Powdered enteral formulae (this should be used when enteral powdered products are supplied)

-E1   Upper left, eyelid

-E2   Lower left, eyelid

-E3   Upper right, eyelid

-E4   Lower right, eyelid

-EJ   Subsequent claim (for epoetin alfa-epo-injection claim only)

-EM   Emergency reserve supply (for ESRD benefit only)

-EP   Service provided as part of medicaid early periodic screening diagnosis and treatment (EPSDT) program

-ET   Emergency treatment (dental procedures performed in emergency situations should show the modifier 'ET')

-F1   Left hand, second digit

-F2   Left hand, third digit

-F3   Left hand, fourth digit

-F4   Left hand, fifth digit

-F5   Right hand, thumb

-F6   Right hand, second digit

-F7   Right hand, third digit

-F8   Right hand, fourth digit

-F9   Right hand, fifth digit

-FA   Left hand, thumb

-FP   Service provided as part of medicaid family planning program

-G1   Most recent URR reading of less than 60

-G2   Most recent URR reading of 60 to 64.9

-G3   Most recent URR reading of 65 to 69.9

-G4   Most recent URR reading of 70 to 74.9

-G5   Most recent URR reading of 75 or greater

-G6   ESRD patient for whom less than six dialysis sessions have been provided in a month

-GA   Waiver of liability statement on file

-GB   Distinct procedural service: the physician may need to indicate that a procedure or service was distinct or separate from other services performed on the same day. This may represent a different session or patient encounter, different procedure or surgery, different site, separate lesion, or separate injury (or area of injury in extensive injuries).

-GC   This service has been performed in part by a resident under the direction of a teaching physician

-GE   This service has been performed by a resident without the presence of a teaching physician under the primary care exception

-GH   Diagnostic mammogram converted from screening mammogram on same day

-GJ   OPT out physician or practitioner emergency or urgent service

-GN   Service delivered personally by a speech-language pathologist or under an outpatient speech-language pathology plan of care

-GO   Service delivered personally by an occupational therapist or under an outpatient occupational therapy plan of care

-GP   Service delivered personally by a physical therapist or under an outpatient physical therapy plan of care

-GT   Via interactive audio and video telecommunication systems

-GX   Service not covered by Medicare

-K0	Lower extremity prosthesis functional level 0 - does not have the ability or potential to ambulate or transfer safely with or without assistance and a prosthesis does not enhance their quality of lefe or mobility.
-K1	Lower extremity prosthesis functional level 1 - has the ability or potential to use a prosthesis for transfers or ambulation on level surfaces at fixed cadence. Typical of the limited and unlimited household ambulator.
-K2	Lower extremity prosthesis functional level 2 - has the ability or potential for ambulation with the ability to traverse low level environmental barriers such as curbs, stairs or uneven surfaces. Typical of the limited community ambulator.
-K3	Lower extremity prosthesis functional level 3 - has the ability or potential for ambulation with variable cadence. Typical of the community ambulator who has the ability to transverse most environmental barriers and may have vocational, therapeutic, or exercise activity that demands prosthetic utilization beyond simple locomotion.
-K4	Lower extremity prosthesis functional level 4 - has the ability or potential for prosthetic ambulation that exceeds the basic ambulation skills, exhibiting high impact, stress, or energy levels, typical of the prosthetic demands of the child, active adult, or athlete.
-KA	Add on option/accessory for wheelchair
-KH	DMEPOS item, initial claim, purchase or first month rental
-KI	DMEPOS item, second or third month rental
-KJ	DMEPOS item, parenteral enteral nutrition (PEN) pump or capped rental, months four to fifteen
-KK	Inhalation solution compounded from an FDA approved formulation
-KL	Product characteristics defined in medical policy are met
-KM	Replacement of facial prosthesis including new impression/moulage
-KN	Replacement of facial prosthesis using previous master model
-KO	Single drug unit dose formulation
-KP	First drug of a multiple drug unit dose formulation
-KQ	Second or subsequent drug of a multiple drug unit dose formulation
-KS	Glucose monitor supply for diabetic beneficiary not treated with insulin
-LC	Left circumflex coronary artery
-LD	Left anterior descending coronary artery
-LL	Lease/rental (use the 'LL' modifier when dme equipment rental is to be applied against the purchase price)
-LR	Laboratory round trip
-LS	FDA-monitored intraocular lens implant
-LT	Left side (used to identify procedures performed on the left side of the body)
-MP	Multiple patients seen (use only in connection with CPT-4 visit codes 90300-90470, visits to skilled nursing, intermediate care and long term care facility and nursing home, boarding home, domiciliary or custodial care medical services
-MS	Six month maintenance and servicing fee for reasonable and necessary parts and labor which are not covered under any manufacturer or supplier warranty
-NR	New when rented (use the 'NR' modifier when DME which was new at the time of rental is subsequently purchased)
-NU	New equipment
-PL	Progressive addition lenses
-Q1	Documentation on file verifying the presence of markedly thickened toenail(s) resulting in soft tissue infection (paronychia) and pain, requiring toenail debridement
-Q2	HCFA/ORD demonstration project procedure/service
-Q3	Live kidney donor: services associated with postoperative medical complications directly related to the donation
-Q4	Service for ordering/referring physician qualifies as a service exemption
-Q5	Service furnished by a substitute physician under a reciprocal billing arrangement
-Q6	Service furnished by a locum tenens physician
-Q7	One class a finding
-Q8	Two class b findings
-Q9	One class b and two class c findings
-QA	FDA investigational device exemption
-QB	Physician providing service in a rural HPSA
-QC	Single channel monitoring
-QD	Recording and storage in solid state memory by a digital recorder
-QE	Prescribed amount of oxygen is less than 1 liter per minute (LPM)
-QF	Prescribed amount of oxygen exceeds 4 liters per minute (LPM) and portable oxygen is prescribed
-QG	Prescribed amount of oxygen is greater than 4 liters per minute (LPM)
-QH	Oxygen conserving device is being used with an oxygen delivery system
-QK	Medical direction of two, three, or four concurrent anesthesia procedures involving qualified individuals
-QL	Patient pronounced dead after ambulance called
-QM	Ambulance service provided under arrangement by a provider of services
-QN	Ambulance service furnished directly by a provider of services

---

▲ Revised code   ● New code   **M** RVSI code or deleted from CPT   **(I)** Interim Value

-QP   Documentation is on file showing that the laboratory test(s) was ordered individually or ordered as a CPT-recognized panel other than automated profile codes 80002-80019, G0058, G0059, and G0060.

-QR   Repeat clinical diagnostic laboratory test performed on the same day to obtain subsequent reportable test value(s) (separate specimens taken in separate encounters)

-QS   Monitored anesthesia care service

-QT   Recording and storage on tape by an analog tape recorder

-QU   Physician providing service in an urban HPSA

-QW   CLIA waived test

-QX   CRNA service: with medical direction by a physician

-QY   Anesthesiologist medically directs one CRNA

-QZ   CRNA service: without medical direction by a physician

-RC   Right coronary artery

-RP   Replacement and repair -RP may be used to indicate replacement of DME, orthotic and prosthetic devices which have been in use for sometime. The claim shows the code for the part, followed by the 'RP' modifier and the charge for the part.

-RR   Rental (use the 'RR' modifier when DME is to be rented)

-RT   Right side (used to identify procedures performed on the right side of the body)

-SF   Second opinion ordered by a professional review organization (PRO) per section 9401, p.l. 99-272 (100% reimbursement - no medicare deductible or coinsurance)

-SG   Ambulatory surgical center (ASC) facility service

-SP   No other patients seen at this facility(use only in connection with CPT-4 visit codes 90300-90470, visits to skilled nursing, intermediate care and long-term care facility and nursing home, boarding home, domiciliary or custodial care medical services)

-T1   Left foot, second digit

-T2   Left foot, third digit

-T3   Left foot, fourth digit

-T4   Left foot, fifth digit

-T5   Right foot, great toe

-T6   Right foot, second digit

-T7   Right foot, third digit

-T8   Right foot, fourth digit

-T9   Right foot, fifth digit

-TA   Left foot, great toe

-TC   Technical component. Under certain circumstances, a charge may be made for the technical component alone. Under those circumstances the technical component charge is identified by adding modifier 'TC' to the usual procedure number. Technical component charges are institutional charges and not billed separately by physicians. However, portable x-ray suppliers only bill for technical component and should utilize modifier TC. The charge data from portable x-ray suppliers will then be used to build customary and prevailing profiles.

-UC   Unclassified ambulance service

-UE   Used durable medical equipment

-VP   Aphakic patient

-YY   Second surgical opinion. See SF for pro-ordered services

-ZZ   Third surgical opinion

HCPCS Section

UPD	Code	Description	Units

Transportation Services Including Ambulance (A0000-A0999)

UPD	Code	Description	Units
	A0021	Ambulance service, outside state per mile, transport (Medicaid only)	—
	A0030	Ambulance service, conventional air service, transport, one way	—
	A0040	Ambulance service, air, helicopter service, transport	—
	A0050	Ambulance service, emergency, water, special transportation services	—
	A0080	Nonemergency transportation: per mile — volunteer, with no vested or personal interest	—
	A0090	Nonemergency transportation: per mile — volunteer, interested individual, neighbor	—
	A0100	Nonemergency transportation: taxi — intracity	—
	A0110	Nonemergency transportation and bus, intra- or interstate carrier systems	—
	A0120	Nonemergency transportation mini-bus, mountain area transports, other non-profit transportation systems	—
	A0130	Nonemergency transportation: wheelchair van	—
	A0140	Nonemergency transportation and air travel (private or commercial), intra- or interstate	—
	A0160	Nonemergency transportation: per mile — caseworker or social worker	BR
	A0170	Nonemergency transportation: ancillary: parking fees, tolls, other	—
	A0180	Nonemergency transportation: ancillary: lodging — recipient	—
	A0190	Nonemergency transportation: ancillary: meals — recipient	—
	A0200	Nonemergency transportation: ancillary: lodging — escort	—
	A0210	Nonemergency transportation: ancillary: meals — escort	—
	A0225	Ambulance service, neonatal transport, base rate, emergency transport, one way	50.0
	A0300	Ambulance service, basic life support (BLS), non-emergency transport, all inclusive (mileage and supplies)	—
	A0302	Ambulance service, BLS, emergency transport, all inclusive (mileage and supplies)	—
	A0304	Ambulance service, advanced life support (ALS), nonemergency transport, no specialized ALS services rendered, all inclusive (mileage and supplies)	—
	A0306	Ambulance service, ALS, nonemergency transport, specialized ALS services rendered, all inclusive (mileage and supplies)	—
	A0308	Ambulance service, ALS, emergency transport, no specialized ALS services rendered, all inclusive (mileage and supplies)	—
	A0310	Ambulance service, ALS, emergency transport, specialized ALS services rendered, all inclusive (mileage and supplies)	—

UPD	Code	Description	Units
	A0320	Ambulance service, BLS, non-emergency transport, supplies included, mileage separately billed	—
	A0322	Ambulance service, BLS, emergency transport, supplies included, mileage separately billed	—
	A0324	Ambulance service, ALS, non-emergency transport, no specialized ALS services rendered, supplies included, mileage separately billed	—
	A0326	Ambulance service, ALS, non-emergency transport, specialized ALS services rendered, supplies included, mileage separately billed	—
	A0328	Ambulance service, ALS, emergency transport, no specialized ALS services rendered, supplies included, mileage separately billed	—
	A0330	Ambulance service, ALS, emergency transport, specialized ALS services rendered, supplies included, mileage separately billed	—
	A0340	Ambulance service, BLS, nonemergency transport, mileage included, disposable supplies separately billed	—
	A0342	Ambulance service, BLS, emergency transport, mileage included, disposable supplies separately billed	—
	A0344	Ambulance service, ALS, nonemergency transport, no specialized ALS services rendered, mileage included, disposable supplies separately billed	—
	A0346	Ambulance service, ALS, nonemergency transport, specialized ALS services rendered, mileage included, disposable supplies separately billed	—
	A0348	Ambulance service, ALS, emergency transport, no specialized ALS services rendered, mileage included, disposable supplies separately billed	—
	A0350	Ambulance service, ALS, emergency transport, specialized ALS services rendered, mileage included, disposable supplies separately billed	—
	A0360	Ambulance service, BLS, nonemergency transport, mileage and disposable supplies separately billed	—
	A0362	Ambulance service, BLS, emergency transport, mileage and disposable supplies separately billed	—
	A0364	Ambulance service, ALS, nonemergency transport, no specialized ALS services rendered, mileage and disposable supplies separately billed	—
	A0366	Ambulance service, ALS, nonemergency transport, specialized ALS services rendered, mileage and disposable supplies separately billed	—
	A0368	Ambulance service, ALS, emergency transport, no specialized ALS services rendered, mileage and disposable supplies separately billed	—
	A0370	Ambulance service, ALS, emergency transport, specialized ALS services rendered, mileage and disposable supplies separately billed	—
	A0380	BLS mileage (per mile)	—
	A0382	BLS routine disposable supplies	—
	A0384	BLS specialized service disposable supplies; defibrillation (used by ALS ambulances and BLS ambulances in jurisdictions where defibrillation is permitted in BLS ambulances)	—
	A0390	ALS mileage (per mile)	—

▲ Revised code   ● New code   M RVSI code or deleted from CPT   (I) Interim Value

UPD		Code	Description	Units
		A0392	ALS specialized service disposable supplies; defibrillation (to be used only in jurisdictions where defibrillation cannot be performed by BLS ambulances)	—
		A0394	ALS specialized service disposable supplies; IV drug therapy	—
		A0396	ALS specialized service disposable supplies; esophageal intubation	—
		A0398	ALS routine disposable supplies	—
		A0420	Ambulance waiting time (ALS or BLS), one-half (1/2) hour increments	—

Waiting Time Table

Units	Time
1	1/2 to1 hr.
2	1to11/2 hrs.
3	11/2 to2 hrs.
4	2to21/2 hrs.
5	21/2 to3 hrs.
6	3to31/2 hrs.
7	31/2 to4 hrs.
8	4to41/2 hrs.
9	41/2 to5 hrs.
10	5to51/2 hrs.

UPD		Code	Description	Units
		A0422	Ambulance (ALS or BLS) oxygen and oxygen supplies, life sustaining situation	—
		A0424	Extra ambulance attendant, ALS or BLS (requires medical review)	—
		A0888	Non-covered ambulance mileage (per mile, e.g., for miles traveled beyond the closest appropriate facility)	—
		A0999	Unlisted ambulance service	BR
98.1	**M**	**A2000**	Code deleted. Use CPT	8.0

Medical and Surgical Supplies (A4000-A8999)

UPD		Code	Description	Units
	▲	**A4206**	Syringe with needle, sterile 1 cc, each	—
	▲	**A4207**	Syringe with needle, sterile 2 cc, each	—
	▲	**A4208**	Syringe with needle, sterile 3 cc, each	—
	▲	**A4209**	Syringe with needle, sterile 5 cc or greater, each	—
		A4210	Needle-free injection device, each	—
		A4211	Supplies for self-administered injections	—
	▲	**A4212**	Non coring needle or stylet with or without catheter	—
	▲	**A4213**	Syringe, sterile, 20 cc or greater, each	—
		A4214	Sterile saline or water, 30 cc vial	—
	▲	**A4215**	Needles only, sterile, any size, each	—
96.1		**A4220**	Refill kit for implantable infusion pump	—
97.1		**A4221**	Supplies for maintenance of drug infusion catheter, per week (list drug separately)	—

▲ Revised code   ● New code   **M** RVSI code or deleted from CPT   **(I)** Interim Value

UPD		Code	Description	Units
97.1		A4222	Supplies for external drug infusion pump, per cassette or bag (list drug separately)	—
96.1		A4230	Infusion set for external insulin pump, non needle cannula type	—
96.1		A4231	Infusion set for external insulin pump, needle type	—
		A4232	Syringe with needle for external insulin pump, sterile, 3cc	—
		A4244	Alcohol or peroxide, per pint	—
	▲	A4245	Alcohol wipes, per box	—
	▲	A4246	Betadine or pHisoHex solution, per pint	—
	▲	A4247	Betadine or iodine swabs/wipes, per box	—
		A4250	Urine test or reagent strips or tablets (100 tablets or strips)	—
96.1		A4253	Blood glucose test or reagent strips for home blood glucose monitor, per 50 strips	—
		A4254	Replacement battery, any type, for use with medically necessary home blood glucose monitor owned by patient	—
97.1		A4255	Platforms for home blood glucose monitor, 50 per box	—
96.1		A4256	Normal, low, and high calibrator solution/chips	—
		A4258	Spring-powered device for lancet, each	—
		A4259	Lancets, per box of 100	—
		A4260	Levonorgestrel (contraceptive) implants system, including implants and supplies	—
98.2	●	A4261	Cervical cap for contraceptive use	—
		A4262	Temporary, absorbable lacrimal duct implant, each	—
		A4263	Permanent, long-term, nondissolvable lacrimal duct implant, each	—
		A4265	Paraffin, per pound	—
		A4270	Disposable endoscope sheath, each	—
96.1		A4300	Implantable access catheter (venous, arterial, epidural, or peritoneal), external access	—
		A4301	Implantable access total system; catheter, port/reservoir (venous, arterial or epidural), percutaneous access	—
		A4305	Disposable drug delivery system, flow rate of 50 ml or greater per hour	—
		A4306	Disposable drug delivery system, flow rate of 5 ml or less per hour	—
		A4310	Insertion tray without drainage bag and without catheter (accessories only)	—
		A4311	Insertion tray without drainage bag with indwelling catheter, Foley type, two-way latex with coating (Teflon, silicone, silicone elastomer or hydrophilic, etc.)	—
		A4312	Insertion tray without drainage bag with indwelling catheter, Foley type, two-way, all silicone	—

UPD	Code	Description	Units
	A4313	Insertion tray without drainage bag with indwelling catheter, Foley type, three-way, for continuous irrigation	—
	A4314	Insertion tray with drainage bag with indwelling catheter, Foley type, two-way latex with coating (Teflon, silicone, silicone elastomer or hydrophilic, etc.)	—
	A4315	Insertion tray with drainage bag with indwelling catheter, Foley type, two-way, all silicone	—
	A4316	Insertion tray with drainage bag with indwelling catheter, Foley type, three-way, for continuous irrigation	—
	A4320	Irrigation tray with bulb or piston syringe, any purpose	—
97.1	A4321	Therapeutic agent for urinary catheter irrigation	—
	A4322	Irrigation syringe, bulb or piston, each	—
	A4323	Sterile saline irrigation solution, 1000 ml	—
	A4326	Male external catheter specialty type (e.g., inflatable, faceplate, etc., each)	—
	A4327	Female external urinary collection device; metal cup, each	—
	A4328	Female external urinary collection device; pouch, each	—
	A4329	External catheter starter set, male/female, includes catheters/urinary collection device, bag/pouch and accessories (tubing, clamps, etc.), seven-day supply	—
	A4330	Perianal fecal collection pouch with adhesive, each	—
	A4335	Incontinence supply; miscellaneous	—
	A4338	Indwelling catheter; Foley type, two-way latex with coating (Teflon, silicone, silicone elastomer, or hydrophilic, etc.), each	—
	A4340	Indwelling catheter; specialty type, (e.g., coude, mushroom, wing, etc.), each	—
	A4344	Indwelling catheter, Foley type, two-way, all silicone, each	—
	A4346	Indwelling catheter; Foley type, three-way for continuous irrigation, each	—
	A4347	Male external catheter with or without adhesive, with or without anti-reflux device; per dozen	—
	A4351	Intermittent urinary catheter; straight tip, each	—
	A4352	Intermittent urinary catheter; coude (curved) tip, each	—
97.1	A4353	Intermittent urinary catheter, with insertion supplies	—
	A4354	Insertion tray with drainage bag but without catheter	—
	A4355	Irrigation tubing set for continuous bladder irrigation through a three-way indwelling Foley catheter, each	—
	A4356	External urethral clamp or compression device (not to be used for catheter clamp), each	—
	A4357	Bedside drainage bag, day or night, with or without anti-reflux device, with or without tube, each	—

▲ Revised code   ● New code   **M** RVSI code or deleted from CPT   **(I)** Interim Value

UPD	Code	Description	Units
	A4358	Urinary leg bag; vinyl, with or without tube, each	—
		Note: See DME section codes E0325 and E0326 for male and female urinals	
	A4359	Urinary suspensory without leg bag, each	—
	A4361	Ostomy faceplate, each	—
	A4362	Skin barrier; solid, four by four or equivalent; each	—
	A4363	Skin barrier; liquid (spray, brush, etc.) powder or paste; per oz.	—
	A4364	Adhesive for ostomy or catheter; liquid (spray, brush, etc.), cement, powder or paste; any composition (e.g., silicone, latex, etc.), per oz.	—
97.1	A4365	Ostomy adhesive remover wipes, 50 per box	—
	A4367	Ostomy belt, each	—
97.1	A4368	Ostomy filter, any type, each	—
	A4397	Irrigation supply; sleeve, each	—
	A4398	Ostomy irrigation supply; bag, each	—
	A4399	Ostomy irrigation supply; cone/catheter, including brush	—
	A4400	Ostomy irrigation set	—
	A4402	Lubricant, per ounce	—
	A4404	Ostomy ring, each	—
	A4421	Ostomy supply; miscellaneous	—
	A4454	Tape, all types, all sizes	—
	A4455	Adhesive remover or solvent (for tape, cement or other adhesive), per ounce	—
	A4460	Elastic bandage, per roll (e.g., compression bandage)	—
98.1	A4462	Abdominal dressing holder/binder, each	—
	A4465	Nonelastic binder for extremity	—
	A4470	Gravlee jet washer	—
	A4480	VABRA aspirator	—
97.1	A4481	Thracheostoma filter, any type, any size, each	—
98.2 ●	A4483	Moisture exchanger, disposable, for use with invasive mechanical ventilation	—
	A4490	Surgical stocking above knee length, each	—
	A4495	Surgical stocking thigh length, each	—
	A4500	Surgical stocking below knee length, each	—
	A4510	Surgical stocking full-length, each	—
	A4550	Surgical trays	—

▲ Revised code   ● New code   **M** RVSI code or deleted from CPT   (I) Interim Value

UPD		Code	Description	Units
		A4554	Disposable underpads, all sizes (e.g., Chux's)	—
		A4556	Electrodes (e.g., apnea monitor)	—
		A4557	Lead wires (e.g., apnea monitor)	—
		A4558	Conductive paste or gel	—
		A4560	Pessary	—
		A4565	Sling	—
		A4570	Splint	—
96.1		A4572	Rib belt	—
		A4575	Topical hyperbaric oxygen chamber, disposable	—
		A4580	Cast supplies (e.g., plaster)	—
96.1		A4590	Special casting material (e.g., fiberglass)	—
		A4611	Battery, heavy duty; replacement for patient-owned ventilator	—
		A4612	Battery cables; replacement for patient-owned ventilator	—
		A4613	Battery charger; replacement for patient-owned ventilator	—
98.2	●	A4614	Peak expiratory flow rate meter, hand held	—
		A4615	Cannula, nasal	—
		A4616	Tubing (oxygen), per foot	—
		A4617	Mouthpiece	—
		A4618	Breathing circuits	—
		A4619	Face tent	—
		A4620	Variable concentration mask	—
		A4621	Tracheostomy mask or collar	—
		A4622	Tracheostomy or laryngectomy tube	—
		A4623	Tracheostomy, inner cannula (replacement only)	—
		A4624	Tracheal suction catheter, any type, each	—
		A4625	Tracheostomy care kit for new tracheostomy	—
		A4626	Tracheostomy cleaning brush, each	—
96.1		A4627	Spacer, bag or reservoir, with or without mask, for use with metered dose inhaler	—
96.1		A4628	Oropharyngeal suction catheter, each	—
		A4629	Tracheostomy care kit for established tracheostomy	—
		A4630	Replacement batteries for medically necessary transcutaneous electrical nerve stimulator (TENS) owned by patient	—

▲ Revised code   ● New code   **M** RVSI code or deleted from CPT   **(I)** Interim Value

UPD	Code	Description	Units
	A4631	Replacement batteries for medically necessary electronic wheelchair owned by patient	—
	A4635	Underarm pad, crutch, replacement, each	—
	A4636	Replacement, handgrip, cane, crutch, or walker, each	—
	A4637	Replacement, tip, cane, crutch, walker, each	—
	A4640	Replacement pad for use with medically necessary alternating pressure pad owned by patient	—
	A4641	Supply of radiopharmaceutical diagnostic imaging agent, not otherwise classified	—
	A4642	Supply of satumomab pendetide, radiopharmaceutical diagnostic imaging agent, per dose	—
	A4643	Supply of additional high dose contrast material(s) during magnetic resonance imaging, e.g., gadoteridol injection	—
	A4644	Supply of low osmolar contrast material (100–199 mg of iodine)	—
	A4645	Supply of low osmolar contrast material (200–299 mg of iodine)	—
	A4646	Supply of low osmolar contrast material (300–399 mg of iodine)	—
	A4647	Supply of paramagnetic contrast material (e.g., gadolinium)	—
	A4649	Surgical supply; miscellaneous	—
	A4650	Centrifuge (includes calibrated microcapillary tubes and sealease)	—
	A4655	Needles and syringes for dialysis	—
	A4660	Sphygmomanometer/blood pressure apparatus with cuff and stethoscope	—
	A4663	Blood pressure cuff only	—
	A4670	Automatic blood pressure monitor	—
	A4680	Activated carbon filters for dialysis	—
	A4690	Dialyzer (artificial kidney) all brands, all sizes, per unit	—
	A4700	Standard dialysate solution, each	—
	A4705	Bicarbonate dialysate solution, each	—
	A4712	Water, sterile	—
	A4714	Treated water (deionized, distilled, reverse osmosis) for use in dialysis system	—
	A4730	Fistula cannulation set for dialysis only	—
	A4735	Local/topical anesthetic for dialysis only	—
	A4740	Shunt accessory for dialysis only	—
	A4750	Blood tubing, arterial or venous, each	—
	A4755	Blood tubing, arterial and venous, combined	—
	A4760	Dialysate standard testing solution, supplies	—

▲ Revised code   ● New code   **M** RVSI code or deleted from CPT   **(I)** Interim Value

UPD	Code	Description	Units
	A4765	Dialysate concentrate additive, each	—
	A4770	Blood testing supplies (e.g., vacutainers and tubes)	—
	A4771	Serum clotting time tube, per box	—
	A4772	Dextrostick or glucose test strips, per box	—
	A4773	Hemostix, per bottle	—
	A4774	Ammonia test paper, per box	—
	A4780	Sterilizing agent for dialysis equipment, per gallon	—
	A4790	Cleansing agent for equipment for dialysis only	—
	A4800	Heparin for dialysis and antidote, any strength, porcine or beef, up to 1,000 units, 10–30 ml	—
	A4820	Hemodialysis kit supply	—
	A4850	Hemostats with rubber tips for dialysis	—
	A4860	Disposable catheter caps	—
	A4870	Plumbing and/or electrical work for home dialysis equipment	—
	A4880	Storage tank utilized in connection with water purification system, replacement tank for dialysis	—
	A4890	Contracts, repair and maintenance, for home dialysis equipment (noncovered)	—
	A4900	Continuous ambulatory peritoneal dialysis (CAPD) supply kit	—
	A4901	Continuous cycling peritoneal dialysis (CCPD) supply kit	—
	A4905	Intermittent peritoneal dialysis (IPD) supply kit	—
	A4910	Nonmedical supplies for dialysis, (i.e., scale, scissors, stop-watch, etc.) Note: For the above procedure (A4910) include the following: Scale, Scissors, Stopwatch, Surgical Brush, Thermometer, Tool Kit, Tourniquet, Tube Occluding Forceps/Clamps	—
	A4912	Gomco drain bottle	—
	A4913	Miscellaneous dialysis supplies, not identified elsewhere, by report	—
	A4914	Preparation kit	—
	A4918	Venous pressure clamp, each	—
	A4919	Dialyzer holder, each	—
	A4920	Harvard pressure clamp, each	—
	A4921	Measuring cylinder, any size, each	—
	A4927	Gloves, sterile or nonsterile, per pair Note: See Also Codes K0419-K0429	—
	A5051	Pouch, closed; with barrier attached (one piece)	—

UPD	Code	Description	Units
	A5052	Pouch, closed; without barrier attached (one piece)	—
	A5053	Pouch, closed; for use on faceplate	—
	A5054	Pouch, closed; for use on barrier with flange (two piece)	—
	A5055	Stoma cap	—
	A5061	Pouch, drainable; with barrier attached (one piece)	—
	A5062	Pouch, drainable; without barrier attached (one piece)	—
	A5063	Pouch, drainable; for use on barrier with flange (two piece system)	—
	A5064	Pouch, drainable; with faceplate attached; plastic or rubber	—
	A5065	Pouch, drainable; for use on faceplate; plastic or rubber	—
	A5071	Pouch, urinary; with barrier attached (one piece)	—
	A5072	Pouch, urinary; without barrier attached (one piece)	—
	A5073	Pouch, urinary; for use on barrier with flange (two piece)	—
	A5074	Pouch, urinary; with faceplate attached; plastic or rubber	—
	A5075	Pouch, urinary; for use on faceplate; plastic or rubber	—
	A5081	Continent device; plug for continent stoma	—
	A5082	Continent device; catheter for continent stoma	—
	A5093	Ostomy accessory; convex insert	—
97.1	A5102	Bedside drainage bottle, with or without tubing, rigid or expandable, each	—
	A5105	Urinary suspensory; with leg bag, with or without tube	—
	A5112	Urinary leg bag; latex	—
	A5113	Leg strap; latex, replacement only, per set	—
	A5114	Leg strap; foam or fabric, replacement only, per set	—
	A5119	Skin barrier; wipes, box per 50	—
	A5121	Skin barrier; solid, 6 x 6 or equivalent, each	—
	A5122	Skin barrier; solid, 8 x 8 or equivalent, each	—
	A5123	Skin barrier; with flange (solid, flexible or accordion), any size, each	—
	A5126	Adhesive; disk or foam pad	—
	A5131	Appliance cleaner, incontinence and ostomy appliances, per 16 oz.	—
	A5149	Incontinence/ostomy supply; miscellaneous	—
98.2 ●	A5200	Percutaneous catheter/tube anchoring device, adhesive skin attachment	—

UPD		Code	Description	Units
		A5500	For diabetics only, fitting (including follow-up) custom preparation and supply of off-the-shelf depth-inlay shoe manufactured to accommodate multi-density insert(s), per shoe	—
		A5501	For diabetics only, fitting (including follow-up) custom preparation and supply of shoe molded from cast(s) of patient's foot (custom molded shoe), per shoe	—
		A5502	For diabetics only, multiple density insert(s), per shoe	—
		A5503	For diabetics only, modification (including fitting) of off-the-shelf depth-inlay shoe or custom molded shoe with roller or rigid rocker bottom, per shoe	—
		A5504	For diabetics only, modification (including fitting) of off-the-shelf depth-inlay shoe or custom molded shoe with wedge(s), per shoe	—
		A5505	For diabetics only, modification (including fitting) of off-the-shelf depth-inlay shoe or custom molded shoe with metatarsal bar, per shoe	—
		A5506	For diabetics only, modification (including fitting) of off-the-shelf depth-inlay shoe or custom molded shoe with off-set heel(s), per shoe	—
96.1		A5507	For diabetics only, not otherwise specified modification (including fitting) of off-the-shelf depth-inlay shoe or custom molded shoe, per shoe	—
	▲	A6020	Collagen based wound dressing, each dressing	—
97.1		A6025	Silicone gel sheet, each	—
97.1		A6154	Wound pouch, each	—
97.1		A6196	Alginate dressing, wound cover, pad size 16 sq. in. or less, each dressing	—
97.1		A6197	Alginate dressing, wound cover, pad size more than 16 sq. in. but less than or equal to 48 sq. in., each dressing	—
97.1		A6198	Alginate dressing, wound cover, pad size more then 48 sq. in., each dressing	—
97.1		A6199	Alginate dressing, wound filler, per 6 inches	—
98.2	●	A6200	Composite dressing, pad size 16 sq. in. or less, without adhesive border, each dressing	—
98.2	●	A6201	Composite dressing, pad size more than 16 sq. in. but less than or equal to 48 sq. in., without adhesive border, each dressing	—
98.2	●	A6202	Composite dressing, pad size more than 48 sq. in., without adhesive border, each dressing	—
97.1		A6203	Composite dressing, pad size 16 sq. in. or less, with any size adhesive border, each dressing	—
97.1		A6204	Composite dressing, pad size more than 16 sq. in. but less than or equal to 48 sq. in., with any size adhesive border, each dressing	—
97.1		A6205	Composite dressing, pad size more than 48 sq. in., with any size adhesive border, each dressing	—
97.1		A6206	Contact layer, 16 sq. in. or less, each dressing	—
97.1		A6207	Contact layer, more than 16 sq. in. but less than or equal to 48 sq. in., each dressing	—
97.1		A6208	Contact layer, more than 48 sq. in., each dressing	—

▲ Revised code   ● New code   M RVSI code or deleted from CPT   (I) Interim Value

UPD	Code	Description	Units
97.1	**A6209**	Foam dressing, wound cover, pad size 16 sq. in. or less, without adhesive border, each dressing	—
97.1	**A6210**	Foam dressing, wound cover, pad size more than 16 sq. in. but less than or equal to 48 sq. in., without adhesive border, each dressing	—
97.1	**A6211**	Foam dressing, wound cover, pad size more then 48 sq. in., without adhesive border, each dressing	—
97.1	**A6212**	Foam dressing, wound cover, pad size 16 sq. in. or less, with any size adhesive border, each dressing	—
97.1	**A6213**	Foam dressing, wound cover, pad size more than 16 sq. in. but less than or equal to 48 sq. in., with any size adhesive border, each dressing	—
97.1	**A6214**	Foam dressing, wound cover, pad size more than 48 sq. in., with any size adhesive border, each dressing	—
97.1	**A6215**	Foam dressing, wound filler, per gram	—
97.1	**A6216**	Gauze, non-impregnated, non-sterile, pad size 16 sq. in. or less, without adhesive border, each dressing	—
97.1	**A6217**	Gauze, non-impregnated, non-sterile, pad size more than 16 sq. in. but less than or equal to 48 sq. in., without adhesive border, each dressing	—
97.1	**A6218**	Gauze, non-impregnated, non-sterile, pad size more than 48 sq. in., without adhesive border, each dressing	—
97.1	**A6219**	Gauze, non-impregnated, pad size 16 sq. in. or less, with any size adhesive border, each dressing	—
97.1	**A6220**	Gauze, non-impregnated, pad size more than 16 sq. in. but less than or equal to 48 sq. in., with any size adhesive border, each dressing	—
97.1	**A6221**	Gauze, non-impregnated, pad size more than 48 sq. in., with any size adhesive border, each dressing	—
97.1	**A6222**	Gauze, impregnated, other than water or normal saline, pad size 16 sq. in. or less, without adhesive border, each dressing	—
97.1	**A6223**	Gauze, impregnated, other than water or normal saline, pad size more than 16 sq. in. but less than or equal to 48 sq. in., without adhesive border, each dressing	—
97.1	**A6224**	Gauze, impregnated, other than water or normal saline, pad size more than 48 sq. in., without adhesive border, each dressing	—
97.1	**A6228**	Gauze, impregnated, water or normal saline, pad size 16 sq. in. or less, without adhesive border, each dressing	—
97.1	**A6229**	Gauze, impregnated, water or normal saline, pad size more than 16 sq. in. but less than or equal to 48 sq. in., without adhesive border, each dressing	—
97.1	**A6230**	Gauze, impregnated, water or normal saline, pad size more than 48 sq. in., without adhesive border, each dressing	—
97.1	**A6234**	Hydrocolloid dressing, wound cover, pad size 16 sq. in. or less, without adhesive border, each dressing	—
97.1	**A6235**	Hydrocolloid dressing, wound cover, pad size more than 16 sq. in. but less than or equal to 48 sq. in., without adhesive border, each dressing	—
97.1	**A6236**	Hydrocolloid dressing, wound cover, pad size more than 48 sq. in., without adhesive border, each dressing	—

▲ Revised code   ● New code   **M** RVSI code or deleted from CPT   **(I)** Interim Value

UPD	Code	Description	Units
97.1	A6237	Hydrocolloid dressing, wound cover, pad size 16 sq. in. or less, with any size adhesive border, each dressing	—
97.1	A6238	Hydrocolloid dressing, wound cover, pad size more than 16 sq. in. but less than or equal to 48 sq. in., with any size adhesive border, each dressing	—
97.1	A6239	Hydrocolloid dressing, wound cover, pad size more than 48 sq. in., with any size adhesive border, each dressing	—
97.1	A6240	Hydrocolloid dressing, wound filler, paste, per fluid ounce	—
97.1	A6241	Hydrocolloid dressing, wound filler, dry form, per gram	—
97.1	A6242	Hydrogel dressing, wound cover, pad size 16 sq. in. or less, without adhesive border, each dressing	—
97.1	A6243	Hydrogel dressing, wound cover, pad size more than 16 sq. in. but less than or equal to 48 sq. in., without adhesive border, each dressing	—
97.1	A6244	Hydrogel dressing, wound cover, pad size more than 48 sq. in., without adhesive border, each dressing	—
97.1	A6245	Hydrogel dressing, wound cover, pad size 16 sq. in. or less, with any size adhesive border, each dressing	—
97.1	A6246	Hydrogel dressing, wound cover, pad size more than 16 sq. in. but less than or equal to 48 sq. in., with any size adhesive border, each dressing	—
97.1	A6247	Hydrogel dressing, wound cover, pad size more than 48 sq. in., with any size adhesive border, each dressing	—
97.1	A6248	Hydrogel dressing, wound filler, gel, per fluid ounce	—
97.1	A6250	Skin sealants, protectants, moisturizers, ointments, any type, any size	—
97.1	A6251	Specialty absorptive dressing, wound cover, pad size 16 sq. in. or less, without adhesive border, each dressing	—
97.1	A6252	Specialty absorptive dressing, wound cover, pad size more than 16 sq. in. but less than or equal to 48 sq. in., without adhesive border, each dressing	—
97.1	A6253	Specialty absorptive dressing, wound cover, pad size more than 48 sq. in., without adhesive border, each dressing	—
97.1	A6254	Specialty absorptive dressing, wound cover, pad size 16 sq. in. or less, with any size adhesive border, each dressing	—
97.1	A6255	Specialty absorptive dressing, wound cover, pad size more than 16 sq. in. but less than or equal to 48 sq. in., with any size adhesive border, each dressing	—
97.1	A6256	Specialty absorptive dressing, wound cover, pad size more than 48 sq. in., with any size adhesive border, each dressing	—
97.1	A6257	Transparent film, 16 sq. in. or less, each dressing	—
97.1	A6258	Transparent film, more than 16 sq. in. but less than or equal to 48 sq. in., each dressing	—
97.1	A6259	Transparent film, more than 48 sq. in., each dressing	—
97.1	A6260	Wound cleansers, any type, any size	—
97.1	A6261	Wound filler, gel/paste, per fluid ounce, not elsewhere classified	—

▲ Revised code   ● New code   **M** RVSI code or deleted from CPT   **(I)** Interim Value

UPD	Code	Description	Units
97.1	A6262	Wound filler, dry form, per gram, not elsewhere classified	—
97.1	A6263	Gauze, elastic, non-sterile, all types, per linear yard	—
97.1	A6264	Gauze, non-elastic, non-sterile, per linear yard	—
97.1	A6265	Tape, all types, per 18 sq. in.	—
97.1	A6266	Gauze, impregnated, other than water or normal saline, any width, per linear yard	—
97.1	A6402	Gauze, non-impregnated, sterile, pad size 16 sq. in. or less, without adhesive border, each dressing	—
97.1	A6403	Gauze, non-impregnated, sterile, pad size more than 16 sq. in. but less than or equal to 48 sq. in., without adhesive border, each dressing	—
97.1	A6404	Gauze, non-impregnated, sterile, pad size more than 48 sq. in., without adhesive border, each dressing	—
97.1	A6405	Gauze, elastic, sterile, all types, per linear yard	—
97.1	A6406	Gauze, non-elastic, sterile, all types, per linear yard	—

Administrative, Miscellaneous, and Investigational (A9000-A9999)

UPD	Code	Description	Units
	A9150	Nonprescription drug	—
	A9160	Noncovered service by podiatrist	—
	A9170	Noncovered service by chiropractor	—
	A9190	Personal comfort item	—
	A9270	Noncovered item or service	—
96.1	A9300	Exercise equipment	—
96.1	A9500	Supply of radiopharmaceutical diagnostic imaging agent, technetium tc 99M sestamibi, per dose	—
97.1	A9503	Supply of radiopharmaceutical diagnostic imaging agent, technetium tc 99M, medronate, up to 30 MCl	—
	A9505	Supply of radiopharmaceutical diagnostic imaging agent, thallous chloride tl 201, per MCl	—

Enteral and Parenteral Therapy (B4000-B9999)

UPD	Code	Description	Units
	B4034	Enteral feeding supply kit; syringe, per day	—
	B4035	Enteral feeding supply kit; pump fed, per day	—
	B4036	Enteral feeding supply kit; gravity fed, per day	—
	B4081	Nasogastric tubing with stylet	—
	B4082	Nasogastric tubing without stylet	—
	B4083	Stomach tube — Levine type	—
96.1	B4084	Gastrostomy/jejunostomy tubing	—

▲ Revised code   ● New code   **M** RVSI code or deleted from CPT   **(I)** Interim Value

UPD	Code	Description	Units
	B4085	Gastronomy tube, silicone with sliding ring, each	—
	B4150	Enteral formulae; category I; semi-synthetic intact protein/protein isolates, 100 calories = 1 unit	—
	B4151	Enteral formulae; category I: natural intact protein/protein isolates, 100 calories = 1 unit	—
	B4152	Enteral formulae; category II: intact protein/protein isolates (calorically dense), 100 calories = 1 unit	—
	B4153	Enteral formulae; category III: hydrolized protein/amino acids, 100 calories = 1 unit	—
	B4154	Enteral formulae; category IV: defined formula for special metabolic need, 100 calories = 1 unit	—
	B4155	Enteral formulae; category V: modular components, 100 calories = 1 unit	—
	B4156	Enteral formulae; category VI: standardized nutrients, 100 calories = 1 unit	—
		Note: See J7042, J7060, J7070 for solution codes for other than parenteral nutrition therapy use.	
	B4164	Parenteral nutrition solution; carbohydrates (dextrose), 50% or less (500 ml = 1 unit) — home mix	—
	B4168	Parenteral nutrition solution; amino acid, 3.5%, (500 ml = 1 unit) — home mix	—
	B4172	Parenteral nutrition solution; amino acid, 5.5% through 7%, (500 ml = 1 unit) — home mix	—
	B4176	Parenteral nutrition solution; amino acid, 7% through 8.5%, (500 ml = 1 unit) — home mix	—
	B4178	Parenteral nutrition solution; amino acid, greater than 8.5% (500 ml = 1 unit) — home mix	—
	B4180	Parenteral nutrition solution; carbohydrates (dextrose), greater than 50% (500 ml = 1 unit) — home mix	—
	B4184	Parenteral nutrition solution; lipids, 10% with administration set (500 ml = 1 unit)	—
	B4186	Parenteral nutrition solution; lipids, 20% with administration set (500 ml = 1 unit)	—
	B4189	Parenteral nutrition solution; compounded amino acid and carbohydrates with electrolytes, trace elements, and vitamins, including preparation, any strength, 10 to 51 grams of protein — premix	—
	B4193	Parenteral nutrition solution; compounded amino acid and carbohydrates with electrolytes, trace elements, and vitamins, including preparation, any strength, 52 to 73 grams of protein — premix	—
	B4197	Parenteral nutrition solution; compounded amino acid and carbohydrates with electrolytes, trace elements and vitamins, including preparation, any strength, 74 to 100 grams of protein — premix	—
	B4199	Parenteral nutrition solution; compounded amino acid and carbohydrates with electrolytes, trace elements and vitamins, including preparation, any strength, over 100 grams of protein — premix	—

▲ Revised code   ● New code   **M** RVSI code or deleted from CPT   **(I)** Interim Value

UPD	Code	Description	Units
	B4216	Parenteral nutrition; additives (vitamins, trace elements, heparin, electrolytes) — home mix, per day	—
	B4220	Parenteral nutrition supply kit; premix, per day	—
	B4222	Parenteral nutrition supply kit; home mix, per day	—
	B4224	Parenteral nutrition administration kit, per day	—
	B5000	Parenteral nutrition solution; compounded amino acid and carbohydrates with electrolytes, trace elements, and vitamins, including preparation, any strength, renal — premix	—
	B5100	Parenteral nutrition solution; compounded amino acid and carbohydrates with electrolytes, trace elements, and vitamins, including preparation, any strength, hepatic — premix	—
	B5200	Parenteral nutrition solution; compounded amino acid and carbohydrates with electrolytes, trace elements, and vitamins, including preparation, any strength, stress (branch chain amino acids) — premix	—
	B9000	Enteral nutrition infusion pump without alarm	—
	B9002	Enteral nutrition infusion pump with alarm	—
	B9004	Parenteral nutrition infusion pump, portable	—
	B9006	Parenteral nutrition infusion pump, stationary	—
	B9998	NOC for enteral supplies	—
	B9999	NOC for parenteral supplies	—

Durable Medical Equipment (E0100-E9999)

UPD	Code	Description	Units
	E0100	Cane, includes canes of all materials, adjustable or fixed, with tip	—
	E0105	Cane, quad or three-prong, includes canes of all materials, adjustable or fixed, with tips	—
	E0110	Crutches, forearm, includes crutches of various materials, adjustable or fixed, pair, complete with tips and handgrips	—
	E0111	Crutch, forearm, includes crutches of various materials, adjustable or fixed, each, with tip and handgrip	—
	E0112	Crutches, underarm, wood, adjustable or fixed, pair, with pads, tips and handgrips	—
	E0113	Crutch, underarm, wood, adjustable or fixed, each, with pad, tip and handgrip	—
	E0114	Crutches, underarm, other than wood, adjustable or fixed, pair, with pads, tips and handgrips	—
	E0116	Crutch, underarm, other than wood, adjustable or fixed, each, with pad, tip and handgrip	—
	E0130	Walker, rigid (pickup), adjustable or fixed height	—
	E0135	Walker, folding (pickup), adjustable or fixed height	—
	E0141	Rigid walker, wheeled, without seat	—

▲ Revised code   ● New code   **M** RVSI code or deleted from CPT   **(I)** Interim Value

UPD	Code	Description	Units
	E0142	Rigid walker, wheeled, with seat	—
	E0143	Folding walker, wheeled, without seat	—
	E0145	Walker, wheeled, with seat and crutch attachments	—
	E0146	Folding walker, wheeled, with seat	—
	E0147	Heavy duty, multiple breaking system, variable wheel resistance walker	—
	E0153	Platform attachment, forearm crutch, each	—
	E0154	Platform attachment, walker, each	—
	E0155	Wheel attachment, rigid pickup walker	—
	E0156	Seat attachment, walker	—
	E0157	Crutch attachment, walker, each	—
	E0158	Leg extensions for a walker	—
97.1	E0159	Brake attachment for wheeled walker, replacement, each	—
	E0160	Sitz type bath or equipment, portable, used with or without commode	—
	E0161	Sitz type bath or equipment, portable, used with or without commode, with faucet attachment/s	—
	E0162	Sitz bath chair	—
	E0163	Commode chair, stationary, with fixed arms	—
	E0164	Commode chair, mobile, with fixed arms	—
	E0165	Commode chair, stationary, with detachable arms	—
	E0166	Commode chair, mobile, with detachable arms	—
	E0167	Pail or pan for use with commode chair	—
	E0175	Foot rest, for use with commode chair, each	—
	E0176	Air pressure pad or cushion, nonpositioning	—
	E0177	Water pressure pad or cushion, nonpositioning	—
	E0178	Gel or gel-like pressure pad or cushion, nonpositioning	—
	E0179	Dry pressure pad or cushion, nonpositioning	—
	E0180	Pressure pad, alternating with pump	—
	E0181	Pressure pad, alternating with pump, heavy duty	—
	E0182	Pump for alternating pressure pad	—
	E0184	Dry pressure mattress	—
	E0185	Gel or gel-like pressure pad for mattress, standard mattress length and width	—
	E0186	Air pressure mattress	—

▲ Revised code   ● New code   **M** RVSI code or deleted from CPT   **(I)** Interim Value

UPD	Code	Description	Units
	E0187	Water pressure mattress	—
	E0188	Synthetic sheepskin pad	—
	E0189	Lambswool sheepskin pad, any size	—
	E0191	Heel or elbow protector, each	—
	E0192	Low pressure and positioning equalization pad, for wheelchair	—
	E0193	Powered air flotation bed (low air loss therapy)	—
	E0194	Air fluidized bed	—
	E0196	Gel pressure mattress	—
	E0197	Air pressure pad for mattress, standard mattress length and width	—
	E0198	Water pressure pad for mattress, standard mattress length and width	—
	E0199	Dry pressure pad for mattress, standard mattress length and width	—
	E0200	Heat lamp, without stand (table model), includes bulb, or infrared element	—
	E0202	Phototherapy (bilirubin) light with photometer	—
	E0205	Heat lamp, with stand, includes bulb, or infrared element	—
	E0210	Electric heat pad, standard	—
	E0215	Electric heat pad, moist	—
97.1	E0217	Water circulating heat pad with pump	—
97.1	E0218	Water circulating cold pad with pump	—
	E0220	Hot water bottle	—
	E0225	Hydrocollator unit, includes pads	—
	E0230	Ice cap or collar	—
	E0235	Paraffin bath unit, portable (see medical supply code A4265 for paraffin)	—
	E0236	Pump for water circulating pad	—
	E0238	Nonelectric heat pad, moist	—
	E0239	Hydrocollator unit, portable	—
	E0241	Bathtub wall rail, each	—
	E0242	Bathtub rail, floor base	—
	E0243	Toilet rail, each	—
	E0244	Raised toilet seat	—
	E0245	Tub stool or bench	—
	E0246	Transfer tub rail attachment	—

UPD	Code	Description	Units
	E0249	Pad for water circulating heat unit	—
	E0250	Hospital bed, fixed height, with any type side rails, with mattress	—
	E0251	Hospital bed, fixed height, with any type side rails, without mattress	—
	E0255	Hospital bed, variable height, hi-lo, with any type side rails, with mattress	—
	E0256	Hospital bed, variable height, hi-lo, with any type side rails, without mattress	—
	E0260	Hospital bed, semi-electric (head and foot adjustment), with any type side rails, with mattress	—
	E0261	Hospital bed, semi-electric (head and foot adjustment), with any type side rails, without mattress	—
	E0265	Hospital bed, total electric (head, foot, and height adjustments), with any type side rails, with mattress	—
	E0266	Hospital bed, total electric (head, foot, and height adjustments), with any type side rails, without mattress	—
	E0270	Hospital bed, institutional type includes: oscillating, circulating and stryker frame, with mattress	—
	E0271	Mattress, inner spring	—
	E0272	Mattress, foam rubber	—
	E0273	Bed board	—
	E0274	Over-bed table	—
	E0275	Bed pan, standard, metal or plastic	—
	E0276	Bed pan, fracture, metal or plastic	—
	E0277	Powered pressure-reducing air mattress	—
	E0280	Bed cradle, any type	—
	E0290	Hospital bed, fixed height, without side rails, with mattress	—
	E0291	Hospital bed, fixed height, without side rails, without mattress	—
	E0292	Hospital bed, variable height, hi-lo, without side rails, with mattress	—
	E0293	Hospital bed, variable height, hi-lo, without side rails, without mattress	—
	E0294	Hospital bed, semi-electric (head and foot adjustment), without side rails, with mattress	—
	E0295	Hospital bed, semi-electric (head and foot adjustment), without side rails, without mattress	—
	E0296	Hospital bed, total electric (head, foot, and height adjustments), without side rails, with mattress	—
	E0297	Hospital bed, total electric (head, foot, and height adjustments), without side rails, without mattress	—
	E0305	Bedside rails, half-length	—

UPD	Code	Description	Units
	E0310	Bedside rails, full-length	—
	E0315	Bed accessory: board, table, or support device, any type	—
	E0325	Urinal; male, jug-type, any material	—
	E0326	Urinal; female, jug-type, any material	—
	E0350	Control unit for electronic bowel irrigation/evacuation system	—
	E0352	Disposable pack (water reservoir bag, speculum, valving mechanism and collection bag/box) for use with the electronic bowel irrigation/evacuation system	—
97.1	E0370	Air pressure elevator for heel	—
98.1	E0371	Nonpowered advanced pressure reducing overlay for mattress, standard mattress length and width	—
98.1	E0372	Powered air overlay for mattress, standard mattress length and width	—
98.1	E0373	Nonpowered advanced pressure reducing mattress	—
	E0424	Stationary compressed gaseous oxygen system, rental; includes contents (per unit), regulator, flowmeter, humidifier, nebulizer, cannula or mask, and tubing; 1 unit = 50 cubic ft	—
	E0425	Stationary compressed gas system, purchase; includes regulator, flowmeter, humidifier, nebulizer, cannula or mask, and tubing	—
	E0430	Portable gaseous oxygen system, purchase; includes regulator, flowmeter, humidifier, cannula or mask, and tubing	—
	E0431	Portable gaseous oxygen system, rental; includes regulator, flowmeter, humidifier, cannula or mask, and tubing	—
	E0434	Portable liquid oxygen system, rental; includes portable container, supply reservoir, humidifier, flowmeter, refill adaptor, contents gauge, cannula or mask, and tubing	—
	E0435	Portable liquid oxygen system, purchase; includes portable container, supply reservoir, flowmeter, humidifier, contents gauge, cannula or mask, tubing, and refill adapter	—
	E0439	Stationary liquid oxygen system, rental; includes use of reservoir, contents (per unit), regulator, flowmeter, humidifier, nebulizer, cannula or mask, and tubing; 1 unit = 10 lbs	—
	E0440	Stationary liquid oxygen system, purchase; includes use of reservoir, contents indicator, regulator, flowmeter, humidifier, nebulizer, cannula or mask, and tubing	—
	E0441	Oxygen contents, gaseous, per unit (for use with owned gaseous stationary systems or when both a stationary and portable gaseous system are owned; 1 unit = 50 cubic ft)	—
	E0442	Oxygen contents, liquid, per unit (for use with owned liquid stationary systems or when both a stationary and portable liquid system are owned; 1 unit = 10 lbs)	—
	E0443	Portable oxygen contents, gaseous, per unit (for use only with portable gaseous systems when no stationary gas or liquid system is used; 1 unit = 5 cubic ft)	—
	E0444	Portable oxygen contents, liquid, per unit (for use only with portable liquid systems when no stationary gas or liquid system is used; 1 unit = 1 lb)	—

▲ Revised code   ● New code   **M** RVSI code or deleted from CPT   **(I)** Interim Value

UPD	Code	Description	Units
	E0450	Volume ventilator, stationary or portable	—
	E0452	Intermittent assist device with continuous positive airway pressure device (cpap)	—
	E0453	Therapeutic ventilator; suitable for use 12 hours or less per day	—
	E0455	Oxygen tent, excluding croup or pediatric tents	—
	E0457	Chest shell (cuirass)	—
	E0459	Chest wrap	—
	E0460	Negative pressure ventilator; portable or stationary	—
	E0462	Rocking bed, with or without side rails	—
	E0480	Percussor, electric or pneumatic, home model	—
	E0500	IPPB machine, all types, with built-in nebulization; manual or automatic valves; internal or external power source	—
	E0550	Humidifier, durable for extensive supplemental humidification during IPPB treatments or oxygen delivery	—
	E0555	Humidifier, durable, glass or autoclavable plastic bottle type, for use with regulator or flowmeter	—
	E0560	Humidifier, durable for supplemental humidification during IPPB treatment or oxygen delivery	—
	E0565	Compressor, air power source for equipment which is not self- contained or cylinder driven	—
	E0570	Nebulizer, with compressor	—
	E0575	Nebulizer, ultrasonic	—
	E0580	Nebulizer, durable, glass or autoclavable plastic, bottle type, for use with regulator or flowmeter	—
	E0585	Nebulizer, with compressor and heater	—
	E0600	Suction pump, home model, portable	—
	E0601	Continuous airway pressure (CPAP) device	—
	E0605	Vaporizer, room type	—
	E0606	Postural drainage board	—
	E0607	Home blood glucose monitor	—
	E0608	Apnea monitor	—
	E0609	Blood glucose monitor with special features (e.g., voice synthesizers, automatic timers, etc.)	—
	E0610	Pacemaker monitor, self-contained, checks battery depletion, includes audible and visible check systems	—
	E0615	Pacemaker monitor, self-contained, checks battery depletion and other pacemaker components, includes digital/visible check systems	—

UPD	Code	Description	Units
	E0621	Sling or seat, patient lift, canvas or nylon	—
	E0625	Patient lift, Kartop, bathroom or toilet	—
	E0627	Seat lift mechanism incorporated into a combination lift-chair mechanism	—
	E0628	Separate seat lift mechanism for use with patient owned furniture — electric	—
	E0629	Separate seat lift mechanism for use with patient owned furniture — nonelectric	—
	E0630	Patient lift, hydraulic, with seat or sling	—
	E0635	Patient lift, electric, with seat or sling	—
	E0650	Pneumatic compressor, nonsegmental home model	—
	E0651	Pneumatic compressor, segmental home model without calibrated gradient pressure	—
	E0652	Pneumatic compressor, segmental home model with calibrated gradient pressure	—
	E0655	Nonsegmental pneumatic appliance for use with pneumatic compressor, half arm	—
	E0660	Nonsegmental pneumatic appliance for use with pneumatic compressor, full leg	—
	E0665	Nonsegmental pneumatic appliance for use with pneumatic compressor, full arm	—
	E0666	Nonsegmental pneumatic appliance for use with pneumatic compressor, half leg	—
	E0667	Segmental pneumatic appliance for use with pneumatic compressor, full leg	—
	E0668	Segmental pneumatic appliance for use with pneumatic compressor, full arm	—
	E0669	Segmental pneumatic appliance for use with pneumatic compressor, half leg	—
	E0671	Segmental gradient pressure pneumatic appliance, full leg	—
	E0672	Segmental gradient pressure pneumatic appliance, full arm	—
	E0673	Segmental gradient pressure pneumatic appliance, half leg	—
	E0690	Ultraviolet cabinet, appropriate for home use	—
	E0700	Safety equipment (e.g., belt, harness or vest)	—
	E0710	Restraint, any type (body, chest, wrist or ankle)	—
	E0720	TENS, two lead, localized stimulation	—
	E0730	TENS, four lead, larger area/multiple nerve stimulation	—
	E0731	Form-fitting conductive garment for delivery of TENS or NMES (with conductive fibers separated from the patient's skin by layers of fabric)	—
	E0740	Incontinence treatment system, pelvic floor stimulator, monitor, sensor and/or trainer	—
	E0744	Neuromuscular stimulator for scoliosis	—
	E0745	Neuromuscular stimulator, electronic shock unit	—
	E0746	Electromyography (EMG), biofeedback device	—

UPD		Code	Description	Units
96.1		**E0747**	Osteogenic stimulator, electrical, noninvasive, other than spinal applications	' —
		E0748	Osteogenic stimulator, electrical, noninvasive, spinal applications	—
		E0749	Osteogenic stimulator, electrical (surgically implanted)	—
		E0751	Implantable neurostimulator pulse generator or combination of external transmitted with implantable receiver (includes extension)	—
	▲	**E0753**	Implantable neurostimulator electrodes, per group of four	—
		E0755	Electronic salivary reflex stimulator (intraoral/noninvasive)	—
97.1		**E0760**	Osteogenesis stimulator, low intensity ultrasound, non-invasive	—
		E0776	IV pole	—
		E0781	Ambulatory infusion pump, single or multiple channels, with administrative equipment, worn by patient	—
		E0782	Infusion pump, implantable, non-programmable	—
96.1		**E0783**	Infusion pump system, implantable, programmable (includes components, e.g., pump catheter, connectors, etc.)	—
		E0784	External ambulatory infusion pump, insulin	—
98.2	●	**E0785**	Implantable intraspinal (epidural/intrathecal) catheter used with implantable infusion pump, replacement	—
		E0791	Parenteral infusion pump, stationary, single or multichannel	—
		E0840	Traction frame, attached to headboard, cervical traction	—
		E0850	Traction stand, freestanding, cervical traction	—
98.1		**E0855**	Cervical traction equipment not requiring additional stand or frame	—
		E0860	Traction equipment, overdoor, cervical	—
		E0870	Traction frame, attached to footboard, extremity traction (e.g., Buck's)	—
		E0880	Traction stand, freestanding, extremity traction (e.g., Buck's)	—
		E0890	Traction frame, attached to footboard, pelvic traction	—
		E0900	Traction stand, freestanding, pelvic traction (e.g., Buck's)	—
		E0910	Trapeze bars, also known as patient helper, attached to bed, with grab bar	—
		E0920	Fracture frame, attached to bed, includes weights	—
		E0930	Fracture frame, freestanding, includes weights	—
		E0935	Passive motion exercise device	—
		E0940	Trapeze bar, freestanding, complete with grab bar	—
		E0941	Gravity assisted traction device, any type	—
		E0942	Cervical head harness/halter	—
		E0943	Cervical pillow	—

UPD	Code	Description	Units
	E0944	Pelvic belt/harness/boot	—
	E0945	Extremity belt/harness	—
	E0946	Fracture, frame, dual with cross bars, attached to bed (e.g., Balken, Four Poster)	—
	E0947	Fracture frame, attachments for complex pelvic traction	—
	E0948	Fracture frame, attachments for complex cervical traction	—
	E0950	Tray	—
	E0951	Loop heel, each	—
	E0952	Loop toe, each	—
	E0953	Pneumatic tire, each	—
	E0954	Semi-pneumatic caster, each	—
	E0958	Wheelchair attachment to convert any wheelchair to one arm drive	—
	E0959	Amputee adapter (device used to compensate for transfer of weight due to lost limbs to maintain proper balance)	—
	E0961	Brake extension, for wheelchair	—
	E0962	One-inch cushion, for wheelchair	—
	E0963	Two-inch cushion, for wheelchair	—
	E0964	Three-inch cushion, for wheelchair	—
	E0965	Four-inch cushion, for wheelchair	—
	E0966	Hook on headrest extension	—
	E0967	Wheelchair hand rims with eight vertical rubber-tipped projections, pair	—
	E0968	Commode seat, wheelchair	—
	E0969	Narrowing device, wheelchair	—
	E0970	No. 2 footplates, except for elevating legrest	—
	E0971	Anti-tipping device, wheelchair	—
	E0972	Transfer board or device	—
	E0973	Adjustable height detachable arms, desk or full-length, wheelchair	—
	E0974	"Grade-aid" (device to prevent rolling back on an incline) for wheelchair	—
	E0975	Reinforced seat upholstery, wheelchair	—
	E0976	Reinforced back, wheelchair, upholstery or other material	—
	E0977	Wedge cushion, wheelchair	—
	E0978	Belt, safety with airplane buckle, wheelchair	—
	E0979	Belt, safety with Velcro closure, wheelchair	—

▲ Revised code   ● New code   **M** RVSI code or deleted from CPT   **(I)** Interim Value

UPD	Code	Description	Units
	E0980	Safety vest, wheelchair	—
	E0990	Elevating leg rest, each	—
	E0991	Upholstery seat	—
	E0992	Solid seat insert	—
	E0993	Back, upholstery	—
	E0994	Armrest, each	—
	E0995	Calf rest, each	—
	E0996	Tire, solid, each	—
	E0997	Caster with fork	—
	E0998	Caster without fork	—
	E0999	Pneumatic tire with wheel	—
	E1000	Tire, pneumatic caster	—
	E1001	Wheel, single	—
	E1031	Rollabout chair, any and all types with casters five inches or greater	—
	E1050	Fully reclining wheelchair; fixed full-length arms, swing-away, detachable, elevating legrests	—
	E1060	Fully reclining wheelchair; detachable arms, desk or full-length, swing-away, detachable, elevating legrests	—
	E1065	Power attachment (to convert any wheelchair to motorized wheelchair, e.g., Solo)	—
	E1066	Battery charger	—
	E1069	Deep cycle battery	—
	E1070	Fully reclining wheelchair; detachable arms, desk or full-length, swing-away, detachable footrests	—
	E1083	Hemi-wheelchair; fixed full-length arms, swing-away, detachable, elevating legrests	—
	E1084	Hemi-wheelchair; detachable arms, desk or full-length, swing-away, detachable, elevating legrests	—
	E1085	Hemi-wheelchair; fixed full-length arms, swing-away, detachable footrests	—
	E1086	Hemi-wheelchair; detachable arms, desk or full-length, swing-away, detachable footrests	—
	E1087	High-strength lightweight wheelchair; fixed full-length arms, swing-away, detachable, elevating legrests	—
	E1088	High-strength lightweight wheelchair; detachable arms, desk or full-length, swing-away, detachable, elevating legrests	—
	E1089	High-strength lightweight wheelchair; fixed-length arms, swing-away, detachable footrests	—

UPD	Code	Description	Units
	E1090	High-strength lightweight wheelchair; detachable arms, desk or full-length, swing-away, detachable footrests	—
	E1091	Youth wheelchair; any type	—
	E1092	Wide, heavy-duty wheelchair; detachable arms, desk or full-length, swing-away, detachable, elevating legrests	—
	E1093	Wide, heavy-duty wheelchair; detachable arms, desk or full-length arms, swing-away, detachable footrests	—
	E1100	Semi-reclining wheelchair; fixed full-length arms, swing-away, detachable, elevating legrests	—
	E1110	Semi-reclining wheelchair; detachable arms, desk or full-length, elevating legrest	—
	E1130	Standard wheelchair; fixed full-length arms, fixed or swing-away, detachable footrests	—
	E1140	Wheelchair; detachable arms, desk or full-length, swing-away, detachable footrests	—
	E1150	Wheelchair; detachable arms, desk or full-length, swing-away, detachable, elevating legrests	—
	E1160	Wheelchair; fixed full-length arms, swing-away, detachable, elevating legrests	—
	E1170	Amputee wheelchair; fixed full-length arms, swing-away, detachable, elevating legrests	—
	E1171	Amputee wheelchair; fixed full-length arms, without footrests or legrests	—
	E1172	Amputee wheelchair; detachable arms, desk or full-length, without footrests or legrests	—
	E1180	Amputee wheelchair; detachable arms, desk or full-length, swing-away, detachable footrests	—
	E1190	Amputee wheelchair; detachable arms, desk or full-length, swing-away, detachable, elevating legrests	—
	E1195	Heavy duty wheelchair; fixed full-length arms, swing-away, detachable, elevating legrests	—
	E1200	Amputee wheelchair; fixed full-length arms, swing-away, detachable footrests	—
	E1210	Motorized wheelchair; fixed full-length arms, swing-away, detachable, elevating legrests	—
	E1211	Motorized wheelchair; detachable arms, desk or full-length, swing-away, detachable, elevating legrests	—
	E1212	Motorized wheelchair; fixed full-length arms, swing-away, detachable footrests	—
	E1213	Motorized wheelchair; detachable arms, desk or full-length, swing-away, detachable footrests	—
	E1220	Wheelchair; specially sized or constructed (indicate brand name, model number, if any, and justification)	—
	E1221	Wheelchair with fixed arm, footrests	—
	E1222	Wheelchair with fixed arm, elevating legrests	—

▲ Revised code   ● New code   **M** RVSI code or deleted from CPT   **(I)** Interim Value

UPD	Code	Description	Units
	E1223	Wheelchair with detachable arms, footrests	—
	E1224	Wheelchair with detachable arms, elevating legrests	—
	E1225	Semi-reclining back for customized wheelchair	—
	E1226	Full reclining back for customized wheelchair	—
	E1227	Special height arms for wheelchair	—
	E1228	Special back height for wheelchair	—
	E1230	Power operated vehicle (three- or four-wheel nonhighway), specify brand name and model number	—
	E1240	Lightweight wheelchair; detachable arms, desk or full-length, swing-away, detachable, elevating legrest	—
	E1250	Lightweight wheelchair; fixed full-length arms, swing-away, detachable footrests	—
	E1260	Lightweight wheelchair; detachable arms, desk or full-length, swing-away, detachable footrests	—
	E1270	Lightweight wheelchair; fixed full-length arms, swing-away, detachable elevating legrests	—
	E1280	Heavy-duty wheelchair; detachable arms, desk or full-length, elevating legrests	—
	E1285	Heavy-duty wheelchair; fixed full-length arms, swing-away, detachable footrests	—
	E1290	Heavy-duty wheelchair; detachable arms, desk or full-length, swing-away, detachable footrests	—
	E1295	Heavy-duty wheelchair; fixed full-length arms, elevating legrests	—
	E1296	Special wheelchair seat height from floor	—
	E1297	Special wheelchair seat depth, by upholstery	—
	E1298	Special wheelchair seat depth and/or width, by construction	—
	E1300	Whirlpool, portable (overtub type)	—
	E1310	Whirlpool, nonportable (built-in type)	—
97.1	E1340	Repair or nonroutine service for durable medical equipment requiring the skill of a technician, labor component, per 15 minutes	—
	E1353	Regulator	—
	E1355	Stand/rack	—
	E1372	Immersion external heater for nebulizer	—
	E1375	Nebulizer portable with small compressor, with limited flow	—
	E1377	Oxygen concentrator, high humidity system equiv. to 244 cu. ft.	—
	E1378	Oxygen concentrator, high humidity system equiv. to 488 cu. ft.	—
	E1379	Oxygen concentrator, high humidity system equiv. to 732 cu. ft.	—
	E1380	Oxygen concentrator, high humidity system equiv. to 976 cu. ft.	—

▲ Revised code   ● New code   **M** RVSI code or deleted from CPT   **(I)** Interim Value

UPD	Code	Description	Units
	E1381	Oxygen concentrator, high humidity system equiv. to 1220 cu. ft.	—
	E1382	Oxygen concentrator, high humidity system equiv. to 1464 cu. ft.	—
	E1383	Oxygen concentrator, high humidity system equiv. to 1708 cu. ft.	—
	E1384	Oxygen concentrator, high humidity system equiv. to 1952 cu. ft.	—
	E1385	Oxygen concentrator, high humidity system equiv. to over 1952 cu. ft.	—
	E1399	Durable medical equipment, miscellaneous	—
	E1400	Oxygen concentrator, manufacturer specified maximum flow rate does not exceed two liters per minute, at 85 percent or greater concentration	—
	E1401	Oxygen concentrator, manufacturer specified maximum flow rate greater than two liters per minute, does not exceed three liters per minute, at 85 percent or greater concentration	—
	E1402	Oxygen concentrator, manufacturer specified maximum flow rate greater than three liters per minute, does not exceed four liters per minute, at 85 percent or greater concentration	—
	E1403	Oxygen concentrator, manufacturer specified maximum flow rate greater than four liters per minute, does not exceed five liters per minute, at 85 percent or greater concentration	—
	E1404	Oxygen concentrator, manufacturer specified maximum flow rate greater than five liters per minute, at 85 percent or greater concentration	—
	E1405	Oxygen and water vapor enriching system with heated delivery	—
	E1406	Oxygen and water vapor enriching system without heated delivery	—
	E1510	Kidney, dialysate delivery system kidney machine, pump recirculating, air removal system, flowrate meter, power off, heater and temp control with alarm, IV poles, pressure gauge, concentrate container	—
	E1520	Heparin infusion pump for dialysis	—
	E1530	Air bubble detector for dialysis	—
	E1540	Pressure alarm for dialysis	—
	E1550	Bath conductivity meter for dialysis	—
	E1560	Blood leak detector for dialysis	—
	E1570	Adjustable chair, for ESRD patients	—
	E1575	Transducer protector/fluid barrier, any size, each	—
	E1580	Unipuncture control system for dialysis	—
	E1590	Hemodialysis machine	—
	E1592	Automatic intermittent peritoneal dialysis system	—
	E1594	Cycler dialysis machine for peritoneal dialysis	—
	E1600	Delivery and/or installation charges for renal dialysis equipment	—
	E1610	Reverse osmosis water purification system	—

▲ Revised code   ● New code   **M** RVSI code or deleted from CPT   **(I)** Interim Value

UPD	Code	Description	Units
	E1615	Deionizer water purification system	—
	E1620	Blood pump for dialysis	—
	E1625	Water softening system	—
	E1630	Reciprocating peritoneal dialysis system	—
	E1632	Wearable artificial kidney	—
	E1635	Compact (portable) travel hemodialyzer system	—
	E1636	Sorbent cartridges, per case	—
	E1640	Replacement components for hemodialysis and/or peritoneal dialysis machines that are owned or being purchased by the patient	—
	E1699	Dialysis equipment, unspecified, by report	—
	E1700	Jaw motion rehabilitation system	—
	E1701	Replacement cushions for jaw motion rehabilitation system, package of six	—
96.1	**E1702**	Replacement measuring scales for jaw motion rehabilitation system, package of 200	—
96.1	**E1800**	Dynamic adjustable elbow extension/flexion device	—
96.1	**E1805**	Dynamic adjustable wrist extension/flexion device	—
96.1	**E1810**	Dynamic adjustable knee extension/flexion device	—
96.1	**E1815**	Dynamic adjustable ankle extension/flexion device	—
96.1	**E1820**	Soft interface material, dynamic adjustable extension/flexion device	—
96.1	**E1825**	Dynamic adjustable finger extension/flexion device	—
	E1830	Dynamic adjustable toe extension/flexion device	—

Procedures/Professional Services (Temporary) (G0000-G9999)

UPD	Code	Description	Units
	G0001	Routine venipuncture for collection of specimen(s)	3.0
	G0002	Office procedure, insertion of temporary indwelling catheter, Foley type (separate procedure)	6.5
98.2	**G0004**	Patient demand single or multiple event recording with pre-symptom memory loop and 24 hour attended monitoring, per 30 day period; includes transmission, physician review and interpretation	(I) 62.0
98.2	**G0005**	Patient demand single or multiple event recording with pre-symptom memory loop and 24 hour attended monitoring, per 30 day period; recording (includes hookup, recording and disconnection)	(I) 10.0
98.2	**G0006**	Patient demand single or multiple event recording with pre-symptom memory loop and 24 hour attended monitoring, per 30 day period; 24 hour attended monitoring, receipt of transmissions, and analysis	(I) 45.0
98.2	**G0007**	Patient demand single or multiple event recording with pre-symptom memory loop and 24 hour attended monitoring, per 30 day period; physician review and interpretation only	(I) 6.0

▲ Revised code   ● New code   **M** RVSI code or deleted from CPT   **(I)** Interim Value

UPD	Code	Description	Units
	G0008	Administration of influenza virus vaccine when no physician fee schedule service on the same day	(I) 3.0
96.1	G0009	Administration of pneumococcal vaccine when no physician fee schedule service on the same day	(I) 6.0
	G0010	Administration of hepatitis B vaccine when no physician fee schedule service on the same day	(I) 6.5
98.2	G0015	Post-symptom telephonic transmission of electrocardiogram rhythm strip(s) and 24 hour attended monitoring, per 30 day period: Tracing only	(I) 46.0
	G0016	Post-symptom telephonic transmission of electrocardiogram rhythm strip(s) and 24 hour attended monitoring, per 30 day period: Physician review and interpretation only	(I) 5.0
96.1	G0025	Collagen skin test kit	(I) 5.0
96.1	G0026	Fecal leukocyte examination	—
96.1	G0027	Semen analysis; presence and/or motility of sperm excluding Huhner test	—
96.1	G0030	PET myocardial perfusion imaging, (following previous PET, G0030–G0047); single study, rest or stress (exercise and/or pharmacologic)	—
96.1	G0031	PET myocardial perfusion imaging, (following previous PET, G0030–G0047); multiple studies, rest or stress (exercise and/or pharmacologic)	—
96.1	G0032	PET myocardial perfusion imaging, (following rest SPECT, 78464); single study, rest or stress (exercise and/or pharmacologic)	—
96.1	G0033	PET myocardial perfusion imaging, (following rest SPECT, 78464); multiple studies, rest or stress (exercise and/or pharmacologic)	—
96.1	G0034	PET myocardial perfusion imaging, (following rest SPECT, 78465); single study, rest or stress (exercise and/or pharmacologic)	—
96.1	G0035	PET myocardial perfusion imaging, (following rest SPECT, 78465); multiple studies, rest or stress (exercise and/or pharmacologic)	—
96.1	G0036	PET myocardial perfusion imaging, (following coronary angiography, 93510–93529); single study, rest or stress (exercise and/or pharmacologic)	—
96.1	G0037	PET myocardial perfusion imaging, (following coronary angiography, 93510–93529); multiple studies, rest or stress (exercise and/or pharmacologic)	—
96.1	G0038	PET myocardial perfusion imaging, (following stress planar myocardial perfusion, 78460); single study, rest or stress (exercise and/or pharmacologic)	—
96.1	G0039	PET myocardial perfusion imaging, (following stress planar myocardial perfusion, 78460); multiple studies, rest or stress (exercise and/or pharmacologic)	—
96.1	G0040	PET myocardial perfusion imaging, (following stress echocardiogram, 93350); single study, rest or stress (exercise and/or pharmacologic)	—
96.1	G0041	PET myocardial perfusion imaging, (following stress echocardiogram, 93350); multiple studies, rest or stress (exercise and/or pharmacologic)	—
96.1	G0042	PET myocardial perfusion imaging, (following stress nuclear ventriculogram, 78481 or 78483); single study, rest or stress (exercise and/or pharmacologic)	—
96.1	G0043	PET myocardial perfusion imaging, (following stress nuclear ventriculogram, 78481 or 78483); multiple studies, rest or stress (exercise and/or pharmacologic)	—

UPD		Code	Description	Units
96.1		**G0044**	PET myocardial perfusion imaging, (following rest ECG, 93000); single study, rest or stress (exercise and/or pharmacologic)	—
96.1		**G0045**	PET myocardial perfusion imaging, (following rest ECG, 93000); multiple studies, rest or stress (exercise and/or pharmacologic)	—
96.1		**G0046**	PET myocardial perfusion imaging, (following stress ECG, 93015); single study, rest or stress (exercise and/or pharmacologic)	—
96.1		**G0047**	PET myocardial perfusion imaging, (following stress ECG, 93015); multiple studies, rest or stress (exercise and/or pharmacologic)	—
98.1	M	**G0051**	G0051 has been deleted. See code 17000	(I) 13.0
98.1	M	**G0052**	G0052 has been deleted. See code 17003	(I) 4.0
98.1	M	**G0053**	G0053 has been deleted. See code 17004	(I) 72.0
98.1	M	**G0064**	G0064 has been deleted. See code 99375	(I) 14.0
98.1	M	**G0065**	G0065 has been deleted. See code 99378	(I) 20.0
98.1	M	**G0066**	G0066 has been deleted. See code 99380	(I) 14.0
98.1	M	**G0071**	G0071 has been deleted. See code 90804	(I) 10.5
98.1	M	**G0072**	G0072 has been deleted. See code 90805	(I) 15.5
98.1	M	**G0073**	G0073 has been deleted. See code 90806	(I) 19.0
98.1	M	**G0074**	G0074 has been deleted. See code 90807	(I) 24.0
98.1	M	**G0075**	G0075 has been deleted. See code 90808	(I) 31.0
98.1	M	**G0076**	G0076 has been deleted. See code 90809	(I) 36.0
98.1	M	**G0077**	G0077 has been deleted. See code 90810	(I) 15.0
98.1	M	**G0078**	G0078 has been deleted. See code 90811	(I) 20.0
98.1	M	**G0079**	G0079 has been deleted. See code 90812	(I) 24.0
98.1	M	**G0080**	G0080 has been deleted. See code 90813	(I) 29.0
98.1	M	**G0081**	G0081 has been deleted. See code 90814	(I) 36.0
98.1	M	**G0082**	G0082 has been deleted. See code 90815	(I) 41.0
98.1	M	**G0083**	G0083 has been deleted. See code 90816	(I) 13.0
98.1	M	**G0084**	G0084 has been deleted. See code 90817	(I) 18.0
98.1	M	**G0085**	G0085 has been deleted. See code 90818	(I) 21.0
98.1	M	**G0086**	G0086 has been deleted. See code 90819	(I) 26.0
98.1	M	**G0087**	G0087 has been deleted. See code 90821	(I) 33.0
98.1	M	**G0088**	G0088 has been deleted. See code 90822	(I) 38.0
98.1	M	**G0089**	G0089 has been deleted. See code 90823	(I) 18.0
98.1	M	**G0090**	G0090 has been deleted. See code 90824	(I) 23.0

UPD		Code	Description	Units	
98.1	M	G0091	G0091 has been deleted. See code 90826	(I) 29.0	
98.1	M	G0092	G0092 has been deleted. See code 90827	(I) 34.0	
98.1	M	G0093	G0093 has been deleted. See code 90828	(I) 41.0	
98.1	M	G0094	G0094 has been deleted. See code 90829	(I) 46.0	
98.2		G0101	Cervical or vaginal cancer screening; pelvic and clinical breast examination	(I) 5.5	
98.2		G0104	Colorectal cancer screening; flexible sigmoidoscopy	(I) 13.0	
98.2		G0105	Colorectal cancer screening; colonoscopy on individual at high risk	(I) 55.0	
98.2		G0106	Colorectal cancer screening; alternative to G0104, screening sigmoidoscopy, barium enema	**Prof.** 10.0	**Total** 28.0
98.2		G0107	Colorectal cancer screening; fecal-occult blood test, 1-3 simultaneous determinations	RNE	
98.2	●	G0108	Diabetes outpatient self-management training services, individual, per session	(I) 12.0	
98.2	●	G0109	Diabetes self-management training services, group session, per individual	(I) 7.0	
98.2		G0110	NETT pulmonary rehabilitation; education/skills training, individual	(I) 9.0	
98.2		G0111	NETT pulmonary rehabilitation; education/skills, group	(I) 4.0	
98.2		G0112	NETT pulmonary rehabilitation; nutritional guidance, initial	(I) 20.0	
98.2		G0113	NETT pulmonary rehabilitation; nutritional guidance, subsequent	(I) 16.0	
98.2		G0114	NETT pulmonary rehabilitation; psychosocial consultation	(I) 12.0	
98.2		G0115	NETT pulmonary rehabilitation; psychological testing	(I) 12.0	
98.2		G0116	NETT pulmonary rehabilitation; psychosocial counselling	(I) 11.5	
98.2		G0120	Colorectal cancer screening; alternative to G0105, screening colonoscopy, barium enema	**Prof.** (I) 10.0	**Total** 28.0
98.2		G0121	Colorectal cancer screening; colonoscopy on individual not meeting criteria for high risk	(I) 55.0	
98.2		G0122	Colorectal cancer screening; barium enema	**Prof.** (I) 10.0	**Total** 28.0
98.2	●	G0123	Screening cytopathology, cervical or vaginal (any reporting system), collected in preservative fluid, automated thin layer preparation, screening by cytotechnologist under physician supervision	RNE	
98.2	●	G0124	Screening cytopathology, cervical or vaginal (any reporting system), collected in preservative fluid, automated thin layer preparation, requiring interpretation by physician	(I) 6.0	
98.2	●	G0125	PET lung imaging of solitary pulmonary nodules, using 2-(fluorine-18)-fluoro-2-deoxy-d-glucose (FDG), following CT (71250/71260 or 71270)	**Prof.** (I) 10.0	**Total** 420.0
98.2	●	G0126	PET lung imaging of solitary pulmonary nodules, using 2-(fluorine-18)-fluoro-2-deoxy-d-glucose (FDG), following CT (71250/71260 or 71270); initial staging of pathologically diagnosed non-small cell lung cancer	**Prof.** (I) 10.0	**Total** 420.0
98.2	●	G0127	Trimming of dystrophic nails, any number	(I) 2.0	

▲ Revised code ● New code M RVSI code or deleted from CPT (I) Interim Value

UPD		Code	Description	Units	
98.2	●	G0128	Direct (face-to-face with patient) skilled nursing services of a registered nurse provided in a comprehensive outpatient rehabilitation facility, each 10 minutes beyond the first 5 minutes	(I) 1.5	
98.2	●	G0130	Single energy x-ray absorptiometry (SEXA) bone density study, one or more sites; appendicular skeleton (peripheral) (e.g., radius, wrist, heel)	**Prof.** (I) 2.0	**Total** 9.0
98.2	●	G0131	Computerized tomography bone mineral density study, one or more sites; axial skeleton (e.g., hips, pelvis, spine)	**Prof.** (I) 3.0	**Total** 25.0
98.2	●	G0132	Computerized tomography bone mineral density study, one or more sites; appendicular skeleton (peripheral) (e.g., radius, wrist, heel)	**Prof.** (I) 2.0	**Total** 9.0
98.2	●	G0141	Screening cytopathology smears, cervical or vaginal, performed by automated system, with manual rescreening, requiring interpretation by physician	RNE	
98.2	●	G0143	Screening cytopathology, cervical or vaginal (any reporting system), collected in preservative fluid, automated thin layer preparation, with manual screening and rescreening by cytotechnologist under physician supervision	—	
98.2	●	G0144	Screening cytopathology, cervical or vaginal (any reporting system), collected in preservative fluid, automated thin layer preparation, with manual screening and computer-assisted rescreening by cytotechnologist under physician supervision	—	
98.2	●	G0145	Screening cytopathology, cervical or vaginal (any reporting system), collected in preservative fluid, automated thin layer preparation, with manual screening and computer-assisted rescreening using cell selection and review under physician supervision	—	
98.2	●	G0147	Screening cytopathology smears, cervical or vaginal, performed by automated system under physician supervision	—	
98.2	●	G0148	Screening cytopathology smears, cervical or vaginal, performed by automated system with manual rescreening	—	
98.1	M	H5300	This code has been deleted.	7.0	

Drugs Administered Other Than Oral Method (J0000-J8999)

UPD		Code	Description	Units
		J0120	Injection, tetracycline, up to 250 mg	—
98.2	●	J0130	Injection abciximab, 10 mg	—
	▲	J0150	Injection, adenosine, 6 mg (not to be used to report any adenosine phosphate compounds, instead use A9270)	—
98.2	●	J0151	Injection, adenosine, 90 mg (not to be used to report any adenosine phosphate compounds, instead use A9270)	—
96.1		J0170	Injection, adrenalin, epinephrine, up to 1 ml ampule	—
		J0190	Injection, biperiden lactate, per 5 mg	—
		J0205	Injection, alglucerase, per 10 units	—
98.1		J0207	Injection, amifostine, 500 mg	—
		J0210	Injection, methyldopate HCl, up to 250 mg	—
	▲	J0256	Injection, alpha 1-proteinase inhibitor — human, 10 mg	—
97.1	▲	J0270	Injection, alprostadil, 1.25 mcg, administered under direct physician supervision, excludes self-administration	—

▲ Revised code　　　● New code　　　M RVSI code or deleted from CPT　　　(I) Interim Value

UPD		Code	Description	Units
98.2	●	J0275	Alprostadil urethral suppository, administered under direct physician supervision, excludes self-administration	—
		J0280	Injection, aminophyllin, up to 250 mg	—
98.2	●	J0285	Injection, amphotericin B, 50 mg	—
	●	J0286	Injection, amphotericin B, any lipid formulation, 50 mg	—
		J0290	Injection, ampicillin sodium, up to 500 mg	—
		J0295	Injection, ampicillin sodium/sulbactam sodium, 1.5 gm	—
		J0300	Injection, amobarbital, up to 125 mg	—
		J0330	Injection, succinylcholine chloride, up to 20 mg	—
		J0340	Injection, nandrolone phenpropionate, up to 50 mg	—
		J0350	Injection, anistreplase, per 30 units	—
		J0360	Injection, hydralazine HCl, up to 20 mg	—
		J0380	Injection, metaraminol bitartrate, per 10 mg	—
		J0390	Injection, chloroquine HCl, up to 250 mg	—
98.2	●	J0395	Injection, arbutamine HCl, 1 mg	—
		J0400	Injection, trimethaphan camsylate, up to 500 mg	—
		J0460	Injection, atropine sulfate, up to 0.3 mg	—
		J0470	Injection, dimercaprol, per 100 mg	—
		J0475	Injection, baclofen, 10 mg	—
98.2	●	J0476	Injection, baclofen, 50 mcg for intrathecal trial	—
		J0500	Injection, dicyclomine HCl, up to 20 mg	—
		J0510	Injection, benzquinamide HCl, up to 50 mg	—
		J0515	Injection, benztropine mesylate, per 1 mg	—
		J0520	Injection, bethanechol chloride mytonachol or urecholine, up to 5 mg	—
		J0530	Injection, penicillin G benzathine and penicillin G procaine, up to 600,000 units	—
		J0540	Injection, penicillin G benzathine and penicillin G procaine, up to 1,200,000 units	—
		J0550	Injection, penicillin G benzathine and penicillin G procaine, up to 2,400,000 units	—
		J0560	Injection, penicillin G benzathine, up to 600,000 units	—
		J0570	Injection, penicillin G benzathine, up to 1,200,000 units	—
		J0580	Injection, penicillin G benzathine, up to 2,400,000 units	—
		J0585	Botulinum toxin type A, per unit	—

▲ Revised code   ● New code   **M** RVSI code or deleted from CPT   **(I)** Interim Value

UPD	Code	Description	Units
	J0590	Injection, ethylnorepinephrine HCl, 1 ml	—
	J0600	Injection, edetate calcium disodium, up to 1000 mg	—
	J0610	Injection, calcium gluconate, per 10 ml	—
	J0620	Injection, calcium glycerophosphate and calcium lactate, per 10 ml	—
	J0630	Injection, calcitonin-salmon, up to 400 units	—
	J0635	Injection, calcitriol, 1 mcg ampule	—
	J0640	Injection, leucovorin calcium, per 50 mg	—
	J0670	Injection, mepivacaine HCl, per 10 ml	—
	J0690	Injection, cefazolin sodium, up to 500 mg	—
	J0694	Injection, cefoxitin sodium, 1 g	—
	J0695	Injection, cefonicid sodium, 1 g	—
	J0696	Injection, ceftriaxone sodium, per 250 mg	—
	J0697	Injection, sterile cefuroxime sodium, per 750 mg	—
	J0698	Cefotaxime sodium, per g	—
	J0702	Injection, betamethasone acetate and betamethasone sodium phosphate, per 3 mg	—
	J0704	Injection, betamethasone sodium phosphate, per 4 mg	—
96.1	J0710	Injection, cephapirin sodium, up to 1 g	—
	J0713	Injection, ceftazidime, per 500 mg	—
	J0715	Injection, ceftizoxime sodium, per 500 mg	—
	J0720	Injection, chloramphenicol sodium succinate, up to 1 g	—
	J0725	Injection, chorionic gonadotropin, per 1,000 USP units	—
	J0730	Injection, chlorpheniramine maleate, per 10 mg	—
98.1	J0735	Injection, clonidine hydrochloride, 1 mg	—
98.1	J0740	Injection, cidofovir, 375 mg	—
	J0743	Injection, cilastatin sodium imipenem, per 250 mg	—
	J0745	Injection, codeine phosphate, per 30 mg	—
	J0760	Injection, colchicine, per 1 mg	—
	J0770	Injection, colistimethate sodium, up to 150 mg	—
	J0780	Injection, prochlorperazine, up to 10 mg	—
	J0800	Injection, corticotropin, up to 40 units	—
	J0810	Injection, cortisone, up to 50 mg	—

▲ Revised code   ● New code   M RVSI code or deleted from CPT   (I) Interim Value

UPD	Code	Description	Units
	J0835	Injection, cosyntropin, per 0.25 mg	—
	J0850	Injection, cytomegalovirus immune globulin intravenous (human), per vial	—
	J0895	Injection, deferoxamine mesylate, 500 mg per 5 cc	—
	J0900	Injection, testosterone enanthate and estradiol valerate, up to 1 cc	—
	J0945	Injection, brompheniramine maleate, per 10 mg	—
	J0970	Injection, estradiol valerate, up to 40 mg	—
	J1000	Injection, depo-estradiol cypionate, up to 5 mg	—
	J1020	Injection, methylprednisolone acetate, 20 mg	—
	J1030	Injection, methylprednisolone acetate, 40 mg	—
	J1040	Injection, methylprednisolone acetate, 80 mg	—
	J1050	Injection, medroxyprogesterone acetate, 100 mg	—
	J1055	Injection, medroxyprogesterone acetate for contraceptive use, 150 mg	—
	J1060	Injection, testosterone cypionate and estradiol cypionate, up to 1 ml	—
	J1070	Injection, testosterone cypionate, up to 100 mg	—
	J1080	Injection, testosterone cypionate, 1 cc, 200 mg	—
96.1	J1090	Injection, testosterone cypionate, 1 cc, 50 mg	—
	J1095	Injection, dexamethasone acetate, per 8 mg	—
	J1100	Injection, dexamethasone sodium phosphate, up to 4 mg/ml	—
	J1110	Injection, dihydroergotamine mesylate, per 1 mg	—
	J1120	Injection, acetazolamide sodium, up to 500 mg	—
	J1160	Injection, digoxin, up to 0.5 mg	—
	J1165	Injection, phenytoin sodium, per 50 mg	—
	J1170	Injection, hydromorphone, up to 4 mg	—
	J1180	Injection, dyphylline, up to 500 mg	—
97.1	J1190	Injection, dexrazoxane hydrochloride, per 250 mg	—
	J1200	Injection, diphenhydramine HCl, up to 50 mg	—
	J1205	Injection, chlorothiazide sodium, per 500 mg	—
	J1212	Injection, DMSO, dimethyl sulfoxide, 50%, 50 ml	—
	J1230	Injection, methadone HCl, up to 10 mg	—
	J1240	Injection, Dimenhydrinate, up to 50 mg	—
96.1	J1245	Injection, dipyridamole, per 10 mg	—

▲ Revised code   ● New code   **M** RVSI code or deleted from CPT   **(I)** Interim Value

UPD		Code	Description	Units
		J1250	Injection, dobutamine HCI, per 250 mg	—
98.2	●	**J1260**	Injection, dolasetron mesylate, 1 mg	—
		J1320	Injection, amitriptyline HCl, up to 20 mg	—
98.1		**J1325**	Injection, epoprostenol, 0.5 mg	—
		J1330	Injection, ergonovine maleate, up to 0.2 mg	—
		J1362	Injection, erythromycin gluceptate, per 250 mg	—
		J1364	Injection, erythromycin lactobionate, per 500 mg	—
		J1380	Injection, estradiol valerate, up to 10 mg	—
		J1390	Injection, estradiol valerate, up to 20 mg	—
		J1410	Injection, estrogen conjugated, per 25 mg	—
		J1435	Injection, estrone, per 1 mg	—
		J1436	Injection, etidronate disodium, per 300 mg	—
		J1440	Injection, filgrastim (G-CSF), 300 mcg	—
		J1441	Injection, filgrastim (G-CSF), 480 mcg	—
		J1455	Injection, foscarnet sodium, per 1,000 mg	—
		J1460	Injection, gamma globulin, intramuscular, 1 cc	—
		J1470	Injection, gamma globulin, intramuscular, 2 cc	—
		J1480	Injection, gamma globulin, intramuscular, 3 cc	—
		J1490	Injection, gamma globulin, intramuscular, 4 cc	—
		J1500	Injection, gamma globulin, intramuscular, 5 cc	—
		J1510	Injection, gamma globulin, intramuscular, 6 cc	—
		J1520	Injection, gamma globulin, intramuscular, 7 cc	—
		J1530	Injection, gamma globulin, intramuscular, 8 cc	—
		J1540	Injection, gamma globulin, intramuscular, 9 cc	—
		J1550	Injection, gamma globulin, intramuscular, 10 cc	—
		J1560	Injection, gamma globulin, intramuscular, over 10 cc	—
		J1561	Injection, immune globulin, intravenous, 500 mg	—
		J1562	Injection, immune globulin, intravenous 5 gms	—
98.1		**J1565**	Injection, respiratory syncytial virus immune globulin, intravenous, 50 mg	—
		J1570	Injection, ganciclovir sodium, 500 mg	—
		J1580	Injection, Garamycin, gentamicin, up to 80 mg	—

▲ Revised code ● New code **M** RVSI code or deleted from CPT **(I)** Interim Value

UPD		Code	Description	Units
		J1600	Injection, gold sodium thiomalate, up to 50 mg	—
		J1610	Injection, glucagon hydrochloride, per 1 mg	—
		J1620	Injection, gonadorelin hydrochloride, per 100 mcg	—
98.1		J1626	Injection, granisetron hydrochloride, 100 mcg	—
		J1630	Injection, haloperidol, up to 5 mg	—
		J1631	Injection, haloperidol decanoate, per 50 mg	—
		J1642	Injection, heparin sodium, (Heparin Lock Flush), per 10 units	—
96.1		J1644	Injection, heparin sodium, per 1,000 units	—
97.1		J1645	Injection dalteparin sodium, per 2500 IU	—
	▲	J1650	Injection, enoxaparin sodium, 10 mg	—
		J1670	Injection, tetanus immune globulin, human, up to 250 units	—
		J1690	Injection, prednisolone tebutate, up to 20 mg	—
		J1700	Injection, hydrocortisone acetate, up to 25 mg	—
		J1710	Injection, hydrocortisone sodium phosphate, up to 50 mg	—
		J1720	Injection, hydrocortisone sodium succinate, up to 100 mg	—
		J1730	Injection, diazoxide, up to 300 mg	—
		J1739	Injection, hydroxyprogesterone caproate, 125 mg/ml	—
		J1741	Injection, hydroxyprogesterone caproate, 250 mg/ml	—
98.1		J1742	Injection, ibutilide fumarate, 1 mg	—
		J1760	Injection, iron dextran, 2 cc	—
		J1770	Injection, iron dextran, 5 cc	—
		J1780	Injection, iron dextran, 10 cc	—
		J1785	Injection, imiglucerase, per unit	—
		J1790	Injection, droperidol, up to 5 mg	—
		J1800	Injection, propranolol HCl, up to 1 mg	—
		J1810	Injection, droperidol and fentanyl citrate, up to 2 ml ampule	—
		J1820	Injection, insulin, up to 100 units	—
98.1	▲	J1825	Injection, interferon beta-1a, 33 mcg, administered under direct physician supervision, excludes self-administration	—
	▲	J1830	Injection interferon beta-1b, 0.25 mg, administered under direct physician supervision, excludes self-administration	—
		J1840	Injection, kanamycin sulfate, up to 500 mg	—
		J1850	Injection, kanamycin sulfate, up to 75 mg	—

▲ Revised code ● New code **M** RVSI code or deleted from CPT **(I)** Interim Value

UPD		Code	Description	Units
		J1885	Injection, ketorolac tromethamine, per 15 mg	—
		J1890	Injection, cephalothin sodium, up to 1 g	—
		J1910	Injection, Kutapressin, up to 2 ml	—
		J1930	Injection, propiomazine HCl, up to 20 mg	—
		J1940	Injection, furosemide, up to 20 mg	—
96.1		J1950	Injection, leuprolide acetate (for depot suspension), per 3.75 mg	—
		J1955	Injection, levocarnitine, per 1 gm	—
98.2	●	J1956	Injection, levofloxacin, 250 mg	—
		J1960	Injection, levorphanol tartrate, up to 2 mg	—
		J1970	Injection, methotrimeprazine, up to 20 mg	—
		J1980	Injection, hyoscyamine sulfate, up to 0.25 mg	—
		J1990	Injection, chlordiazepoxide HCl, up to 100 mg	—
		J2000	Injection, lidocaine HCl, 50 cc	—
		J2010	Injection, lincomycin HCl, up to 300 mg	—
		J2060	Injection, lorazepam, 2 mg	—
		J2150	Injection, mannitol, 25% in 50 ml	—
		J2175	Injection, meperidine HCl, per 100 mg	—
		J2180	Injection, meperidine and promethazine HCl, up to 50 mg	—
		J2210	Injection, methylergonovine maleate, up to 0.2 mg	—
96.1		J2240	Injection, metocurine iodide, up to 2 mg	—
		J2250	Injection, midazolam HCl, per 1 mg	—
		J2260	Injection, milrinone lactate, per 5 ml	—
		J2270	Injection, morphine sulfate, up to 10 mg	—
98.2	●	J2271	Injection, morphine sulfate, 100 mg	—
96.1		J2275	Injection, morphine sulfate (preservative-free sterile solution), per 10 mg	—
96.1		J2300	Injection, nalbuphine HCl, per 10 mg	—
		J2310	Injection, naloxone HCl, per 1 mg	—
		J2320	Injection, nandrolone decanoate, up to 50 mg	—
		J2321	Injection, nandrolone decanoate, up to 100 mg	—
		J2322	Injection, nandrolone decanoate, up to 200 mg	—
		J2330	Injection, thiothixene, up to 4 mg	—

UPD		Code	Description	Units
		J2350	Injection, niacinamide, niacin, up to 100 mg	—
98.2	●	J2355	Injection, oprelvekin, 5 mg	—
		J2360	Injection, orphenadrine citrate, up to 60 mg	—
		J2370	Injection, phenylephrine HCl, up to 1 ml	—
		J2400	Injection, chloroprocaine HCl, per 30 ml	—
		J2405	Injection, ondansetron HCl, per 1 mg	—
		J2410	Injection, oxymorphone HCl, up to 1 mg	—
		J2430	Injection, pamidronate disodium, per 30 mg	—
		J2440	Injection, papaverine HCl, up to 60 mg	—
		J2460	Injection, oxytetracycline HCl, up to 50 mg	—
		J2480	Injection, hydrochlorides of opium alkaloids, up to 20 mg	—
		J2510	Injection, penicillin G procaine, aqueous, up to 600,000 units	—
		J2512	Injection, pentagastrin, per 2 ml	—
		J2515	Injection, pentobarbital sodium, per 50 mg	—
		J2540	Injection, penicillin G potassium, up to 600,000 units	—
		J2545	Pentamidine isethionate, inhalation solution, per 300 mg, administered through a DME	—
		J2550	Injection, promethazine HCl, up to 50 mg	—
		J2560	Injection, phenobarbital sodium, up to 120 mg	—
96.1		J2590	Injection, oxytocin, up to 10 units	—
		J2597	Injection, desmopressin acetate, per 1 mcg	—
		J2640	Injection, prednisolone sodium phosphate, up to 20 mg	—
		J2650	Injection, prednisolone acetate, up to 1 ml	—
		J2670	Injection, tolazoline HCl, up to 25 mg	—
		J2675	Injection, progesterone, (Gesterol 50, Progestaject) per 50 mg	—
		J2680	Injection, fluphenazine decanoate, up to 25 mg	—
		J2690	Injection, procainamide HCl, up to 1 g	—
		J2700	Injection, oxacillin sodium, up to 250 mg	—
		J2710	Injection, neostigmine methylsulfate, up to 0.5 mg	—
		J2720	Injection, protamine sulfate, per 10 mg	—
		J2725	Injection, protirelin, per 250 mcg	—
		J2730	Injection, pralidoxime chloride, up to 1 g	—

▲ Revised code   ● New code   **M** RVSI code or deleted from CPT   **(I)** Interim Value

UPD		Code	Description	Units
		J2760	Injection, phentolamine mesylate, up to 5 mg	—
		J2765	Injection, metoclopramide HCl, up to 10 mg	—
		J2790	Injection, Rho (D) immune globulin, human, one dose package	—
98.2	●	J2792	Injection, rho D immune globulin, intravenous, human, solvent detergent, 100 I.U.	—
		J2800	Injection, methocarbamol, up to 10 ml	—
		J2810	Injection, theophylline, per 40 mg	—
		J2820	Injection, sargramostim (GM-CSF), 50 mcg	—
		J2860	Injection, secobarbital sodium, up to 250 mg	—
		J2910	Injection, aurothioglucose, up to 50 mg	—
		J2912	Injection, sodium chloride, 0.9%, per 2 ml	—
		J2920	Injection, methylprednisolone sodium succinate, up to 40 mg	—
		J2930	Injection, methylprednisolone sodium succinate, up to 125 mg	—
		J2950	Injection, promazine HCl, up to 25 mg	—
		J2970	Injection, methicillin sodium, up to 1 g	—
98.2	●	J2994	Injection reteplase, 37.6 mg (two single use vials)	—
		J2995	Injection, streptokinase, per 250,000 IU	—
		J2996	Injection, alteplase recombinant, per 10 mg	—
		J3000	Injection, streptomycin, up to 1 g	—
		J3010	Injection, fentanyl citrate, up to 2 ml	—
	▲	J3030	Injection, sumatriptan succinate, 6 mg, administered under direct physician supervision, excludes self-administration	—
		J3070	Injection, pentazocine HCl, up to 30 mg	—
		J3080	Injection, chlorprothixene, up to 50 mg	—
		J3105	Injection, terbutaline sulfate, up to 1 mg	—
		J3120	Injection, testosterone enanthate, up to 100 mg	—
		J3130	Injection, testosterone enanthate, up to 200 mg	—
		J3140	Injection, testosterone suspension, up to 50 mg	—
		J3150	Injection, testosterone propionate, up to 100 mg	—
		J3230	Injection, chlorpromazine HCl, up to 50 mg	—
		J3240	Injection, thyrotropin, up to 10 IU	—
		J3250	Injection, trimethobenzamide HCl, up to 200 mg	—
96.1		J3260	Injection, tobramycin sulfate, up to 80 mg	—

UPD	Code	Description	Units
	J3265	Injection, torsemide, 10 mg/ml	—
	J3270	Injection, imipramine HCl, up to 25 mg	—
	J3280	Injection, thiethylperazine maleate, up to 10 mg	—
	J3301	Injection, triamcinolone acetonide, per 10 mg	—
	J3302	Injection, triamcinolone diacetate, per 5 mg	—
96.1	J3303	Injection, triamcinolone hexacetonide, per 5 mg	—
	J3305	Injection, trimetrexate glucoronate, per 25 mg	—
	J3310	Injection, perphenazine, up to 5 mg	—
	J3320	Injection, spectinomycin dihydrochloride, up to 2 g	—
	J3350	Injection, urea, up to 40 g	—
	J3360	Injection, diazepam, up to 5 mg	—
	J3364	Injection, urokinase, 5,000 IU vial	—
	J3365	Injection, IV, urokinase, 250,000 IU vial	—
	J3370	Injection, vancomycin HCl, up to 500 mg	—
	J3390	Injection, methoxamine HCl, up to 20 mg	—
	J3400	Injection, triflupromazine HCl, up to 20 mg	—
	J3410	Injection, hydroxyzine HCl, up to 25 mg	—
	J3420	Injection, vitamin B-12 cyanocobalamin, up to 1,000 mcg	—
	J3430	Injection, phytonadione (vitamin K), per 1 mg	—
	J3450	Injection, mephentermine sulfate, up to 30 mg	—
96.1	J3470	Injection, hyaluronidase, up to 150 units	—
96.1	J3475	Injection, magnesium sulphate, per 500 mg	—
	J3480	Injection, potassium chloride, per 2 mEq	—
	J3490	Unclassified drugs	—
	J3520	Edetate disodium	—
	J3530	Nasal vaccine inhalation	—
	J3535	Drug administered through a metered dose inhaler	—
	J3570	Laetrile, amygdalin, vitamin B-17	—
	J7030	Infusion, normal saline solution, 1,000 cc	—
	J7040	Infusion, normal saline solution, sterile (500 ml = 1 unit)	—
	J7042	5% dextrose/normal saline (500 ml = 1 unit)	—

▲ Revised code   ● New code   M RVSI code or deleted from CPT   (I) Interim Value

UPD		Code	Description	Units
		J7050	Infusion, normal saline solution, 250 cc	—
		J7051	Sterile saline or water, up to 5 cc	—
		J7060	5% dextrose/water (500 ml = 1 unit)	—
		J7070	Infusion, D-5-W, 1,000 cc	—
		J7100	Infusion, dextran 40, 500 ml	—
		J7110	Infusion, dextran 75, 500 ml	—
		J7120	Ringer's lactate infusion, up to 1,000 cc	—
		J7130	Hypertonic saline solution, 50 or 100 meq, 20 cc vial	—
96.1	▲	**J7190**	Factor VIII (antihemophilic factor, human) per I.U.	—
		J7191	Factor VIII (anti-hemophilic factor (porcine)), per I.U.	—
	▲	**J7192**	Factor VIII (antihemophilic factor, recombinant) per I.U.	—
		J7194	Factor IX complex, per IU	—
		J7196	Other hemophilia clotting factors (e.g., anti-inhibitors), per IU	—
		J7197	Antithrombin III (human), per IU	—
97.1		**J7300**	Intrauterine copper contraceptive	—
	●	**J7315**	Sodium hyaluronate, 20 mg, for intra-articular injection	—
	●	**J7320**	Hylan G-F 20, 16 mg, for intra-articular injection	—
		J7500	Azathioprine, oral, tab, 50 mg, 100s ea	—
		J7501	Azathioprine, parenteral, vial, 100 mg, 20 ml ea	—
		J7503	Cyclosporine, parenteral, per 50 mg	—
		J7504	Lymphocyte immune globulin, anti-thymocyte globulin, parenteral, amp, 50 mg/ml, 5 ml ea	—
		J7505	Monoclonal antibodies - parenteral, 5 mg	—
		J7506	Prednisone, oral, per 5 mg	—
		J7507	Tacrolimus, oral, per 1 mg	—
96.1		**J7508**	Tacrolimus, oral, per 5 mg	—
96.1		**J7509**	Methylprednisolone, oral, per 4 mg	—
96.1		**J7510**	Prednisolone, oral, per 5 mg	—
		J7599	Immunosuppressive drug, not otherwise classified	—
		J7610	Acetylcysteine, 10%, per ml, inhalation solution administered through DME	—
		J7625	Albuterol sulfate, 0.5%, per ml, inhalation solution administered through DME	—
		J7627	Bitolterol mesylate, 0.2%, per 10 ml, inhalation solution administered through DME	—

▲ Revised code   ● New code   **M** RVSI code or deleted from CPT   **(I)** Interim Value

UPD	Code	Description	Units
	J7630	Cromolyn sodium, per 20 mg, inhalation solution administered through DME	—
	J7640	Epinephrine, 2.25%, per ml, inhalation solution administered through DME	—
	J7645	Ipratropium bromide 0.02%, per ml, inhalation solution, administered through a DME	—
	J7650	Isoetharine HCl, 0.1%, per ml, inhalation solution administered through DME	—
	J7651	Isoetharine HCl, 0.125%, per ml, inhalation solution administered through DME	—
	J7652	Isoetharine HCl, 0.167%, per ml, inhalation solution administered through DME	—
	J7653	Isoetharine HCl, 0.2%, per ml, inhalation solution administered through DME	—
	J7654	Isoetharine HCl, 0.25%, per ml, inhalation solution administered through DME	—
	J7655	Isoetharine HCl, 1.0%, per ml, inhalation solution administered through DME	—
	J7660	Isoproterenol HCl, 0.5%, per ml, inhalation solution administered through DME	—
	J7665	Isoproterenol HCl, 1.0%, per ml, inhalation solution administered through DME	—
	J7670	Metaproterenol sulfate, 0.4%, per 2.5 ml, inhalation solution administered through DME	—
	J7672	Metaproterenol sulfate, 0.6%, per 2.5 ml, inhalation solution administered through DME	—
	J7675	Metaproterenol sulfate, 5.0%, per ml, inhalation solution administered through DME	—
	J7699	NOC drugs, inhalation solution administered through DME	—
	J7799	NOC drugs, other than inhalation drugs, administered through DME	—
	J8499	Prescription drug, oral, nonchemotherapeutic, not otherwise specified	—
	J8530	Cyclophosphamide, oral, 25 mg	—
	J8560	Etoposide, oral, 50 mg	—
	J8600	Melphalan, oral 2 mg	—
	J8610	Methotrexate, oral, 2.5 mg	—
	J8999	Prescription drug, oral, chemotherapeutic, not otherwise specified	—

Chemotherapy Drugs (J9000-J9999)

UPD	Code	Description	Units
	J9000	Doxorubicin HCl, 10 mg	—
	J9015	Aldesleukin, per single use vial	—
	J9020	Asparaginase, 10,000 units	—
	J9031	BCG live (intravesical), per installation	—
	J9040	Bleomycin sulfate, 15 units	—
	J9045	Carboplatin, 50 mg	—

▲ Revised code   ● New code   **M** RVSI code or deleted from CPT   **(I)** Interim Value

UPD		Code	Description	Units
		J9050	Carmustine, 100 mg	—
		J9060	Cisplatin, powder or solution, per 10 mg	—
		J9062	Cisplatin, 50 mg	—
		J9065	Injection, cladribine, per 1 mg	—
		J9070	Cyclophosphamide, 100 mg	—
		J9080	Cyclophosphamide, 200 mg	—
		J9090	Cyclophosphamide, 500 mg	—
		J9091	Cyclophosphamide, 1 g	—
		J9092	Cyclophosphamide, 2 g	—
		J9093	Cyclophosphamide, lyophilized, 100 mg	—
		J9094	Cyclophosphamide, lyophilized, 200 mg	—
		J9095	Cyclophosphamide, lyophilized, 500 mg	—
		J9096	Cyclophosphamide, lyophilized, 1 g	—
		J9097	Cyclophosphamide, lyophilized, 2 g	—
		J9100	Cytarabine, 100 mg	—
		J9110	Cytarabine, 500 mg	—
		J9120	Dactinomycin, 0.5 mg	—
		J9130	Dacarbazine, 100 mg	—
		J9140	Dacarbazine, 200 mg	—
		J9150	Daunorubicin HCl, 10 mg	—
98.2	●	J9151	Daunorubicin citrate, liposomal formulation, 10 mg	—
		J9165	Diethylstilbestrol diphosphate, 250 mg	—
98.1		J9170	Docetaxel, 20 mg	—
		J9181	Etoposide, 10 mg	—
		J9182	Etoposide, 100 mg	—
		J9185	Fludarabine phosphate, 50 mg	—
		J9190	Fluorouracil, 500 mg	—
		J9200	Floxuridine, 500 mg	—
98.1		J9201	Gemcitabine HCl, 200 mg	—
		J9202	Goserelin acetate implant, per 3.6 mg	—
98.1		J9206	Irinotecan, 20 mg	—

▲ Revised code   ● New code   **M** RVSI code or deleted from CPT   **(I)** Interim Value

UPD		Code	Description	Units
		J9208	Ifosfamide, per 1 gm	—
		J9209	Mesna, 200 mg	—
		J9211	Idarubicin HCl, 5 mg	—
		J9213	Interferon alfa-2A, recombinant, 3 million units	—
		J9214	Interferon alfa-2B, recombinant, 1 million units	—
		J9215	Interferon alfa-N3, (human leukocyte derived), 250,000 IU	—
		J9216	Interferon gamma-1B, 3 million units	—
		J9217	Leuprolide acetate (for depot suspension), 7.5 mg	—
		J9218	Leuprolide acetate, per 1 mg	—
		J9230	Mechlorethamine HCl, (nitrogen mustard), 10 mg	—
		J9245	Injection, melphalan HCl, 50 mg	—
		J9250	Methotrexate sodium, 5 mg	—
		J9260	Methotrexate sodium, 50 mg	—
		J9265	Paclitaxel, 30 mg	—
		J9268	Pentostatin, per 10 mg	—
		J9270	Plicamycin, 2,500 mcg	—
		J9280	Mitomycin, 5 mg	—
		J9290	Mitomycin, 20 mg	—
		J9291	Mitomycin, 40 mg	—
		J9293	Injection, mitoxantrone HCl, per 5 mg	—
98.2	●	J9310	Rituximab, 100 mg	—
		J9320	Streptozocin, 1 gm	—
		J9340	Thiotepa, 15 mg	—
98.1		J9350	Topotecan, 4 mg	—
		J9360	Vinblastine sulfate, 1 mg	—
		J9370	Vincristine sulfate, 1 mg	—
		J9375	Vincristine sulfate, 2 mg	—
96.1		J9380	Vincristine sulfate, 5 mg	—
		J9390	Vinorelbine tartrate, per 10 mg	—
98.1		J9600	Porfimer sodium, 75 mg	—
		J9999	Not otherwise classified, antineoplastic drug	—

▲ Revised code   ● New code   M RVSI code or deleted from CPT   (I) Interim Value

UPD	Code	Description	Units
		K Codes (Temporary) (K0000-K9999)	
	K0001	Standard wheelchair	—
	K0002	Standard hemi (low seat) wheelchair	—
	K0003	Lightweight wheelchair	—
	K0004	High strength, lightweight wheelchair	—
	K0005	Ultralightweight wheelchair	—
	K0006	Heavy-duty wheelchair	—
	K0007	Extra heavy-duty wheelchair	—
	K0008	Custom manual wheelchair/base	—
	K0009	Other manual wheelchair/base	—
	K0010	Standard-weight frame motorized/power wheelchair	—
	K0011	Standard-weight frame motorized/power wheelchair with programmable control parameters for speed adjustment, tremor dampening, acceleration control and braking	—
	K0012	Lightweight portable motorized/power wheelchair	—
	K0013	Custom motorized/power wheelchair base	—
	K0014	Other motorized/power wheelchair base	—
	K0015	Detachable, nonadjustable height armrest, each	—
	K0016	Detachable, adjustable height armrest, complete assembly, each	—
	K0017	Detachable, adjustable height armrest, base, each	—
	K0018	Detachable, adjustable height armrest, upper portion, each	—
	K0019	Arm pad, each	—
	K0020	Fixed, adjustable height armrest, pair	—
	K0021	Antitipping device, each	—
	K0022	Reinforced back upholstery	—
	K0023	Solid back insert, planar back, single density foam, attached with straps	—
	K0024	Solid back insert, planar back, single density foam, with adjustable hook-on hardware	—
	K0025	Hook-on headrest extension	—
	K0026	Back upholstery for ultralightweight or high-strength lightweight wheelchair	—
	K0027	Back upholstery for wheelchair type other than ultralightweight or high-strength lightweight wheelchair	—
	K0028	Fully reclining back	—

▲ Revised code   ● New code   **M** RVSI code or deleted from CPT   **(I)** Interim Value

UPD	Code	Description	Units
	K0029	Reinforced seat upholstery	—
	K0030	Solid seat insert, planar seat, single density foam	—
	K0031	Safety belt/pelvic strap	—
	K0032	Seat upholstery for ultralightweight or high-strength lightweight wheelchair	—
	K0033	Seat upholstery for wheelchair type other than ultralightweight or high-strength lightweight wheelchair	—
	K0034	Heel loop, each	—
	K0035	Heel loop with ankle strap, each	—
	K0036	Toe loop, each	—
	K0037	High mount flip-up footrest, each	—
	K0038	Leg strap, each	—
	K0039	Leg strap, H style, each	—
	K0040	Adjustable angle footplate, each	—
	K0041	Large size footplate, each	—
	K0042	Standard size footplate, each	—
	K0043	Footrest, lower extension tube, each	—
	K0044	Footrest, upper hanger bracket, each	—
	K0045	Footrest, complete assembly	—
	K0046	Elevating legrest, lower extension tube, each	—
	K0047	Elevating legrest, upper hanger bracket, each	—
	K0048	Elevating legrest, complete assembly	—
	K0049	Calf pad, each	—
	K0050	Ratchet assembly	—
	K0051	Cam release assembly, footrest or leg rest, each	—
	K0052	Swingaway, detachable footrests, each	—
	K0053	Elevating footrests, articulating (telescoping), each	—
	K0054	Seat width of 10, 11, 12, 15, 17, or 20 inches for a high-strength, lightweight or ultralightweight wheelchair	—
	K0055	Seat depth of 15, 17, or 18 inches for a high strength, lightweight or ultralightweight wheelchair	—
▲	**K0056**	Seat height less than 17" or equal to or greater than 21" for a high strength, lightweight, or ultralightweight wheelchair	—
	K0057	Seat width 19 or 20 inches for heavy duty or extra heavy-duty chair	—
	K0058	Seat depth 17 or 18 inches for a motorized/power wheelchair	—

UPD	Code	Description	Units
	K0059	Plastic coated handrim, each	—
	K0060	Steel handrim, each	—
	K0061	Aluminum handrim, each	—
	K0062	Handrim with 8 to 10 vertical or oblique projections, each	—
	K0063	Handrim with 12 to 16 vertical or oblique projections, each	—
	K0064	Zero pressure tube (flat free insert), any size, each	—
	K0065	Spoke protectors	—
	K0066	Solid tire, any size, each	—
	K0067	Pneumatic tire, any size, each	—
	K0068	Pneumatic tire tube, each	—
	K0069	Rear wheel assembly, complete, with solid tire, spokes or molded, each	—
	K0070	Rear wheel assembly, complete with pneumatic tire, spokes or molded, each	—
	K0071	Front caster assembly, complete, with pneumatic tire, each	—
	K0072	Front caster assembly, complete, with semipneumatic tire, each	—
	K0073	Caster pin lock, each	—
	K0074	Pneumatic caster tire, any size, each	—
	K0075	Semipneumatic caster tire, any size, each	—
	K0076	Solid caster tire, any size, each	—
	K0077	Front caster assembly, complete, with solid tire, each	—
	K0078	Pneumatic caster tire tube, each	—
	K0079	Wheel lock extension, pair	—
	K0080	Antirollback device, pair	—
	K0081	Wheel lock assembly, complete, each	—
	K0082	22 NF deep cycle lead acid battery, each	—
	K0083	22 NF gel cell battery, each	—
	K0084	Group 24 deep cycle lead acid battery, each	—
	K0085	Group 24 gel cell battery, each	—
	K0086	U-1 lead acid battery, each	—
	K0087	U-1 gel cell battery, each	—
	K0088	Battery charger, lead acid or gel cell	—
	K0089	Battery charger, dual mode	—

▲ Revised code   ● New code   **M** RVSI code or deleted from CPT   **(I)** Interim Value

UPD	Code	Description	Units
	K0090	Rear wheel tire for power wheelchair, any size, each	—
	K0091	Rear wheel tire tube other than zero pressure for power wheelchair, any size, each	—
	K0092	Rear wheel assembly for power wheelchair, complete, each	—
	K0093	Rear wheel zero pressure tire tube (flat free insert) for power wheelchair, any size, each	—
	K0094	Wheel tire for power base, any size, each	—
	K0095	Wheel tire tube other than zero pressure for each base, any size, each	—
	K0096	Wheel assembly for power base, complete, each	—
	K0097	Wheel zero pressure tire tube (flat free insert) for power base, any size, each	—
	K0098	Drive belt for power wheelchair	—
	K0099	Front caster for power wheelchair	—
	K0100	Amputee adapter, pair	—
	K0101	One-arm drive attachment	—
	K0102	Crutch and cane holder	—
	K0103	Transfer board, less than 25 inches	—
	K0104	Cylinder tank carrier	—
	K0105	IV hanger	—
	K0106	Arm trough, each	—
	K0107	Wheelchair tray	—
	K0108	Other accessory	—
	K0109	Customization of wheelchair base frame (option or accessory)	—
	K0112	Trunk support device, vest type, with inner frame, prefabricated	—
	K0113	Trunk support device, vest type, without inner frame, prefabricated	—
	K0114	Back support system for use with a wheelchair, with inner frame, prefabricated	—
	K0115	Seating system, back module, posterior-lateral control, with or without lateral supports, custom fabricated for attachment to wheelchair base	—
	K0116	Seating system, combined back and seat module, custom fabricated for attachment to wheelchair base	—
	K0119	Azathioprine, oral, tab, 50 mg	—
	K0120	Azathioprine, parenteral, 100 mg	—
	K0122	Cyclosporine, parenteral, 250 mg	—
	K0123	Lymphocyte immune globulin, antithmocyte globulin, parenteral, 250 mg	—
	K0137	Skin barrier; liquid (spray, brush, etc.), per oz.	—

▲ Revised code   ● New code   M RVSI code or deleted from CPT   (I) Interim Value

UPD		Code	Description	Units
		K0138	Skin barrier; paste, per oz.	—
		K0139	Skin barrier; powder, per oz.	—
		K0168	Administration set, small volume nonfiltered pneumatic nebulizer, disposable	—
		K0169	Small volume nonfiltered pneumatic nebulizer, disposable	—
		K0170	Administration set, small volume nonfiltered pneumatic nebulizer, non-disposable	—
		K0171	Administration set, small volume filtered pneumatic nebulizer	—
		K0172	Large volume nebulizer, disposable, unfilled, used with aerosol compressor	—
		K0173	Large volume nebulizer, disposable, prefilled, used with aerosol compressor	—
		K0174	Reservoir bottle, non-disposable, used with large volume ultrasonic nebulizer	—
		K0175	Corrugated tubing, disposable, used with large volume nebulizer, 100 feet	—
		K0176	Corrugated tubing, non-disposable, used with large volume nebulizer, 100 feet	—
		K0177	Water collection device, used with large volume nebulizer	—
		K0178	Filter, disposable, used with aerosol compressor	—
		K0179	Filter, non-disposable, used with aerosol compressor or ultrasonic generator	—
		K0180	Aerosol mask, used with DME nebulizer	—
		K0181	Dome and mouthpiece, used with small volume ultrasonic nebulizer	—
		K0182	Water, distilled, used with large volume nebulizer, 1000 ml	—
	▲	K0183	Nasal application device used with positive airway pressure device	—
		K0184	Nasal pillows/seals, replacement for nasal application device, pair	—
	▲	K0185	Headgear used with positive airway pressure device	—
	▲	K0186	Chin strap used with positive airway pressure device	—
	▲	K0187	Tubing used with positive airway pressure device	—
	▲	K0188	Filter, disposable, used with positive airway pressure device	—
	▲	K0189	Filter, nondisposable, used with positive airway pressure device	—
		K0190	Canister, disposable, used with suction pump	—
		K0191	Canister, non-disposable, used with suction pump	—
		K0192	Tubing, used with suction pump	—
		K0193	Continuous positive airway pressure (CPAP) device, with humidifier	—
		K0194	Intermittent assist device with continuous positive airway pressure (CPAP), with humidifier	—
98.1		K0195	Elevating leg rest, pair (for use with capped rental wheelchair base)	—
	▲	K0268	Humidifier, nonheated, used with positive airway pressure device	—

UPD	Code	Description	Units
	K0269	Aerosol compressor, adjustable pressure, light duty for intermittent use	—
98.1	**K0270**	Ultrasonic generator with small volume ultrasonic nebulizer	—
	K0277	Skin barrier; solid 4 x 4 or equivalent, with built-in convexity, each	—
	K0278	Skin barrier; with flange (solid, flexible or accordion) with built-in convexity, any size, each	—
	K0279	Skin barrier; with flange (solid, flexible or accordion) extended wear, with built-in convexity, any size, each	—
	K0280	Extension drainage tubing, any type, any length, with connector/adaptor, for use with urinary leg bag or urostomy pouch, each	—
	K0281	Lubricant, individual sterile packet, for insertion of urinary catheter, each	—
	K0283	Saline solution, per 10 ml, metered dose dispenser, for use with inhalation drugs	—
	K0284	External infusion pump, mechanical, reusable, for extended drug infusion	—
96.1	**K0400**	Adhesive skin support attachment for use with external breast prosthesis, each	—
96.1	**K0401**	For diabetics only, deluxe feature of off-the-shelf depth inlay shoe or custom molded shoe, per shoe	—
96.1	**K0407**	Urinary catheter anchoring device, adhesive skin attachment	—
96.1	**K0408**	Urinary catheter anchoring device, leg strap	—
96.1	**K0409**	Sterile water irrigation solution, 1000 ml	—
96.1	**K0410**	Male external catheter, with adhesive coating, each	—
96.1	**K0411**	Male external catheter, with adhesive strip, each	—
	K0412	Mycophenolate mofetil, oral, 250 mg (CellCept)	—
97.1	**K0415**	Prescription antiemetic drug, oral, per 1 mg, for use in conjunction with oral anti-cancer drug, not otherwise specified	—
97.1	**K0416**	Prescription antiemetic drug, rectal, per 1 mg, for use in conjunction with oral anti-cancer drug, not otherwise specified	—
97.1	**K0417**	External infusion pump, mechanical, reusable, for short term drug infusion	—
97.1	**K0418**	Cyclosporin, oral, per 100 mg (Sandimmune)	—
97.1	**K0419**	Pouch, drainable, with faceplate attached, plastic, each	—
97.1	**K0420**	Pouch, drainable, with faceplate attached, rubber, each	—
97.1	**K0421**	Pouch, drainable, for use on faceplate, plastic, each	—
97.1	**K0422**	Pouch, drainagle, for use on faceplate, rubber, each	—
97.1	**K0423**	Pouch, urinary, with faceplate attached, plastic, each	—
97.1	**K0424**	Pouch, urinary, with faceplate attached, rubber, each	—
97.1	**K0425**	Pouch, urinary, for use on faceplate, plastic, each	—
97.1	**K0427**	Pouch, urinary, for use on faceplate, rubber, each	—

▲ Revised code   ● New code   **M** RVSI code or deleted from CPT   **(I)** Interim Value

UPD		Code	Description	Units
97.1		**K0428**	Ostomy faceplate equivalent, silicone ring, each	—
97.1		**K0429**	Skin barrier, solid 4x4 or equivalent, extended wear, without built-in convexity, each	—
97.1		**K0430**	Skin barrier, with flange (solid, flexible or accordion), extended wear, without built-in convexity, any size, each	—
97.1		**K0431**	Pouch, closed, with standard wear barrier attached, with built-in convexity (1 piece), each	—
97.1		**K0432**	Pouch, drainable, with extended wear barrier attached, without built-in convexity (1 piece), each	—
97.1		**K0433**	Pouch, drainable, with standard wear barrier attached, with built-in convexity (1 piece), each	—
97.1		**K0434**	Pouch, drainable, with extended wear barrier attached, with built-in convexity (1 piece), each	—
97.1		**K0435**	Pouch, urinary, with extended wear barrier attached, without built-in convexity (1 piece), each	—
97.1		**K0436**	Pouch, urinary, with standard wear barrier attached, with built-in convexity (1 piece), each	—
97.1		**K0437**	Pouch, urinary, with extended wear barrier attached, with built-in convexity (1 piece), each	—
97.1		**K0438**	Ostomy deodorant for use in ostomy pouch, liquid, per fluid ounce	—
97.1		**K0439**	Ostomy deodorant for use in ostomy pouch, solid, per tablet	—
97.1		**K0440**	Nasal prosthesis, provided by a non-physician	—
97.1		**K0441**	Midfacial prosthesis, provided by a non-physician	—
97.1		**K0442**	Orbital prosthesis, provided by a non-physician	—
97.1		**K0443**	Upper facial prosthesis, provided by a non-physician	—
97.1		**K0444**	Hemi-facial prosthesis, provided by a non-physician	—
97.1		**K0445**	Auricular prosthesis, provided by a non-physician	—
97.1		**K0446**	Partial facial prosthesis, provided by a non-physician	—
97.1		**K0447**	Nasal septal prosthesis, provided by a non-physician	—
97.1		**K0448**	Unspecified maxillofacial prosthesis, by report, provided by a non-physician	—
97.1		**K0449**	Repair or modification of maxillofacial prosthesis, labor component, 15 minute increments, provided by a non-physician	—
97.1		**K0450**	Adhesive liquid, for use with facial prosthesis only, per ounce	—
97.1		**K0451**	Adhesive remover, wipes, for use with facial prosthesis, per box of 50	—
97.1		**K0452**	Wheelchair bearings, any type	—
98.1		**K0455**	Infusion pump used for uninterrupted administration of epoprostenol	—
98.2	●	**K0456**	Hospital bed, heavy duty, extra wide, with any type side rails, with mattress	—

UPD		Code	Description	Units
98.2	●	K0457	Extra wide/heavy duty commode chair, each	—
98.2	●	K0458	Heavy duty walker, without wheels, each	—
98.2	●	K0459	Heavy duty wheeled walker, each	—
98.2	●	K0460	Power add-on, to convert manual wheelchair to motorized wheelchair, joystick control	—
98.2	●	K0461	Power add-on, to convert manual wheelchair to power operated vehicle, tiller control	—
98.1		K0503	Acetylcysteine, inhalation solution administered through DME, unit dose form, per gram	—
98.1		K0504	Albuterol, inhalation solution administered through DME, concentrated form, per milligram	—
98.1		K0505	Albuterol, inhalation solution administered through DME, unit dose form, per milligram	—
98.1		K0506	Atropine, inhalation solution administered through DME, concentrated form, per milligram	—
98.1		K0507	Atropine, inhalation solution administered through DME, unit dose form, per milligram	—
98.1		K0508	Bitolterol mesylate, inhalation solution administered through DME, concentrated form, per milligram	—
98.1		K0509	Bitolterol mesylate, inhalation solution administered through DME, unit dose form, per milligram	—
98.1		K0511	Cromolyn sodium, inhalation solution administered through DME, unit dose form, per 10 milligrams	—
98.1		K0512	Dexamethasone, inhalation solution administered through DME, concentrated form, per milligram	—
98.1		K0513	Dexamethasone, inhalation solution administered through DME, unit dose form, per milligram	—
98.1		K0514	Dornase alpha, inhalation solution administered through DME, unit dose form, per milligram	—
98.1		K0515	Glycopyrrolate, inhalation solution administered through DME, concentrated form, per milligram	—
98.1		K0516	Glycopyrrolate, inhalation solution administered through DME, unit dose form, per milligram	—
98.1		K0518	Ipratropium bromide, inhalation solution administered through DME, unit dose form, per milligram	—
98.1		K0519	Isoetharine HCl, inhalation solution administered through DME, concentrated form, per milligram	—
98.1		K0520	Isoetharine HCl, inhalation solution administered through DME, unit dose form, per milligram	—
98.1		K0521	Isoproterenol HCl, inhalation solution administered through DME, concentrated form, per milligram	—

▲ Revised code　　　　● New code　　　　M RVSI code or deleted from CPT　　　　(I) Interim Value

UPD	Code	Description	Units
98.1	**K0522**	Isoproterenol HCl, inhalation solution administered through DME, unit dose form, per milligram	—
98.1	**K0523**	Metaproterenol sulfate, inhalation solution administered through DME, concentrated form, per 10 milligrams	—
98.1	**K0524**	Metaproterenol sulfate, inhalation solution administered through DME, unit dose form, per 10 milligrams	—
98.1	**K0525**	Terbutaline sulfate, inhalation solution administered through DME, concentrated form, per milligram	—
98.1	**K0526**	Terbutaline sulfate, inhalation solution administered through DME, unit dose form, per milligram	—
98.1	**K0527**	Triamcinolone, inhalation solution administered through DME, concentrated form, per milligram	—
98.1	**K0528**	Triamcinolone, inhalation solution administered through DME, unit dose form, per milligram	—
98.1	**K0529**	Sterile water or sterile saline, 1,000 ml, used with large volume nebulizer	—
98.1	**K0530**	Nebulizer, durable, glass, or autoclavable plastic, bottle type, not used with oxygen	—

Orthotic Procedures (L0000-L4999)

UPD	Code	Description	Units
	L0100	Cervical, craniostenosis, helmet molded to patient model	—
	L0110	Cervical, craniostenosis, helmet, nonmolded	—
	L0120	Cervical, flexible, nonadjustable (foam collar)	—
	L0130	Cervical, flexible, thermoplastic collar, molded to patient	—
	L0140	Cervical, semi-rigid, adjustable (plastic collar)	—
	L0150	Cervical, semi-rigid, adjustable molded chin cup (plastic collar with mandibular/occipital piece)	—
	L0160	Cervical, semi-rigid, wire frame occipital/mandibular support	—
	L0170	Cervical, collar, molded to patient model	—
	L0172	Cervical, collar, semi-rigid thermoplastic foam, two piece	—
	L0174	Cervical, collar, semi-rigid, thermoplastic foam, two piece with thoracic extension	—
	L0180	Cervical, multiple post collar, occipital/mandibular supports, adjustable	—
	L0190	Cervical, multiple post collar, occipital/mandibular supports, adjustable cervical bars (Somi, Guilford, Taylor types)	—
	L0200	Cervical, multiple post collar, occipital/mandibular supports, adjustable cervical bars, and thoracic extension	—
	L0210	Thoracic, rib belt	—
	L0220	Thoracic, rib belt, custom fabricated	—
	L0300	TLSO, flexible (dorso-lumbar surgical support)	—

UPD	Code	Description	Units
	L0310	TLSO, flexible (dorso-lumbar surgical support), custom fabricated	—
	L0315	TLSO, flexible (dorso-lumbar surgical support), elastic type, with rigid posterior panel	—
	L0317	TLSO, flexible (dorso-lumbar surgical support), hyperextension, elastic type, with rigid posterior panel	—
	L0320	TLSO, anterior-posterior control (Taylor type), with apron front	—
	L0330	TLSO, anterior-posterior-lateral control (Knight-Taylor type), with apron front	—
	L0340	TLSO, anterior-posterior-lateral-rotary control (Arnold, Magnuson, Steindler types), with apron front	—
	L0350	TLSO, anterior-posterior-lateral-rotary control, flexion compression jacket, custom fitted	—
	L0360	TLSO, anterior-posterior-lateral-rotary control, flexion compression jacket molded to patient model	—
	L0370	TLSO, anterior-posterior-lateral-rotary control, hyperextension (Jewett, Lennox, Baker, Cash types)	—
	L0380	TLSO, anterior-posterior-lateral-rotary control, with extensions	—
	L0390	TLSO, anterior-posterior-lateral control molded to patient model	—
	L0400	TLSO, anterior-posterior-lateral control molded to patient model, with interface material	—
	L0410	TLSO, anterior-posterior-lateral control, two-piece construction, molded to patient model	—
	L0420	TLSO, anterior-posterior-lateral control, two-piece construction, molded to patient model, with interface material	—
	L0430	TLSO, anterior-posterior-lateral control, with interface material, custom fitted	—
	L0440	TLSO, anterior-posterior-lateral control, with overlapping front section, spring steel front, custom fitted	—
	L0500	LSO, flexible (lumbo-sacral surgical support)	—
	L0510	LSO, flexible (lumbo-sacral surgical support), custom fabricated	—
	L0515	LSO, flexible (lumbo-sacral surgical support) elastic type, with rigid posterior panel	—
	L0520	LSO, anterior-posterior-lateral control (Knight, Wilcox types), with apron front	—
	L0530	LSO, anterior-posterior control (Macausland type), with apron front	—
	L0540	LSO, lumbar flexion (Williams flexion type)	—
	L0550	LSO, anterior-posterior-lateral control, molded to patient model	—
	L0560	LSO, anterior-posterior-lateral control, molded to patient model, with interface material	—
	L0565	LSO, anterior-posterior-lateral control, custom fitted	—
	L0600	Sacroiliac, flexible (sacroiliac surgical support)	—

UPD	Code	Description	Units
	L0610	Sacroiliac, flexible (sacroiliac surgical support), custom fabricated	—
	L0620	Sacroiliac, semi-rigid (Goldthwaite, Osgood types), with apron front	—
	L0700	CTLSO, anterior-posterior-lateral control, molded to patient model (Minerva type)	—
	L0710	CTLSO, anterior-posterior-lateral control, molded to patient model, with interface material (Minerva type)	—
	L0810	Halo procedure, cervical halo incorporated into jacket vest	—
	L0820	Halo procedure, cervical halo incorporated into plaster body jacket	—
	L0830	Halo procedure, cervical halo incorporated into Milwaukee type orthosis	—
	L0860	Addition to halo procedure, magnetic resonance image compatible system	—
	L0900	Torso support, ptosis support	—
	L0910	Torso support, ptosis support, custom fabricated	—
	L0920	Torso support, pendulous abdomen support	—
	L0930	Torso support, pendulous abdomen support, custom fabricated	—
	L0940	Torso support, postsurgical support	—
	L0950	Torso support, postsurgical support, custom fabricated	—
	L0960	Torso support, postsurgical support, pads for postsurgical support	—
	L0970	TLSO, corset front	—
	L0972	LSO, corset front	—
	L0974	TLSO, full corset	—
	L0976	LSO, full corset	—
	L0978	Axillary crutch extension	—
	L0980	Peroneal straps, pair	—
	L0982	Stocking supporter grips, set of four (4)	—
	L0984	Protective body sock, each	—
98.1	**L0999**	Addition to spinal orthosis, not otherwise specified	—
	L1000	CTLSO (Milwaukee), inclusive of furnishing initial orthosis, including model	—
	L1010	Addition to CTLSO or scoliosis orthosis, axilla sling	—
	L1020	Addition to CTLSO or scoliosis orthosis, kyphosis pad	—
	L1025	Addition to CTLSO or scoliosis orthosis, kyphosis pad, floating	—
	L1030	Addition to CTLSO or scoliosis orthosis, lumbar bolster pad	—
	L1040	Addition to CTLSO or scoliosis orthosis, lumbar or lumbar rib pad	—
	L1050	Addition to CTLSO or scoliosis orthosis, sternal pad	—

UPD	Code	Description	Units
	L1060	Addition to CTLSO or scoliosis orthosis, thoracic pad	—
	L1070	Addition to CTLSO or scoliosis orthosis, trapezius sling	—
	L1080	Addition to CTLSO or scoliosis orthosis, outrigger	—
	L1085	Addition to CTLSO or scoliosis orthosis, outrigger, bilateral with vertical extensions	—
	L1090	Addition to CTLSO or scoliosis orthosis, lumbar sling	—
	L1100	Addition to CTLSO or scoliosis orthosis, ring flange, plastic or leather	—
	L1110	Addition to CTLSO or scoliosis orthosis, ring flange, plastic or leather, molded to patient model	—
	L1120	Addition to CTLSO, scoliosis orthosis, cover for upright, each	—
	L1200	TLSO, inclusive of furnishing initial orthosis only	—
	L1210	Addition to TLSO, (low profile), lateral thoracic extension	—
	L1220	Addition to TLSO, (low profile), anterior thoracic extension	—
	L1230	Addition to TLSO, (low profile), Milwaukee type superstructure	—
	L1240	Addition to TLSO, (low profile), lumbar derotation pad	—
	L1250	Addition to TLSO, (low profile), anterior ASIS pad	—
	L1260	Addition to TLSO, (low profile), anterior thoracic derotation pad	—
	L1270	Addition to TLSO, (low profile), abdominal pad	—
	L1280	Addition to TLSO, (low profile), rib gusset (elastic), each	—
	L1290	Addition to TLSO, (low profile), lateral trochanteric pad	—
	L1300	Other scoliosis procedure, body jacket molded to patient model	—
	L1310	Other scoliosis procedure, postoperative body jacket	—
	L1499	Spinal orthosis, not otherwise specified	—
	L1500	THKAO, mobility frame (Newington, Parapodium types)	—
	L1510	THKAO, standing frame	—
	L1520	THKAO, swivel walker	—
	L1600	HO, abduction control of hip joints, flexible, Frejka type with cover	—
	L1610	HO, abduction control of hip joints, flexible, (Frejka cover only)	—
	L1620	HO, abduction control of hip joints, flexible, (Pavlik harness)	—
	L1630	HO, abduction control of hip joints, semi-flexible (Von Rosen type)	—
	L1640	HO, abduction control of hip joints, static, pelvic band or spreader bar, thigh cuffs	—
	L1650	HO, abduction control of hip joints, static, adjustable (Ilfled type)	—

UPD	Code	Description	Units
	L1660	HO, abduction control of hip joints, static, plastic	—
	L1680	HO, abduction control of hip joints, dynamic, pelvic control, adjustable hip motion control, thigh cuffs (Rancho hip action type)	—
	L1685	HO, abduction control of hip joint, postoperative hip abduction type, custom fabricated	—
	L1686	HO, abduction control of hip joint, postoperative hip abduction type	—
	L1700	Legg Perthes orthosis, (Toronto type)	—
	L1710	Legg Perthes orthosis, (Newington type)	—
	L1720	Legg Perthes orthosis, trilateral, (Tachdijan type)	—
	L1730	Legg Perthes orthosis, (Scottish Rite type)	—
	L1750	Legg Perthes orthosis, Legg Perthes sling (Sam Brown type)	—
	L1755	Legg Perthes orthosis, (Patten bottom type)	—
	L1800	KO, elastic with stays	—
	L1810	KO, elastic with joints	—
	L1815	KO, elastic or other elastic type material with condylar pad(s)	—
	L1820	KO, elastic with condylar pads and joints	—
	L1825	KO, elastic knee cap	—
	L1830	KO, immobilizer, canvas longitudinal	—
	L1832	KO, adjustable knee joints, positional orthosis, rigid support	—
	L1834	KO, without knee joint, rigid, molded to patient model	—
	L1840	KO, derotation, medial-lateral, anterior cruciate ligament, custom fabricated to patient model	—
98.1	L1843	KO, single upright, thigh and calf, with adjustable flexion and extension joint, medial-lateral and rotation control, custom fitted	—
	L1844	KO, single upright, thigh and calf, with adjustable flexion and extension joint, medial-lateral and rotation control, molded to patient model	—
	L1845	KO, double upright, thigh and calf, with adjustable flexion and extension joint, medial-lateral and rotation control, custom fitted	—
	L1846	KO, double upright, thigh and calf, with adjustable flexion and extension joint, medial-lateral and rotation control, molded to patient model	—
	L1850	KO, Swedish type	—
	L1855	KO, molded plastic, thigh and calf sections, with double upright knee joints, molded to patient model	—
	L1858	KO, molded plastic, polycentric knee joints, pneumatic knee pads (CTI)	—
	L1860	KO, modification of supracondylar prosthetic socket, molded to patient model (SK)	—

UPD	Code	Description	Units
	L1870	KO, double upright, thigh and calf lacers, molded to patient model with knee joints	—
96.1	L1880	KO, double upright, nonmolded thigh and calf cuffs/lacers with knee joints	—
	L1885	KO, single or double upright, thigh and calf, with funtional active resistance control	—
	L1900	AFO, spring wire, dorsiflexion assist calf band	—
	L1902	AFO, ankle gauntlet	—
	L1904	AFO, molded ankle gauntlet, molded to patient model	—
	L1906	AFO, multiligamentus ankle support	—
	L1910	AFO, posterior, single bar, clasp attachment to shoe counter	—
	L1920	AFO, single upright with static or adjustable stop (Phelps or Perlstein type)	—
	L1930	AFO, plastic	—
	L1940	AFO, molded to patient model, plastic	—
	L1945	AFO, molded to patient model, plastic, rigid anterior tibial section (floor reaction)	—
	L1950	AFO, spiral, molded to patient model (IRM type), plastic	—
	L1960	AFO, posterior solid ankle, molded to patient model, plastic	—
	L1970	AFO, plastic molded to patient model, with ankle joint	—
	L1980	AFO, single upright free plantar dorsiflexion, solid stirrup, calf band/cuff (single bar "BK" orthosis)	—
	L1990	AFO, double upright free plantar dorsiflexion, solid stirrup, calf band/cuff (double bar "BK" orthosis)	—
	L2000	KAFO, single upright, free knee, free ankle, solid stirrup, thigh and calf bands/cuffs (single bar "AK" orthosis)	—
	L2010	KAFO, single upright, free ankle, solid stirrup, thigh and calf bands/cuffs (single bar "AK" orthosis), without knee joint	—
	L2020	KAFO, double upright, free knee, free ankle, solid stirrup, thigh and calf bands/cuffs (double bar "AK" orthosis)	—
	L2030	KAFO, double upright, free ankle, solid stirrup, thigh and calf bands/cuffs, (double bar "AK" orthosis), without knee joint	—
98.1	L2035	KAFO, full plastic, static, prefabricated (pediatric size)	—
	L2036	KAFO, full plastic, double upright, free knee, molded to patient model	—
	L2037	KAFO, full plastic, single upright, free knee, molded to patient model	—
	L2038	KAFO, full plastic, without knee joint, multiaxis ankle, molded to patient model (Lively orthosis or equal)	—
97.1	L2039	KAFO, full plastic, single upright, poly-axial hinge, medial lateral rotation control, molded to patient model	—

▲ Revised code   ● New code   **M** RVSI code or deleted from CPT   **(I)** Interim Value

UPD	Code	Description	Units
	L2040	HKAFO, torsion control, bilateral rotation straps, pelvic band/belt	—
	L2050	HKAFO, torsion control, bilateral torsion cables, hip joint, pelvic band/belt	—
	L2060	HKAFO, torsion control, bilateral torsion cables, ball bearing hip joint, pelvic band/ belt	—
	L2070	HKAFO, torsion control, unilateral rotation straps, pelvic band/belt	—
	L2080	HKAFO, torsion control, unilateral torsion cable, hip joint, pelvic band/belt	—
	L2090	HKAFO, torsion control, unilateral torsion cable, ball bearing hip joint, pelvic band/belt	—
	L2102	AFO, fracture orthosis, tibial fracture cast orthosis, plaster type casting material, molded to patient	—
	L2104	AFO, fracture orthosis, tibial fracture cast orthosis, synthetic type casting material, molded to patient	—
	L2106	AFO, fracture orthosis, tibial fracture cast orthosis, thermoplastic type casting material, molded to patient	—
	L2108	AFO, fracture orthosis, tibial fracture cast orthosis, molded to patient model	—
	L2112	AFO, fracture orthosis, tibial fracture orthosis, soft	—
	L2114	AFO, fracture orthosis, tibial fracture orthosis, semi-rigid	—
	L2116	AFO, fracture orthosis, tibial fracture orthosis, rigid	—
	L2122	KAFO, fracture orthosis, femoral fracture cast orthosis, plaster type casting material, molded to patient	—
	L2124	KAFO, fracture orthosis, femoral fracture cast orthosis, synthetic type casting material, molded to patient	—
	L2126	KAFO, fracture orthosis, femoral fracture cast orthosis, thermoplastic type casting material, molded to patient	—
	L2128	KAFO, fracture orthosis, femoral fracture cast orthosis, molded to patient model	—
	L2132	KAFO, fracture orthosis, femoral fracture cast orthosis, soft	—
	L2134	KAFO, fracture orthosis, femoral fracture cast orthosis, semi-rigid	—
	L2136	KAFO, fracture orthosis, femoral fracture cast orthosis, rigid	—
	L2180	Addition to lower extremity fracture orthosis, plastic shoe insert with ankle joints	—
	L2182	Addition to lower extremity fracture orthosis, drop lock knee joint	—
	L2184	Addition to lower extremity fracture orthosis, limited motion knee joint	—
	L2186	Addition to lower extremity fracture orthosis, adjustable motion knee joint, Lerman type	—
	L2188	Addition to lower extremity fracture orthosis, quadrilateral brim	—
	L2190	Addition to lower extremity fracture orthosis, waist belt	—

UPD	Code	Description	Units
	L2192	Addition to lower extremity fracture orthosis, hip joint, pelvic band, thigh flange, and pelvic belt	—
	L2200	Addition to lower extremity, limited ankle motion, each joint	—
	L2210	Addition to lower extremity, dorsiflexion assist (plantar flexion resist), each joint	—
	L2220	Addition to lower extremity, dorsiflexion and plantar flexion assist/resist, each joint	—
	L2230	Addition to lower extremity, split flat caliper stirrups and plate attachment	—
	L2240	Addition to lower extremity, round caliper and plate attachment	—
	L2250	Addition to lower extremity, foot plate, molded to patient model, stirrup attachment	—
	L2260	Addition to lower extremity, reinforced solid stirrup (Scott-Craig type)	—
	L2265	Addition to lower extremity, long tongue stirrup	—
	L2270	Addition to lower extremity, varus/valgus correction ("T") strap, padded/lined or malleolus pad	—
	L2275	Addition to lower extremity, varus/vulgus correction, plastic modification, padded/lined	—
	L2280	Addition to lower extremity, molded inner boot	—
	L2300	Addition to lower extremity, abduction bar (bilateral hip involvement), jointed, adjustable	—
	L2310	Addition to lower extremity, abduction bar, straight	—
	L2320	Addition to lower extremity, nonmolded lacer	—
	L2330	Addition to lower extremity, lacer molded to patient model	—
	L2335	Addition to lower extremity, anterior swing band	—
	L2340	Addition to lower extremity, pretibial shell, molded to patient model	—
	L2350	Addition to lower extremity, prosthetic type, (BK) socket, molded to patient model, (used for "PTB," "AFO" orthoses)	—
	L2360	Addition to lower extremity, extended steel shank	—
	L2370	Addition to lower extremity, Patten bottom	—
	L2375	Addition to lower extremity, torsion control, ankle joint and half solid stirrup	—
	L2380	Addition to lower extremity, torsion control, straight knee joint, each joint	—
	L2385	Addition to lower extremity, straight knee joint, heavy duty, each joint	—
	L2390	Addition to lower extremity, offset knee joint, each joint	—
	L2395	Addition to lower extremity, offset knee joint, heavy duty, each joint	—
	L2397	Addition to lower extremity orthosis, suspension sleeve	—
	L2405	Addition to knee joint, drop lock, each joint	—

▲ Revised code   ● New code   **M** RVSI code or deleted from CPT   **(I)** Interim Value

UPD	Code	Description	Units
	L2415	Addition to knee joint, cam lock (Swiss, French, bail types) each joint	—
	L2425	Addition to knee joint, disc or dial lock for adjustable knee flexion, each joint	—
97.1	**L2430**	Addition to knee joint, ratchet lock for active and progressive knee extension, each joint	—
	L2435	Addition to knee joint, polycentric joint, each joint	—
	L2492	Addition to knee joint, lift loop for drop lock ring	—
	L2500	Addition to lower extremity, thigh/weight bearing, gluteal/ischial weight bearing, ring	—
	L2510	Addition to lower extremity, thigh/weight bearing, quadri-lateral brim, molded to patient model	—
	L2520	Addition to lower extremity, thigh/weight bearing, quadri-lateral brim, custom fitted	—
	L2525	Addition to lower extremity, thigh/weight bearing, ischial containment/narrow M-L brim molded to patient model	—
	L2526	Addition to lower extremity, thigh/weight bearing, ischial containment/narrow M-L brim, custom fitted	—
	L2530	Addition to lower extremity, thigh/weight bearing, lacer, nonmolded	—
	L2540	Addition to lower extremity, thigh/weight bearing, lacer, molded to patient model	—
	L2550	Addition to lower extremity, thigh/weight bearing, high roll cuff	—
	L2570	Addition to lower extremity, pelvic control, hip joint, Clevis type, two position joint, each	—
	L2580	Addition to lower extremity, pelvic control, pelvic sling	—
	L2600	Addition to lower extremity, pelvic control, hip joint, Clevis type, or thrust bearing, free, each	—
	L2610	Addition to lower extremity, pelvic control, hip joint, Clevis or thrust bearing, lock, each	—
	L2620	Addition to lower extremity, pelvic control, hip joint, heavy-duty, each	—
	L2622	Addition to lower extremity, pelvic control, hip joint, adjustable flexion, each	—
	L2624	Addition to lower extremity, pelvic control, hip joint, adjustable flexion, extension, abduction control, each	—
	L2627	Addition to lower extremity, pelvic control, plastic, molded to patient model, reciprocating hip joint and cables	—
	L2628	Addition to lower extremity, pelvic control, metal frame, reciprocating hip joint and cables	—
	L2630	Addition to lower extremity, pelvic control, band and belt, unilateral	—
	L2640	Addition to lower extremity, pelvic control, band and belt, bilateral	—
	L2650	Addition to lower extremity, pelvic and thoracic control, gluteal pad, each	—
	L2660	Addition to lower extremity, thoracic control, thoracic band	—

▲ Revised code   ● New code   **M** RVSI code or deleted from CPT   **(I)** Interim Value

UPD	Code	Description	Units
	L2670	Addition to lower extremity, thoracic control, paraspinal uprights	—
	L2680	Addition to lower extremity, thoracic control, lateral support uprights	—
	L2750	Addition to lower extremity orthosis, plating chrome or nickel, per bar	—
97.1	L2755	Addition to lower extremity orthosis, carbon graphite lamination	—
	L2760	Addition to lower extremity orthosis, extension, per extension, per bar (for lineal adjustment for growth)	—
	L2770	Addition to lower extremity orthosis, any material, per bar or joint	—
	L2780	Addition to lower extremity orthosis, noncorrosive finish, per bar	—
	L2785	Addition to lower extremity orthosis, drop lock retainer, each	—
	L2795	Addition to lower extremity orthosis, knee control, full kneecap	—
	L2800	Addition to lower extremity orthosis, knee control, kneecap, medial or lateral pull	—
	L2810	Addition to lower extremity orthosis, knee control, condylar pad	—
	L2820	Addition to lower extremity orthosis, soft interface for molded plastic, below knee section	—
	L2830	Addition to lower extremity orthosis, soft interface for molded plastic, above knee section	—
	L2840	Addition to lower extremity orthosis, tibial length sock, fracture or equal, each	—
	L2850	Addition to lower extremity orthosis, femoral length sock, fracture or equal, each	—
	L2860	Addition to lower extremity joint, knee or ankle, concentric adjustable torsion style mechanism, each	—
	L2999	Lower extremity orthoses, not otherwise specified	—
	L3000	Foot insert, removable, molded to patient model, "UCB" type, Berkeley shell, each	—
	L3001	Foot insert, removable, molded to patient model, Spenco, each	—
	L3002	Foot insert, removable, molded to patient model, Plastazote or equal, each	—
	L3003	Foot insert, removable, molded to patient model, silicone gel, each	—
	L3010	Foot insert, removable, molded to patient model, longitudinal arch support, each	—
	L3020	Foot insert, removable, molded to patient model, longitudinal/metatarsal support, each	—
	L3030	Foot insert, removable, formed to patient foot, each	—
	L3040	Foot, arch support, removable, premolded, longitudinal, each	—
	L3050	Foot, arch support, removable, premolded, metatarsal, each	—
	L3060	Foot, arch support, removable, premolded, longitudinal/metatarsal, each	—
	L3070	Foot, arch support, nonremovable, attached to shoe, longitudinal, each	—

▲ Revised code   ● New code   M RVSI code or deleted from CPT   (I) Interim Value

UPD	Code	Description	Units
	L3080	Foot, arch support, nonremovable, attached to shoe, metatarsal, each	—
	L3090	Foot, arch support, nonremovable, attached to shoe, longitudinal/metatarsal, each	—
	L3100	Hallus-Valgus night dynamic splint	—
	L3140	Foot, abduction rotation bar, including shoes	—
	L3150	Foot, abduction rotation bar, without shoes	—
	L3160	Foot, adjustable shoe-styled positioning device	—
	L3170	Foot, plastic heel stabilizer	—
	L3201	Orthopedic shoe, oxford with supinator or pronator, infant	—
	L3202	Orthopedic shoe, oxford with supinator or pronator, child	—
	L3203	Orthopedic shoe, oxford with supinator or pronator, junior	—
	L3204	Orthopedic shoe, hightop with supinator or pronator, infant	—
	L3206	Orthopedic shoe, hightop with supinator or pronator, child	—
	L3207	Orthopedic shoe, hightop with supinator or pronator, junior	—
	L3208	Surgical boot, each, infant	—
	L3209	Surgical boot, each, child	—
	L3211	Surgical boot, each, junior	—
	L3212	Benesch boot, pair, infant	—
	L3213	Benesch boot, pair, child	—
	L3214	Benesch boot, pair, junior	—
	L3215	Orthopedic footwear, woman's shoes, oxford	—
	L3216	Orthopedic footwear, woman's shoes, depth inlay	—
	L3217	Orthopedic footwear, woman's shoes, hightop, depth inlay	—
	L3218	Orthopedic footwear, woman's surgical boot, each	—
	L3219	Orthopedic footwear, man's shoes, oxford	—
	L3221	Orthopedic footwear, man's shoes, depth inlay	—
	L3222	Orthopedic footwear, man's shoes, hightop, depth inlay	—
	L3223	Orthopedic footwear, man's surgical boot, each	—
	L3224	Orthopedic footwear, woman's shoe, oxford, used as an integral part of a brace (orthosis)	—
	L3225	Orthopedic footwear, man's shoe, oxford, used as an integral part of a brace (orthosis)	—
	L3230	Orthopedic footwear, custom shoes, depth inlay	—

UPD	Code	Description	Units
	L3250	Orthopedic footwear, custom molded shoe, removable inner mold, prosthetic shoe, each	—
	L3251	Foot, shoe molded to patient model, silicone shoe, each	—
	L3252	Foot, shoe molded to patient model, Plastazote (or similar), custom fabricated, each	—
	L3253	Foot, molded shoe Plastazote (or similar), custom fitted, each	—
	L3254	Nonstandard size or width	—
	L3255	Nonstandard size or length	—
	L3257	Orthopedic footwear, additional charge for split size	—
	L3260	Ambulatory surgical boot, each	—
	L3265	Plastazote sandal, each	—
	L3300	Lift, elevation, heel, tapered to metatarsals, per inch	—
	L3310	Lift, elevation, heel and sole, neoprene, per inch	—
	L3320	Lift, elevation, heel and sole, cork, per inch	—
	L3330	Lift, elevation, metal extension (skate)	—
	L3332	Lift, elevation, inside shoe, tapered, up to one-half inch	—
	L3334	Lift, elevation, heel, per inch	—
	L3340	Heel wedge, SACH	—
	L3350	Heel wedge	—
	L3360	Sole wedge, outside sole	—
	L3370	Sole wedge, between sole	—
	L3380	Clubfoot wedge	—
	L3390	Outflare wedge	—
	L3400	Metatarsal bar wedge, rocker	—
	L3410	Metatarsal bar wedge, between sole	—
	L3420	Full sole and heel wedge, between sole	—
	L3430	Heel, counter, plastic reinforced	—
	L3440	Heel, counter, leather reinforced	—
	L3450	Heel, SACH cushion type	—
	L3455	Heel, new leather, standard	—
	L3460	Heel, new rubber, standard	—
	L3465	Heel, Thomas with wedge	—
	L3470	Heel, Thomas extended to ball	—

UPD		Code	Description	Units
		L3480	Heel, pad and depression for spur	—
		L3485	Heel, pad, removable for spur	—
	▲	L3500	Orthopedic shoe addition, insole, leather	—
	▲	L3510	Orthopedic shoe addition, insole, rubber	—
	▲	L3520	Orthopedic shoe addition, insole, felt covered with leather	—
	▲	L3530	Orthopedic shoe addition, sole, half	—
	▲	L3540	Orthopedic shoe addition, sole, full	—
	▲	L3550	Orthopedic shoe addition, toe tap, standard	—
	▲	L3560	Orthopedic shoe addition, toe tap, horseshoe	—
	▲	L3570	Orthopedic shoe addition, special extension to instep (leather with eyelets)	—
	▲	L3580	Orthopedic shoe addition, convert instep to velcro closure	—
	▲	L3590	Orthopedic shoe addition, convert firm shoe counter to soft counter	—
	▲	L3595	Orthopedic shoe addition, March bar	—
		L3600	Transfer of an orthosis from one shoe to another, caliper plate, existing	—
		L3610	Transfer of an orthosis from one shoe to another, caliper plate, new	—
		L3620	Transfer of an orthosis from one shoe to another, solid stirrup, existing	—
		L3630	Transfer of an orthosis from one shoe to another, solid stirrup, new	—
		L3640	Transfer of an orthosis from one shoe to another, Dennis Browne splint (Riveton), both shoes	—
	▲	L3649	Orthopedic shoe, modification, addition or transfer, not otherwise specified	—
		L3650	SO, figure of eight design abduction restrainer	—
		L3660	SO, figure of eight design abduction restrainer, canvas and webbing	—
		L3670	SO, acromio/clavicular (canvas and webbing type)	—
98.2	●	L3675	SO, vest type abduction restrainer, canvas webbing type, or equal	—
		L3700	EO, elastic with stays	—
		L3710	EO, elastic with metal joints	—
		L3720	EO, double upright with forearm/arm cuffs, free motion	—
		L3730	EO, double upright with forearm/arm cuffs, extension/flexion assist	—
		L3740	EO, double upright with forearm/arm cuffs, adjustable position lock with active control	—
		L3800	WHFO, short opponens, no attachment	—
		L3805	WHFO, long opponens, no attachment	—
		L3810	WHFO, addition to short and long opponens, thumb abduction ("C") bar	—

▲ Revised code   ● New code   **M** RVSI code or deleted from CPT   **(I)** Interim Value

UPD	Code	Description	Units
	L3815	WHFO, addition to short and long opponens, second M.P. abduction assist	—
	L3820	WHFO, addition to short and long opponens, I.P. extension assist, with M.P. extension stop	—
	L3825	WHFO, addition to short and long opponens, M.P. extension stop	—
	L3830	WHFO, addition to short and long opponens, M.P. extension assist	—
	L3835	WHFO, addition to short and long opponens, M.P. spring extension assist	—
	L3840	WHFO, addition to short and long opponens, spring swivel thumb	—
	L3845	WHFO, addition to short and long opponens, thumb I.P. extension assist, with M.P. stop	—
	L3850	WHO, addition to short and long opponens, action wrist, with dorsiflexion assist	—
	L3855	WHFO, addition to short and long opponens, adjustable M.P. flexion control	—
	L3860	WHFO, addition to short and long opponens, adjustable M.P. flexion control and I.P.	—
	L3890	Addition to upper extremity joint, wrist or elbow, concentric adjustable torsion style mechanism, each	—
	L3900	WHFO, dynamic flexor hinge, reciprocal wrist extension/flexion, finger flexion/extension, wrist or finger driven	—
	L3901	WHFO, dynamic flexor hinge, reciprocal wrist extension/flexion, finger flexion/extension, cable driven	—
	L3902	WHFO, external powered, compressed gas	—
	L3904	WHFO, external powered, electric	—
	L3906	WHO, wrist gauntlet, molded to patient model	—
	L3907	WHFO, wrist gauntlet with thumb spica, molded to patient model	—
	L3908	WHO, wrist extension control cock-up, nonmolded	—
	L3910	WHFO, Swanson design	—
	L3912	HFO, flexion glove with elastic finger control	—
	L3914	WHO, wrist extension cock-up	—
	L3916	WHFO, wrist extension cock-up, with outrigger	—
	L3918	HFO, knuckle bender	—
	L3920	HFO, knuckle bender, with outrigger	—
	L3922	HFO, knuckle bender, two segment to flex joints	—
	L3924	WHFO, Oppenheimer	—
	L3926	WHFO, Thomas suspension	—
	L3928	HFO, finger extension, with clock spring	—
	L3930	WHFO, finger extension, with wrist support	—

▲ Revised code   ● New code   **M** RVSI code or deleted from CPT   **(I)** Interim Value

UPD	Code	Description	Units
	L3932	FO, safety pin, spring wire	—
	L3934	FO, safety pin, modified	—
	L3936	WHFO, Palmer	—
	L3938	WHFO, dorsal wrist	—
	L3940	WHFO, dorsal wrist, with outrigger attachment	—
	L3942	HFO, reverse knuckle bender	—
	L3944	HFO, reverse knuckle bender, with outrigger	—
	L3946	HFO, composite elastic	—
	L3948	FO, finger knuckle bender	—
	L3950	WHFO, combination Oppenheimer, with knuckle bender and two attachments	—
	L3952	WHFO, combination Oppenheimer, with reverse knuckle and two attachments	—
	L3954	HFO, spreading hand	—
97.1	L3956	Addition of joint to upper extremity orthosis, any material; per joint	—
	L3960	SEWHO, abduction positioning, airplane design	—
	L3962	SEWHO, abduction positioning, Erbs palsey design	—
	L3963	SEWHO, molded shoulder, arm, forearm, and wrist, with articulating elbow joint	—
	L3964	SEO, mobile arm support attached to wheelchair, balanced, adjustable	—
	L3965	SEO, mobile arm support attached to wheelchair, balanced, adjustable Rancho type	—
	L3966	SEO, mobile arm support attached to wheelchair, balanced, reclining	—
	L3968	SEO, mobile arm support attached to wheelchair, balanced, friction arm support (friction dampening to proximal and distal joints)	—
	L3969	SEO, mobile arm support, monosuspension arm and hand support, overhead elbow forearm hand sling support, yoke type arm suspension support	—
	L3970	SEO, addition to mobile arm support, elevating proximal arm	—
	L3972	SEO, addition to mobile arm support, offset or lateral rocker arm with elastic balance control	—
	L3974	SEO, addition to mobile arm support, supinator	—
	L3980	Upper extremity fracture orthosis, humeral	—
	L3982	Upper extremity fracture orthosis, radius/ulnar	—
	L3984	Upper extremity fracture orthosis, wrist	—
	L3985	Upper extremity fracture orthosis, forearm, hand with wrist hinge	—
	L3986	Upper extremity fracture orthosis, combination of humeral, radius/ulnar, wrist (example: Colles' fracture)	—

▲ Revised code   ● New code   **M** RVSI code or deleted from CPT   **(I)** Interim Value

UPD	Code	Description	Units
	L3995	Addition to upper extremity orthosis, sock, fracture or equal, each	—
	L3999	Upper limb orthosis, not otherwise specified	—
	L4000	Replace girdle for Milwaukee orthosis	—
	L4010	Replace trilateral socket brim	—
	L4020	Replace quadrilateral socket brim, molded to patient model	—
	L4030	Replace quadrilateral socket brim, custom fitted	—
	L4040	Replace molded thigh lacer	—
	L4045	Replace nonmolded thigh lacer	—
	L4050	Replace molded calf lacer	—
	L4055	Replace nonmolded calf lacer	—
	L4060	Replace high roll cuff	—
	L4070	Replace proximal and distal upright for KAFO	—
	L4080	Replace metal bands KAFO, proximal thigh	—
	L4090	Replace metal bands KAFO-AFO, calf or distal thigh	—
	L4100	Replace leather cuff KAFO, proximal thigh	—
	L4110	Replace leather cuff KAFO-AFO, calf or distal thigh	—
	L4130	Replace pretibial shell	—
97.1	L4205	Repair of orthotic device, labor component, per 15 minutes	—
	L4210	Repair of orthotic device, repair or replace minor parts	—
	L4350	Pneumatic ankle control splint (e.g., aircast)	—
	L4360	Pneumatic walking splint (e.g., aircast)	—
	L4370	Pneumatic full leg splint (e.g., aircast)	—
	L4380	Pneumatic knee splint (e.g., aircast)	—
97.1	L4392	Replace soft interface material, ankle contracture splint	—
97.1	L4394	Replace soft interface material, foot drop splint	—
97.1	L4396	Ankle contracture splint	—
97.1 ▲	L4398	Foot drop splint, recumbent positioning device	—

Prosthetic Procedures (L5000-L9999)

UPD	Code	Description	Units
	L5000	Partial foot, shoe insert with longitudinal arch, toe filler	—
	L5010	Partial foot, molded socket, ankle height, with toe filler	—
	L5020	Partial foot, molded socket, tibial tubercle height, with toe filler	—

▲ Revised code   ● New code   **M** RVSI code or deleted from CPT   **(I)** Interim Value

UPD	Code	Description	Units
	L5050	Ankle, Symes, molded socket, SACH foot	—
	L5060	Ankle, Symes, metal frame, molded leather socket, articulated ankle/foot	—
	L5100	Below knee, molded socket, shin, SACH foot	—
	L5105	Below knee, plastic socket, joints and thigh lacer, SACH foot	—
	L5150	Knee disarticulation (or through knee), molded socket, external knee joints, shin, SACH foot	—
	L5160	Knee disarticulation (or through knee), molded socket, bent knee configuration, external knee joints, shin, SACH foot	—
	L5200	Above knee, molded socket, single axis constant friction knee, shin, SACH foot	—
	L5210	Above knee, short prosthesis, no knee joint ("stubbies"), with foot blocks, no ankle joints, each	—
	L5220	Above knee, short prosthesis, no knee joint ("stubbies"), with articulated ankle/foot, dynamically aligned, each	—
	L5230	Above knee, for proximal femoral focal deficiency, constant friction knee, shin, SACH foot	—
	L5250	Hip disarticulation, Canadian type; molded socket, hip joint, single axis constant friction knee, shin, SACH foot	—
	L5270	Hip disarticulation, tilt table type; molded socket, locking hip joint, single axis constant friction knee, shin, SACH foot	—
	L5280	Hemipelvectomy, Canadian type; molded socket, hip joint, single axis constant friction knee, shin, SACH foot	—
	L5300	Below knee, molded socket, SACH foot, endoskeletal system, including soft cover and finishing	—
	L5310	Knee disarticulation (or through knee), molded socket, SACH foot endoskeletal system, including soft cover and finishing	—
	L5320	Above knee, molded socket, open end, SACH foot, endoskeletal system, single axis knee, including soft cover and finishing	—
	L5330	Hip disarticulation, Canadian type; molded socket, endo-skeletal system, hip joint, single axis knee, SACH foot, including soft cover and finishing	—
	L5340	Hemipelvectomy, Canadian type; molded socket, endoskeletal system, hip joint, single axis knee, SACH foot, including soft cover and finishing	—
	L5400	Immediate postsurgical or early fitting, application of initial rigid dressing, including fitting, alignment, suspension, and one cast change, below knee	—
	L5410	Immediate postsurgical or early fitting, application of initial rigid dressing, including fitting, alignment and suspension, below knee, each additional cast change and realignment	—
	L5420	Immediate postsurgical or early fitting, application of initial rigid dressing, including fitting, alignment and suspension and one cast change "AK" or knee disarticulation	—
	L5430	Immediate postsurgical or early fitting, application of initial rigid dressing, including fitting, alignment and suspension, "AK" or knee disarticulation, each additional cast change and realignment	—

UPD	Code	Description	Units
	L5450	Immediate postsurgical or early fitting, application of nonweight bearing rigid dressing, below knee	—
	L5460	Immediate postsurgical or early fitting, application of nonweight bearing rigid dressing, above knee	—
	L5500	Initial, below knee "PTB" type socket, non-alignable system, pylon, no cover, SACH foot, plaster socket, direct formed	—
	L5505	Initial, above knee — knee disarticulation, ischial level socket, non-alignable system, pylon, no cover, SACH foot plaster socket, direct formed	—
	L5510	Preparatory, below knee "PTB" type socket, non-alignable system, pylon, no cover, SACH foot, plaster socket, molded to model	—
	L5520	Preparatory, below knee "PTB" type socket, non-alignable system, pylon, no cover, SACH foot, thermoplastic or equal, direct formed	—
	L5530	Preparatory, below knee "PTB" type socket, non-alignable system, pylon, no cover, SACH foot, thermoplastic or equal, molded to model	—
	L5535	Preparatory, below knee "PTB" type socket, non-alignable system, pylon, no cover, SACH foot, prefabricated, adjustable open end socket	—
	L5540	Preparatory, below knee "PTB" type socket, non-alignable system, pylon, no cover, SACH foot, laminated socket, molded to model	—
	L5560	Preparatory, above knee — knee disarticulation, ischial level socket, non-alignable system, pylon, no cover, SACH foot, plaster socket, molded to model	—
	L5570	Preparatory, above knee — knee disarticulation, ischial level socket, non-alignable system, pylon, no cover, SACH foot, thermoplastic or equal, direct formed	—
	L5580	Preparatory, above knee — knee disarticulation, ischial level socket, non-alignable system, pylon, no cover, SACH foot, thermoplastic or equal, molded to model	—
	L5585	Preparatory, above knee — knee disarticulation, ischial level socket, non-alignable system, pylon, no cover, SACH foot, prefabricated adjustable open end socket	—
	L5590	Preparatory, above knee — knee disarticulation, ischial level socket, non-alignable system, pylon, no cover, SACH foot, laminated socket, molded to model	—
	L5595	Preparatory, hip disarticulation — hemipelvectomy, pylon, no cover, SACH foot, thermoplastic or equal, molded to patient model	—
	L5600	Preparatory, hip disarticulation — hemipelvectomy, pylon, no cover, SACH foot, laminated socket, molded to patient model	—
	L5610	Addition to lower extremity, endoskeletal system, above knee, hydracadence system	—
	L5611	Addition to lower extremity, endoskeletal system, above knee — knee disarticulation, 4-bar linkage, with friction swing phase control	—
	L5613	Addition to lower extremity, endoskeletal system, above knee — knee disarticulation, 4-bar linkage, with hydraulic swing phase control	—
	L5614	Addition to lower extremity, endoskeletal system, above knee — knee disarticulation, 4-bar linkage, with pneumatic swing phase control	—

▲ Revised code   ● New code   **M** RVSI code or deleted from CPT   **(I)** Interim Value

UPD	Code	Description	Units
96.1	L5616	Addition to lower extremity, endoskeletal system, above knee, universal multiplex system, friction swing phase control	—
	L5617	Addition to lower extremity, quick change self-aligning unit, above or below knee, each	—
	L5618	Addition to lower extremity, test socket, Symes	—
	L5620	Addition to lower extremity, test socket, below knee	—
	L5622	Addition to lower extremity, test socket, knee disarticulation	—
	L5624	Addition to lower extremity, test socket, above knee	—
	L5626	Addition to lower extremity, test socket, hip disarticulation	—
	L5628	Addition to lower extremity, test socket, hemipelvectomy	—
	L5629	Addition to lower extremity, below knee, acrylic socket	—
	L5630	Addition to lower extremity, Symes type, expandable wall socket	—
	L5631	Addition to lower extremity, above knee or knee disarticulation, acrylic socket	—
	L5632	Addition to lower extremity, Symes type, "PTB" brim design socket	—
	L5634	Addition to lower extremity, Symes type, posterior opening (Canadian) socket	—
	L5636	Addition to lower extremity, Symes type, medial opening socket	—
	L5637	Addition to lower extremity, below knee, total contact	—
	L5638	Addition to lower extremity, below knee, leather socket	—
	L5639	Addition to lower extremity, below knee, wood socket	—
	L5640	Addition to lower extremity, knee disarticulation, leather socket	—
	L5642	Addition to lower extremity, above knee, leather socket	—
	L5643	Addition to lower extremity, hip disarticulation, flexible inner socket, external frame	—
	L5644	Addition to lower extremity, above knee, wood socket	—
	L5645	Addition to lower extremity, below knee, flexible inner socket, external frame	—
	L5646	Addition to lower extremity, below knee, air cushion socket	—
	L5647	Addition to lower extremity, below knee, suction socket	—
	L5648	Addition to lower extremity, above knee, air cushion socket	—
	L5649	Addition to lower extremity, ischial containment/narrow M-L socket	—
	L5650	Addition to lower extremity, total contact, above knee or knee disarticulation socket	—
	L5651	Addition to lower extremity, above knee, flexible inner socket, external frame	—
	L5652	Addition to lower extremity, suction suspension, above knee or knee disarticulation socket	—

UPD	Code	Description	Units
	L5653	Addition to lower extremity, knee disarticulation, expandable wall socket	—
	L5654	Addition to lower extremity, socket insert, Symes (Kemblo, Pelite, Aliplast, Plastazote or equal)	—
	L5655	Addition to lower extremity, socket insert, below knee (Kemblo, Pelite, Aliplast, Plastazote or equal)	—
	L5656	Addition to lower extremity, socket insert, knee disarticulation (Kemblo, Pelite, Aliplast, Plastazote or equal)	—
	L5658	Addition to lower extremity, socket insert, above knee (Kemblo, Pelite, Aliplast, Plastazote or equal)	—
	L5660	Addition to lower extremity, socket insert, Symes, silicone gel or equal	—
	L5661	Addition to lower extremity, socket insert, multidurometer, Symes	—
	L5662	Addition to lower extremity, socket insert, below knee, silicone gel or equal	—
	L5663	Addition to lower extremity, socket insert, knee disarticulation, silicone gel or equal	—
	L5664	Addition to lower extremity, socket insert, above knee, silicone gel or equal	—
	L5665	Addition to lower extremity, socket insert, multidurometer, below knee	—
	L5666	Addition to lower extremity, below knee, cuff suspension	—
	L5667	Addition to lower extremity, below knee/above knee, socket insert, suction suspension with locking mechanism	—
	L5668	Addition to lower extremity, below knee, molded distal cushion	—
	L5669	Addition to lower extremity, below knee/above knee, socket insert, suction suspension without locking mechanism	—
	L5670	Addition to lower extremity, below knee, molded supracondylar suspension ("PTS" or similar)	—
	L5672	Addition to lower extremity, below knee, removable medial brim suspension	—
	L5674	Addition to lower extremity, below knee, latex sleeve suspension or equal, each	—
	L5675	Addition to lower extremity, below knee, latex sleeve suspension or equal, heavy duty, each	—
	L5676	Addition to lower extremity, below knee, knee joints, single axis, pair	—
	L5677	Addition to lower extremity, below knee, knee joints, polycentric, pair	—
	L5678	Addition to lower extremity, below knee joint covers, pair	—
	L5680	Addition to lower extremity, below knee, thigh lacer, nonmolded	—
	L5682	Addition to lower extremity, below knee, thigh lacer, gluteal/ischial, molded	—
	L5684	Addition to lower extremity, below knee, fork strap	—
	L5686	Addition to lower extremity, below knee, back check (extension control)	—
	L5688	Addition to lower extremity, below knee, waist belt, webbing	—

UPD	Code	Description	Units
	L5690	Addition to lower extremity, below knee, waist belt, padded and lined	—
	L5692	Addition to lower extremity, above knee, pelvic control belt, light	—
	L5694	Addition to lower extremity, above knee, pelvic control belt, padded and lined	—
	L5695	Addition to lower extremity, above knee, pelvic control, sleeve suspension, neoprene or equal, each	—
	L5696	Addition to lower extremity, above knee or knee disarticulation, pelvic joint	—
	L5697	Addition to lower extremity, above knee or knee disarticulation, pelvic band	—
	L5698	Addition to lower extremity, above knee or knee disarticulation, Silesian bandage	—
	L5699	All lower extremity prostheses, shoulder harness	—
	L5700	Replacement, socket, below knee, molded to patient model	—
	L5701	Replacement, socket, above knee/knee disarticulation, including attachment plate, molded to patient model	—
	L5702	Replacement, socket, hip disarticulation, including hip joint, molded to patient model	—
	L5704	Replacement, custom shaped protective cover, below knee	—
	L5705	Replacement, custom shaped protective cover, above knee	—
	L5706	Replacement, custom shaped protective cover, knee disarticulation	—
	L5707	Replacement, custom shaped protective cover, hip disarticulation	—
	L5710	Addition, exoskeletal knee-shin system, single axis, manual lock	—
	L5711	Addition, exoskeletal knee-shin system, single axis, manual lock, ultra-light material	—
	L5712	Addition, exoskeletal knee-shin system, single axis, friction swing and stance phase control (safety knee)	—
	L5714	Addition, exoskeletal knee-shin system, single axis, variable friction swing phase control	—
	L5716	Addition, exoskeletal knee-shin system, polycentric, mechanical stance phase lock	—
	L5718	Addition, exoskeletal knee-shin system, polycentric, friction swing and stance phase control	—
	L5722	Addition, exoskeletal knee-shin system, single axis, pneumatic swing, friction stance phase control	—
	L5724	Addition, exoskeletal knee-shin system, single axis, fluid swing phase control	—
	L5726	Addition, exoskeletal knee-shin system, single axis, external joints, fluid swing phase control	—
	L5728	Addition, exoskeletal knee-shin system, single axis, fluid swing and stance phase control	—
	L5780	Addition, exoskeletal knee-shin system, single axis, pneumatic/hydra pneumatic swing phase control	—

UPD		Code	Description	Units
		L5785	Addition, exoskeletal system, below knee, ultra-light material (titanium, carbon fiber or equal)	—
		L5790	Addition, exoskeletal system, above knee, ultra-light material (titanium, carbon fiber or equal)	—
		L5795	Addition, exoskeletal system, hip disarticulation, ultra-light material (titanium, carbon fiber or equal)	—
		L5810	Addition, endoskeletal knee-shin system, single axis, manual lock	—
		L5811	Addition, endoskeletal knee-shin system, single axis, manual lock, ultra-light material	—
		L5812	Addition, endoskeletal knee-shin system, single axis, friction swing and stance phase control (safety knee)	—
97.1		L5814	Addition, endoskeletal knee-shin system, polycentric, hydraulic swing phase control, mechanical stance phase lock	—
		L5816	Addition, endoskeletal knee-shin system, polycentric, mechanical stance phase lock	—
		L5818	Addition, endoskeletal knee-shin system, polycentric, friction swing and stance phase control	—
		L5822	Addition, endoskeletal knee-shin system, single axis, pneumatic swing, friction stance phase control	—
		L5824	Addition, endoskeletal knee-shin system, single axis, fluid swing phase control	—
98.1	▲	L5826	Addition, endoskeletal knee-shin system, single axis, hydraulic swing phase control, with miniature high activity frame	—
		L5828	Addition, endoskeletal knee-shin system, single axis, fluid swing and stance phase control	—
		L5830	Addition, endoskeletal knee-shin system, single axis, pneumatic/swing phase control	—
96.1	▲	L5840	Addition, endoskeletal knee-shin system, 4-bar linkage or multiaxial, pneumatic swing phase control	—
96.1		L5845	Addition, endoskeletal knee-shin system, stance flexion feature, adjustable	—
		L5846	Addition, endoskeletal knee-shin system, microprocessor control feature, swing phase only	—
		L5850	Addition, endoskeletal system, above knee or hip disarticulation, knee extension assist	—
		L5855	Addition, endoskeletal system, hip disarticulation, mechanical hip extension assist	—
		L5910	Addition, endoskeletal system, below knee, alignable system	—
		L5920	Addition, endoskeletal system, above knee or hip disarticulation, alignable system	—
96.1		L5925	Addition, endoskeletal system, above knee, knee disarticulationor hip disarticulation, manual lock	—
		L5930	Addition, endoskeletal system, high activity knee control frame	—

▲ Revised code   ● New code   M RVSI code or deleted from CPT   (I) Interim Value

UPD		Code	Description	Units
		L5940	Addition, endoskeletal system, below knee, ultra-light material (titanium, carbon fiber or equal)	—
		L5950	Addition, endoskeletal system, above knee, ultra-light material (titanium, carbon fiber or equal)	—
		L5960	Addition, endoskeletal system, hip disarticulation, ultra-light material (titanium, carbon fiber or equal)	—
		L5962	Addition, endoskeletal system, below knee, flexible protective outer surface covering system	—
		L5964	Addition, endoskeletal system, above knee, flexible protective outer surface covering system	—
		L5966	Addition, endoskeletal system, hip disarticulation, flexible protective outer surface covering system	—
98.2	●	**L5968**	All lower extremity prosthesis, ankle, multiaxial shock absorbing system	—
		L5970	All lower extremity prostheses, foot, external keel, SACH foot	—
		L5972	All lower extremity prostheses, flexible keel foot (Safe, Sten, Bock Dynamic or equal)	—
		L5974	All lower extremity prostheses, foot, single axis ankle/foot	—
98.2	●	**L5975**	All lower extremity prosthesis, combination single axis ankle and flexible keel foot	—
		L5976	All lower extremity prostheses, energy storing foot (Seattle Carbon Copy II or equal)	—
		L5978	All lower extremity prostheses, foot, multi-axial ankle/foot	—
		L5979	All lower extremity prostheses, multi-axial ankle/foot, dynamic response	—
		L5980	All lower extremity prostheses, flex-foot system	—
		L5981	All lower extremity prostheses, flex-walk system or equal	—
		L5982	All exoskeletal lower extremity prostheses, axial rotation unit	—
96.1		**L5984**	All endoskeletal lower extremity prostheses, axial rotation unit	—
		L5985	All endoskeletal lower extremity prostheses, dynamic prosthetic pylon	—
		L5986	All lower extremity prostheses, multi-axial rotation unit ("MCP" or equal)	—
97.1		**L5987**	All lower extremity prosthesis, shank foot system with vertical loading pylon	—
98.2	●	**L5988**	All lower extremity prosthesis, combination vertical shock and multiaxial rotation/torsional force reducing pylon	—
		L5999	Lower extremity prosthesis, not otherwise specified	—
		L6000	Partial hand, Robin-Aids, thumb remaining (or equal)	—
		L6010	Partial hand, Robin-Aids, little and/or ring finger remaining (or equal)	—
		L6020	Partial hand, Robin-Aids, no finger remaining (or equal)	—
		L6050	Wrist disarticulation, molded socket, flexible elbow hinges, triceps pad	—

▲ Revised code   ● New code   **M** RVSI code or deleted from CPT   **(I)** Interim Value

UPD	Code	Description	Units
	L6055	Wrist disarticulation, molded socket with expandable interface, flexible elbow hinges, triceps pad	—
	L6100	Below elbow, molded socket, flexible elbow hinge, triceps pad	—
	L6110	Below elbow, molded socket (Muenster or Northwestern suspension types)	—
	L6120	Below elbow, molded double wall split socket, step-up hinges, half cuff	—
	L6130	Below elbow, molded double wall split socket, stump activated locking hinge, half cuff	—
	L6200	Elbow disarticulation, molded socket, outside locking hinge, forearm	—
	L6205	Elbow disarticulation, molded socket with expandable interface, outside locking hinges, forearm	—
	L6250	Above elbow, molded double wall socket, internal locking elbow, forearm	—
	L6300	Shoulder disarticulation, molded socket, shoulder bulkhead, humeral section, internal locking elbow, forearm	—
	L6310	Shoulder disarticulation, passive restoration (complete prosthesis)	—
	L6320	Shoulder disarticulation, passive restoration (shoulder cap only)	—
	L6350	Interscapular thoracic, molded socket, shoulder bulkhead, humeral section, internal locking elbow, forearm	—
	L6360	Interscapular thoracic, passive restoration (complete prosthesis)	—
	L6370	Interscapular thoracic, passive restoration (shoulder cap only)	—
	L6380	Immediate postsurgical or early fitting, application of initial rigid dressing, including fitting alignment and suspension of components, and one cast change, wrist disarticulation or below elbow	—
	L6382	Immediate postsurgical or early fitting, application of initial rigid dressing including fitting alignment and suspension of components, and one cast change, elbow disarticulation or above elbow	—
	L6384	Immediate postsurgical or early fitting, application of initial rigid dressing including fitting alignment and suspension of components, and one cast change, shoulder disarticulation or interscapular thoracic	—
	L6386	Immediate postsurgical or early fitting, each additional cast change and realignment	—
	L6388	Immediate postsurgical or early fitting, application of rigid dressing only	—
	L6400	Below elbow, molded socket, endoskeletal system, including soft prosthetic tissue shaping	—
	L6450	Elbow disarticulation, molded socket, endoskeletal system, including soft prosthetic tissue shaping	—
	L6500	Above elbow, molded socket, endoskeletal system, including soft prosthetic tissue shaping	—
	L6550	Shoulder disarticulation, molded socket, endoskeletal system, including soft prosthetic tissue shaping	—
	L6570	Interscapular thoracic, molded socket, endoskeletal system, including soft prosthetic tissue shaping	—

▲ Revised code   ● New code   **M** RVSI code or deleted from CPT   (I) Interim Value

UPD	Code	Description	Units
	L6580	Preparatory, wrist disarticulation or below elbow, single wall plastic socket, friction wrist, flexible elbow hinges, figure of eight harness, humeral cuff, Bowden cable control, "USMC" or equal pylon, no cover, molded to patient model	—
	L6582	Preparatory, wrist disarticulation or below elbow, single wall socket, friction wrist, flexible elbow hinges, figure of eight harness, humeral cuff, Bowden cable control, "USMC" or equal pylon, no cover, direct formed	—
	L6584	Preparatory, elbow disarticulation or above elbow, single wall plastic socket, friction wrist, locking elbow, figure of eight harness, fair lead cable control, "USMC" or equal pylon, no cover, molded to patient model	—
	L6586	Preparatory, elbow disarticulation or above elbow, single wall socket, friction wrist, locking elbow, figure of eight harness, fair lead cable control, "USMC" or equal pylon, no cover, direct formed	—
	L6588	Preparatory, shoulder disarticulation or interscapular thoracic, single wall plastic socket, shoulder joint, locking elbow, friction wrist, chest strap, fair lead cable control, "USMC" or equal pylon, no cover, molded to patient model	—
	L6590	Preparatory, shoulder disarticulation or interscapular thoracic, single wall socket, shoulder joint, locking elbow, friction wrist, chest strap, fair lead cable control, "USMC" or equal pylon, no cover, direct formed	—
	L6600	Upper extremity additions, polycentric hinge, pair	—
	L6605	Upper extremity additions, single pivot hinge, pair	—
	L6610	Upper extremity additions, flexible metal hinge, pair	—
	L6615	Upper extremity addition, disconnect locking wrist unit	—
	L6616	Upper extremity addition, additional disconnect insert for locking wrist unit, each	—
	L6620	Upper extremity addition, flexion-friction wrist unit	—
	L6623	Upper extremity addition, spring assisted rotational wrist unit with latch release	—
	L6625	Upper extremity addition, rotation wrist unit with cable lock	—
	L6628	Upper extremity addition, quick disconnect hook adapter, Otto Bock or equal	—
	L6629	Upper extremity addition, quick disconnect lamination collar with coupling piece, Otto Bock or equal	—
	L6630	Upper extremity addition, stainless steel, any wrist	—
	L6632	Upper extremity addition, latex suspension sleeve, each	—
	L6635	Upper extremity addition, lift assist for elbow	—
	L6637	Upper extremity addition, nudge control elbow lock	—
	L6640	Upper extremity additions, shoulder abduction joint, pair	—
	L6641	Upper extremity addition, excursion amplifier, pulley type	—
	L6642	Upper extremity addition, excursion amplifier, lever type	—
	L6645	Upper extremity addition, shoulder flexion-abduction joint, each	—

UPD	Code	Description	Units
	L6650	Upper extremity addition, shoulder universal joint, each	—
	L6655	Upper extremity addition, standard control cable, extra	—
	L6660	Upper extremity addition, heavy duty control cable	—
	L6665	Upper extremity addition, Teflon, or equal, cable lining	—
	L6670	Upper extremity addition, hook to hand, cable adapter	—
	L6672	Upper extremity addition, harness, chest or shoulder, saddle type	—
	L6675	Upper extremity addition, harness, figure of eight type, for single control	—
	L6676	Upper extremity addition, harness, figure of eight type, for dual control	—
	L6680	Upper extremity addition, test socket, wrist disarticulation or below elbow	—
	L6682	Upper extremity addition, test socket, elbow disarticulation or above elbow	—
	L6684	Upper extremity addition, test socket, shoulder disarticulation or interscapular thoracic	—
	L6686	Upper extremity addition, suction socket	—
	L6687	Upper extremity addition, frame type socket, below elbow or wrist disarticulation	—
	L6688	Upper extremity addition, frame type socket, above elbow or elbow disarticulation	—
	L6689	Upper extremity addition, frame type socket, shoulder disarticulation	—
	L6690	Upper extremity addition, frame type socket, interscapular-thoracic	—
	L6691	Upper extremity addition, removable insert, each	—
	L6692	Upper extremity addition, silicone gel insert or equal, each	—
	L6700	Terminal device, hook, Dorrance or equal, model #3	—
	L6705	Terminal device, hook, Dorrance or equal, model #5	—
	L6710	Terminal device, hook, Dorrance or equal, model #5X	—
	L6715	Terminal device, hook, Dorrance or equal, model #5XA	—
	L6720	Terminal device, hook, Dorrance or equal, model #6	—
	L6725	Terminal device, hook, Dorrance or equal, model #7	—
	L6730	Terminal device, hook, Dorrance or equal, model #7LO	—
	L6735	Terminal device, hook, Dorrance or equal, model #8	—
	L6740	Terminal device, hook, Dorrance or equal, model #8X	—
	L6745	Terminal device, hook, Dorrance or equal, model #88X	—
	L6750	Terminal device, hook, Dorrance or equal, model #10P	—
	L6755	Terminal device, hook, Dorrance or equal, model #10X	—

UPD	Code	Description	Units
	L6765	Terminal device, hook, Dorrance or equal, model #12P	—
	L6770	Terminal device, hook, Dorrance or equal, model #99X	—
	L6775	Terminal device, hook, Dorrance or equal, model #555	—
	L6780	Terminal device, hook, Dorrance or equal, model #SS555	—
	L6790	Terminal device, hook, Accu hook or equal	—
	L6795	Terminal device, hook, 2 load or equal	—
	L6800	Terminal device, hook, APRL VC or equal	—
	L6805	Terminal device, modifier wrist flexion unit	—
	L6806	Terminal device, hook, TRS Grip, Grip III, VC, or equal	—
	L6807	Terminal device, hook, Grip I, Grip II, VC, or equal	—
	L6808	Terminal device, hook, TRS Adept, infant or child, VC, or equal	—
	L6809	Terminal device, hook, TRS Super Sport, passive	—
	L6810	Terminal device, pincher tool, Otto Bock or equal	—
	L6825	Terminal device, hand, Dorrance, VO	—
	L6830	Terminal device, hand, APRL, VC	—
	L6835	Terminal device, hand, Sierra, VO	—
	L6840	Terminal device, hand, Becker Imperial	—
	L6845	Terminal device, hand, Becker Lock Grip	—
	L6850	Terminal device, hand, Becker Plylite	—
	L6855	Terminal device, hand, Robin-Aids, VO	—
	L6860	Terminal device, hand, Robin-Aids, VO soft	—
	L6865	Terminal device, hand, passive hand	—
	L6867	Terminal device, hand, Detroit Infant Hand (mechanical)	—
	L6868	Terminal device, hand, passive infant hand, Steeper, Hosmer or equal	—
	L6870	Terminal device, hand, child mitt	—
	L6872	Terminal device, hand, NYU child hand	—
	L6873	Terminal device, hand, mechanical infant hand, Steeper or equal	—
	L6875	Terminal device, hand, Bock, VC	—
	L6880	Terminal device, hand, Bock, VO	—
	L6890	Terminal device, glove for above hands, production glove	—
	L6895	Terminal device, glove for above hands, custom glove	—

UPD	Code	Description	Units
	L6900	Hand restoration (casts, shading and measurements included), partial hand, with glove, thumb or one finger remaining	—
	L6905	Hand restoration (casts, shading and measurements included), partial hand, with glove, multiple fingers remaining	—
	L6910	Hand restoration (casts, shading and measurements included), partial hand, with glove, no fingers remaining	—
	L6915	Hand restoration (shading and measurements included), replacement glove for above	—
	L6920	Wrist disarticulation, external power, self-suspended inner socket, removable forearm shell, Otto Bock or equal switch, cables, two batteries and one charger, switch control of terminal device	—
	L6925	Wrist disarticulation, external power, self-suspended inner socket, removable forearm shell, Otto Bock or equal electrodes, cables, two batteries and one charger, myoelectronic control of terminal device	—
	L6930	Below elbow, external power, self-suspended inner socket, removable forearm shell, Otto Bock or equal switch, cables, two batteries and one charger, switch control of terminal device	—
	L6935	Below elbow, external power, self-suspended inner socket, removable forearm shell, Otto Bock or equal electrodes, cables, two batteries and one charger, myoelectronic control of terminal device	—
	L6940	Elbow disarticulation, external power, molded inner socket, removable humeral shell, outside locking hinges, forearm, Otto Bock or equal switch, cables, two batteries and one charger, switch control of terminal device	—
	L6945	Elbow disarticulation, external power, molded inner socket, removable humeral shell, outside locking hinges, forearm, Otto Bock or equal electrodes, cables, two batteries and one charger, myoelectronic control of terminal device	—
	L6950	Above elbow, external power, molded inner socket, removable humeral shell, internal locking elbow, forearm, Otto Bock or equal switch, cables, two batteries and one charger, switch control of terminal device	—
	L6955	Above elbow, external power, molded inner socket, removable humeral shell, internal locking elbow, forearm, Otto Bock or equal electrodes, cables, two batteries and one charger, myoelectronic control of terminal device	—
	L6960	Shoulder disarticulation, external power, molded inner socket, removable shoulder shell, shoulder bulkhead, humeral section, mechanical elbow, forearm, Otto Bock or equal switch, cables, two batteries and one charger, switch control of terminal device	—
	L6965	Shoulder disarticulation, external power, molded inner socket, removable shoulder shell, shoulder bulkhead, humeral section, mechanical elbow, forearm, Otto Bock or equal electrodes, cables, two batteries and one charger, myoelectronic control of terminal device	—
	L6970	Interscapular-thoracic, external power, molded inner socket, removable shoulder shell, shoulder bulkhead, humeral section, mechanical elbow, forearm, Otto Bock or equal switch, cables, two batteries and one charger, switch control of terminal device	—
	L6975	Interscapular-thoracic, external power, molded inner socket, removable shoulder shell, shoulder bulkhead, humeral section, mechanical elbow, forearm, Otto Bock or equal electrodes, cables, two batteries and one charger, myoelectronic control of terminal device	—

▲ Revised code   ● New code   **M** RVSI code or deleted from CPT   **(I)** Interim Value

UPD	Code	Description	Units
	L7010	Electronic hand, Otto Bock, Steeper or equal, switch controlled	—
	L7015	Electronic hand, System Teknik, Variety Village or equal, switch controlled	—
	L7020	Electronic greifer, Otto Bock or equal, switch controlled	—
	L7025	Electronic hand, Otto Bock or equal, myoelectronically controlled	—
	L7030	Electronic hand, System Teknik, Variety Village or equal, myoelectronically controlled	—
	L7035	Electronic greifer, Otto Bock or equal, myoelectronically controlled	—
	L7040	Prehensile actuator, Hosmer or equal, switch controlled	—
	L7045	Electronic hook, child, Michigan or equal, switch controlled	—
	L7170	Electronic elbow, Hosmer or equal, switch controlled	—
	L7180	Electronic elbow, Boston, Utah or equal, myoelectronically controlled	—
	L7185	Electronic elbow, adolescent, Variety Village or equal, switch controlled	—
	L7186	Electronic elbow, child, Variety Village or equal, switch controlled	—
	L7190	Electronic elbow, adolescent, Variety Village or equal, myoelectronically controlled	—
	L7191	Electronic elbow, child, Variety Village or equal, myoelectronically controlled	—
	L7260	Electronic wrist rotator, Otto Bock or equal	—
	L7261	Electronic wrist rotator, for Utah arm	—
	L7266	Servo control, Steeper or equal	—
	L7272	Analogue control, UNB or equal	—
	L7274	Proportional control, 6-12 volt, Liberty, Utah or equal	—
	L7360	Six volt battery, Otto Bock or equal, each	—
	L7362	Battery charger, six volt, Otto Bock or equal	—
	L7364	Twelve volt battery, Utah or equal, each	—
	L7366	Battery charger, twelve volt, Utah or equal	—
	L7499	Upper extremity prosthesis, not otherwise specified	—
	L7500	Repair of prosthetic device, hourly rate	—
	L7510	Repair of prosthetic device, repair or replace minor parts	—
97.1	**L7520**	Repair prosthetic device, labor component, per 15 minutes	—
97.1	**L7900**	Vacuum erection system	—
	L8000	Breast prosthesis, mastectomy bra	—
	L8010	Breast prosthesis, mastectomy sleeve	—
98.2 ●	**L8015**	External breast prosthesis garment, with mastectomy form, post-mastectomy	—

UPD		Code	Description	Units
		L8020	Breast prosthesis, mastectomy form	—
		L8030	Breast prosthesis, silicone or equal	—
98.2	●	**L8035**	Custom breast prosthesis, post mastectomy, molded to patient model	—
98.1		**L8039**	Breast prosthesis, not otherwise specified	—
	▲	**L8100**	Gradient compression stocking, below knee, 18-30 mmhg, each	—
	▲	**L8110**	Gradient compression stocking, below knee, 30-40 mmhg, each	—
	▲	**L8120**	Gradient compression stocking, below knee, 40-50 mmhg, each	—
	▲	**L8130**	Gradient compression stocking, thigh length, 18-30 mmhg, each	—
	▲	**L8140**	Gradient compression stocking, thigh length, 30-40 mmhg, each	—
	▲	**L8150**	Gradient compression stocking, thigh length, 40-50 mmhg, each	—
	▲	**L8160**	Gradient compression stocking, full length/chap style, 18-30 mmhg, each	—
	▲	**L8170**	Gradient compression stocking, full length/chap style, 30-40 mmhg, each	—
	▲	**L8180**	Gradient compression stocking, full length/chap style, 40-50 mmhg, each	—
	▲	**L8190**	Gradient compression stocking, waist length, 18-30 mmhg, each	—
98.2	●	**L8195**	Gradient compression stocking, waist length, 30-40 mmhg, each	—
	▲	**L8200**	Gradient compression stocking, waist length, 40-50 mmhg, each	—
	▲	**L8210**	Gradient compression stocking, custom made	—
	▲	**L8220**	Gradient compression stocking, lymphedema	—
	▲	**L8230**	Gradient compression stocking, garter belt	—
98.1	▲	**L8239**	Gradient compression stocking, not otherwise specified	—
		L8300	Truss, single with standard pad	—
		L8310	Truss, double with standard pads	—
		L8320	Truss, addition to standard pad, water pad	—
		L8330	Truss, addition to standard pad, scrotal pad	—
		L8400	Prosthetic sheath, below knee, each	—
		L8410	Prosthetic sheath, above knee, each	—
		L8415	Prosthetic sheath, upper limb, each	—
97.1		**L8417**	Prosthetic sheath/sock, including a gel cushion layer, below knee or above knee, each	—
	▲	**L8420**	Prosthetic sock, multiple ply, below knee, each	—
	▲	**L8430**	Prosthetic sock, multiple ply, above knee, each	—
	▲	**L8435**	Prosthetic sock, multiple ply, upper limb, each	—

▲ Revised code   ● New code   **M** RVSI code or deleted from CPT   **(I)** Interim Value

UPD		Code	Description	Units
		L8440	Prosthetic shrinker, below knee, each	—
		L8460	Prosthetic shrinker, above knee, each	—
		L8465	Prosthetic shrinker, upper limb, each	—
	▲	**L8470**	Prosthetic sock, single ply, fitting, below knee, each	—
	▲	**L8480**	Prosthetic sock, single ply, fitting, above knee, each	—
	▲	**L8485**	Prosthetic sock, single ply, fitting, upper limb, each	—
		L8490	Addition to prosthetic sheath/sock, air seal suction retention system	—
		L8499	Unlisted procedure for miscellaneous prosthetic services	—
		L8500	Artificial larynx, any type	—
		L8501	Tracheostomy speaking valve	—
		L8600	Implantable breast prosthesis, silicone or equal	—
		L8603	Collagen implant, urinary tract, per 2.5 cc syringe, includes shipping and necessary supplies	—
97.1		**L8610**	Ocular implant	—
		L8612	Aqueous shunt	—
97.1		**L8613**	Ossicula implant	—
		L8614	Cochlear device/system	—
98.1	M	**L8619**	Cochlear implant external speech processor, replacement	—
97.1		**L8630**	Metacarpophalangeal joint implant	—
97.1		**L8641**	Metatarsal joint implant	—
		L8642	Hallux implant	—
97.1		**L8658**	Interphalangeal joint implant	—
97.1		**L8670**	Vascular graft material, synthetic, implant	—
98.1		**L8699**	Prosthetic implant, not otherwise specified	—

Medical Services (M0000-M0302)

UPD		Code	Description	Units
98.1	M	**M0005**	This code has been deleted.	8.0
98.1	M	**M0006**	This code has been deleted.	1.5
98.1	M	**M0007**	This code has been deleted.	9.0
98.1	M	**M0008**	This code has been deleted.	3.0
		M0064	Brief office visit for the sole purpose of monitoring or changing drug prescriptions used in the treatment of mental psychoneurotic and personality disorders	4.5
		M0075	Cellular therapy	—

▲ Revised code   ● New code   **M** RVSI code or deleted from CPT   **(I)** Interim Value

UPD	Code	Description	Units
	M0076	Prolotherapy	—
	M0100	Intragastric hypothermia using gastric freezing (MNP)	—
	M0300	IV chelation therapy (chemical endarterectomy)	—
	M0301	Fabric wrapping of abdominal aneurysm (MNP)	—
	M0302	Assessment of cardiac output by electrical bioimpedance	—

Pathology and Laboratory Services (P0000-P9999)

UPD	Code	Description	Units
	P2028	Cephalin floculation, blood	—
	P2029	Congo red, blood	—
	P2031	Hair analysis (excluding arsenic)	4.7
	P2033	Thymol turbidity, blood	—
96.1	**P2038**	Mucoprotein, blood (seromucoid) (medical necessity procedure)	—
	P3000	Screening Papanicolaou smear, cervical or vaginal, up to three smears, by technician under physician supervision	(I) 3.0
	P3001	Screening Papanicolaou smear, cervical or vaginal, up to three smears, requiring interpretation by physician	—
	P7001	Culture, bacterial, urine; quantitative, sensitivity study	2.0
	P9010	Blood (whole), for transfusion, per unit	—
	P9011	Blood (split unit), specify amount	—
	P9012	Cryoprecipitate, each unit	—
	P9013	Fibrinogen unit	—
	P9016	Leukocyte poor blood, each unit	—
	P9017	Plasma, single donor, fresh frozen, each unit	—
	P9018	Plasma, protein fraction, each unit	—
	P9019	Platelet concentrate, each unit	—
	P9020	Platelet rich plasma, each unit	—
	P9021	Red blood cells, each unit	—
	P9022	Washed red blood cells, each unit	—
	P9603	Travel allowance one way in connection with medically necessary laboratory specimen collection drawn from homebound or nursing home bound patient; prorated miles actually travelled	—
	P9604	Travel allowance one way in connection with medically necessary laboratory specimen collection drawn from homebound or nursing home bound patient; prorated trip charge	—
	P9610	P9610 has been deleted	6.5

▲ Revised code   ● New code   **M** RVSI code or deleted from CPT   **(I)** Interim Value

UPD		Code	Description	Units
		P9615	Catheterization for collection of specimen(s) (multiple patients)	BR

Q Codes (Temporary) (Q0000–Q9999)

UPD		Code	Description	Units
96.1		**Q0034**	Administration of influenza vaccine to Medicare beneficiaries by participating demonstration sites	—
		Q0068	Extracorporeal plasmapheresis: immunoabsorption with staphylococcal protein A columns	(I) 26.0
		Q0081	Infusion therapy, using other than chemotherapeutic drugs, per visit	—
		Q0082	Activity therapy furnished in connection with partial hospitalization (e.g., music, dance, art or play therapies that are not primarily recreational), per visit	—
		Q0083	Chemotherapy administration by other than infusion technique only (e.g., subcutaneous, intramuscular, push), per visit	—
		Q0084	Chemotherapy administration by infusion technique only, per visit	—
		Q0085	Chemotherapy administration by both infusion technique and other technique(s) (e.g., subcutaneous, intramuscular, push), per visit	—
		Q0086	Physical therapy evaluation/treatment, per visit	—
		Q0091	Screening Papanicolaou smear; obtaining, preparing and conveyance of cervical or vaginal smear to laboratory	(I) 2.8
		Q0092	Set-up portable x-ray equipment	(I) 2.6
98.1	M	**Q0103**	This code has been deleted.	(I) 12.5
98.1	M	**Q0104**	This code has been deleted.	(I) 4.5
98.1	M	**Q0109**	This code has been deleted.	(I) 12.5
98.1	M	**Q0110**	This code has been deleted.	(I) 4.5
		Q0111	Wet mounts, including preparations of vaginal, cervical or skin specimens	—
		Q0112	All potassium hydroxide (KOH) preparations	—
		Q0113	Pinworm examination	—
		Q0114	Fern test	—
		Q0115	Post-coital direct, qualitative examinations of vaginal or cervical mucous	—
97.1		**Q0132**	Dispensing fee for covered drug administered through DME nebulizer	—
		Q0136	Injection, epoetin alpha, (for non ESRD use), per 1,000 units	—
97.1		**Q0144**	Azithromycin dihydrate, oral, capsules/powder, 1 gram (Zithromax)	—
97.1		**Q0156**	Infusion, albumin (human), 5%, 500 ml	—
97.1		**Q0157**	Infusion, albumin (human), 25%, 50 ml	—
98.2	●	**Q0160**	Factor IX (antihemophilic factor, purified, non-recombinant) per I.U.	—
98.2	●	**Q0161**	Factor IX (antihemophilic factor, recombinant) per I.U.	—

UPD		Code	Description	Units
98.2	●	**Q0163**	Diphenhydramine hydrochloride, 50 mg, oral, FDA approved prescription anti-emetic, for use as a complete therapeutic substitute for an IV anti-emetic at time of chemotherapy treatment not to exceed a 48-hour dosage regimen	—
98.2	●	**Q0164**	Prochlorperazine maleate, 5 mg, oral, FDA approved prescription anti-emetic, for use as a complete therapeutic substitute for an IV anti-emetic at the time of chemotherapy treatment, not to exceed a 48-hour dosage regimen	—
98.2	●	**Q0165**	Prochlorperazine maleate, 10 mg, oral, FDA approved prescription anti-emetic, for use as a complete therapeutic substitute for an IV anti-emetic at the time of chemotherapy treatment, not to exceed a 48-hour dosage regimen	—
98.2	●	**Q0166**	Granisetron hydrochloride, 1 mg, oral, FDA approved prescription anti-emetic, for use as a complete therapeutic substitute for an IV anti-emetic at the time of chemotherapy treatment, not to exceed a 24-hour dosage regimen	—
98.2	●	**Q0167**	Dronabinol, 2.5 mg, oral, FDA approved prescription anti-emetic, for use as a complete therapeutic substitute for an IV anti-emetic at the time of chemotherapy treatment, not to exceed a 48-hour dosage regimen	—
98.2	●	**Q0168**	Dronabinol, 5 mg, oral, FDA approved prescription anti-emetic, for use as a complete therapeutic substitute for an IV anti-emetic at the time of chemotherapy treatment, not to exceed a 48-hour dosage regimen	—
98.2	●	**Q0169**	Promethazine hydrochloride, 12.5 mg, oral, FDA approved prescription anti-emetic, for use as a complete therapeutic substitute for an IV anti-emetic at the time of chemotherapy treatment, not to exceed a 48-hour dosage regimen	—
98.2	●	**Q0170**	Promethazine hydrochloride, 25 mg, oral, FDA approved prescription anti-emetic, for use as a complete therapeutic substitute for an IV anti-emetic at the time of chemotherapy treatment, not to exceed a 48-hour dosage regimen	—
98.2	●	**Q0171**	Chlorpromazine hydrochloride, 10 mg, oral, FDA approved prescription anti-emetic, for use as a complete therapeutic substitute for an IV anti-emetic at the time of chemotherapy treatment, not to exceed a 48-hour dosage regimen	—
98.2	●	**Q0172**	Chlorpromazine hydrochloride, 25 mg, oral, FDA approved prescription anti-emetic, for use as a complete therapeutic substitute for an IV anti-emetic at the time of chemotherapy treatment, not to exceed a 48-hour dosage regimen	—
98.2	●	**Q0173**	Trimethobenzamide hydrochloride, 250 mg, oral, FDA approved prescription anti-emetic, for use as a complete therapeutic substitute for an IV anti-emetic at the time of chemotherapy treatment, not to exceed a 48-hour dosage regimen	—
98.2	●	**Q0174**	Thiethylperazine maleate, 10 mg, oral, FDA approved prescription anti-emetic, for use as a complete therapeutic substitute for an IV anti-emetic at the time of chemotherapy treatment, not to exceed a 48-hour dosage regimen	—
98.2	●	**Q0175**	Perphenzaine, 4 mg, oral, FDA approved prescription anti-emetic, for use as a complete therapeutic substitute for an IV anti-emetic at the time of chemotherapy treatment, not to exceed a 48-hour dosage regimen	—
98.2	●	**Q0176**	Perphenzaine, 8mg, oral, FDA approved prescription anti-emetic, for use as a complete therapeutic substitute for an IV anti-emetic at the time of chemotherapy treatment, not to exceed a 48-hour dosage regimen	—
98.2	●	**Q0177**	Hydroxyzine pamoate, 25 mg, oral, FDA approved prescription anti-emetic, for use as a complete therapeutic substitute for an IV anti-emetic at the time of chemotherapy treatment, not to exceed a 48-hour dosage regimen	—
98.2	●	**Q0178**	Hydroxyzine pamoate, 50 mg, oral, FDA approved prescription anti-emetic, for use as a complete therapeutic substitute for an IV anti-emetic at the time of chemotherapy treatment, not to exceed a 48-hour dosage regimen	—

▲ Revised code   ● New code   **M** RVSI code or deleted from CPT   **(I)** Interim Value

UPD		Code	Description	Units
98.2	●	Q0179	Ondansetron hydrochloride 8 mg, oral, FDA approved prescription anti-emetic, for use as a complete therapeutic substitute for an IV anti-emetic at the time of chemotherapy treatment, not to exceed a 48-hour dosage regimen	—
98.2	●	Q0180	Dolasetron mesylate, 100 mg, oral, FDA approved prescription anti-emetic, for use as a complete therapeutic substitute for an IV anti-emetic at the time of chemotherapy treatment, not to exceed a 24-hour dosage regimen	—
98.2	●	Q0181	Unspecified oral dosage form, FDA approved prescription anti-emetic, for use as a complete therapeutic substitute for an IV anti-emetic at the time of chemotherapy treatment, not to exceed a 48-hour dosage regimen	—
98.2	●	Q0183	Dermal tissue, of human origin, with and without other bioengineered or processed elements, but without metabolically active elements, per square centimeter	—
98.2	●	Q0184	Dermal tissue, of human origin, with or without other bioengineered or processed elements, with metabolically active elements, per square centimeter	—
98.2	●	Q0185	Dermal and epidermal tissue, of human origin, with or without bioengineered or processed elements, with metabolically active elements, per square centimeter	—
		Q9920	Injection of EPO, per 1000 units, at patient HCT of 20 or less	—
		Q9921	Injection of EPO, per 1000 units, at patient HCT of 21	—
		Q9922	Injection of EPO, per 1000 units, at patient HCT of 22	—
		Q9923	Injection of EPO, per 1000 units, at patient HCT of 23	—
		Q9924	Injection of EPO, per 1000 units, at patient HCT of 24	—
		Q9925	Injection of EPO, per 1000 units, at patient HCT of 25	—
		Q9926	Injection of EPO, per 1000 units, at patient HCT of 26	—
		Q9927	Injection of EPO, per 1000 units, at patient HCT of 27	—
		Q9928	Injection of EPO, per 1000 units, at patient HCT of 28	—
		Q9929	Injection of EPO, per 1000 units, at patient HCT of 29	—
		Q9930	Injection of EPO, per 1000 units, at patient HCT of 30	—
		Q9931	Injection of EPO, per 1000 units, at patient HCT of 31	—
		Q9932	Injection of EPO, per 1000 units, at patient HCT of 32	—
		Q9933	Injection of EPO, per 1000 units, at patient HCT of 33	—
		Q9934	Injection of EPO, per 1000 units, at patient HCT of 34	—
		Q9935	Injection of EPO, per 1000 units, at patient HCT of 35	—
		Q9936	Injection of EPO, per 1000 units, at patient HCT of 36	—
		Q9937	Injection of EPO, per 1000 units, at patient HCT of 37	—
		Q9938	Injection of EPO, per 1000 units, at patient HCT of 38	—
		Q9939	Injection of EPO, per 1000 units, at patient HCT of 39	—
		Q9940	Injection of EPO, per 1000 units, at patient HCT of 40 or above	—

▲ Revised code   ● New code   **M** RVSI code or deleted from CPT   **(I)** Interim Value

UPD	Code	Description	Units

Diagnostic Radiology Services (R0000-R5999)

UPD	Code	Description	Units
	R0070	Transportation of portable x-ray equipment and personnel to home or nursing home, per trip to facility or location, one patient seen	—
	R0075	Transportation of portable x-ray equipment and personnel to home or nursing home, per trip to facility or location, more than one patient seen, per patient	—
	R0076	Transportation of portable EKG to facility or location, per patient	—

Vision Services (V0000-V2999)

UPD	Code	Description	Units
	V2020	Frames, purchases	BR
	V2025	Deluxe frame	BR
	V2100	Sphere, single vision, plano to plus or minus 4.00, per lens	—
	V2101	Sphere, single vision, plus or minus 4.12 to plus or minus 7.00d, per lens	—
	V2102	Sphere, single vision, plus or minus 7.12 to plus or minus 20.00d, per lens	—
	V2103	Spherocylinder, single vision, plano to plus or minus 4.00d sphere, 0.12 to 2.00d cylinder, per lens	—
	V2104	Spherocylinder, single vision, plano to plus or minus 4.00d sphere, 2.12 to 4.00d cylinder, per lens	—
	V2105	Spherocylinder, single vision, plano to plus or minus 4.00d sphere, 4.25 to 6.00d cylinder, per lens	—
	V2106	Spherocylinder, single vision, plano to plus or minus 4.00d sphere, over 6.00d cylinder, per lens	—
	V2107	Spherocylinder, single vision, plus or minus 4.25 to plus or minus 7.00 sphere, 0.12 to 2.00d cylinder, per lens	—
	V2108	Spherocylinder, single vision, plus or minus 4.25d to plus or minus 7.00d sphere, 2.12 to 4.00d cylinder, per lens	—
	V2109	Spherocylinder, single vision, plus or minus 4.25 to plus or minus 7.00d sphere, 4.25 to 6.00d cylinder, per lens	—
	V2110	Spherocylinder, single vision, plus or minus 4.25 to 7.00d sphere, over 6.00d cylinder, per lens	—
	V2111	Spherocylinder, single vision, plus or minus 7.25 to plus or minus 12.00d sphere, 0.25 to 2.25d cylinder, per lens	—
	V2112	Spherocylinder, single vision, plus or minus 7.25 to plus or minus 12.00d sphere, 2.25d to 4.00d cylinder, per lens	—
	V2113	Spherocylinder, single vision, plus or minus 7.25 to plus or minus 12.00d sphere, 4.25 to 6.00d cylinder, per lens	—
	V2114	Spherocylinder, single vision sphere over plus or minus 12.00d, per lens	—
	V2115	Lenticular (myodisc), per lens, single vision	—
	V2116	Lenticular lens, nonaspheric, per lens, single vision	—
	V2117	Lenticular, aspheric, per lens, single vision	—

▲ Revised code   ● New code   M RVSI code or deleted from CPT   (I) Interim Value

UPD	Code	Description	Units
	V2118	Aniseikonic lens, single vision	—
	V2199	Not otherwise classified, single vision lens	—
	V2200	Sphere, bifocal, plano to plus or minus 4.00d, per lens	—
	V2201	Sphere, bifocal, plus or minus 4.12 to plus or minus 7.00d, per lens	—
	V2202	Sphere, bifocal, plus or minus 7.12 to plus or minus 20.00d, per lens	—
	V2203	Spherocylinder, bifocal, plano to plus or minus 4.00d sphere, 0.12 to 2.00d cylinder, per lens	—
	V2204	Spherocylinder, bifocal, plano to plus or minus 4.00d sphere, 2.12 to 4.00d cylinder, per lens	—
	V2205	Spherocylinder, bifocal, plano to plus or minus 4.00d sphere, 4.25 to 6.00d cylinder, per lens	—
	V2206	Spherocylinder, bifocal, plano to plus or minus 4.00d sphere, over 6.00d cylinder, per lens	—
	V2207	Spherocylinder, bifocal, plus or minus 4.25 to plus or minus 7.00d sphere, 0.12 to 2.00d cylinder, per lens	—
	V2208	Spherocylinder, bifocal, plus or minus 4.25 to plus or minus 7.00d sphere, 2.12 to 4.00d cylinder, per lens	—
	V2209	Spherocylinder, bifocal, plus or minus 4.25 to plus or minus 7.00d sphere, 4.25 to 6.00d cylinder, per lens	—
	V2210	Spherocylinder, bifocal, plus or minus 4.25 to plus or minus 7.00d sphere, over 6.00d cylinder, per lens	—
	V2211	Spherocylinder, bifocal, plus or minus 7.25 to plus or minus 12.00d sphere, 0.25 to 2.25d cylinder, per lens	—
	V2212	Spherocylinder, bifocal, plus or minus 7.25 to plus or minus 12.00d sphere, 2.25 to 4.00d cylinder, per lens	—
	V2213	Spherocylinder, bifocal, plus or minus 7.25 to plus or minus 12.00d sphere, 4.25 to 6.00d cylinder, per lens	—
	V2214	Spherocylinder, bifocal, sphere over plus or minus 12.00d, per lens	—
	V2215	Lenticular (myodisc), per lens, bifocal	—
	V2216	Lenticular, nonaspheric, per lens, bifocal	—
	V2217	Lenticular, aspheric lens, bifocal	—
	V2218	Aniseikonic, per lens, bifocal	—
	V2219	Bifocal seg width over 28mm	—
	V2220	Bifocal add over 3.25d	—
	V2299	Specialty bifocal (by report)	—
	V2300	Sphere, trifocal, plano to plus or minus 4.00d, per lens	—
	V2301	Sphere, trifocal, plus or minus 4.12 to plus or minus 7.00d per lens	—

▲ Revised code ● New code **M** RVSI code or deleted from CPT **(I)** Interim Value

UPD	Code	Description	Units
	V2302	Sphere, trifocal, plus or minus 7.12 to plus or minus 20.00, per lens	—
	V2303	Spherocylinder, trifocal, plano to plus or minus 4.00d sphere, 0.12 to 2.00d cylinder, per lens	—
	V2304	Spherocylinder, trifocal, plano to plus or minus 4.00d sphere, 2.25 to 4.00d cylinder, per lens	—
	V2305	Spherocylinder, trifocal, plano to plus or minus 4.00d sphere, 4.25 to 6.00 cylinder, per lens	—
	V2306	Spherocylinder, trifocal, plano to plus or minus 4.00d sphere, over 6.00d cylinder, per lens	—
	V2307	Spherocylinder, trifocal, plus or minus 4.25 to plus or minus 7.00d sphere, 0.12 to 2.00d cylinder, per lens	—
	V2308	Spherocylinder, trifocal, plus or minus 4.25 to plus or minus 7.00d sphere, 2.12 to 4.00d cylinder, per lens	—
	V2309	Spherocylinder, trifocal, plus or minus 4.25 to plus or minus 7.00d sphere, 4.25 to 6.00d cylinder, per lens	—
	V2310	Spherocylinder, trifocal, plus or minus 4.25 to plus or minus 7.00d sphere, over 6.00d cylinder, per lens	—
	V2311	Spherocylinder, trifocal, plus or minus 7.25 to plus or minus 12.00d sphere, 0.25 to 2.25d cylinder, per lens	—
	V2312	Spherocylinder, trifocal, plus or minus 7.25 to plus or minus 12.00d sphere, 2.25 to 4.00d cylinder, per lens	—
	V2313	Spherocylinder, trifocal, plus or minus 7.25 to plus or minus 12.00d sphere, 4.25 to 6.00d cylinder, per lens	—
	V2314	Spherocylinder, trifocal, sphere over plus or minus 12.00d, per lens	—
	V2315	Lenticular (myodisc), per lens, trifocal	—
	V2316	Lenticular nonaspheric, per lens, trifocal	—
	V2317	Lenticular, aspheric lens, trifocal	—
	V2318	Aniseikonic lens, trifocal	—
	V2319	Trifocal seg width over 28 mm	—
	V2320	Trifocal add over 3.25d	—
	V2399	Specialty trifocal (by report)	—
	V2410	Variable asphericity lens, single vision, full field, glass or plastic, per lens	—
	V2430	Variable asphericity lens, bifocal, full field, glass or plastic, per lens	—
	V2499	Variable sphericity lens, other type	—
	V2500	Contact lens, PMMA, spherical, per lens	—
	V2501	Contact lens, PMMA, toric or prism ballast, per lens	—
	V2502	Contact lens, PMMA, bifocal, per lens	—

UPD	Code	Description	Units
	V2503	Contact lens, PMMA, color vision deficiency, per lens	—
	V2510	Contact lens, gas permeable, spherical, per lens	—
	V2511	Contact lens, gas permeable, toric, prism ballast, per lens	—
	V2512	Contact lens, gas permeable, bifocal, per lens	—
	V2513	Contact lens, gas permeable, extended wear, per lens	—
	V2520	Contact lens, hydrophilic, spherical, per lens	—
	V2521	Contact lens, hydrophilic, toric, or prism ballast, per lens	—
	V2522	Contact lens, hydrophilic, bifocal, per lens	—
	V2523	Contact lens, hydrophilic, extended wear, per lens	—
96.1	**V2530**	Contact lens, scleral, gas impermeable, per lens (for contact lens modification, see CPT Level I code 92325)	—
	V2531	Contact lens, scleral, gas permeable, per lens (for contact lens modification, see CPT Level I code 92325)	—
	V2599	Contact lens, other type	—
	V2600	Hand held low vision aids and other nonspectacle mounted aids	—
	V2610	Single lens spectacle mounted low vision aids	—
96.1	**V2615**	Telescopic and other compound lens system, including distance vision telescopic, near vision telescopes and compound microscopic lens system	—
	V2623	Prosthetic eye, plastic, custom	—
	V2624	Polishing/resurfacing of ocular prosthesis	—
	V2625	Enlargement of ocular prosthesis	—
	V2626	Reduction of ocular prosthesis	—
	V2627	Scleral cover shell	—
	V2628	Fabrication and fitting of ocular conformer	—
	V2629	Prosthetic eye, other type	—
	V2630	Anterior chamber intraocular lens	—
	V2631	Iris supported intraocular lens	—
	V2632	Posterior chamber intraocular lens	—
	V2700	Balance lens, per lens	—
	V2710	Slab off prism, glass or plastic, per lens	—
	V2715	Prism, per lens	—
	V2718	Press-on lens, Fresnell prism, per lens	—
	V2730	Special base curve, glass or plastic, per lens	—

UPD	Code	Description	Units
	V2740	Tint, plastic, rose 1 or 2, per lens	—
	V2741	Tint, plastic, other than rose 1 or 2, per lens	—
	V2742	Tint, glass, rose 1 or 2, per lens	—
	V2743	Tint, glass, other than rose 1 or 2, per lens	—
	V2744	Tint, photochromatic, per lens	—
	V2750	Antireflective coating, per lens	—
	V2755	U-V lens, per lens	—
	V2760	Scratch resistant coating, per lens	—
	V2770	Occluder lens, per lens	—
96.1	**V2780**	Oversize lens, per lens	—
	V2781	Progressive lens, per lens	—
	V2785	Processing, preserving and transporting corneal tissue	—
	V2799	Vision service, miscellaneous	—

Hearing Services (V5000-V5999)

UPD	Code	Description	Units
	V5008	Hearing screening	—
	V5010	Assessment for hearing aid	—
	V5011	Fitting/orientation/checking of hearing aid	—
	V5014	Repair/modification of a hearing aid	—
	V5020	Conformity evaluation	—
	V5030	Hearing aid, monaural, body worn, air conduction	—
	V5040	Hearing aid, monaural, body worn, bone conduction	—
	V5050	Hearing aid, monaural, in the ear	—
	V5060	Hearing aid, monaural, behind the ear	—
	V5070	Glasses, air conduction	—
	V5080	Glasses, bone conduction	—
	V5090	Dispensing fee, unspecified hearing aid	—
	V5100	Hearing aid, bilateral, body worn	—
	V5110	Dispensing fee, bilateral	—
	V5120	Binaural, body	—
	V5130	Binaural, in the ear	—
	V5140	Binaural, behind the ear	—

UPD	Code	Description	Units
	V5150	Binaural, glasses	—
	V5160	Dispensing fee, binaural	—
	V5170	Hearing aid, CROS, in the ear	—
	V5180	Hearing aid, CROS, behind the ear	—
	V5190	Hearing aid, CROS, glasses	—
	V5200	Dispensing fee, CROS	—
	V5210	Hearing aid, BICROS, in the ear	—
	V5220	Hearing aid, BICROS, behind the ear	—
	V5230	Hearing aid, BICROS, glasses	—
	V5240	Dispensing fee, BICROS	—
	V5299	Hearing service, miscellaneous	—
	V5336	Repair/modification of augmentative communicative system or device (excludes adaptive hearing aid)	—
	V5362	Speech screening	—
	V5363	Language screening	—
	V5364	Dysphagia screening	—

Procedural Index

This index is intended to direct the user to a general area. Please refer to your CPT index for a more specific procedural description and/or code reference.

Heart & Pericardium

Aortic anomalies 33800–33853
Arterial grafting 33533–33545
Arterial-venous grafting 33517–33530
Cardiac assist 33960–33978
Cardiac tumor 33120–33130
Cardiac valves 33400–33478
Coronary artery anomalies 33500–33506
Coronary endarterectomy 33572
Heart/lung transplant 33930–33945
Unlisted procedure, cardiac surgery 33999
Pacemaker or defibrillator 33200–33261
Pericardium 33010–33050
Pulmonary artery 33910–33924
Pulmonary venous drainage 33730–33732
Septal defect 33641–33697
Shunting procedures 33735–33767
Single ventricle & other anomalies 33600–33619
Sinus of valsalva 33702–33722
Thoracic aortic aneurysm 33860–33877
Transposition of the great vessels 33770–33781
Truncus arteriosus 33786–33788
Venous grafting 33510–33516
Wounds of heart & vessels 33300–33335
Hematology and coagulation 85002–85999
Home services 99341–99350

Hospital inpatient services

Hospital discharge services 99238–99239
Initial hospital care 99221–99223
Subsequent hospital care 99231–99233

Hospital observation services

Initial observation care 99218–99220
Observation care discharge services 99217

Humerus (upper arm) & elbow

Amputation 24900–24940
Athrodesis 24800–24802
Excision 24065–24155
Fracture and-or dislocation 24500–24685
Incision 23930–24006
Introduction or removal 24160–24220
Miscellaneous 24999
Repair, revision or reconstruction 24301–24498
Immunization injections 90700–90749
Immunology 86000–86804
Intersex surgery 55970–55980

Intestine

Endoscopy 44360–44394
Enterostomy-external fistulization 44300–44346
Excision 44100–44160
Incision 44005–44055
Introduction 44500
Repair 44602–44799

Kidney

Endoscopy 50551–50580
Excision 50200–50290
Incision 50010–50135
Introduction 50390–50398
Other procedure 50590
Renal transplant 50300–50380
Repair 50400–50540
Laparoscopy/peritoneoscopy/
    hysteroscopy 56300–56399

Larynx

Destruction 31595
Endoscopy 31505–31579
Excision 31300–31420
Introduction 31500–31502
Other 31599
Repair 31580–31590

Leg & Ankle Joint

Amputation 27880–27889
Athrodesis 27870–27871
Excision 27613–27647
Fracture and-or dislocation 27750–27848
Incision 27600–27612
Introduction or removal 27648
Manipulation 27860
Miscellaneous 27892–27899
Repair, revision or reconstruction 27650–27745

Lips

Excision 40490–40530
Other procedures 40799
Repair 40650–40761

Liver

Excision 47100–47136
Incision 47000–47015
Repair 47300–47362
Other Procedures 47399

Lungs & Pleura

Endoscopy 32601–32665
Excision 32310–32540
Incision 32000–32225
Lung transplantation 32850–32854
Repair 32800–32820
Surgical collapse 32900–32999

Lymph nodes & Lymphatic channels

Excision 38500–38555
Incision 38300–38382
Introduction 38790–38999
Limited lymphadenectomy for staging . . 38562–38564
Radical lymphadenectomy 38700–38780

Palatae, Uvula
Excision 42100–42160
Incision. 42000
Repair 42180–42281

Pancreas
Endoscopy 43260–43272
Excision 48100–48180
Incision. 48000–48020
Introduction 48400
Repair 48500–48547
Unlisted procedure, pancreas 48999
Transplantation 48550–48556
Parathyroid, thymus, adrenal glands,
    & carotid body 60500–60699

Pelvis & hip joint
Amputation 27290–27295
Athrodesis. 27280–27286
Excision 27040–27080
Fracture and-or dislocation 27193–27266
Incision. 26990–27036
Introduction or removal. 27086–27095
Manipulation 27275
Miscellaneous. 27299
Repair, revision or reconstruction 27097–27187

Penis
Destruction. 54050–54065
Excision 54100–54161
Incision. 54000–54015
Introduction 54200–54250
Manipulation 54450
Repair. 54300–54440

Pharynx, adenoids, & tonsils
Excision 42800–42894
Incision. 42700–42725
Other procedures 42955–42999
Repair. 42900–42953

Physical medicine
Modalities. 97010–97039
Other procedures 97799
Procedures 97110–97546
Tests and measurements. 97703–97750

Preventive medicine services
Evaluation 99401–99429
Counseling and/or risk factor
    reduction intervention 99381–99397

Prolonged services
Prolonged physician service with direct
    (face-to-face) patient contact 99354–99357
Prolonged physician service without direct
    (face-to-face) patient contact 99358–99360

Prostate
Excision. 55801–55865
Incision 55700–55725
Other procedures. 55870–55899

Psychiatry
General clinical psychiatric diagnostic or
    evaluative interview procedures. . . . 90801–90802
Psychiatric therapeutic procedures 90804–90899
Pulmonary. 94010–94799

Radiation oncology
Clinical treatment planning
    (external and internal sources) 77261–77299
Medical radiation physics, dosimetry,
    treatment devices and special
    services 77300–77399
Radiation treatment delivery. 77401–77417

Rectum
Destruction 45190
Endoscopy. 45300–45385
Excision. 45100–45170
Incision 45000–45020
Manipulation. 45900–45915
Repair 45500–45825

Salivary gland & ducts
Excision. 42400–42450
Incision 42300–42340
Other Procedures 42550–42699
Repair 42500–42510

Scrotum
Excision. 55150
Incision 55100–55120
Repair 55175–55180

Seminal vesicles
Excision. 55650–55680
Incision 55600–55605

Shoulder
Amputation 23900–23921
Athrodesis 23800–23802
Excision. 23065–23222
Fracture and-or dislocation. 23500–23680
Incision 23000–23044
Introduction or removal 23330–23350
Manipulation. 23700
Miscellaneous 23929
Repair, revision or reconstruction. 23395–23491

Skin, subcutaneous & accessory structures
Adjacent tissue transfer or
    rearrangement 14000–14350
Biopsy 11100–11101